APPLIED
PHARMACOLOGY
FOR THE
DENTAL HYGIENIST

APPLIED
PHARMACOLOGY
FOR THE
DENTAL HYGIENIST

Sixth Edition

Elena Bablenis Haveles, BS Pharm, PharmD
Adjunct Associate Professor of Pharmacology
Gene W. Hirschfeld School of Dental Hygiene
College of Health Sciences
Old Dominion University
Norfolk, Virginia

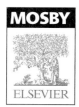

3251 Riverport Lane
Maryland Heights, Missouri 63043

APPLIED PHARMACOLOGY FOR
THE DENTAL HYGIENIST

ISBN-13: 978-0-323-06558-0

Notice

Knowledge and best practice in this field are constantly changing. As new research and experience broaden our knowledge, changes in practice, treatment and drug therapy may become necessary or appropriate. Readers are advised to check the most current information provided (i) on procedures featured or (ii) by the manufacturer of each product to be administered, to verify the recommended dose or formula, the method and duration of administration, and contraindications. It is the responsibility of the practitioner, relying on their own experience and knowledge of the patient, to make diagnoses, to determine dosages and the best treatment for each individual patient, and to take all appropriate safety precautions. To the fullest extent of the law, neither the Publisher nor the Author assumes any liability for any injury and/or damage to persons or property arising out of or related to any use of the material contained in this book.

The Publisher

Library of Congress Cataloging-in-Publication Data
Haveles, Elena B. (Bablenis)
   Applied pharmacology for the dental hygienist / Elena Bablenis Haveles. — 6th ed.
       p. ; cm.
   Includes bibliographical references and index.
   ISBN 978-0-323-06558-0 (pbk. : alk. paper)   1. Dental pharmacology.   2. Dental hygiene.   I. Title.
   [DNLM: 1. Pharmacology, Clinical.   2. Dental Hygienists.   QV 50 H384a 2011]
   RK701.R46 2011
   617.6′01—dc22

                                                                                    2009043308

Vice President and Publisher: Linda Duncan
Executive Editor: John Dolan
Managing Editor: Kristin Hebberd
Publishing Services Manager: Catherine Jackson
Project Manager: David Stein
Designer: Teresa McBryan

Printed in the United States.

Last digit is print number: 9 8 7 6 5 4 3 2 1

Reviewers

Barbara Bennett, CDA, RDH, MS
Department Chair
Dental Hygiene and Dental Assisting Programs
Co-Division Director
Health Programs
Texas State Technical College
Harlingen, Texas

Karen M. Bratus, DDS
Faculty
Department of Dental Hygiene
Baker College of Auburn Hills
Auburn Hills, Michigan

Deborah P. Milliken, DMD
Supervising Dentist
Professor, Dental Hygiene
South Florida Community College
Avon Park, Florida

Dr. Ron Swisher
Professor
Department of Natural Sciences
Program in Health Sciences
Oregon Institute of Technology
Klamath Falls, Oregon

To my husband Paul and
sons Andrew and Harry

Preface

Knowledge of pharmacology is imperative to the success of a dental hygiene student. *Applied Pharmacology for the Dental Hygienist,* Sixth Edition, is written with the specific needs of the dental hygienist in mind to help ensure your success in this subject matter.

Society is information-conscious, and it is expected that the dental hygienist be knowledgeable about medications. Dental hygienists are called on to complete medication and health histories, administer certain medications, provide counseling about oral hygiene, and, in some states, prescribe medication and provide counseling about medications.

The primary goal of this book remains to produce safe and effective dental practitioners and to offer them the tools that they need to continue to learn throughout their lifetimes. This textbook provides the dental hygienist with the necessary knowledge of pharmacology to assess for medical illness, adverse reactions, and drug interactions that may affect oral health care and treatment. It is not intended that the dental hygienist take the place of the dentist in providing the patient with information about the various medications but that he or she will work with the dentist in providing appropriate patient care.

INTENDED AUDIENCE

The primary intended audience of this specific textbook is the dental hygiene student. However, practicing dental hygienists and dentists may find this book useful for a quick review of pharmacology, and the information may also benefit dental students as a classroom text or resource.

IMPORTANCE TO THE PROFESSION

Continual learning after the completion of a formal education is especially critical in the dynamic area of pharmacology. New drugs are constantly being discovered and synthesized. New effects of old drugs are identified. New diseases and drugs for the treatment of those diseases are being studied. Today's dental hygiene student will need to be able to access new information about new drugs in the future and intelligently communicate with others (professionals and patients) using the unique medical and pharmacologic vocabularies. It is hoped that this textbook will also help dental hygiene students to accomplish the following goals:

1. Students should achieve an understanding of the need and importance of obtaining and using appropriate reference material when needed. When confronted with a patient taking a new or unfamiliar drug, the professional will use the appropriate references to learn about the effects of the drug. Pharmacology is a field in which new information is constantly becoming available.

2. Students should develop the ability to find the necessary information about drugs with which they are not familiar. The textbook encourages the use of the current reference sources that will be available where dental hygienists practice.

3. Students should develop the ability to apply that information to their clinical dental patients within a reasonable time.

ORGANIZATION

The material has been organized to create a readable and clinically applicable resource in pharmacology that specifically addresses the needs of the dental hygiene student. The textbook is divided into four sections:

PART ONE: General Principles of Pharmacology includes general information about pharmacology, pharmacokinetics, drug action and handling, adverse reactions, prescription writing, autonomic pharmacology, the role of the dental hygienist, and pharmacology in oral health care.

PART TWO: Drugs Used in Dentistry includes the pharmacology of nonopioid analgesics, opioid analgesics, antibiotics, antifungals, antiviral drugs, local anesthetics, general anesthetics with a special emphasis on nitrous oxide, and vitamins and minerals. It also has chapters on the treatment of oral conditions and dental hygiene–related disorders. Each chapter focuses on dental-related adverse effects, how the drug may affect oral health care, and the specific dental hygiene considerations.

PART THREE: Drugs that May Alter Dental Treatment includes the more common disease states or medical conditions that patients may present with, as well as how those medications or the disease states themselves can affect oral health care. Each chapter also focuses on dental-related adverse effects, how the drug may affect oral health care, and specific dental hygiene considerations.

PART FOUR: Special Situations includes significant information on treating emergency situations, women who are pregnant or lactating, patients with substance abuse issues, and those patients self-treating with herbal remedies or supplements. Each chapter also focuses on dental-related adverse effects, how the drug may affect oral health care, and specific dental hygiene considerations.

KEY FEATURES

This book includes many features and learning aids to assist the student studying pharmacology:

- *Dental Focus:* Although pharmacologic basics are covered overall and for specific types of drugs, interactions of clinical interest in dentistry are incorporated throughout the book. These sections offer explanations on why certain drugs are used or contraindicated in a dental treatment plan, providing students with targeted information they will need for practice.

- *Consistent Presentation:* Information about each drug varies, but all drugs are presented using a similar format so that sections can be easily identified. Each drug group is discussed and includes the group's indications (for what purpose the drugs are used), pharmacokinetics (how the body handles the drugs), pharmacologic effects (what the drugs do), adverse reactions (bad things the drugs do), drug interactions (how the drugs react with other drugs in the body), and the dosage of the drugs (how much is indicated).
- *Clinical Skills Assessment:* Review questions are included at the end of each chapter, with answers available to instructors. These questions help students assess their knowledge and gauge comprehension of chapter material.
- *Key Terminology:* Key terms are bolded throughout and appear in color within chapter discussions; each term is defined in a back-of-book glossary. The language of pharmacology is new to many dental hygiene students, and the in-text highlights draw students' attention to terms they may need to review. The glossary provides a centralized, quick, and handy reference.
- *Summary Tables and Boxes:* Throughout, concepts are summarized in boxes and tables to accompany narrative discussions, providing easy-to-read versions of text discussions that support visual learners and serve as useful tools for review and study.
- *Note Boxes:* Boxes are interspersed throughout text discussions to briefly convey important concepts, indications, contraindications, memory tools, warnings, and more. They are easy to see and provide quick statements or phrases that are easy to remember.
- *Reference Citations:* Chapters contain bibliographical information as necessary, directing students to targeted sources of information where additional dental-related information can be located.
- *Appendixes:* Resources such as the top 200 drugs, *What If ...* scenarios that quickly outline situations in which relatively quick assessments and decisions are required, and the calculation of children's dosages highlight additional information that proves useful in the clinical environment.
- *Drug Index:* A separate index covers the mention of all the drugs discussed within the book, allowing readers to quickly access targeted information about specific drugs or drug classes.

NEW TO THIS EDITION

- *Chapter on Hygiene-Related Oral Disorders:* Oral hygiene is highlighted, specifically in terms of the prevention of dental caries, gingivitis, and hypersensitivity. Both pharmacologic and nonpharmacologic therapies are discussed, and the role of the dental hygienist in patient education is emphasized.
- *Chapter on Natural/Herbal Products and Dietary Supplements:* Herbal medicine is explored, including its regulation, package labeling, safety and potential drug interactions, manufacturing, and standardization. Several of the most common supplements are outlined, with specific information provided on adverse effects and dental hygiene implications.

- *Dental Hygiene Considerations Boxes:* Each chapter concludes with a compilation of the most relevant dental-specific information, which is summarized in terms of how that chapter's content specifically relates to the day-to-day practice of dental hygiene. These sections help explain to students the need for an understanding of pharmacology and its importance in helping them achieve maximal oral health for their patients.
- *Writing Level:* Certain content areas and tables throughout the book have been simplified to better explain difficult concepts, such as receptors and metabolism. Pharmacology is a complex subject matter, and this book attempts to present information in a way that helps ensure that students can fully comprehend the content and apply it to the practice of dental hygiene.
- *Art Program:* Approximately one third of the images are new to this edition, and many of those that appeared in the previous edition have been updated and improved. The new images are more targeted and visually appealing and help support text discussions so that students can see key concepts at work.
- *Chapter Objectives:* Each chapter begins with a list of learning objectives that the student should master on completion. The objectives help students set goals for what they will accomplish and also serve as checkpoints for comprehension and study tools in the preparation for examinations.
- *Textbook Design:* A new design incorporates more graphics and a more modern look to help readers engage in the content.

ANCILLARIES

A companion Evolve website has been created specifically for *Applied Pharmacology for the Dental Hygienist* and can be accessed directly from http://evolve.elsevier.com/Haveles/pharmacology. The following resources are provided:

For the Instructor

- *Test Bank:* Approximately 900 objective-style questions—multiple-choice, true/false, matching, and short-answer—are provided, with accompanying rationales for correct answers and page-number references for remediation.
- *Image Collection:* All the book's images, organized by chapter with correlating figure numbers to the textbook, are available for download into PowerPoint or other presentations and materials.
- *Animations:* Three-dimensional narrated visualizations of basic body system workings provide foundational anatomical and physiological information to support pharmacologic concepts.
- *PowerPoint Presentations:* Lecture slides are included for each chapter.
- *Case Studies:* Case presentations are followed by thought questions that deal with drug indications, contraindications, interactions, and more. Answers are provided.
- *Chapter Features:* A detailed chapter outline, listing of key terms, chapter objectives, and *Dental Hygiene Considerations* are compiled for each chapter to support lesson planning.
- *Color Pill Atlas:* A labeled color image is provided for some of the most commonly prescribed medications.

- *Answers to Clinical Skills Assessments:* Answers and rationales are provided for each end-of-chapter review question.

For the Student

- *Practice Quizzes:* Approximately 350 questions are provided in an instant-feedback format to allow students to assess their understanding of content and prepare for examinations. Rationales and page-number references are provided for remediation.
- *Labeling Exercises:* Drag-and-drop matching exercises are created from many of the book's illustrations to reinforce and help students visualize concepts.

- *Glossary Exercises:* Crossword puzzles are created from the book's glossary to help students master key terminology.
- *Drug Guides:* The major groups and specific drugs covered within each chapter are organized and summarized in terms of classification and mechanism of action for a quick study tool.

Elena Bablenis Haveles

Acknowledgments

Thank you to my peers and administrators at the Gene W. Hirschfeld School of Dental Hygiene, Old Dominion University, for their support.

To my children, Andrew and Harry, many thanks for allowing Mom to work on this book when we would rather have done so many other things together.

To my husband, Paul, thank you for your guidance and support as I try to juggle this and everything else in our lives. I love you.

EBH

How to Be Successful in Pharmacology

Before the lecture, read the syllabus outline for the subject to be covered during the class period. Become familiar with the vocabulary. Guess what might be said about the various topics. Think of what has been said in pharmacology about the topic; look at your pharmacology notes to see what you already know about the topic. Skim the textbook chapter(s) assigned to identify areas to be covered.

Attend class, take notes in your syllabus, and ask yourself questions about what was said. Compare what was said with what you previously thought about the topic.

Reread your lecture notes before the next class. Add and complete things you remember from class. Ask fellow classmates for clarification if you have questions. Reread notes from previous classes.

Read the textbook assignment. Note especially those areas discussed in class. Let the textbook assignment answer questions you might have had in class. Answer general course objectives in the front of your syllabus for the drug group covered.

Look up in a medical dictionary any words for which you don't know the meaning. Construct a vocabulary list for each subject. Pay attention to the derivatives of the unknown medical word—its stem, prefixes, and suffixes.

Use active learning when studying. Be able to determine what portion of your study time is spent in active learning. Use the examples below to classify your study methods.

- *Active:* Writing things down, making up flash cards, speaking out loud, discussing the concepts with classmates, asking each other questions, giving a lecture (to your parrot) without notes, making a video or audio tape recording of your performances (for your own practice), or writing everything you know about a drug on an empty blackboard.
- *Not active:* Looking over notes, reading the book, listening in lecture, and reviewing your notes.

Did you answer the Clinical Skills Assessment questions? These questions are included at the end of each chapter so the learner can check to see if he or she knows the answers to these questions. It is a review for your benefit. Answers are only available through your instructor.

Did you think about what the information may mean to the dental hygienist? Trying to understand why things happen will make learning more efficient and more fun, too. What problems might be encountered when treating a patient taking this medication? How can the chance that something untoward will happen be minimized?

Did you think of examples in "real life"? By thinking of real-life examples, readers can transform a topic into a picture in their brain. For example, the "fight or flight" response associated with the sympathetic nervous system can be visualized as a caveman, his eyes big and his heart pounding, being chased by a hungry tiger.

USE OF OBJECTIVES TO FOCUS STUDYING

Find out what the objectives are for your pharmacology class. These are some objectives that may give you an idea about the organization of the material.

Goals for **commonly prescribed dental drugs** include the following:

- State the therapeutic use(s) for each drug group.
- Discuss the mechanism of action of the drug, when applicable.
- Explain the important pharmacokinetics for the drug group.
- List and describe the major pharmacologic effects associated with the drug group. State and discuss the important adverse reactions or side effects and their management or minimization.
- Describe any contraindications/cautions to the use of the drug group.
- Recognize clinically significant drug–drug, drug–disease, and drug–food interactions.
- Describe "patient instructions" for each drug group that could be prescribed.

Goals for agents patients may be taking that can alter dental treatment:

- Determine the "dental implications" of each drug group for the management of dental patients taking [drug group name].
- Determine whether any dental drugs are likely to have drug interactions with these groups.
- State change(s) in the treatment plans that would be required for patients taking medications.

Contents

GENERAL PRINCIPLES

1

Information, Sources, Regulatory Agencies, Drug Legislation, and Prescription Writing

LEARNING OBJECTIVES

1. Discuss the history of pharmacology and its relationship to the oral health care provider.
2. Define the ways in which drugs are named and the significance of each.
3. Describe the acts and agencies within the federal government designed to regulate drugs.
4. Identify the four phases of clinical evaluation involved in drug approval and the five schedules of drugs.
5. Describe the elements of a drug prescription.

Pharmacology is derived from the Greek prefix *pharmaco-,* meaning "drug" or "medicine," and the Greek suffix *-logy,* meaning "study." Therefore pharmacology is the study of drugs. *Dorland's Illustrated Medical Dictionary* defines the term drug as follows:

> Any chemical compound used on or administered to humans or animals as an aid in the diagnosis, treatment, or prevention of disease or other abnormal condition, for the relief of pain or suffering, or to control or improve any physiologic or pathologic condition.

Others define a *drug* as any chemical substance that affects biologic systems. These definitions, however, are not complete. For example, birth control pills are indicated in the treatment of which disease? Is pregnancy a disease? Another problem with the current definition of pharmacology is that there is a large group of substances (drugs?) that are categorized as "dietary supplements." These agents include herbs, vitamins, minerals, and amino acids. Although these substances may have pharmacologic effects on the body, by law they are not classified as drugs. This classification avoids the Food and Drug Administration (FDA) approval for efficacy and safety required for drugs.

HISTORY

In the beginning, plants found in the jungle were discovered to produce beneficial effects.

Pharmacology had its beginning when human ancestors noticed that ingesting certain plants altered body functions or awareness. The first pharmacologist was a person who became more astute in observing and remembering which plant products produced predictable results. From this humble beginning, a huge industrial and academic community concerned with the study and development of drugs has evolved. Plants from the rain forest and chemicals from tar have been searched for the presence of drugs. The agents discovered and found to be useful are then prescribed and dispensed through the practice of medicine, dentistry, pharmacy, and nursing. Health care providers who can write prescriptions include physicians (for humans), veterinarians (for animals), dentists (for dental problems), and optometrists (for eye problems). Physicians' assistants, nurse practitioners, and pharmacists can prescribe drugs under certain guidelines and in certain states.

PHARMACOLOGY AND ORAL HEALTH CARE PROVIDERS

The American Dental Association (ADA) and American Dental Hygienists' Association (ADHA) have been analyzing tasks that oral health care providers should be able to perform during the practice of their professions. In education, these activities are termed competencies.

> What knowledge is needed to perform the functions of a dental professional?

To perform each competency (meaning to do something), certain facts or concepts (meaning something you know) must be accessed (find it) by the dental professional. The facts or concepts needed include didactic information (something learned from a book) relative to the task being performed (a dental procedure). Decisions that surround performing the competency rely on a body of information, termed the *foundation knowledge*. Each content area is then analyzed to determine what relationship exists among the course content, the competencies, and the appropriate foundation knowledge. Examples of questions that would need to be answered to perform a certain dental procedure (the foundation knowledge required to determine the pros and cons of performing a certain dental procedure on a certain patient with certain diseases) could include the questions shown in Table 1-1.

From the example in Table 1-1, it can be seen that the dental health care worker cannot practice by doing "something" to "someone" with "some problem." Thought, facts, reasoning, and problem solving are involved in making decisions about each patient seen in the dental office. Dental professionals are not robots; they use clinical judgment to make the best decisions about each patient.

Table 1-1 illustrates the relationship among the professional, the task, and the foundation knowledge. Because the dental and dental hygiene professions require knowledge and decision making, the "explanation behind the task" is important.

Specific topics to be covered in each discipline are determined by this process. In the best educational situation, the process would be patient specific and produce learning issues and content that cross multiple disciplines. However, in the meantime, educational experiences are still often organized in discipline-based units. This textbook is also arranged in this manner.

Knowledge of pharmacology is imperative for the dental professional to perform important functions such as the following:

- *Obtaining a health history.* To obtain a complete and useful health history, a knowledge of commonly prescribed drugs is required. Patients with systemic diseases unrelated to their dental health are often taking medications prescribed by their physician. An understanding of the actions, indications, adverse reactions, and therapeutic uses of these drugs can help determine potential effects on dental treatment. Comparing the medical conditions of the patient with the medications he or she is taking often raises questions in the interview. Examples of this would include patients taking calcium channel blockers for hypertension and the risk of xerostomia or patients taking an aspirin each day to prevent a heart attack or stroke and the increased risk of gingival bleeding.
- *Administering drugs in the office.* Because both the dentist and the dental hygienist administer certain drugs in the office, knowledge of these agents is crucial. For example, the oral health care provider commonly applies topical fluoride, and in some states, both the dentist and the dental hygienist administer local anesthetics and nitrous oxide. In-depth knowledge of these agents is especially important because of their frequent use.
- *Handling emergency situations.* The ability to recognize and assist in dental emergencies requires knowledge of certain drugs. The indications for these drugs and their adverse reactions must be considered. For example, a patient having an anaphylactic reaction must have epinephrine administered quickly.
- *Planning appointments.* Patients taking medication for systemic diseases may require special handling in the dental office. For example, asthmatic patients should have afternoon appointments, whereas diabetic patients usually have fewer problems with a morning appointment. Certain patients may need to take medication before their appointment. Patients with rheumatic heart disease need to be premedicated with antibiotics before some of their dental or dental hygiene appointments.
- *Nonprescription medication.* Often, nonprescription or over-the-counter (OTC) products may be recommended for the patient. The study of pharmacology will assist the oral health care provider in an intelligent selection of an appropriate OTC product.
- *Nutritional or herbal supplements.* Many patients self-treat or are prescribed nutritional or herbal supplements for any number of disease states. Although the vast majority of these supplements do not carry FDA approval for treating disease states, patients still use them. These supplements are drugs and can cause adverse effects and interact with different drugs.
- *Discussing drugs.* When drugs are discussed with either the patient or another health professional, proper terminology is needed. Drugs prescribed by the dentist can cause adverse effects in patients; patients often ask the oral health care

TABLE 1-1	RELATIONSHIP AMONG TASKS PERFORMED IN PRACTICE AND INFORMATION LEARNED IN PHARMACOLOGY	
Professional	Competency (Ability)	Foundation Knowledge
Dental hygienist	1. Remove calculus and plaque. 2. Administer local anesthetics.	Treatment modifications based on existing medical conditions or current medications.
Dentist	"Restore" a carious lesion	Same as above

provider questions about their medications. Knowledge of the terms used to describe adverse reactions can facilitate discussions with the patient, dentist, or physician. For example, the term *allergy* refers to an allergic response to a drug (e.g., hives from aspirin). Patients, however, often confuse the term allergy with the term *side effects*. Side effects refer to predictable responses to drugs that act on nontarget organs (e.g., stomach upset). The correct knowledge of these terms can help clarify a patient's symptoms. Understanding the difference between the two effects of aspirin aids in determining whether a nonsteroidal antiinflammatory drug (e.g., ibuprofen) can be used for dental discomfort in a particular patient. When the health history is taken and the drugs the patient is taking are listed, it is important that treatment does not begin until the drugs are checked for any problems relating to dentistry.

- *Life-long learning.* Because it is impossible to remember everything learned about current drugs and because new drugs are always being discovered and marketed, appropriate reference sources should be available and consulted. To be able to evaluate the information retrieved from reference sources, understanding of the terminology of pharmacology and its global organization is essential.

SOURCES OF INFORMATION

There are many different medications available, and it is important for the dental hygienist to know where to look for information about prescription medications, nonprescription medications, and herbal supplements. There are many sources, including reference texts, association journals, and the internet, where pertinent drug information can be found. Table 1-2 reviews the different sources of information.

Each publication type may be judged on its lack of bias, its publication date (when the current edition was released), its readability (vocabulary, simplicity of explanations, and presence of visual aids), its degree of detail (all you want to know and much more, just the right amount of information, or not enough to understand what is being said), and its price.

Every dental office should have at least one reference book that lists the names of both prescription and OTC drugs. Further, a standard pharmacology textbook would be helpful in understanding the reference books. Because of the release of new drugs, a recent edition (not more than 1 to 2 years old) of a reference book is needed. Table 1-3 compares properties of different reference sources.

Although books serve as the usual source of information on drugs, computer software and even Internet-based services are becoming more readily available. In addition, the practicing pharmacist can be a source of information. It is particularly important for the dental professional to establish a professional relationship with a local pharmacist, who may assist him or her in understanding the possible effects of a new drug on a patient.

DRUG NAMES

It is important for the dentist and the dental hygienist to understand the ways in which a drug can be named because he or she must be able to discuss drugs with both the patient and the

provider of the patient's care. The ability to refer to a drug's name(s) is complicated by the fact that all drugs have at least two names, and many have more.

When a particular drug is being investigated by a company, it is identified by its chemical name, which is determined by its chemical structure. If the structure is unknown at the time of investigation, a code name, usually a combination of letters and numbers, is assigned to the product (e.g., RU-486). Often, the code name is used even when the chemical structure is identified and named. It is much easier to speak and write the code name than the full name of the chemical structure.

> Each drug has only one generic name but may have several trade names.

If a compound is found to be useful and it is determined that the compound will be marketed commercially, the pharmaceutical company discovering the drug gives the drug a trade name (e.g., Coke). This name, which is capitalized, is usually chosen so that it can be easily remembered and promoted commercially. This trade name, registered as a trademark under the Federal Trademark Law, is the property of the registering company. The trade name is protected by the Federal Patent Law for 20 years from the earliest claimed filing date, plus patent term extensions. Although the brand name is technically the name of the company marketing the product, it is often used interchangeably with the trade name.

Before any drug is marketed, it is given a generic name that becomes the "official" name of the drug. For each drug, there is only one generic name (e.g., cola) selected by the United States Adopted Name Council, and the name is not capitalized. This council selects a generic name that hopefully does not conflict with other drug names. Recently, the names of several marketed drugs were changed because they were confused with the name of another drug that had already been marketed.

An example of the many names a product can have is provided by lidocaine, a local anesthetic commonly used in dentistry. Figure 1-1 compares the generic and trade names of lidocaine.

After the original manufacturer's patents have expired, other companies can market the generic drug under a trade name of their choosing (e.g., Pepsi). When lidocaine first appeared on the market, it was manufactured by Astra and was available only as Xylocaine, but when its patent expired, other companies started making the drug, and each company gave it their own brand name (e.g., Octocaine). When a patient states an allergy to Xylocaine, the oral health care provider must be aware that lidocaine is the generic name of this drug and that the patient should not be given lidocaine under another trade name such as Octocaine.

Drugs prescribed by physicians cause a similar problem. Patients often know these drugs by the trade name. If a patient reports an allergic reaction to Amoxil (the trade name), the oral health care provider must be aware that this patient should not take other brands of amoxicillin (the generic name) or any other type of penicillin.

This book uses generic names when discussing drugs because there is only one generic name for each drug. Trade names (also known as *proprietary names*) appear in parentheses after the generic name. Most reference books include indexes that allow a drug to be accessed using either the generic or trade name. Newer drugs are usually referred to by their trade names. Old and traditional drugs are often referred to by their generic names.

TABLE 1-2   SELECTED DRUG INFORMATION REFERENCES

Reference	Brief Description
American Health-Systems Formulary Service	Detailed reference source that provides an unbiased guide to all aspects of a drug's properties. It is updated yearly, and quarterly supplements are provided. The detail in this book is especially valuable when a specific drug fact is needed. CD-ROM available.
United States Pharmacopeia-Drug Information (USP DI)	Volume 1: *Drug Information for the Health Care Provider* provides the health professional with necessary information regarding basic pharmacology and pharmacokinetics, dosing, adverse reactions, and drug interactions. Volume 2: *Advice for the Patient* is written for the patient and includes appropriate information on pharmacology, pharmacokinetics, dosing, adverse reactions, and drug interactions. The USP DI is published annually with quarterly updates via CD-ROM. Monthly updates are available for those with the online USP DI.
Drug Facts and Comparisons	Contains the most complete listing of currently available drugs, including prescription and OTC medications and is arranged by pharmacologic class. It is available in a loose-leaf binder (updated monthly), annual hardback book, online, or as CD-ROM.
Physicians' Desk Reference (PDR)	Most common reference book in the dental office because of its historically inexpensive price. New drugs are added annually, and, often, older drugs are removed from the book to make space for newer drugs. Information provided comes directly from the manufacturer's package insert. The manufacturers are listed alphabetically, and drugs are listed alphabetically within each manufacturer's section. CD-ROM is available.
Handbook of Nonprescription Drugs: An Interactive Approach to Self-Care (OTC Handbook)	Published every 3 years by the American Pharmaceutical Association. This textbook provides the reader with detailed information about all classes of nonprescription drugs available in the United States. It also reviews the pathophysiology of different disease states and their treatments. There are several chapters that pertain to oral health care, and one chapter devoted to nicotine-related products.
PDR for Nonprescription Drugs, Supplements, and Herbs	This reference book provides information on OTC drugs, supplements, and herbs and is organized alphabetically by manufacturers or product name. It also provides complete descriptions of commonly used OTC medications; useful, at-a-glance information such as ingredients, indications, and interactions on hundreds of drugs; administration and dosage recommended for symptomatic relief; and color photographs of OTC drugs for quick identification.
PDR for Herbal Medicines	The fourth edition of this book provides health care professionals with an updated reference so they can better advise patients who ask about specific herbal remedies. The information presented in this reference book provides the latest scientific data in the most comprehensive herbal reference compiled, including Commission E indications, which is the closest thing to an approved usage guide in the world of herbal medicines. Key monographs have been updated to include recent scientific findings on efficacy, safety, and potential interactions; clinical trials (including abstracts); case reports; and meta-analysis results. There are also updated sections on enhanced patient management techniques and nutritional supplements.
Natural Products: A Case-Based Approach for Health Care Professionals	Written by Karen Shapiro and published by the American Pharmaceutical Association, this reference book offers practitioners guidelines for integrating natural products—including vitamins, soy and whey protein supplements, fish oils, dong quai, evening primrose oil, pygeum, stinging nettle, etc—into their treatment plan for a variety of common conditions and goals. The most common conditions discussed include dementia, osteoarthritis, menopause, depression, erectile dysfunction, diabetes, cold and flu, weight loss, and performance enhancement. This book is intended for classroom use.
Merck Manual for Medical Information	Published every 5 to 6 years by Merck Research Labs, this reference book provides the reader with general information on disease states and drug therapy. Online version and CD-ROM available.
Drug Interaction Facts	Published yearly with monthly updates, this book provides information on reported drug interactions and rates clinical significance of those interactions. Online version and CD-ROM available.
Mosby's Dental Drug Reference	Provides access to information on drugs commonly taken by patients. Drugs are presented alphabetically by generic name and include indications, contraindications, dental considerations, and pharmacologic classification. An alphabetic cross-index offers access to both brand and generic name drugs. Fact tables are located on the inside covers and in the appendixes. Images of pathologic conditions, a color pill atlas, and patient education sheets are available on a CD ROM and/or a companion website. Updated every 2 years.
Lexi-Comp's Drug Information Handbook for Dentistry	Contains concise lists of drug attributes and sections relevant to dentistry for each drug. The book is written by dentists and covers over 7600 drugs and herbal products. Each monograph contains up to 32 fields of information, including dosage, local anesthetic/vasoconstrictor precautions, drug interactions, and effects on dental treatment.
Goodman and Gilman's The Pharmacologic Basis of Therapeutics	This pharmacology textbook, published every 5 years, is the standard pharmacology textbook for pharmacy and medicine. It provides the reader with in-depth information regarding the chemistry, mechanism of action, pharmacologic effects, pharmacokinetics, adverse reactions, and therapeutic uses of drugs. Also available on CD-ROM.

TABLE 1-3   COMPARISONS AMONG REFERENCE SOURCES

Reference*	Organization	Bias	Price	Update Frequency	Comments
DDR	Alphabetic by generic drug name	N	$	Every 2 years	Dental implications, brief
LCD	Alphabetic by generic drug name	N	$$	1/year; CD = 4/year	Dental implications, brief
PDR	Alphabetic by manufacturer's name; within that list, alphabetic by trade name	Y	$$	1/year; 4/year; CD = 4/year	Package insert, not often updated, contains selected drugs
F & C	By therapeutic class	N	$$$$	1/year; 12/year (paper); CD = 4/year	Has many tables; includes most prescriptions and OTC drugs
AHFS	Alphabetic by pharmacologic class	N	$$$	1/year; CD = 4/year	Detailed coverage; useful to answer specific questions
USP DI	Alphabetic by pharmacologic class	N	$$$	1/year; 12/year; CD = 4/year	Extensive list of properties of drugs

N, No; Y, yes; OTC, over the counter; $, least expensive; $$, moderately expensive; $$$, expensive; $$$$, most expensive.
DDR, Mosby's Dental Drug Reference (Mosby); LCD, Lexi-Comp's Drug Information Handbook for Dentistry (Lexi-Comp); PDR, Physicians' Desk Reference (Thomson Reuters); F & C, Drug Facts and Comparisons (Wolters Kluwer); AHFS, AHFS Drug Information (American Society of Health-System Pharmacists); USP DI, United States Pharmacopeia-Drug Information (Thomson Reuters).

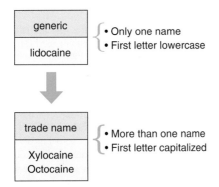

FIGURE 1-1
A comparison between the trade and generic drug names of lidocaine.

A problem occurs in naming multiple-entity drugs, which are drugs with several ingredients. These drugs are difficult to discuss by their generic names because they contain several ingredients.

Drug Substitution

> For dental drugs, generic substitution provides equivalent therapeutic results at a cost savings.

In the discussion of generic and trade names, the question of generic equivalence and substitution arises. Are the various different generic products equivalent? After 17 years, the patent of the original drug expires, and other companies can market the same compound under a generic name. In 1984, Congress passed the Drug Price Competition and Patent Term Restoration Act, which allowed generic drugs to receive expedited approval. The FDA still requires that the active ingredient of the generic product enter the bloodstream at the same rate as the trade name product. The variation allowed for the generic name product is the same as for the reformulations of the brand name product. For the few drugs that are difficult to formulate and have narrow therapeutic indexes, no differences exist between the trade name product and the generic product; therefore generic substitution drugs give equivalent therapeutic results and provide a cost savings to the patient.

Drugs can be judged "similar" in several ways. When two formulations of a drug meet the chemical and physical standards established by the regulatory agencies, they are termed *chemically equivalent.* If the two formulations produce similar concentrations of the drug in the blood and tissues, they are termed *biologically equivalent.* If they prove to have an equal therapeutic effect in a clinical trial, they are termed *therapeutically equivalent.* A preparation can be chemically equivalent yet not biologically or therapeutically equivalent. These products are said to differ in their bioavailability. Before generic drugs are marketed, they must be shown to be biologically equivalent, which would make them therapeutically equivalent.

Top 200 Drugs

Appendix A lists the 200 drugs most often prescribed in 2008 and their pharmacologic group. In the right column of the appendix the rank order appears. This number represents the position that the drug appears in the top 200. The rank of 1 is the most often prescribed drug for that year. Both generic and trade names appear on the list, depending on how the prescription is written. The oral health care provider must become familiar with these names because patients may know the names of the drugs they are taking but not know how the names are spelled. By referring to the list of the top 200 drugs, the oral health care provider can check the patient's medications and spell them accurately so that they can be accessed in reference sources. This textbook discusses most of the agents included in this list.

FEDERAL REGULATIONS AND REGULATORY AGENCIES

Many agencies are involved in regulating the production, marketing, advertising, labeling, and prescribing of drugs.

Harrison Narcotic Act

In 1914 the Harrison Narcotic Act established regulations governing the use of opium, opiates, and cocaine. Marijuana laws were added in 1937. Before this law, mixtures sold OTC could

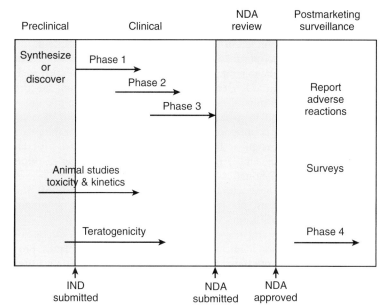

FIGURE 1-2
Development of a new drug. *IND*, Investigational new drug; *NDA*, new drug application.

contain opium and cocaine. These mixtures were promoted to be effective for many "problems."

Food and Drug Administration

The FDA of the Department of Health and Human Services (DHHS) grants approval so that drugs can be marketed in the United States. Before a drug can be approved by the FDA, it must be determined to be both safe and effective. The FDA requires physical and chemical standards for specific products and quality control in drug manufacturing plants. It determines what drugs may be sold by prescription and OTC and regulates the labeling and advertising of prescription drugs. Because the FDA is often more stringent than regulatory bodies in other countries, drugs are often marketed in Europe and South America before they are available in the United States.

Federal Trade Commission

The Federal Trade Commission (FTC) regulates the trade practices of drug companies and prohibits the false advertising of foods, nonprescription (OTC) drugs, and cosmetics.

Drug Enforcement Administration

The Drug Enforcement Administration (DEA) of the Department of Justice administers the Controlled Substances Act of 1970. This federal agency regulates the manufacture and distribution of substances that have a potential for abuse, including opioids (narcotics), stimulants, and sedatives.

Omnibus Budget Reconciliation Act

The newest federal regulation concerning drugs is the Omnibus Budget Reconciliation Act (OBRA) of 1990. It mandates that, beginning January 1, 1993, pharmacists must provide patient counseling and a prospective drug utilization review (DUR) for Medicaid patients. Although this federal law covers only Medicaid patients, State Boards of Pharmacy are interpreting this law to apply to all patients. Dental patients who have their prescriptions filled at a pharmacy should receive counseling from the pharmacist about their prescriptions.

CLINICAL EVALUATION OF A NEW DRUG

If a discovered or synthesized compound becomes a marketed drug, it must pass through many steps before it is approved (Figure 1-2). Animal studies begin by measuring both the acute and chronic toxicity. The median lethal dose is determined for several species of animals. Long-term animal studies continue, including a search for teratogenic effects. Toxicity and pharmacokinetic properties are also noted. An investigational new drug application (INDA) must be filled before any clinical trials can be performed. Human studies of drugs involve the following four phases:

- *Phase 1:* Small and then increasing doses are administered to a limited number of healthy human volunteers, primarily to determine safety. This phase determines the biologic effects, metabolism, safe dose range in humans, and toxic effects of the drug.
- *Phase 2:* Larger groups of humans are given the drug and any adverse reactions are reported to the FDA. The main purpose of phase 2 is to test effectiveness.
- *Phase 3:* More clinical evaluation takes place involving a large number of patients who have the condition for which the drug is indicated. During this phase, both safety and efficacy must be demonstrated. Dosage is also determined during this phase.
- *Phase 4:* This phase involves postmarketing surveillance. The toxicity of the drug that occurs in patients taking the drug after it is released is recorded. Several drugs in recent years have been removed from the market only after phase 4 has shown serious toxicity.

DRUG LEGISLATION
History

The Food and Drug Act of 1906 was the first federal law to regulate interstate commerce in drugs. The Harrison Narcotic Act of 1914 and its amendments provided federal control over narcotic drugs and required registration of all practitioners prescribing narcotics.

The Food and Drug Act was rewritten and became the Food, Drug and Cosmetic Act of 1938. This law and its subsequent amendments prohibit interstate commerce of drugs that have not been shown to be safe and effective. The Durham-Humphrey Law of 1952 is a particularly important amendment to the Food, Drug and Cosmetic Act because it requires that certain types of drugs be sold by prescription only. This law requires that these drugs be labeled as follows: "Caution: Federal law prohibits dispensing without prescription." This law also prohibits the refilling of a prescription unless directions to the contrary are indicated on the prescription. The Drug Amendments of 1962 (Kefauver-Harris Bill) made major changes in the Food, Drug and Cosmetic Act. Under these amendments, manufacturers were required to demonstrate the effectiveness of drugs, to follow strict rules in testing, and to submit to the FDA any reports of adverse effects from drugs already on the market. Manufacturers were also required to list drug ingredients by generic name in labeling and advertising and to state adverse effects, contraindications, and efficacy of a drug.

The Drug Abuse Control Amendments of 1965 required accounting for drugs with a potential for abuse such as barbiturates and amphetamines.

The Controlled Substance Act of 1970 replaced the Harrison Narcotic Act and the Drug Abuse Control Amendments to the Food, Drug and Cosmetic Act. The Controlled Substances Act is extremely important because it sets current requirements for writing prescriptions for drugs often prescribed in dental practice.

Scheduled Drugs

Federal law divides controlled substances into five schedules according to their abuse potential (Table 1-4). The rules for prescribing these agents, whether prescriptions can be telephoned to the pharmacist, and whether refills are allowed differ depending on the drug's schedule. New drug entities are evaluated and added to the appropriate schedule. Drugs on the market may be moved from one schedule to another if changes in abuse patterns are discovered.

The current requirements for prescribing controlled drugs (Controlled Substance Act of 1970) are as follows:

- Any prescription for a controlled substance requires a DEA number.
- All Schedule II through IV drugs require a prescription.
- Any prescription for Schedule II drugs must be written in pen or indelible ink or typed. A designee of the dentist, such as the dental hygienist, may write the prescription, but the prescriber must personally sign the prescription in ink and is responsible for what any designee has written.
- Schedule II prescriptions cannot be telephoned to the pharmacist (except at the discretion of the pharmacist for an emergency supply to be followed by a written prescription within 72 hours).
- Because Schedule II prescriptions cannot be refilled, the patient must obtain a new written prescription to obtain more medication.
- Certain states require the use of "triplicate" or "duplicate" prescription blanks for Schedule II drugs. These blanks, provided by the state, are requested by the dentist. After a prescription is written, the dentist keeps one copy and gives two copies to the patient. The patient presents these two copies to the pharmacist, who must file one copy and send the other to the State Board of Pharmacy. These consecutively numbered blank prescription pads provide additional control for Schedule II drugs.
- Prescriptions for Schedule III and IV drugs may be telephoned to the pharmacist and may be refilled no more than five times in 6 months, if so noted on the prescription.

PRESCRIPTION WRITING

Dental practitioners need to become familiar with the basics of prescription writing for the following reasons:

- If prescriptions are written correctly, it will save the time of the office personnel, dentist, and pharmacist who must call to clarify prescriptions.
- Prescriptions written carefully are less likely to result in mistakes.
- With extra effort when unusual prescriptions are written, the dentist can save the patient's and pharmacist's time. For example, if the unusual is explained on the prescription, problems will be minimized. Sometimes it may be expedient

TABLE 1-4	SCHEDULES OF CONTROLLED SUBSTANCES		
Schedule	Abuse Potential	Examples	Handling
I	Highest	Heroin, LSD, marijuana, hallucinogens	No accepted medical use; experimental use, only in research
II	High	Oxycodone, morphine, amphetamine, secobarbital	Written prescription with provider's signature only; no refills
III	Moderate	Codeine mixtures (Tylenol #3), hydrocodone mixtures (Vicodin)	Prescriptions may be telephoned; no more than five prescriptions in 6 months
IV	Less	Diazepam (Valium), dextropropoxyphene forms (Darvon)	Prescriptions may be telephoned; no more than five prescriptions in 6 months
V	Least	Some codeine-containing cough syrups	Can be bought OTC in some states

LSD, Lysergic acid diethylamide; *OTC*, over the counter.

to call the prescription to the pharmacy so that the unusual use can be explained and a reference given.

Measurement

♦ METRIC SYSTEM

The metric system is based on multiples of 10.

In pharmacy, the primary measuring system is the metric system. Scientific calculations use a base of 10. Consequently, the metric system, which is based on 10, is the language of scientific measurement. Only metric units should be used in prescription writing.

The basic metric unit for the measurement of weight is the kilogram (kg). The basic metric unit for volume is the liter (L). One milliliter (ml), one one-thousandth of a liter, is exactly 1 cubic centimeter (cc). Because the various units of the metric system are based on multiples of 10, several prefixes can apply to units of both weight and volume (Table 1-5).

Solid drugs are dispensed by weight (milligrams [mg]) and liquid drugs by volume (milliliters [ml]). It is rarely necessary to use units other than the milligram or the milliliter in prescription writing; occasionally, grams (gm) or micrograms (μg) are used. In addition to the milliliter, the liter is also used to measure volume.

TABLE 1-5 COMMON ABBREVIATIONS

Abbreviations	English
a or $\bar{a}$	before
ac	before meals
bid	twice a day
$\bar{c}$	with
cap	capsule
d	day
disp	dispense
gm	gram
gr	grain
gtt	drop
h	hour
hs	at bedtime
$\bar{p}$	after
pc	after meals
PO	by mouth
prn	as required, if needed
q	every
qid	4 times a day
$\bar{s}$	without
sig	write (label)
$\bar{ss}$	one-half
stat	immediately (now)
tab	tablet
tid	3 times a day
ud	as directed

♦ HOUSEHOLD MEASURES

Although clinicians will direct the pharmacist to dispense a liquid preparation in milliliters, it is generally converted by the pharmacist into a convenient household unit of measurement to be included in the directions to the patient. Liquids are converted into teaspoonfuls (tsp or t; 1 tsp equals 5 ml) and tablespoonfuls (tbsp or T; 1 tbsp equals 15 ml). This is because the average American does not use the metric system of measurement in daily life. The pharmacist will give a calibrated oral syringe or dropper for infants and younger children. Most liquid dose forms come with calibrated dosing cups for both adults and children. Household utensils should not be used. The dosing cups are available in 2.5-, 5-, and 10-ml volumes with milliliters marked along the length.

Prescriptions

♦ FORMAT

The parts of the prescription are divided into three sections. They are the heading, body, and closing (Figure 1-3).

Heading. The heading of the prescription contains the following information:

- Name, address, and telephone number of the prescriber (printed on the prescription blank)
- Name, address, age, and telephone number of the patient (written)
- Date of prescription (not a legal prescription unless filled in with date); often missing

The name, address, and telephone number of the prescriber are important when the pharmacist must contact the prescribing clinician for verification or questions. The date is particularly important because it allows the pharmacist to intercept prescriptions that may not have been filled at the time of writing. For example, a prescription for an antibiotic written 3 months before being presented to the pharmacist might be used for a different reason than the dentist originally intended. Likewise, a prescription for a pain medication that is even a few days old requires the pharmacist to question the patient as to why the prescription is being filled so long after it was written. The age of the patient enables the pharmacist to check for the proper dose.

Body. The body of the prescription contains the following information:

- The Rx symbol
- Name and dose size or concentration (liquids) of the drug
- Amount to be dispensed
- Directions to the patient

The first entry after the Rx symbol is the name of the drug being prescribed. This is followed by the size (milligrams) of the tablet or capsule desired. In the case of liquids, the name of the drug is followed by its concentration (milligrams per milliliter [mg/ml]). The second entry is the quantity to be dispensed, that is, the number of capsules or tablets or milliliters of liquid. In the case of tablets and capsules, the word "Dispense" is often replaced with #, the symbol for a number. When writing prescriptions for opioids or other controlled substances, the prescriber should add in parentheses the number of tablets or capsules written out in Roman numerals or in longhand after the Arabic number of tablets or capsules. This reduces the possibility of an intended 8 becoming an 18 or 80 at the discretion

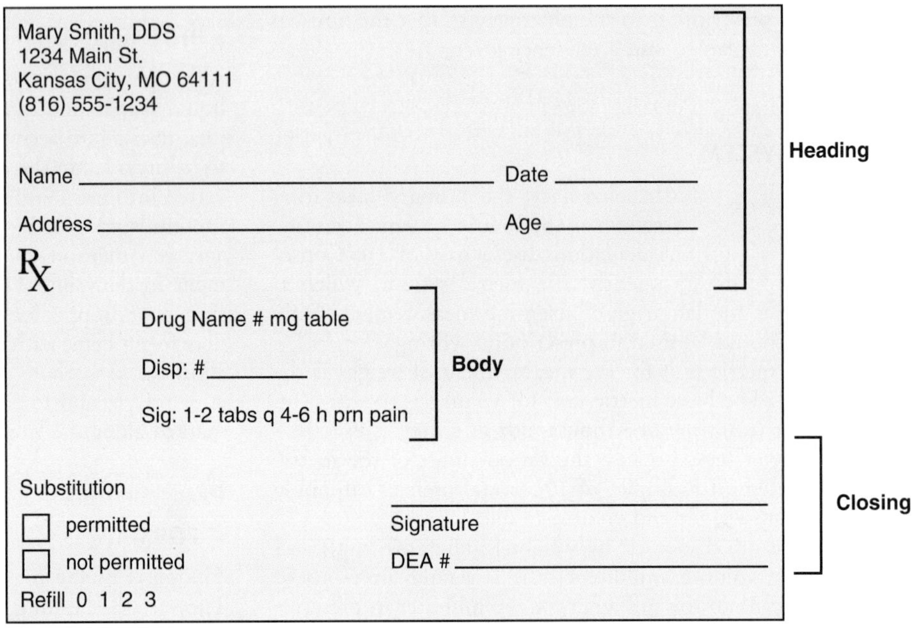

FIGURE 1-3
A typical prescription form.

BOX 1-1 COMMON METRIC PREFIXES

Weight
1 *kilo*gram (kg) = 1000 grams (g or gm)
1 gram (g) = 10 *deci*grams (dg)
1 gram = 100 *centi*grams (cg)
1 gram = 1000 *milli*grams (mg)
1 gram = 1,000,000 *micro*grams (μg or mcg)

Volume
1 liter (L) = 10 *deci*liters (dl)
1 liter = 100 *centi*liters (cl)
1 liter = 1000 *milli*liters (ml)
1 liter = 1,000,000 *micro*liters (μl)

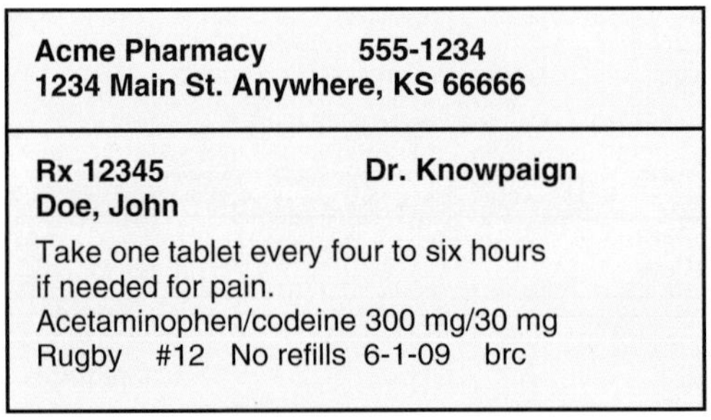
Acme Pharmacy 555-1234
1234 Main St. Anywhere, KS 66666
Rx 12345 Dr. Knowpaign
Doe, John
Take one tablet every four to six hours
if needed for pain.
Acetaminophen/codeine 300 mg/30 mg
Rugby #12 No refills 6-1-09 brc

FIGURE 1-4
Sample of a typical prescription label.

of an enterprising patient. Directions to the patient are preceded by the abbreviation "Sig:" (Latin for *signa*, "write"). The directions to the patient must be completely clear and explicit and should include the amount of medication and the time, frequency, and route of administration. The pharmacist will transcribe any Latin abbreviations (Box 1-1) into English on the label when the prescription is filled. The use of ud ("as directed") does not provide the proper information on the label for the patient. Often with ud prescriptions, the patient does not remember how to take the medicine. To clarify for the patient without adequate written instructions, the pharmacist must contact the prescriber for clarification (this wastes dentist, pharmacist, and patient time). After a few months, the patient will forget the quick instructions given verbally in the dental office after a dental appointment. Even prescriptions for chlorhexidine should be specific for amount, time, other activities to perform, and when water can be used.

Closing. The closing of the prescription contains the following:

- Prescriber's signature
- DEA number, if required
- Refill instructions

After the body of the prescription, space is provided for the prescriber's signature. Certain states have more than one place to sign. Certain institutions also provide a space on which to print the prescriber's name. This is not necessary for dentists with their own prescription blanks. If there are several dentists in one office, the names of all the dentists in the practice should be included on the prescription blanks. Then the individual dentist should check a box or circle his or her name so the pharmacist will know who signed the prescription.

In addition, the law requires that all prescriptions must be labeled with the name of the medication and its strength. Figure 1-4 is a sample prescription label. This allows easy identification by other practitioners or quick identification in emergency situations. One should note that the name, address, and telephone number of the pharmacy; the patient's and dentist's names; the directions for use; the name and strength of the medication; and the original date and the date filled (refilled) are required. The quantity of medication dispensed (number of tablets) and the number of refills remaining may be noted as well. If a generic drug is prescribed, then the generic name of the drug and the manufacturer is required on the label. If the trade drug is used, only the trade name is required on the label.

In most states, before a dentist can legally write a prescription for a patient, the following two criteria must be met:

- *Patient of record:* The person for whom the prescription is being written is a patient of record (no next-door neighbors or relatives, unless they are also patients of record).
- *Dental condition:* The condition for which the prescription is being prescribed is a dental-related condition (no birth control pills or thyroid replacement drugs).

Abbreviations. A few abbreviation forms are used in prescription writing to save time. The abbreviations also make alteration of a prescription by the patient more difficult. In some cases they are necessary to get all the required information into the space on the prescription form. Some abbreviations that may be useful are shown in Table 1-5. If abbreviations are used on a prescription, they should be clearly written. For example, the three abbreviations qd (every day), qod (every other day), and qid (four times a day) can look quite similar, and choosing the wrong one could be disastrous.

Explanations Accompanying Prescriptions

The dental health care worker should be able to answer the patient's questions about the prescription and should make sure that the patient knows how to take the medication prescribed (how long and when), what precautions to observe (drug interactions, possible side effects, driving limitations), and the reason for taking the medication. Information about the consequences of noncompliance should be included. By informing the patient about the medication, the likelihood that the patient will comply with the prescription instructions increases. The dental office should either keep a copy of each prescription written in the patient's record or record the medication, dose, and number prescribed. A patient should never get home and not know which drug is the antibiotic (for infection) and which is the analgesic (for pain). Side effects, such as drowsiness (for Schedule II drugs) or stomach upset, should be noted on the label. Some drug abusers ("shoppers") search for dental offices that might provide them with prescriptions for controlled substances or prescription blanks that they can use to forge their own prescriptions. Every dental office should keep prescription blanks in a secure place. The prescriber's DEA number should not be printed on the prescription blanks but should be written in only when needed.* The dental health care worker should watch to see that prescription blanks are not scattered around the office. If the dentist practices in a state that requires "triplicate" or "duplicate" prescription blanks for Schedule II prescriptions, then those pads must be stored under lock and key to prevent them from being stolen.

---

*Because of the use of DEA numbers to file insurance claims, there may come a time when including the DEA number on the prescription blank becomes commonplace.

CLINICAL SKILLS ASSESSMENT

1. Define the term *pharmacology.*
2. Explain why the oral health care provider should have a knowledge of pharmacology.
3. Explain the importance of conducting health/medication histories.
4. Why should a dental practice keep more than one type of reference book?
5. Discuss the most important features of a good reference book.
6. Define and give an example of the following terms:
   a. Chemical name
   b. Trade name
   c. Brand name
   d. Generic name
7. Explain why a list of the most current drugs should be available in every dental office.
8. Name three federal regulatory agencies and state the major responsibility of each.
9. Explain the various stages of testing through which a drug must pass before it is marketed for the general public.
10. List the information required in a prescription.
11. Explain two precautions that should be taken in the dental office to discourage drug abusers.
12. List the components of the Controlled Substance Act.

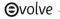

Drug Action and Handling

LEARNING OBJECTIVES

1. Differentiate dose, potency, and efficacy in the context of the actions of drugs.
2. Explain the pharmacologic effect of a drug.
3. Discuss the major steps of pharmacokinetics: absorption, distribution, metabolism, and excretion.
4. Summarize the various routes of drug administration.
5. Provide example of factors that may alter the effect of a drug.

To discuss the drugs used in dentistry or those that patients may be taking when they come to the dental office, the dental health care worker must be familiar with some basic principles of pharmacology. This chapter discusses the action of drugs in the body and methods of drug administration. Chapter 3 considers the problems or adverse reactions these drugs can cause. By understanding how drugs work, what effects they can have, and what problems they can cause, the dental health care worker can better communicate with the patient and other health care providers about medications the patient may be taking or may need to have prescribed for dental treatment.

Drugs are broadly defined as chemical substances used for the diagnosis, prevention, or treatment of disease or for the prevention of pregnancy. Most drugs are differentiated from inert chemicals and chemicals necessary for the maintenance of life processes (e.g., vitamins) by their ability to act selectively in biologic systems to accomplish a desired effect. Historically, drugs were discovered by randomly searching for active components among plants, animals, minerals, and the soil. Today, organic synthetic chemistry researchers are primarily responsible for developing new drugs. Parent compounds that exhibit known pharmacologic activity are chemically modified to produce congeners or analogs: agents of a similar chemical structure with a similar pharmacologic effect. This technique of modifying a chemical molecule to provide more useful therapeutic agents has evolved from studies of the relationship between the chemical structure and the biologic activity called *structure-activity relationship* (SAR).

CHARACTERIZATION OF DRUG ACTION

Dose-response curve, potency, and *efficacy* are terms used to measure drug response or action.

Log Dose Effect Curve

When a drug exerts an effect on biologic systems, the effect can be related quantitatively to the dose of the drug given. If the dose of the drug is plotted against the intensity of the effect, a curve will result (Figure 2-1). If this curve is replotted using the log of the dose (log dose) versus the response, another curve is produced from which the potency and efficacy of a drug's action may be determined (Figure 2-2).

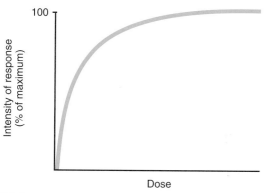

FIGURE 2-1

Dose effect curve. The x-axis (horizontal) is an increasing dose of the drug, and the y-axis (vertical) is an increasing effect of the drug.

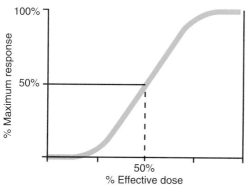

FIGURE 2-2

Log dose effect curve. As the dose is increased (going to the right on the x-axis), the effect (the y-axis) is zero at first, then there is a small effect, and finally the effect quickly increases. Around the dose where the line is increasing sharply is the therapeutic range of the compound. Finally, the curve plateaus (flattens out). This is the maximum response a drug can exhibit.

Potency

Potency—related to the amount of drug needed to produce an effect
---

The potency of a drug is a function of the amount of drug required to produce an effect. The potency of a drug is shown by the location of that drug's curve along the log-dose axis (x-axis). The curves in Figure 2-3 illustrate two drugs with different potencies. The potency of drug *A* is greater because the dose required to produce its effect is smaller. The potency of *B* is less than *A* because *B* requires a larger dose to produce its effect.

As an example of different potencies, three alcoholic beverages are compared: bourbon, beer, and wine cooler (or spritzer). One ounce of bourbon contains the same amount of alcohol as one beer (12 oz) or as one wine cooler or spritzer (16 oz [depends on dilution]). All of these drinks could equally inebriate an individual (produce adverse reactions). To produce a similarly drunk individual, the same amount of alcohol would have to be ingested. However, this amount would be contained in a different volume of fluid, depending on its concentration (or potency).* Therefore, when someone says "I'm not drunk

---
*Ignoring the effect on the stomach of different nonalcoholic fluids or food ingested.

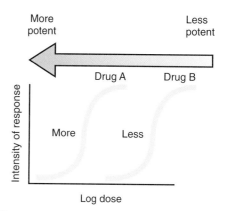

FIGURE 2-3

Potency of agent. The arrow is shaded proportional to increasing potency. (*Dark shading,* very potent; *light shading,* low potency.)

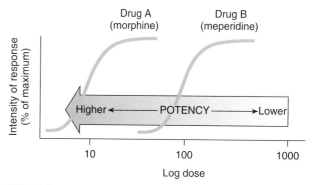

FIGURE 2-4

Comparison of log dose effect curves for morphine and meperidine.

because I just drank beer," the statement is false. The absolute potency of a drug is immaterial as long as an appropriate dose is administered. Both meperidine and morphine have the ability to treat severe pain, but approximately 100 mg of meperidine would be required to produce the same action as 10 mg of morphine. Thus the absolute potency of oral morphine is 10 times that of oral meperidine, or meperidine is one-tenth as potent as morphine, even though both agents can relieve intense pain (equal efficacy, as explained next). In Figure 2-4, the curve for drug *B* (meperidine) is to the right of the curve for drug *A* (morphine) because the dose of meperidine needed to produce pain relief is larger (10 times larger) than that for morphine. The potency of different drugs that elicit similar effects can be compared by observing the dose that produces 50% (drop a vertical line down from the center of the curve) of the total, or maximum, effect.

Efficacy

Efficacy—related to the maximal effect of a drug, regardless of dose
---

Efficacy is the maximum intensity of effect or response that can be produced by a drug. Administering more drug will not increase the efficacy of the drug but can often increase the probability of an adverse reaction. The efficacy of a drug increases as the height of the curve increases (Figure 2-5). The efficacy of the drugs whose curves are illustrated in Figure 2-5 are shown by the height of the curve when it plateaus (levels out horizontally). It is shaded from least (light) to most (dark) potent. The efficacy of any drug is a major descriptive characteristic indicating its action. For example, the efficacy of drug *B* (meperidine) and drug *A* (morphine) is about the same because both drugs relieve severe pain.

If one "drink" of both bourbon (1 oz) and beer (12 oz) were ingested, they could produce equal "silliness" in an individual. If very large doses of either agent were ingested, unconsciousness could be produced. Both are equally efficacious, but they differ in their potency. *The efficacy and the potency of a drug are unrelated.*

Because death is the endpoint when measuring the lethal dose, the median lethal dose (LD_{50}) is the dose when one-half of the subjects die. For obvious reasons, the LD_{50} is only determined in animals.

Chemical Signaling Among Cells

For the autonomic nervous system to function, messages from the brain must be transmitted to many parts of the body commanding the parts to "do something" (e.g., enlarge pupil or sweat). Complex mechanisms for transmitting these messages allow for amplification or damping of the effect, depending on a multitude of factors. The complexity allows for very fine tuning of the body's functions. Neurotransmitters are chemicals responsible for transporting a wide variety of messages across the synapse (space between nerve and receptor). Chemical signaling involves release of neurotransmitters, local substances, and hormone secretion.

◆ NEUROTRANSMITTERS

The messengers that move the electrical impulses from a nerve are transmitted across the synapse via neurotransmitters. The

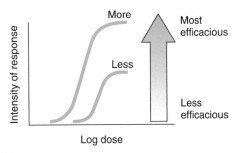

FIGURE 2-5
Efficacy of agent.

neurotransmitters are released and quickly travel across the synapse to the receptor (Figure 2-6). There are at least 50 different agents that transmit messages. Examples of neurotransmitters include acetylcholine, norepinephrine/epinephrine, dopamine, serotonin, γ-aminobutyric acid (GABA), and histamine.

◆ LOCAL

Some organs secrete chemicals that work near them. These chemicals are not released into the systemic circulation. Prostaglandins and histamine are examples. For example, a person wears a nickel-containing watch and a red spot appears on the skin beneath the watch. This localized allergic reaction is caused by release of inflammation-producing substances, such as histamine, at that point on the skin. Because the reaction is localized, the patient's nose does not begin to run. Prostaglandins contract the uterine muscles and become important as a baby is born. When prostaglandins are released in the uterus, they produce menstrual "cramps," and when released in the stomach, they protect its lining.

◆ HORMONES

Hormones are secreted to produce effects throughout the body. Examples include insulin, thyroid hormone, and adrenocorticosteroids. These reactions are usually slower than the ones associated with the neurotransmitters.

MECHANISM OF ACTION OF DRUGS

After drugs have been distributed to their site of action, they elicit a pharmacologic effect. The pharmacologic effect occurs because of a modulation in the function of an organism. Drugs do not impart a new function to the organism; they merely produce either the same action as an endogenous agent or block the action of an endogenous agent. This signaling mechanism has two functions: amplification of the signal and flexible regulation. The presence of very fine controls to modulate the body's function allows the regulation of certain reactions, slowing or speeding them.

Nerve Transmission

Within a nerve, the transmission of impulses travels along the nerve, producing a nerve action potential. The action potential

FIGURE 2-6
For the neurotransmitter (or drug acting like a neurotransmitter) to complete the message, it must get inside the cell. After the drug binds with its receptor, the reaction often opens a channel so that the message can get inside the cell.

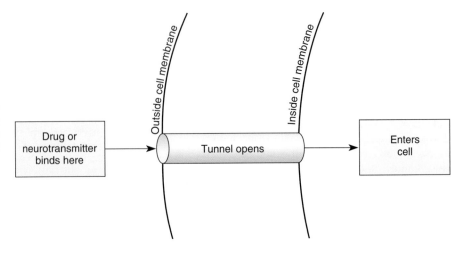

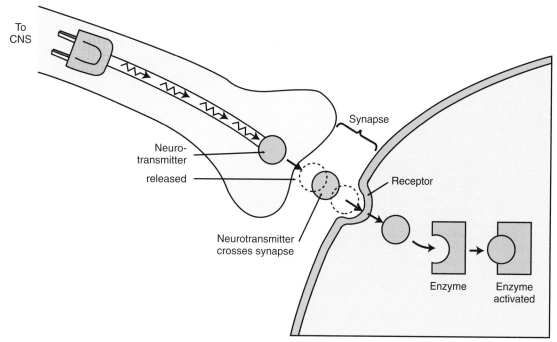

FIGURE 2-7
The neurotransmitter is transmitting the message (like electricity) across the synapse (space where nerve is absent). The neurotransmitter then interacts with the receptor (shaped to fit together), which then may signal an enzyme to be synthesized or activated.

is triggered by the neurotransmitter released at the previous synapse. Drugs that interfere with this process, such as local anesthetics (see Chapter 10), block messages from being sent. The processes involved in the drug's effect begin the drug-receptor interaction. The receptors, macromolecular chemical structures, interact with both endogenous substances and drugs. This drug-receptor interaction results in a conformational (shape) change, which may allow the drug inside the cell to produce its effect or may cause the release of a second messenger, which then produces the effect. Many of the effects involve altering enzyme-regulated reactions or regulatory processes for protein synthesis after a series of reactions, similar to a chain reaction. These steps in the process of communicating are briefly discussed.

Receptors

Once a drug passes through the biologic membrane, it is carried to many different areas of the body, or site of action, to exert its therapeutic effect or adverse effect. For the drug to exert its effects, it must bind with the receptor site on the cell membrane. Drug receptors appear to consist of many large molecules that exist either on the cell membrane or within the cell itself (Figure 2-7). More than one receptor type or identical receptors can be found at the site of action. Usually, a specific drug will bind with a specific receptor in a lock-and-key fashion. Many drug-receptor interactions consist of weak chemical bonds, and the energy formed during this interaction is very low. As a result, the bonds can be formed and broken easily. Once a bond is broken, another drug molecule immediately binds to the receptor.

Different drugs often compete for the same receptor sites. The drug with the stronger affinity for the receptor will bind to more receptors than the drug with the weaker affinity (Figure 2-8). More of the drug with the weaker affinity will be required

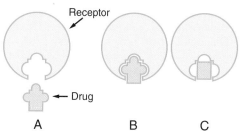

FIGURE 2-8
A, Drugs act by forming a chemical bond with specific receptor sites, similar to a lock and key. **B,** The better the "fit," the better the response. Drugs with complete attachment and response are called *agonists*. **C,** Drugs that attach but do not elicit a response are called *antagonists*. (From Clayton BD, Stock YN, Harroun RD: *Basic pharmacology for nurses,* ed 14, St Louis, 2007, Mosby.)

to produce a pharmacologic response. Drugs with a stronger affinity for receptor sites are more potent than drugs with weaker affinities for the same site.

◆ AGONISTS AND ANTAGONISTS

When a drug combines with a receptor, it alters the function of the organism. It may produce enhancement or inhibition of the function. Drugs that combine with the receptor may be classified as either agonists or antagonists (Figure 2-9).

Agonist. An agonist is a drug that (1) has affinity for a receptor, (2) combines with the receptor, and (3) produces an effect. Naturally occurring neurotransmitters are agonists.

Antagonist. An antagonist counteracts the action of the agonist. The following are three different types of antagonists:
- A *competitive antagonist* is a drug that (1) has affinity for a receptor, (2) combines with the receptor, and (3) produces

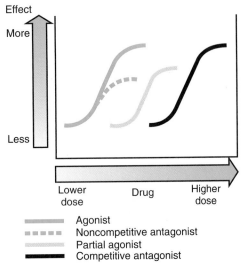

FIGURE 2-9
Agonists and antagonists and their interactions.

Legend:
— Agonist
- - - Noncompetitive antagonist
······ Partial agonist
— Competitive antagonist

no effect. This causes a shift to the right in the dose-response curve (see Figure 2-9). The antagonist competes with the agonist for the receptor, and the outcome depends on the relative affinity and concentrations of each agent. If the concentration of the agonist is increased, the competitive antagonism can be overcome and vice versa.

- *Noncompetitive antagonists* bind to a receptor site that is different from the binding site for the agonist. This reduces the maximal response of the agonist (see Figure 2-9).
- A *physiologic antagonist* has affinity for a different receptor site than the agonist. This decreases the maximal response of the agonist by producing an opposite effect via different receptors.

Transport carriers are systems that are available for moving neurotransmitters or drugs into the cell. In the process of making a neurotransmitter, the precursors (chemical to make a neurotransmitter) must be taken into the cell by an active transport pump (requires adenosine triphosphatase [ATPase]). For example, the precursor for norepinephrine is tyramine, so it must be pumped into the cell. After the neurotransmitter is synthesized, it is placed in little "suitcases" called *granules*. These go to the membranes and await the signal to "dump" their contents into the synapse. After the neurotransmitter is released, there are three paths that it can take. It can be broken down by enzymes designed to terminate the neurotransmitter's effect, it can migrate to the receptor and interact to produce an effect, or it can be taken up by the presynaptic nerve ending (reuptake). Reuptake is an easy way (requires little energy) to recover the neurotransmitter for future use because it is as easy as vacuuming up dirt.

PHARMACOKINETICS

Pharmacokinetics is the study of how a drug enters the body, circulates within the body, is changed by the body, and leaves the body. Factors that influence the movement of a drug are divided into four major steps: absorption, distribution, metabolism, and excretion (ADME).

Passage Across Body Membranes

The amount of drug passing through a cell membrane and the rate at which a drug moves are important in describing the time course of action and the variation in individual response to a drug. Before a drug is absorbed, transported, distributed to body tissues, metabolized, and subsequently eliminated from the body, it must pass through various membranes such as cellular membranes, blood capillary membranes, and intracellular membranes. Although these membranes have variable functions, they share certain physicochemical characteristics that influence the passage of drugs across their borders.

These membranes are composed of lipids (fats), proteins, and carbohydrates. The membrane lipids make the membrane relatively impermeable to ions and polar molecules. Membrane proteins make up the structural components of the membrane and help move the molecules across the membrane during the transport process. Membrane carbohydrates are combined with either proteins or lipids. The lipid molecules orient themselves so that they form a fluid bimolecular leaflet structure with the hydrophobic (lipophilic) ends of the molecules shielded from the surrounding aqueous environment and the hydrophilic ends in contact with the water. The various proteins are embedded in and layered onto this fluid lipid bilayer, forming a mosaic. Studies of the ability of substances to penetrate this membrane have indicated the presence of a system of pores or holes through which lower-molecular-weight and smaller size chemicals can pass.

The physicochemical properties of drugs that influence the passage of drugs across biologic membranes are lipid solubility, degree of ionization, and molecular size and shape. The mechanisms of drug transfer across biologic membranes are passive transfer and specialized transport.

♦ PASSIVE TRANSFER

Lipid-soluble substances move across the lipoprotein membrane by a passive transfer process called *simple diffusion*. This type of transfer is directly proportional to the concentration gradient (difference) of the drug across the membrane and the degree of lipid solubility. For example, a highly lipid-soluble compound will attain a higher concentration at the membrane site and will readily diffuse across the membrane into an area of lower concentration (Figure 2-10). A water-soluble agent will have difficulty passing through a membrane.

Water-soluble molecules small enough to pass through the membrane pores may be carried through the pores by the bulk flow of water. This process of filtration through single-cell membranes may occur with drugs having molecular weights of 200 or less. However, drugs with molecular weights of 60,000 can "filter" through capillary membranes.

♦ SPECIALIZED TRANSPORT

Certain substances are transported across cell membranes by processes that are more complex than simple diffusion or filtration. These processes include the following:

- **Active transport** is a process by which a substance is transported against a concentration gradient or electrochemical gradient. This action is blocked by metabolic inhibitors. Active transport is believed to be mediated by transport "carriers" that furnish energy for the transportation of the drug.
- **Facilitated diffusion** does not move against a concentration gradient. This phenomenon involves the transport of some

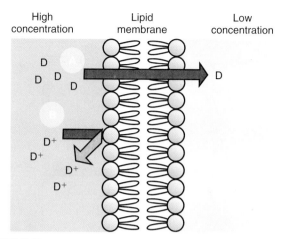

High concentration — Lipid membrane — Low concentration

FIGURE 2-10

Passage of drug and metabolite through membranes. **A,** Lipid soluble, nonionized: drug easily passes through the cell membrane from area of high to low drug concentration. **B,** Water soluble, ionized: drug cannot pass through the cell membrane. *D,* Drug.

substances, such as glucose, into cells. It has been suggested that the process of pinocytosis may explain the passage of macromolecular substances into the cells.

Absorption

Absorption is the process by which drug molecules are transferred from the site of administration to the circulating blood. This process requires the drug to pass through biologic membranes.

The following factors influence the rate of absorption of a drug:

- The physicochemical factors discussed previously.
- The site of absorption, which is determined by the route of administration. For example, one advantage of the oral route is the large absorbing area presented by the intestinal mucosa.
- The drug's solubility. Drugs in solution are more rapidly absorbed than insoluble drugs.

◆ EFFECT OF IONIZATION

Drugs that are weak electrolytes dissociate in solution and equilibrate into a nonionized form and an ionized form. The nonionized, or uncharged, portion acts like a nonpolar, lipid-soluble compound that readily crosses body membranes (see Figure 2-10). The ionized portion will traverse these membranes with greater difficulty because it is less lipid soluble.

The pH of the tissues at the site of administration and the dissociation characteristics (pKa) of the drug will determine the amount of drug present in the ionized and nonionized state. The proportion in each state will determine the ease with which the drug will penetrate the tissues.

Weak Acids. When the pH at the site of absorption increases, the hydrogen ion concentration simply falls. This results in an increase in the ionized form (A⁻), which cannot easily penetrate tissues.

Conversely, if the pH of the site falls, the hydrogen ion concentration will rise. This results in an increase in the unionized form (HA), which can more easily penetrate tissues.

Weak Bases. If the pH of the site rises, the hydrogen ion concentration will fall. This results in an increase in the un-

ionized form (B), which can more easily penetrate tissues. Conversely, if the pH of the site falls, the hydrogen ion concentration will rise. This results in an increase in the ionized form (BH⁺), which cannot easily penetrate tissues. In summary, weak acids are better absorbed when the pH is less than the pKa, whereas weak bases are better absorbed when the pH is greater than the pKa.

This dissociation also explains the fact that in the presence of infection the acidity of the tissue increases (and the pH decreases) and the effect of local anesthetics decreases. In the presence of infection, the [H⁺] increases because of accumulating waste products in the infected area. The increase in [H⁺] (decrease in pH) leads to an increase in ionization and a decrease in penetration of the membrane. This reduced penetration reduces the clinical effect of the local anesthetic.

◆ ORAL ABSORPTION

The dose form of a drug is an important factor influencing absorption of drugs administered via the oral route. Unless the drug is administered as a solution, the absorption of the drug in the gastrointestinal tract involves a release from a dose form such as a tablet or capsule. This release requires the following steps before absorption can take place:

- *Disruption:* The initial disruption of a tablet coating or capsule shell is necessary.
- *Disintegration:* The tablet or capsule contents must disintegrate (break apart).
- *Dispersion:* The concentrated drug particles must be dispersed (spread) throughout the stomach or intestines.
- *Dissolution:* The drug must be dissolved (in solution) in the gastrointestinal fluid.

A drug in solution skips these four steps, so it usually has a quicker onset of action.

◆ ABSORPTION FROM INJECTION SITE

Absorption of a drug from the site of injection depends on the solubility of the drug and the blood flow at that site. For example, drugs with low water solubility, such as some penicillin salts, are absorbed very slowly after intramuscular injection. Absorption at injection sites is also affected by the dose form. Drugs in suspension are absorbed much more slowly than those in solution. Certain insulin preparations are formulated in suspension form to decrease their absorption rate and prolong their action. Drugs that are least soluble will have the longest duration of action.

Distribution

◆ BASIC PRINCIPLES

All drugs occur in two forms in the blood: bound to plasma proteins and the free drug. The free drug is the form that exerts the pharmacologic effect. The bound drug is a reservoir (place to store) for the drug. The proportion of drug in each form depends on the properties of that specific drug (percent protein bound). Within each compartment (e.g., blood, brain), the drug is split between the bound drug and the free drug. Only the free drug can pass across cell membranes.

For a drug to exert its activity, it must be made available at its site of action in the body. The mechanism by which this is accomplished is distribution, which is the passage of drugs into various body fluid compartments such as plasma, interstitial

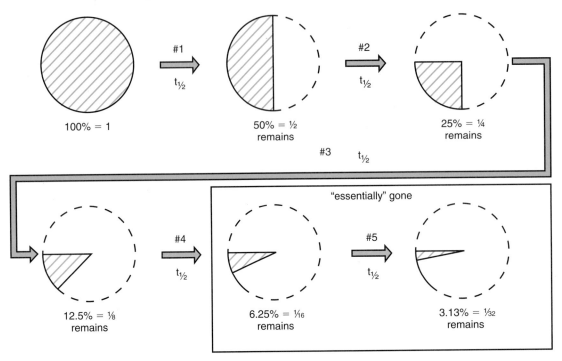

FIGURE 2-11
First-order kinetics. Half-life constant throughout usual doses. Half of the dose of the drug in the body is removed with each half-life. *#1, #2 ... #5*, Number of half-lives that have passed.

fluids, and intracellular fluids. The manner in which a drug is distributed in the body will determine how rapidly it produces the desired response; the duration of that response; and in some cases, whether a response will be elicited at all.

Drug distribution occurs when a drug moves to various sites in the body, including its site of action in specific tissues. However, drugs are also distributed to areas where no action is desired (nonspecific tissues). Some drugs, because of their characteristics, are poorly distributed to certain regions of the body. Other drugs are distributed to their site of action and then redistributed to another tissue site. The distribution of a drug is determined by several factors such as the size of the organ, the blood flow to the organ, the solubility of the drug, the plasma protein-binding capacity, and the presence of certain barriers (blood-brain barrier, placenta).

♦ **DISTRIBUTION BY PLASMA**

After a drug is absorbed from its site of administration, it is distributed to its site of action by the blood plasma. Therefore the biologic activity of a drug is related to the concentration of the free, or unbound, drug in the plasma. Drugs are bound reversibly to plasma proteins such as albumin and globulin. The drug that is bound to the protein does not contribute to the intensity of the drug action because only the unbound form is biologically active. The bound drug is considered a storage site. If one drug is highly bound, another administered drug that is highly bound may displace the first drug from its plasma protein-binding sites, increasing the effect of the first drug. This is one mechanism of drug interaction.

Half-Life

The half-life ($t_{1/2}$) of a drug is the amount of time that passes for the concentration of a drug to fall to one-half of its blood

level (Figure 2-11). When the half-life of a drug is short, it is quickly removed from the body and its duration of action is short. When the half-life of a drug is long, it is slowly removed from the body and its duration of action is long.

Figure 2-11 shows the percent of a drug remaining after each of four and five half-lives. Because only 3% to 6% remains after four or five half-lives, respectively, we can say that the drug is essentially gone. Conversely, it takes about four or five half-lives of repeated dosing for a drug's level to build up to a steady state (level amount) in the body. If the half-life of a drug is 1 hour, then in 4 or 5 hours the drug would be mostly gone from the body. In 4 hours, 94% of the drug would be gone. However, if the half-life of a drug is 60 hours, then it would take 240 (10 days) to 300 hours (12 days) for that drug to be eliminated from the body. Even after discontinuing a drug with a long half-life, its effect can take several days to dissipate, depending on its half-life.

Blood-Brain Barrier

The tissue sites of distribution should be considered before administration. For example, for drugs to penetrate the central nervous system (CNS), they must cross the blood-brain barrier. The passage of a drug across this barrier is related to the drug's lipid solubility and degree of ionization. The endothelium of this barrier contains a cell layer and a basement membrane. The welding of the endothelial cells together prevents the formation of clefts, gaps, or pores that might allow the penetration of certain drugs. To diffuse transcellularly, the drug must penetrate the epithelial and basement membrane cells. Thiopental, a highly lipid-soluble, nonionized drug, easily penetrates the blood-brain barrier to gain access to the cerebrospinal fluid and induce sleep within seconds after intravenous administration. In contrast, a highly ionized compound such as hexamethonium would not be likely to cross this barrier and therefore would produce few if any effects on the brain.

♦ PLACENTA

The passage of drugs across the placenta involves simple diffusion in accordance with their degree of lipid solubility. Although the placenta may act as a selective barrier against a few drugs, most drugs pass easily across the placental barrier. Lipid-soluble drugs penetrate this membrane most easily. Therefore when agents are administered to the mother, they are concomitantly administered to the fetus. The term *barrier* is a misnomer.

♦ ENTEROHEPATIC CIRCULATION

Drugs are typically absorbed via the intestines, are distributed through the serum, pass to specific and nonspecific sites of action, come to the liver, and are metabolized before being excreted via the kidneys. When a drug undergoes enterohepatic circulation, the process varies. The steps are the same until the drug is metabolized. At that point, the metabolite is secreted via the bile into the intestine. The metabolite is broken down by enzymes and releases the drug. The drug is then absorbed again, and the process continues. After being taken up by the liver the second time, these drugs are again secreted into the bile. This circular pattern continues with some drug escaping with each passing. This process prolongs the effect of a drug. If enterohepatic circulation is blocked, the level of the drug in the serum will fall.

Redistribution

Redistribution of a drug is the movement of a drug from the site of action to nonspecific sites of action. A drug's duration of action can be affected by redistribution of the drug from one organ to another. If redistribution occurs between specific sites and nonspecific sites, a drug's action will be terminated. For example, thiopental produces sleep within seconds, but the effect is terminated within a few minutes. This is because the drug is first distributed to the CNS (sleep), subsequently redistributed through the plasma to the muscle (action terminated), and finally reaches the fat depots of the body (no action still).

Metabolism (Biotransformation)

> Drug metabolism produces compounds that are more polar (ionized) and more easily excreted.

Metabolism, which is also known as biotransformation, is the body's way of changing a drug so that it can be more easily excreted by the kidneys. Many drugs undergo metabolic transformation or change, most commonly in the liver. The metabolite (metabolic product) formed is usually more polar (ionized) and less lipid soluble than its parent compound. This means that renal tubular reabsorption of the metabolite will be reduced because reabsorption favors lipid-soluble compounds. Metabolites are also less likely to bind to plasma or tissue proteins and less likely to be stored in fat tissue. Decreased renal tubular reabsorption, decreased binding to the plasma or tissue proteins, and decreased fat storage cause the metabolite to be excreted more easily. Drug metabolism is an enzyme-dependent process that has developed through evolution.

Drugs can be metabolized in one of three of the following different means (Figure 2-12):

* *Active to inactive:* By metabolism, an inactive compound may be formed from an active parent drug. This is the most

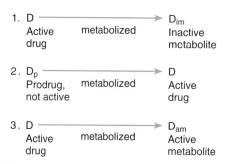

FIGURE 2-12
Metabolism mechanisms.

common type of reaction in drug biotransformation. Agents that interfere with the metabolism of certain drugs will increase the blood level of the drugs whose metabolism is inhibited. An example of this is doxycycline. Doxycycline itself is the active compound and is metabolized by the liver into a metabolite without activity.

* *Inactive to active:* An inactive parent drug may be transformed into an active compound. The inactive compound is then termed a *prodrug*. Interference with the metabolism of this drug will delay its onset of action because it will be harder for the active compound to be formed. For example, acyclovir is an antiviral agent. To be effective, it must be taken into the cell and converted to its active metabolite.

* *Active to active:* An active parent drug may be converted to a second active compound, which is then converted to an inactive product. The total effect of such a drug would be the addition of the effect of the parent drug plus the effect of the active drug metabolite. When an active metabolite is formed, the action of the drug is prolonged. For example, diazepam (Valium), an active antianxiety agent, is metabolized into its active metabolite, desmethyldiazepam. Diazepam's action is prolonged because of its own effect combined with that of its active metabolite.

Although the rates and pathways of drug metabolism vary among species, most studies indicate that drug biotransformation in laboratory animals is similar to that in humans. Many synthetic mechanisms of drug metabolism occur in the body to form metabolites.

♦ FIRST-PASS EFFECT

Metabolism of drugs may be divided into two general types: phase I and phase II. If a drug has no functional groups with which to combine, then the drug must undergo a phase I reaction.

Phase I. In phase I reactions, lipid molecules are metabolized by the three processes of oxidation, reduction, and hydrolysis.

Oxidation. When a drug is administered that does not possess an appropriate functional group suitable for combining with body acids (conjugation), the body has more difficulty detoxifying that drug. An enzyme system responsible for the oxidative metabolism of many drugs is located in the liver. The enzymes are located in the endoplasmic reticulum and are termed *microsomal enzymes* because they are found in the microsomal fraction as prepared from liver homogenates. A variety of oxidative reactions, such as hydroxylation or the incorporation of oxygen into the substrate molecule, occur in these hepatic microsomal enzymes.

Oxidative processes involving enzymes other than those of the hepatic microsomal enzymes can take place. Some compounds are oxidatively deaminated by enzymes located in the liver, kidney, and nervous tissue. Other agents are detoxified by specific oxidative enzymes.

Hydrolysis. Some ester compounds are metabolized by hydrolysis. Hydrolytic enzymes, which are found in plasma and a variety of tissues, break up esters and add water. The ester local anesthetics are inactivated by plasma cholinesterases.

Reduction. Many reduction reactions are mediated by the enzymes found in the hepatic microsomes.

Microsomal Enzymes. Phase I reactions are carried out by the microsomal or cytochrome P-450 enzymes, which are also known as the *mixed function oxidases* in the liver. The concentration of these enzymes can be affected by drugs and environmental substances. Phase I metabolism may be affected by other drugs that alter microsomal enzyme inhibition or induction.

Induction. The P-450 hepatic microsomal enzymes can be induced (the amount of enzyme increased) by some drugs and by smoking tobacco. Because drugs that cause enzyme induction cause other drugs to be more quickly metabolized, the metabolized drugs will have reduced pharmacologic effects. More recent evidence has discovered that the hepatic enzymes can be divided into many categories called *isoenzymes.* Examples of isoenzymes include cytochrome P-450 2D6 and 3A4. Table 2-1 lists samples of drugs that are substrates of these enzymes and drugs that either induce or inhibit these isoenzymes. For example, phenobarbital stimulates the production of microsomal enzymes that normally metabolize the anticoagulant warfarin. Thus administering phenobarbital to a patient taking warfarin can decrease warfarin's anticoagulant response because the metabolism of the anticoagulant is stimulated by phenobarbital (Figure 2-13).

Some drugs, such as valproate and carbamazepine (anticonvulsants), can also stimulate their own metabolism. The tolerance that patients develop to certain drugs can be explained, at least in part, by an increased ability to metabolize the drug because of stimulation of microsomal enzymes.

Inhibition. Inhibition of the metabolism of certain drugs may occur through several mechanisms. With inhibition, the blood levels and action of the drugs metabolized by these enzymes will be increased. Examples of drugs that inhibit the metabolism of other drugs are erythromycin and cimetidine. Inhibiting the microsomal enzymes would result in an increase in the effect of the drugs metabolized by the liver enzymes (see Table 2-1).

Phase II. Phase II reactions involve conjugation with the following agents: glucuronic acid, sulfuric acid, acetic acid, or an amino acid. The most common conjugation occurs with glucuronic acid. This conjugation is termed glucuronidation. Glucuronic acid, which is a substance normally occurring in the body, may be transferred to a drug molecule that has an appropriate functional group to accept it. Functional groups that may be involved include ethers, alcohols, aromatic amines, and carboxylic acid. This mechanism, either alone or in combination with a phase I reaction, allows the body to convert a lipid-soluble drug to a more polar compound. The enzymes that mediate the conjugation are termed transferases.

◆ EXCRETION

Although drugs may be excreted by any of several routes that have direct access to the external environment, renal (kidney)

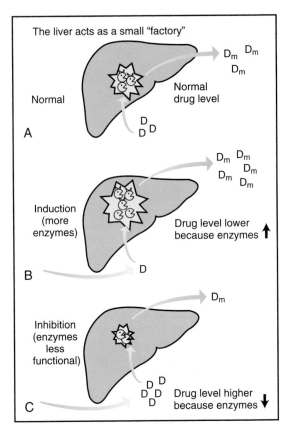

FIGURE 2-13

Alteration of drug metabolism induction and inhibition. Enzyme induction and inhibition alter the blood levels of drugs metabolized by the hepatic enzymes. **A,** Normal. The liver is metabolizing drugs at the normal rate producing the normal effects. **B,** Induction. With enzyme induction (stimulation), increase in the enzymes causes the drug to be more quickly metabolized, and blood level of the drug and its effect are decreased (assume that metabolite is inactive). Induction = effect. **C,** Inhibition. With enzyme inhibition, the metabolism of drugs is slower (weaker enzymes) and the blood level of the drug that is metabolized is increased. Inhibition = effect.

excretion is the most important. Extrarenal routes include the lungs, bile, gastrointestinal tract, sweat, saliva, and milk. Drugs may be excreted unchanged or as metabolites.

Kinetics. Kinetics is the mathematical representation of the way in which drugs are removed from the body. The most common mechanism is first-order kinetics (see Figure 2-11).

A few drugs, such as aspirin and alcohol, exhibit zero-order kinetics. With zero-order kinetics, the rate of metabolism remains constant over time, and the same amount of drug is metabolized per unit of time regardless of dose. Zero-order kinetics occurs because the enzymes that metabolize these drugs can become saturated at usual therapeutic doses. If the dose of the drug is increased, the metabolism cannot increase above its maximum rate. With small doses, drugs with zero-order kinetics can metabolize the drug without buildup. With high doses, the metabolism of the drug cannot increase and the duration of action of the drug can be greatly prolonged (Figure 2-14). Small changes in the dose of these drugs may produce a large change in the serum concentration, leading to unexpected toxicity.

Renal Route. Elimination of substances in the kidney can occur by the following three routes:

TABLE 2-1 SELECTED CYP-450 ISOENZYMES SUBSTRATES, INHIBITORS, AND INDUCERS

Number	Substrate	Inhibitors	Inducers
CYP 1A2	Antidepressants, tricyclic d-Warfarin Theophylline	Fluoroquinolones	Barbiturates Carbamazepine
CYP 2C8/9/10	Anticonvulsants NSAIDs s-Warfarin	Anticonvulsants Antidepressants, SSRI	Cimetidine Omeprazole
CYP 2C18/19	Antidepressants Naproxen Propranolol Proton pump inhibitors	Antidepressants, SSRI Imidazoles Omeprazole	Barbiturates Rifampin
CYP 2D6	Antiarrhythmics Antidepressants Antipsychotics Opioids	Antidepressants, SSRI Antipsychotics Cimetidine	Not susceptible
CYP 2E1	Alcohol	Alcohol intoxication	Alcohol, abuse (person sober)
CYP 3A3	Erythromycin	Cimetidine	
CYP 3A4	Antidepressants Benzodiazepines Calcium channel blockers Carbamazepine HMG-CoA reductase inhibitors Imidazoles Macrolides	Antidepressants Corticosteroids Grapefruit juice Imidazoles Macrolides Omeprazole	Anticonvulsants
CYP 3A5	Lovastatin Midazolam Nifedipine		

CYP, Cytochrome; HMG-CoA, 3-hydroxy-3-methylglutaryl-coenzyme A; NSAIDs, nonsteroidal antiinflammatory drugs; SSRI, selective serotonin reuptake inhibitor.

1. *Glomerular filtration:* Either the unchanged drug or its metabolites are filtered through the glomeruli and concentrated in the renal tubular fluid. This filtration process depends on the amount of plasma protein binding and the glomerular filtration rate. Bound drugs cannot be filtered and remain in the systemic circulation. Most drugs are managed by this mechanism.

2. *Active tubular secretion:* Active secretion transports the drug from the bloodstream across the renal tubular epithelial cells and into the renal tubular fluid. Glomerular filtration and active tubular secretion are relatively nonselective, and several compounds, both exogenous and endogenous (naturally occurring), can compete for transport.

3. *Passive tubular diffusion:* With most drugs, passive tubular diffusion (also termed *passive reabsorption*) plays a part in regulating the amount of drug in the tubular fluid. This process favors the reabsorption of nonionized, lipid-soluble compounds. The more ionized, less lipid-soluble metabolites have more difficulty penetrating the cell membranes of the renal tubules and are likely to be retained in the tubular fluid and eliminated in the urine. This process is also influenced by the urinary pH, which affects the amount of ionized and nonionized drug in the tubular fluid. By altering the pH of the urine, drug excretion can be favored in cases of poisoning or can be inhibited when a prolongation of the drug effect is desired. Weakly ionized acids or bases are excreted in the following fashion:

- *Alkaline urine:* When the tubular urinary pH is more alkaline than the plasma, weak acids are excreted more rapidly and weak bases are excreted more slowly.
- *Acid urine:* When tubular urine is more acid, weak acids are excreted more slowly and weak bases are excreted more rapidly.

Extrarenal Routes. Certain drugs may be partially or completely eliminated via routes other than the kidney by the lungs. Gases used in general anesthesia are excreted across the lung tissue by a process of simple diffusion. Alcohol is also partially excreted from the lungs. (One can smell alcohol on someone's breath if they have been drinking alcohol.) This fact is used when testing a driver's breath for the presence of alcohol (Breathalyzer).

Biliary Excretion. Biliary excretion is the major route by which systemically absorbed drugs enter the gastrointestinal tract and are eliminated in the feces. Drugs excreted in the bile may also be reabsorbed from the intestines. Thus enterohepatic circulation, discussed earlier, prolongs a drug's action.

Other. Two minor routes of elimination are in the milk and the sweat. The distribution of drugs in milk may be a potential source of undesirable effects for the nursing infant. Chapter 25 discusses dental drugs that can be given to nursing mothers.

Saliva. Drugs can also be excreted into the saliva. After drugs are excreted in the saliva, they are usually swallowed and their fate is the same as drugs ingested orally. The following drugs have been detected at significant levels in saliva after oral

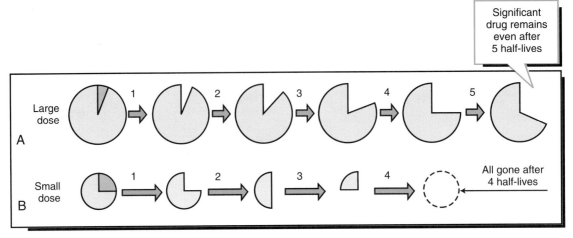

FIGURE 2-14

Zero-order kinetics. Large dose **(A).** Small dose **(B).** Disappearance of a drug whose metabolism is saturable: With small dose **(B),** the drug is metabolized more quickly than when a large dose **(A)** is given. With large dose the metabolism cannot increase, so it takes a long time for the body to clear the drug. The half-life varies with the dose of the drug.

ingestion: aspirin, phenytoin, ampicillin, diazepam, penicillin VK, and phenobarbital. Present evidence suggests that most drugs that are secreted in the salivary glands enter saliva by simple diffusion, and their passage depends mainly on the lipid solubility of the drug. Thus a drug with high lipid solubility at plasma and salivary pH will readily enter saliva from plasma.

Drug levels in saliva have been studied to see if they can be used to monitor therapy with certain agents. For example, antiepileptic drug monitoring is essential for the rational treatment of epilepsy, and the measurement of these drugs in plasma is now routine. Assay of salivary concentrations of these drugs may become a reliable method that is not invasive for predicting plasma levels. More study is needed before salivary levels can replace measuring the blood levels of the drug.

Gingival Crevicular Fluid. Drugs may also be excreted in the gingival crevicular fluid (GCF). Drugs excreted in the GCF produce a higher level of drug in the gingival crevices, which can increase their usefulness in the treatment of periodontal disease. Some drugs, such as the tetracyclines, are concentrated in the GCF. This means that the drug level of tetracycline in the GCF will be several times (four or more times) higher than the blood level. This property makes the systemic use of a drug more effective within the gingival sulcus than one that is not concentrated.

ROUTES OF ADMINISTRATION AND DOSE FORMS
Routes of Administration

Route—various ways a drug can be administered

The route of administration of a drug affects both the onset and duration of response. *Onset* refers to the time it takes for the drug to begin to have its effect. *Duration* is the length of a drug's effect. The routes of administration can be classified as enteral or parenteral. Drugs given by the enteral route are placed directly into the gastrointestinal tract by oral or rectal administration. Parenteral administration bypasses the gastrointestinal tract and includes various injection routes, inhalation, and topical administration. In practice, the term *parenteral* usually refers to an injection.

Although oral administration is considered the safest, least expensive, and most convenient route, the parenteral route has certain advantages. The injection results in fast absorption, which produces a rapid onset and a more predictable response than oral administration. The parenteral route is useful for emergencies, unconsciousness, lack of cooperation, or nausea. Some drugs must be administered by injection to remain active. The disadvantages of the parenteral route include the facts that asepsis must be maintained to prevent infection, an intravascular injection can occur by accident, administration by injection is more painful, it is difficult to remove the drug, adverse effects may be more pronounced, and self-medication is difficult. Parenteral therapy is also more dangerous and more expensive than oral medication. Figure 2-15 illustrates several common forms of drug administration.

◆ ORAL ROUTE

Oral—most common and most popular route of administration

The oral route of administration is the simplest way to introduce a drug into the body. It allows the use of many different dose forms to obtain the desired results; tablets, capsules, and liquids are conveniently given. An advantage of this route is the large absorbing area present in the small intestine. Oral administration produces a slower onset of action than parenterally administered agents. One disadvantage of this route is that stomach and intestinal irritation may result in nausea and vomiting. Another disadvantage is that certain drugs, such as insulin, are inactivated by gastrointestinal tract acidity or enzymes.

When drugs are given orally, they are absorbed through the intestinal wall and then pass through the hepatic (liver) portal circulation, which can inactivate some drugs. This is termed the *first-pass effect* because the drug passes through the liver first before it circulates in the systemic circulation. During the drug's first pass through the liver, it is metabolized (amount metabolized varies) and the amount of drug available to produce a systemic effect is reduced. Drugs with a high first-pass effect have a larger oral-to-parenteral dose ratio. This means that the dose required for an equivalent effect orally is much greater than the dose needed when used parenterally. Because morphine has a high first-pass effect, the oral dose needed to produce an equivalent effect is much larger than its parenteral dose.

Blood levels obtained after oral administration are less predictable than those obtained parenterally. The presence of food in the stomach, the pathologic condition of the gastrointestinal tract, the effects of gastric acidity, and passage through the hepatic portal circulation can alter blood levels. Drug interactions can occur when two drugs are present in the stomach. The oral route necessitates greater patient cooperation.

◆ RECTAL ROUTE

Drugs may be given rectally as suppositories, creams, or enemas. Rectal administration can be used if a patient is vomiting or unconscious. This route may be used for either a local (e.g., hemorrhoids) or a systemic (e.g., antiemetic) effect. Because

most drugs are poorly and irregularly absorbed rectally, this route is not often used to achieve a systemic drug effect. In addition, patient acceptance of this route is poor.

◆ INTRAVENOUS ROUTE

Intravenous administration produces the most rapid drug response, with an almost immediate onset of action. Because the injection is made directly into the blood, the absorption phase is bypassed. Another advantage of the intravenous route is that it produces a more predictable response than oral administration because factors that affect drug absorption have been eliminated. It is also the route of choice for an emergency situation. The disadvantages of administration include phlebitis caused by local irritation, drug irretrievability (cannot get it back), allergy, and side effects related to high plasma concentrations of the drug.

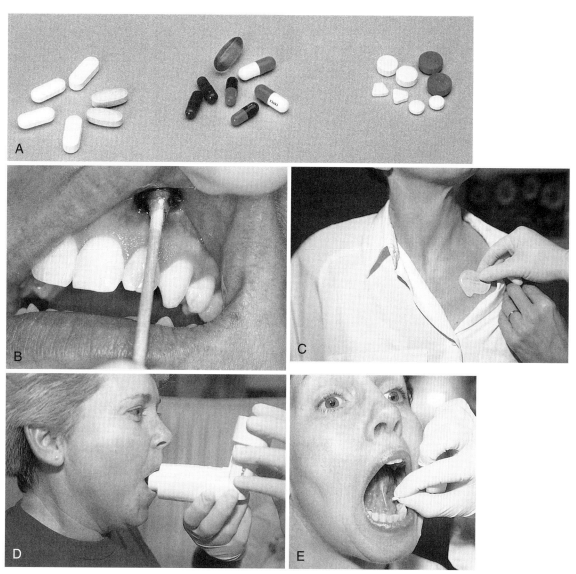

FIGURE 2-15

Routes of drug administration. **A,** Oral route in the form of pills, tablets, capsules, or liquids. **B,** Topical route by applying on the surface of the mucosa or skin. **C,** Transdermal route through a patch that continuously releases a controlled quantity of a medication through the skin. **D,** Inhalation route by breathing in a gaseous substance. **E,** Sublingual route by placing medication under the tongue (absorption takes place through the oral mucosa).

Continued

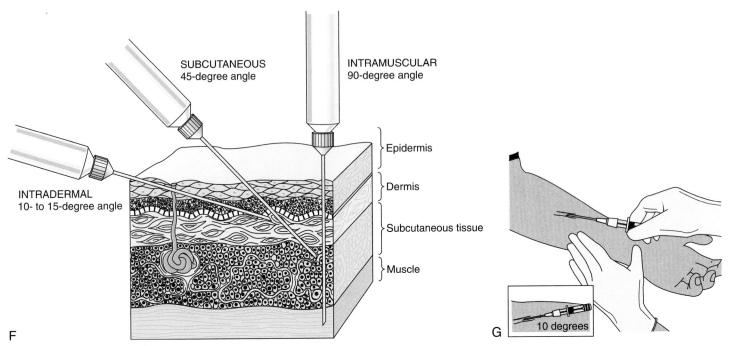

FIGURE 2-15, cont'd

F, Injection route. The type of drug determines how the injection is given: subcutaneous, directly under the skin; intramuscular, into a muscle; intradermal, into the skin. (**G,** Example of an intravenous push medication administration. (**A,** From Young AP, Proctor DB: *Kinn's the medical assistant: an applied learning approach,* ed 10, St. Louis, 2007, Saunders; **B,** from Daniel SJ, Harfst SA, Wilder RS: *Mosby's dental hygiene: concepts, cases, and competencies,* ed 2, St. Louis, 2008, Mosby; **C-F,** from Chester GA: *Modern medical assisting,* Philadelphia, 1998, Saunders; **G,** from Clayton BD, Stock YN, Harroun RD: *Basic pharmacology for nurses,* ed 14, St Louis, 2007, Mosby.)

◆ INTRAMUSCULAR ROUTE

Absorption of drugs injected into the muscle occurs because of the high blood flow through skeletal muscles. Somewhat irritating drugs may be tolerated if given by the intramuscular route. This route may also be used for injection of suspensions to provide a sustained effect. Injections are usually made in the deltoid region or gluteal mass.

◆ SUBCUTANEOUS ROUTE

The subcutaneous route involves the injection of solutions or suspensions of drugs into the subcutaneous areolar tissue to gain access to the systemic circulation. If irritating solutions are injected, sterile abscesses may result. Insulin is commonly administered by this route.

◆ INTRADERMAL ROUTE

Small amounts of drugs, such as local anesthetics, can be injected into the epidermis of the skin to provide local anesthesia. With this type of injection, a small bump (bleb) rises as the liquid is injected just under the skin. The tuberculosis skin test is performed using the intradermal route.

◆ INTRATHECAL ROUTE

Intrathecal administration involves the injection of solutions into the spinal subarachnoid space. This may be used for spinal anesthesia or for the treatment of certain forms of meningitis.

◆ INTRAPERITONEAL ROUTE

The intraperitoneal route involves placing fluid into the peritoneal cavity, where exchange of substances can occur. A drug may be absorbed through the mesenteric veins. This route of administration is also used for peritoneal dialysis. In this case, the substances are passing from the body to the fluid. Large volumes of fluids are slowly run into the peritoneal cavity. A waiting period of several hours allows the waste products from the body to be exchanged with the fluid in the peritoneal cavity. The fluid is removed, and the body's waste products are carried out in the fluid. This process is used as a substitute for the failing kidney to manage patients with renal failure.

◆ INHALATION ROUTE

> Inhalation route—used for local or systemic effects

The inhalation route may be used in the administration of the gaseous, microcrystalline, liquid, or powdered form of drugs. This route of administration may be used for either local or systemic effects. An example of inhalers being used for their local effects are those used to treat asthma. After inhalation, the drug is deposited on the bronchiolar endothelium and exerts its action by producing bronchodilation or reducing inflammation. Inhalation of aerosolized liquid in fine droplets also produces a local effect. Today's oral metered dose inhalers contain hydrofluorocarbons that do not harm the ozone. These inhalers contain finely powdered drugs that are also inhaled into the lungs. One advantage of the use of the powdered form is that inhalation must continue until the visible powder is gone. General anesthetics in the form of volatile liquids, such as isoflurane, or gases, such as nitrous oxide (N_2O) and oxygen, are examples of the use of the inhalation route for systemic effects. This route of administration is popular for the abuse of many drugs (smoked or even inhaled) because of the quick onset of action and the lack of need for needles.

◆ TOPICAL ROUTE

Topical routes consist of application to body surfaces. Topical applications are administered to the skin, the oral mucosa, and even sublingually (under the tongue). The inhalation route could even be called topical. Drugs used topically may be intended to produce either local or systemic effects.

Because most drugs do not penetrate intact skin, application to the skin is generally used for local effects. Corticosteroids are applied to inflamed or irritated skin. Intravaginal creams or suppositories or solutions or suspensions instilled into the eye or ear are other ways to administer topical agents to produce local effects.

Rarely, systemic side effects (unintended) can occur from the topical administration of drugs for their local effect. One example is the administration of topical corticosteroids over a large proportion of the body, resulting in symptoms of systemic toxicity (Cushing's syndrome). If an occlusive dressing (commercial plastic wrap or a plastic suit) is used or if the surface is abraded, inflamed, or sloughing, the chance of side effects increases dramatically. In the oral cavity, interruptions in the mucous membranes or mucosal inflammation increase the likelihood of a systemic effect. Local anesthetics sprayed into the mouth may be adsorbed and produce a blood level equivalent to that produced by intravenous administration.

Examples of drugs applied topically for a systemic effect include transdermal patches and sublingual spray or tablet administration. Drugs that often produce allergic reactions should not be administered topically because sensitization occurs more readily than when used orally.

Subgingival Strips and Gels. A dental-specific topical application involves the placement of drug-impregnated strips or gels subgingivally. Systemic effects are minimized because small doses can be used when drugs are administered via this route. Doxycycline gel (Atridox) and a chlorhexidine-containing chip (PerioChip) are examples of agents administered into the gingival crevice.

Transdermal Patch. Transdermal drug delivery systems (drug patches) are designed to provide continuous controlled release of medication through a semipermeable membrane over a given period after application of drug to the intact skin. This eliminates the need for repeated oral dosing. Examples of patches on the market include scopolamine (Transderm-Scop), nitroglycerin (Transderm-Nitro, Nitrodisc, Nitro-Dur), clonidine (Catapres-TTS), estrogens (Estraderm, Climara), fentanyl (Duragesic), and nicotine transdermal patches (NicoDerm, Nicobid).

Most patches consist of several layers. Beginning with the skin, the layers are as follows: adhesive (to stick to the skin), membrane (to control the rate of drug release), drug reservoir (where the drug is stored), and a backing that is impenetrable to the drug (to keep the drug from evaporating into the air) (Figure 2-16). Before use, the protective backing must be removed. The most common problems with transdermal patches are local irritation, erythema, and edema. These problems can be minimized by rotating the location of the patch. Patches are designed to be changed daily, every few days, or weekly, depending on the drug.

Topical Anesthesia. Topical anesthetics are applied directly to the mucous membranes and rapidly absorbed into the systemic

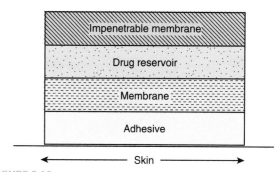

FIGURE 2-16
Layers of a transdermal patch.

circulation, providing the patient with injection-free local anesthesia. An example of this type of anesthesia is the combination of lidocaine and prilocaine (Oraqix).

> SL—"under the tongue" for systemic effects

Sublingual and Buccal Routes. Two ways in which drugs can be applied topically are sublingual (SL) and buccal routes. The mucous membranes of the oral cavity provide a convenient absorbing surface for the systemic administration of drugs, which can be placed under the tongue (sublingual) or on other areas of the oral mucosa (buccal pouch). Absorption of many drugs into the systemic circulation occurs rapidly. An example of this effect is the fast onset of action of nitroglycerin sublingual tablets to treat acute anginal pain. Drugs that are susceptible to degradation by the gastrointestinal tract and even by the liver, such as testosterone, are safely administered as sublingual tablets because they avoid both the first-pass effect and gastrointestinal acid and enzymes.

◆ OTHER ROUTES

Drugs, such as progestins (Norplant), can be implanted under the skin to release a drug over a prolonged duration (5 years). Pumps that deliver drugs intravenously can be implanted in the body. When insulin pumps are used, they can be programmed externally using a calculator-like keyboard.

Dose Forms

Table 2-2 lists the usual dose forms. The most commonly used dose forms in dentistry are the tablet and capsule given orally. Liquid solutions or suspensions are often prescribed for children. Sometimes drugs are given in solution or suspension when a liquid form is desired. Liquid forms of a drug are often used for children. For injection, the drug may be in solution, such as a local anesthetic, or it may be in a suspension, such as procaine penicillin G, when a longer duration of action is desired. Mouthwashes containing alcohol are also recommended by dental health care workers. Elixirs (contain alcohol) and syrups (contain sugar) are children's dose forms.

FACTORS THAT ALTER DRUG EFFECTS

When a drug is administered, the following factors may influence or modify the drug's effect:

* *Patient compliance:* Through either lack of understanding or lack of motivation, patients often take medication incorrectly or not at all. Sometimes this may result from faulty com-

TABLE 2-2   DOSAGE FORMS

Form	Definition	Example
Tablet	Molded or compressed medicinal substance with inert binder included to make a hard mass	Acetaminophen tablet
Capsule	Gelatin shell that disintegrates in water to administer solids or liquids	Tetracycline capsule
Pill	Globular or ovoid dose form made by incorporating medicinal agents with other binders to make a plastic mass; obsolete	Ferrous carbonate pill
Lozenge, troche	Flavored dose form designed to be held in the mouth to dissolve or disintegrate slowly	Cough drop
Suppository	Single-dose medication in waxy or fatty conical or ovoid shape that liberates active ingredient after insertion into the rectum or vagina for local or systemic effects	Glycerin suppository
Solution	One-phase system of two or more chemical components	Saline water
Elixir	Sweetened hydroalcoholic solution containing flavoring materials	Acetaminophen and codeine elixir; diphenhydramine
Syrup	Nearly saturated aqueous solution of sugar	Dextromethorphan syrup
Tincture	Alcoholic or hydroalcoholic solution of drugs	Iodine tincture
Spirit	Solution of volatile substance in alcohol	Aromatic ammonia spirit
Lotion	Liquid suspension that can be protective	Hand lotion
Emulsion	Preparation of two immiscible liquids, usually water and oil, one dispersed as small globules in the other	Liquid petrolatum emulsion
Suspension	Dispersion containing finely divided insoluble material suspended in a liquid medium	Amoxicillin suspension
Cream	Emulsions that contain an oily and aqueous phase; external phase aqueous	Hydrocortisone cream
Ointment	Semisolid preparation for external use that is a consistency that can be applied by rubbing; external phase oily	Hydrocortisone ointment, A+D ointment
Transdermal patch	A permeable polymer membrane backed with a drug reservoir designed to provide controlled release of medication over a given period after application to intact skin	Nitroglycerin, scopolamine, fentanyl, nicotine
Aerosol spray	Solution of volatile liquids with a propellant that delivers drugs to area	Albuterol inhaler, foot spray
Intradermal implant	Small pellets implanted under skin that allow drugs to be released slowly	Norplant
Micropump	An implanted pump that delivers drug via a needle	Insulin pump

munication, inadequate patient education, or the patient's health belief system. Thus poor patient compliance can be an important factor in a therapeutic failure.

- *Psychologic factors:* The attitude of the prescriber and the dental staff can affect the efficacy of the drug prescribed. A placebo is a dose form that looks like the active agent but contains no active ingredients (the "sugar pill"). The magnitude of the placebo effect depends on the patient's perception, and there is large individual variation. Health care providers can maximize the drug's effect to achieve an improved therapeutic result by talking up the drug. This may account for the popularity of herbs and plants.

- *Tolerance:* A patient may exhibit tolerance to many drugs, including the sedative-hypnotics and the opioids. Drug tolerance is defined as the need for an increasingly larger dose of the drug to obtain the same effects as the original dose or the decreased effect produced after repeated administration of a given dose of the drug. When a patient becomes tolerant to one drug, tolerance to other drugs with similar pharmacologic actions occurs. This is termed *cross-tolerance.* If toler-

ance develops, a normal sensitivity to the drug's effect may be restored by ceasing administration of the drug. Tachyphylaxis is the very rapid development of tolerance, often within hours.

- *Pathologic state:* Diseased patients may respond to the administration of medication differently than other patients. For example, patients with hyperthyroidism are extremely sensitive to the toxic effects of epinephrine. Hepatic or renal disease influences the metabolism and excretion of drugs, potentially leading to an increased duration of drug action. With repeated doses in diseased patients, the serum level of a drug may become toxic.

- *Time of administration:* The time a drug is administered, especially in relation to meals, alters the response to that drug. Certain drugs with a sedative action are best administered at bedtime to minimize the sedation experienced by the patient.

- *Route of administration:* The effect of the route of administration on the onset and duration of action of a drug was discussed previously.

- *Sex:* The sex of the patient can alter a drug's effect. Women may be more sensitive than men to certain drugs, perhaps because of their smaller size or their hormones. Pregnancy alters the effect of certain drugs. Women of child-bearing age should avoid teratogenic drugs, and the oral health care provider should determine whether the patient is pregnant before administering any agent.
- *Genetic variation:* Many differences in patient response to drugs have been associated with variations in ability to metabolize certain drugs. This difference may account for the fact that certain populations have a higher incidence of adverse effects to some drugs—a genetic predisposition.
- *Drug interactions:* A drug's effect may be modified by previous or concomitant administration of another drug. There are many mechanisms by which drug interactions may modify a patient's treatment.
- *Age and weight:* The dose of a drug administered to children should be reduced from the adult dose. Age or weight has been suggested as a method of calculating a child's dose. Because of the great variability of weight in relation to age, the child's weight should be used to determine the child's dose. Because a child is not just a small adult, the manufacturer's recommendations for children's dosing would be best. Older adults may respond differently to drugs than younger patients. Whether this is solely because of changes in renal or liver function or whether being elderly patients predisposes this sensitivity is controversial.
- *Environment:* The environment contains many substances that may affect the action of drugs. Smoking induces enzymes, so higher doses of benzodiazepines are needed to produce the same effect as compared to nonsmokers. Some chemical contaminants, such as pesticides or solvents, can have an effect on a drug's action.
- *Other:* The action of drugs can be altered by the patient-provider interaction. If the patient "believes" in the substance or process (drug/herb//incantation) being used, the patient's opinion will enhance the drug's effect. The attitude of both the patient and the provider can alter the physiology of the body. These actions may account for the positive effect of many mental exercises (e.g., meditation).

DENTAL HYGIENE CONSIDERATIONS

1. Various factors can affect drug absorption. The dental hygienist should be aware of them.
2. The most common factors affecting drug absorption include patient compliance or adherence to medication therapy. Lack of health insurance, misunderstanding of the reason for the medication, or a lack of faith in the health care system can lead to noncompliance.
3. Patient age and pathologic state can affect drug metabolism. As a result, lower doses and slower dose increases may be necessary. All of this can be attained by knowing the patient's age and during a health history.
4. Lower protein stores can lead to less medication being stored in protein, which puts the patient at risk for toxicity. This is most common in elderly patients, who by virtue of their age have lower protein stores.
5. The dental hygienist should also understand drug potency so that the appropriate medication and dose are prescribed.

CLINICAL SKILLS ASSESSMENT

1. Define and differentiate between the potency and efficacy of a drug.
2. Describe the dose-response curve using the terms ED_{50} (effective dose) and LD_{50} (lethal dose).
3. Define the term *pharmacokinetics.* Name the four categories involved.
4. Define the major routes of drug administration, including the following:
   a. Oral
   b. Intravenous
   c. Inhalation
   d. Topical
5. State the dose forms most often used in dentistry.
6. Explain the influence of pH on the dissociation characteristics of weak acids and weak bases.
7. Explain each of the steps involved in oral absorption, including the following:
   a. Disruption
   b. Disintegration
   c. Dispersion
   d. Dissolution
8. Define the $t_{1/2}$, or half-life, of a drug and state its significance.
9. Though an elderly patient appears healthy and weighs 110 pounds, what are your concerns regarding drug distribution?
10. Define the following terms:
    a. Agonist
    b. Competitive antagonist
    c. Physiologic antagonist
    d. Isomers
    e. Chirals
11. What are the different ways that drugs can be metabolized?
12. State the major route of drug excretion.
13. Explain how metabolism can be altered by an effect on liver microsomal enzymes.

⊖volve

Please visit http://evolve.elsevier.com/Haveles/pharmacology for review questions and additional practice and reference materials.

3

Adverse Reactions

LEARNING OBJECTIVES

1. Define an adverse drug reaction and name five categories of reaction.
2. Discuss the risk-to-benefit ratio of the use of a drug for therapeutic effect and its potential adverse reactions.
3. Explain how the toxic effects of drugs are evaluated.

Although drugs may act on biologic systems to accomplish a desired effect, they lack absolute specificity in that they can act on many different organs or tissues. This lack of specificity is the reason for undesirable or adverse drug reactions. No drug is free from producing some adverse effects in a certain number of patients. It is estimated that between 5% and 10% of the patients hospitalized annually in the United States are admitted because of adverse reactions to drugs. While hospitalized, 10% to 20% of patients experience adverse reactions caused by drugs.

The dental health care worker is in a good position to observe any adverse reactions or undesirable effects caused by drugs administered in the dental office. Adverse reactions to drugs prescribed by the patient's physician can be identified in the health history. The dental health care worker should question the patient about any potential oral manifestations of drugs. For example, if the patient is taking phenytoin (Dilantin), questions about enlargement of the patient's gums should be explored. Because many drugs can produce xerostomia, complaints of dry mouth should direct the dental health care worker to examine the patient's medications. Knowledge of the typical adverse drug reactions can help dental office personnel identify, minimize, or prevent these types of reactions. Because of the rapport between a patient and the dental health care worker, the patient will often reveal important facts about the health history or ask questions concerning medications prescribed. The dental health care worker must know the terms used to describe adverse reactions to discuss a drug's undesirable effect accurately with other health professionals. For example, allergy refers to a specific type of reaction to a drug but does not include a complaint of excessive gas, or flatulence.

DEFINITIONS AND CLASSIFICATIONS

Unfortunately, every drug has more than one action. The clinically desirable actions are termed *therapeutic effects,* and the undesirable reactions are termed adverse effects. Dividing a drug's effects into two categories is artificial because it depends on the indication for which the drug is being used. For example, when an antihistamine used to relieve hay fever causes drowsiness, the drowsiness can be considered an adverse effect. However, if the antihistamine were being used to induce sleep (over-the-counter [OTC] sleep aid), drowsiness would be considered the therapeutic effect.

An adverse drug reaction is a response to a drug that is not desired, is potentially harmful, and occurs at usual therapeutic doses. It may be an exaggeration of the desired response, an expected but undesired response, an allergic reaction, a cytotoxic reaction, or an effect on the fetus. Often, adverse drug reactions are divided into the following categories:

• *Toxic reaction:* A toxic reaction is an extension of the pharmacologic effect resulting from a drug's effect on the target organs. In this instance, the amount of the desired effect is excessive.

• *Side effect:* A side effect is a dose-related reaction that is not part of the desired therapeutic outcome. It occurs when a drug acts on nontarget organs to produce undesirable effects. The terms *side effect* and *adverse reaction* often are used interchangeably. The upset stomach produced by ibuprofen is an adverse reaction when ibuprofen is given to manage pain.

• *Idiosyncratic reaction:* An idiosyncratic reaction is a genetically related abnormal drug response. Certain populations, because of their genetic constitution, are more susceptible to certain adverse reactions to specific drugs. Eskimos metabolize certain drugs faster than other populations; therefore a larger dose of those drugs would be needed in that population (e.g., isoniazid).

• *Drug allergy:* A drug allergy is an immunologic response to a drug resulting in a reaction such as a rash or anaphylaxis. This response accounts for less than 5% of all adverse reactions. Unlike other adverse reactions, allergic reactions are neither predictable nor dose related.

• *Interference with natural defense mechanisms:* Certain drugs, such as adrenocorticosteroids, can reduce the body's ability to fight infection. Drugs that interfere with the body's defenses cause a patient to get infections more easily and have more trouble fighting them.

The importance of distinguishing between different types of adverse effects can be seen using aspirin as an example. Aspirin can produce adverse reactions such as gastric upset or pain. At higher doses, aspirin can predictably produce toxicity such as tinnitus and hyperthermia (elevated temperature). Another type of reaction to aspirin is allergic, often involving a rash or difficulty in breathing (asthma-like reaction). These differences are significant and become pertinent when discussing an adverse reaction with another health professional. Patients who experience allergic reactions to a medication should not receive that medication or similar medications. Side effects such as gastrointestinal upset, although bothersome, are not reasons to avoid prescribing a medication. It can be given. However, if the gastrointestinal upset is too much for the patient, another drug should be considered. It is important to describe in the patient's chart the patient's "problem" in enough detail so that side effects can be separated from allergic reactions. Figure 3-1 describes the

types of adverse reactions and notes whether they are predictable or dose dependent.

CLINICAL MANIFESTATIONS OF ADVERSE REACTIONS

Before a drug is used, there must be an assessment of its risk against its benefits (risk-to-benefit ratio). This means that the beneficial effect of the drug must be weighed against its potential for adverse reactions. For example, one would compare the drug's therapeutic effect (e.g., controlling seizures) with its potential to cause an adverse reaction (e.g., birth defects). In a real-life example, one should compare the therapeutic effect of certain drugs to produce weight loss to their potential for the serious adverse reactions of primary pulmonary hypertension (which is fatal in 50% of patients) or cardiac valvular damage.

Exaggerated Effect on Target Tissues

An exaggerated effect on its target tissue or organ is considered an extension of the therapeutic effect caused by the overreaction of a sensitive patient or by the use of a dose that is too large. For example, a patient may experience exaggerated hypoglycemia when given a therapeutic dose of an oral hypoglycemic agent for the treatment of diabetes. The patient's blood sugar may fall too low, either because of an unusual sensitivity to the drug or because the dose administered was too high for that patient. Occasionally, this type of adverse reaction may result from liver or kidney disease. Because the disease interferes with the drug's metabolism or excretion, the drug's action may be enhanced or prolonged.

Effect on Nontarget Tissues

The effect on nontarget organs or tissues is caused by the nontherapeutic action of the drug. These reactions can occur at usual doses, but they appear more often at higher doses. For example, aspirin may produce gastric upset in usual therapeutic doses, but with higher doses salicylism, characterized by tinnitus, disturbances in the acid-base balance, and confusion, can result. Toxic reactions can affect many parts of the body. A reduction in the dose of a drug usually reduces these adverse reactions.

Effect on Fetal Development (Teratogenic Effect)

The word *teratogenic* comes from the Greek prefix *terato-,* meaning "monster," and the suffix *-genic,* meaning "producing," or "producing a malformed fetus." The relationship between drugs and congenital abnormalities has been recognized since the middle of the twentieth century. In 1961, thalidomide, an OTC drug marketed in Europe, was found to produce phocomelia (short arms and legs) in the exposed fetus. In some cases, only one dose of this drug produced the effect. This incident reinforced the fact that more studies were needed to determine the effect of drugs on pregnant women. For new drugs, there are many more studies on animals and their reproductive capacity before the drugs are placed on the market. Although more information is now available about the safety of drugs in pregnant women, sufficient information is still lacking.

The Food and Drug Administration (FDA) has attempted to address the concerns about the lack of adequate knowledge of drugs by defining five FDA pregnancy categories: A, B, C, D, and X, ranked from least risky to most risky. (See Table 25-2

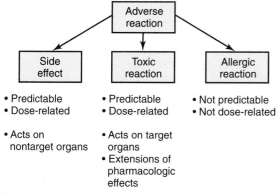

FIGURE 3-1
Classification of common adverse reactions.

for a discussion of the meaning of these categories.) They are similar to school grades: A is the "best" or least teratogenic and X is equivalent to F or not ever to be used if someone might get pregnant. Some older drugs may be classified as C because there are insufficient data to place them in higher categories.

Although no drug can be considered "completely safe" for administration to a pregnant woman, many of the drugs used in dentistry are considered to be among the safest. These include the antibiotics penicillin and erythromycin, the pain medication acetaminophen (Tylenol), and the local anesthetic lidocaine. Even these drugs should be administered only if there is a clear need. Elective dental procedures should be conservatively addressed. Drugs that are used in dentistry that are contraindicated during pregnancy include tetracycline, nonsteroidal antiinflammatory agents, the benzodiazepines, and metronidazole. The teratogenic potential for dental drugs is discussed in Chapter 25.

Many drug manufacturers, especially those that produce some of the older drugs, continue to place in their package inserts such statements as the following:
- "There are no adequate and well-controlled studies in pregnant women."
- "Risks must be balanced against the uncontrolled disease."
- "Safety during pregnancy has not been established; use requires that potential benefits be weighed against its possible hazard to the mother and child."
- "Animal reproductive studies are not always indicative of human effects."
- "Animal reproduction studies have not been conducted with …"
- "… potential benefit must be weighed against the possible hazards to the mother and fetus."

Encouragement of increased information, especially for newer agents, has resulted in more information about use during pregnancy such as the following statements:
- "Pregnancy category D"
- "Shown to decrease fetal birth weight when given at 50 times the dose recommended for humans."
- "No evidence of birth abnormalities or impaired fertility in doses two times the usual human dose."

However, there are still plenty of statements such as the following:

> With regard to teratogenesis, it is important to remember that the risk to the fetus must always be considered when considering the benefit to the mother.

In addition, dental patients do not always announce that they are pregnant, so it is important to ask any woman of childbearing age (between approximately 11 and 63 years of age [a 63-year-old French woman gave birth in 1997]) if she is pregnant. Problem drugs should be avoided as early as possible during the pregnancy. The greatest risk from exposure to drugs occurs before the pregnancy status is known.

Local Effect

Local reactions are characterized by local tissue irritation. Occasionally, injectable drugs can produce irritation, pain, and tissue **necrosis** at the site of injection. Topically applied agents can produce irritation at the site of application. Drugs taken orally can produce gastrointestinal symptoms, such as nausea or **dyspepsia**, because of their local actions on the gastrointestinal tract.

Drug Interactions

A drug interaction can occur when the effect of one drug is altered by another drug. These interactions may result in undesirable effects such as toxicity or lack of efficacy. Drug interactions can also produce beneficial effects. Whenever prescribing or suggesting a drug to a dental patient, the chance of drug interactions must be considered. The likelihood that a drug interaction would occur increases with the number of drugs that a patient is taking. Drug-food and drug-disease interactions may also occur.

Hypersensitivity (Allergic Reaction)

Hypersensitivity reactions occur when the **immune system** of an individual responds to the drug administered or applied. One example of an allergic (hypersensitivity) reaction is when a patient is given a drug and develops hives. For a drug to produce an allergic reaction, it must act as an antigen and react with an antibody in a previously sensitized patient. This reaction is neither dose dependent nor predictable. For an allergic reaction to occur, an ingested drug may be metabolized to a reactive metabolite known as a **hapten**. This hapten can act as an antigen after combining with proteins in the body. The antigen formed then stimulates the production of an antibody. With subsequent exposure to the drug, the antibodies formed will react with the antigen (drug or metabolite) administered and elicit an antigen-antibody reaction. This reaction triggers a series of biochemical and physiologic events that can be life threatening.

Drug allergy can be divided into the following four types of reactions, depending on the type of antibody produced or the cell mediating the reaction (Table 3-1):
- *Type I* reactions are mediated by immunoglobulin E (IgE) antibodies. When a drug antigen binds to IgE antibody, histamine, leukotrienes, and prostaglandins are released, producing vasodilation, edema, and the inflammatory response. The targets of this reaction are the bronchioles, resulting in **anaphylactic shock**; the respiratory system, resulting in rhinitis and asthma; and the skin, resulting in **urticaria** and dermatitis. Because these reactions can occur relatively quickly after drug exposure, they are known as immediate hypersensitivity reactions. **Anaphylaxis** is an acute, life-threatening allergic reaction characterized by **hypotension, bronchospasm**, laryngeal edema, and cardiac arrhythmias that can occur within a few minutes after drug administration. Drugs used in dentistry that have produced fatal anaphylaxis include the penicillins, ester local anesthetics, and aspirin. Unexpected anaphylaxis may occur such as after a patient has been given a dose of penicillin by injection. Oral penicillin can also produce anaphylaxis, but it is much less common.
- *Type II*, or cytotoxic/cytolytic, reactions are complement-dependent reactions involving either immunoglobulin G (IgG) or immunoglobulin M (IgM) antibodies. The antigen-antibody complex is fixed to a circulating blood cell, resulting in lysis. Examples of this reaction are penicillin-induced hemolytic anemia and methyldopa-induced autoimmune hemolytic anemia.
- *Type III*, or **Arthus**, reactions are mediated by IgG. In these reactions, the drug antigen-antibody complex fixes complement and deposits in the vascular endothelium. The reaction is manifested as serum sickness and includes urticarial skin eruptions, **arthralgia**, arthritis, lymphadenopathy,

TABLE 3-1 HYPERSENSITIVITY REACTIONS

Type	Mediator	Reaction	Example
I (immediate, anaphylactic)	Antibody	IgE antibody is induced by allergen and binds via its Fc receptor to mast cells and basophils. After encountering the antigen again, the fixed IgE becomes cross-linked, inducing degranulation and release of mediators (e.g., histamine).	Anaphylaxis to penicillin
II (cytotoxic)	Antibody	Antigens on a cell surface combine with antibody; this leads to complement-mediated lysis (e.g., transfusion of Rh reactions or autoimmune hemolytic anemia).	Quinine lyses platelets, resulting in thrombocytopenia
III (immune complex)	Antibody	Antigen-antibody immune complexes are deposited in tissues, complement is activated, and polymorphonuclear cells are attracted to the site, causing tissue damage.	Serum sickness
IV (delayed)	Cell	Helper T lymphocytes sensitized by an antigen release lymphokines on second contact with the same antigen. The lymphokines induce inflammation and activate macrophages that in turn release various mediators.	Poison ivy, TB tests

From Levinson WE: *Review of medical microbiology and immunology,* ed 10, New York, 2008, McGraw-Hill Medical.
Ig, Immunoglobulin; *TB,* tuberculosis.

and fever. This reaction can be caused by the penicillins and sulfonamides.

- *Type IV,* or delayed hypersensitivity, reactions are mediated by sensitized T lymphocytes and macrophages. When the cells contact the antigen, an inflammatory reaction is produced by lymphokines, neutrophils, and macrophages. An example of a type IV reaction is allergic contact dermatitis caused by topical application of drugs. Topical benzocaine, penicillin, poison oak, and poison ivy can produce this type of reaction. Reaction to "cheap" jewelry is another example.

Idiosyncrasy

An idiosyncratic reaction is a reaction that is neither the drug's side effect nor an allergic reaction. Some idiosyncrasies have been found to be genetically determined abnormal reactions, whereas others may be the result of an immunologic mechanism. About 10% of black males can develop severe hemolytic anemia when given the antimalarial drug primaquine. This is because of a deficiency in an enzyme, glucose-6-phosphate dehydrogenase.

Interference with Natural Defense Mechanisms

A drug's effect on the body's defense mechanisms can result in an adverse reaction. Long-term systemic administration of corticosteroids can result in decreased resistance to infection. Because periodontal disease involves both infection and an immune response, drugs that are immunosuppressive could exacerbate a patient's poor oral health.

TOXICOLOGIC EVALUATION OF DRUGS

> LD_{50} kills one half of the subjects.
> ED_{50} produces a response in one half of the subjects.

Optimally, evaluations of the toxic effects of drugs are based on experiments that are performed with lower animals and clinical trials conducted in humans. Animal experiments can often elicit adverse reactions that could occur in humans, but unfortunately, drug reactions in animals do not

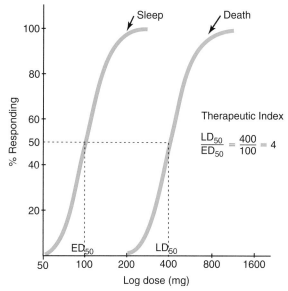

FIGURE 3-2
Dose-response curve and therapeutic index.

always predict reactions in humans. The lethal dose (LD_{50}), one measure of the toxicity of a drug, is the dose of a drug that kills 50% of the experimental animals. The median effective dose (ED_{50}) is the dose required to produce a specified intensity of effect in 50% of the animals. Figure 3-2 shows a plot of the dose of a drug against the percentage of maximum response (sleep or death) in animals. A dose-response curve is then obtained. The value on the dose axis that corresponds to the 50% intensity level on the response axis can be read directly from the curve. This figure illustrates the ED_{50} and LD_{50}.

Because all drugs are toxic at some dose, the LD_{50} is meaningless unless the ED_{50} is also known. The ratio LD_{50}/ED_{50} is the therapeutic index (TI) of a drug:

$$TI = \frac{LD_{50}}{ED_{50}}$$

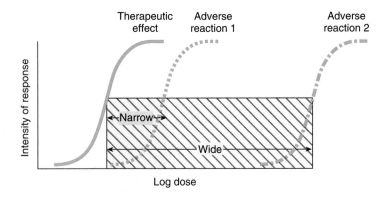

FIGURE 3-3
Difference between narrow and wide therapeutic indexes.

If the value of the TI is small (narrow TI), then toxicity is more likely. If the TI is large (wide TI), then the drug will be safer (Figure 3-3). A drug with a wide TI will have a large LD_{50} and a small ED_{50} (the distance between these curves is large). A TI of greater than 10 is usually needed to produce a therapeutically useful drug. The TI derived from animal studies determines both the LD_{50} and the ED_{50} from a variety of animals.

DENTAL HYGIENE CONSIDERATIONS

1. Know the difference between a side effect, toxic effect, and allergic reaction.
2. Always ask the patient to explain what happened if the patient has stated that he or she has had an allergic reaction to a medication.
3. Remember that an allergic reaction to a medication usually means that the patient should not receive that medication or any other medication in the same chemical class.
4. Side effects, although bothersome, usually do not prevent the patient from taking the medication. The medication may have to be given with food or milk or taken at bedtime. If the patient cannot tolerate the side effect, then switch the patient to another drug.
5. Make sure that the patient understands how to take the medication in order to avoid toxic reactions.
6. Always explain what adverse effects the patient can experience and what the patient should do if he or she experiences them.
7. Always ask female patients from puberty to menopause if there is a possibility that they may be pregnant. This is to avoid exposing the developing fetus to medications.

CLINICAL SKILLS ASSESSMENT

1. Name four classifications of adverse drug reactions.
2. Describe the problem with identifying teratogenic agents (see also Chapter 25).
3. Describe the types of adverse reactions.
4. Explain the four mechanisms by which an allergic reaction can occur.
5. Describe why the risk-to-benefit ratio is important and helpful in deciding whether to administer a drug to a patient.

⊖volve ───────────────────────

Please visit http://evolve.elsevier.com/Haveles/pharmacology for review questions and additional practice and reference materials.

DRUGS USED IN DENTISTRY

4 Autonomic Drugs

LEARNING OBJECTIVES

1. Identify the major components and functional organization of the autonomic nervous system.
2. Discuss the pharmacologic effects, adverse reactions, contraindications, and dental considerations of cholinergic agents.
3. Discuss the pharmacologic effects, adverse reactions, contraindications, and dental considerations of anticholinergic agents.
4. Identify the major components of the sympathetic nervous system.
5. Discuss the pharmacologic effects, adverse reactions, contraindications, and dental considerations of adrenergic agents.
6. Explain the workings of adrenergic blocking agents and neuromuscular blocking agents.

The dentist and the dental hygienist should become familiar with the autonomic nervous system (ANS) drugs for three reasons. First, certain ANS drugs are used in dentistry. For example, both the vasoconstrictors added to some local anesthetic solutions and the drugs used to increase salivary flow are ANS drugs. Second, some ANS drugs produce oral adverse reactions. For example, the anticholinergics produce xerostomia.

> Autonomic nervous system (ANS) drug effects are important because many other drugs have the same effects.

Third, members of other drug groups have effects similar to the ANS drugs. Antidepressants and antipsychotics are drug groups with autonomic side effects, specifically anticholinergic effects. An understanding of the effects of the autonomic drugs on the body will facilitate an understanding of the action of other drug groups that have autonomic effects. Before the ANS drugs can be understood, the normal functioning of the ANS must be reviewed. A review of the physiology of the ANS is helpful in understanding these drugs.

AUTONOMIC NERVOUS SYSTEM

The ANS functions largely as an automatic modulating system for many bodily functions, including the regulation of blood pressure and heart rate, gastrointestinal tract motility, salivary gland secretions, and bronchial smooth muscle. This system relies on specific neurotransmitters (chemicals that are released to send messages) and a variety of receptors to initiate functional responses in the target tissues. Before ANS pharmacology is discussed, the anatomy and physiology of this system are reviewed.

Anatomy

The ANS has two divisions, the sympathetic autonomic nervous system (SANS) and the parasympathetic autonomic nervous system (PANS). Each consists of afferent (sensory) fibers (What's happening?), central integrating areas (Let's coordinate all this info! Hey, what did you find out?), efferent (peripheral) motor preganglionic fibers, and postganglionic motor fibers (Begin sweating! Heart begin palpitating!).

The preganglionic neuron (Figure 4-1) originates in the central nervous system (CNS) and passes out to form the ganglia at the synapse with the postganglionic neuron. The space between the preganglionic and postganglionic fibers is termed the *synapse* or synaptic cleft. The postganglionic neuron originates in the ganglia and innervates the effector organ or tissue.

Parasympathetic Autonomic Nervous System

Cell bodies in the CNS give rise to the preganglionic fibers of the parasympathetic division. They originate in the nuclei of the third, seventh, ninth, and tenth cranial nerves (CN III, VII, IX, and X) and the second through the fourth sacral segments (S2 to S4) of the spinal cord. The preganglionic fibers of the PANS are relatively long and extend near to or into the innervated organ. The distribution is relatively simple for the third, seventh, and ninth cranial nerves, whereas the tenth or vagus nerve has a complex distribution. There usually is a low ratio of synaptic connections between preganglionic and postganglionic neurons, which leads to a discrete response when the PANS is stimulated. The postganglionic fibers, originating in the ganglia, are usually short and terminate on the innervated tissue.

Sympathetic Autonomic Nervous System

The cell bodies that give origin to the preganglionic fibers of the SANS span from the thoracic (T1) to the lumbar (L2) portion of the spinal cord (sometimes referred to as the "in between" distribution, that is, between the two locations of the innervation of the PANS). This produces a more diffuse effect in the SANS. The preganglionic fibers exit the cord to enter the sympathetic chain located along each side of the vertebral column. Once a part of the sympathetic chain (groups of nerves a few inches from the vertebral column), preganglionic fibers form multiple synaptic connections with postganglionic cell bodies located up and down the sympathetic chain. Thus a single SANS preganglionic fiber often synapses with numerous postganglionic neurons. This produces a more diffuse effect in the SANS. The postganglionic fibers then terminate at the effector organ or tissues.

The adrenal medulla is also innervated by the sympathetic preganglionic fibers. It functions much like a large sympathetic ganglion, with the glands in the medulla representing the postganglionic component. When the SANS is stimulated, the adrenal medulla releases primarily epinephrine and a small amount of norepinephrine (NE) into the systemic circulation.

A diffuse response is produced when the SANS is stimulated because of the high ratio of synaptic connections between the preganglionic and postganglionic fibers and because epinephrine is released by the adrenal medulla, into the bloodstream, when stimulated.

Functional Organization

> Divisions of the parasympathetic autonomic nervous system (PANS) and sympathetic autonomic nervous system (SANS) often produce opposite effects like the yin and yang.

In general, the divisions of the ANS, the parasympathetic and the sympathetic, tend to act in opposite directions (Figure 4-2). The parasympathetic division of the ANS is concerned with the conservation of the body processes. Both digestion and intestinal tract motility are greatly influenced by the PANS. The sympathetic division is designed to cope with sudden emergencies such as the "fright or flight" or "fight or flight" situation. In most but not all instances, the actions produced by each system are opposite: one increases the heart rate and the other decreases it; one dilates the pupils of the eye and the other constricts them. The receptors being innervated for each function may be different. For example, both the PANS and the SANS stimulate muscles in the eye that change the size of the pupil. The SANS stimulates the radial smooth muscles (out from the pupil like sun rays), producing an increase in pupil size. When the pupils are dilated the effect is termed *mydriasis*). The PANS stimulates the circular smooth muscles (like a bull's-eye), producing a decrease in pupil size. When pupils are constricted the effect is termed *miosis*.

Almost all body tissues are innervated by the ANS, with many but not all, organs receiving both parasympathetic and sympathetic innervation. The response of a specific tissue to stimuli at any one time will be equal to the sum of the excitatory and inhibitory influences of the two divisions of the ANS (if a tissue receives both innervations). Table 4-1 summarizes the effects of the ANS on major tissues and organ systems.

In addition to the dual innervation of tissues, there is another way in which the two divisions of the ANS can interact. Sensory fibers in one division can influence the motor fibers in the other. Thus, although in an isolated tissue preparation the stimulation of one of the divisions would produce a specific response, in the intact body a more complex and integrated response can be expected. The net effect would be a combination of the direct and indirect effects.

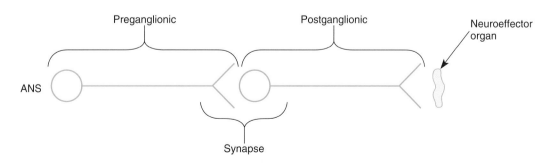

FIGURE 4-1
Typical efferent nerve. The preganglionic fiber originates in the brain. It ends at the synapse, where the neurotransmitter carries the message to the postganglionic fiber. A group of synapses make up a ganglia. The postganglionic fiber releases a neurotransmitter to send the message to an effector organ.

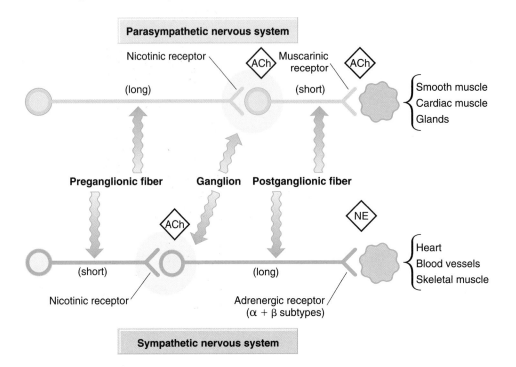

FIGURE 4-2

The parasympathetic and sympathetic nervous systems and their relationship to each other. *ACh,* Acetylcholine; *NE,* norepinephrine. (From Lilley LL, Harrington S, Snyder JS: *Pharmacology and the nursing process,* ed 5, St Louis, 2007, Mosby.)

Neurotransmitters

Neurotransmitters are like carrier pigeons: they carry messages.

Communication between nerves or between nerves and effector tissue takes place by the release of chemical neurotransmitters across the synaptic cleft. Neurotransmitters are released in response to the nerve action potential (or pharmacologic agents in certain cases) to interact with a specific membrane component: the receptor. Receptors are usually found on the postsynaptic fiber and the effector organ but may be located on the presynaptic membrane as well (Table 4-2). The interaction between neurotransmitter and receptor is specific and is rapidly terminated by disposition of the neurotransmitter substance. There are several specific mechanisms by which the neurotransmitter produces an effect on the receptor.

Disposition occurs most often by either reuptake into the presynaptic nerve terminal or enzymatic breakdown of the transmitter. Nerves in the ANS contain the necessary enzyme systems and other metabolic processes to synthesize, store, and release neurotransmitters. Thus drugs can modify ANS activity by altering any of the events associated with neurotransmitters: (1) synthesis, (2) storage, (3) release, (4) receptor interaction, and (5) disposition. The specificity of the neurotransmitters and receptors dictates the tissue response, which occurs as follows:

- Between the preganglionic and postganglionic nerves: Acetylcholine is the neurotransmitter in the synapse (ganglia) formed between the preganglionic and postganglionic nerves. Nerves that release acetylcholine are termed *cholinergic*. Because this synapse is also stimulated by nicotine, it is also termed *nicotinic* in response.
- Between postganglionic nerves and the effector tissues:

  - *PANS:* The neurotransmitter released from the postganglionic nerve terminal is acetylcholine; it is also termed *cholinergic*. Because the postsynaptic tissue responds to muscarine, it is identified as muscarinic. Thus the cholinergic synapses are distinguished from one another.
  - *SANS:* NE is the transmitter substance released by the postganglionic nerves and is designated as adrenergic.
  - *Neuromuscular junction:* Although not within the ANS, the neuromuscular junction (Figure 4-3) of skeletal muscle releases the neurotransmitter acetylcholine and is termed *cholinergic*. The neuromuscular junction is part of the somatic system and is also discussed in Chapter 11. Figures 4-4, 4-5, and 4-6 illustrate the PANS, SANS, and neuromuscular junction.

Drug Groups

The four drug groups in the ANS exert their effects primarily on the organs or tissues innervated by the ANS. (They are just doing the same thing that the body would normally do when it is working.) Each of the divisions of the nervous system, the PANS and the SANS, can be affected. The action of each of the divisions of the ANS can be increased or decreased.

These four functions divide the ANS drugs into four groups: P+, P−, S+, and S−. Stimulation of the PANS can be abbreviated P+, and blocking of the PANS can be abbreviated P−. Stimulation of the SANS can be abbreviated S+, and blocking of the SANS can be abbreviated S−. These abbreviations are not routinely used in the literature but are helpful with note taking, outlines, and discussions. The groups are named by several methods, but the basic concepts of naming include the following:

- A drug that acts at the location where acetylcholine is released as the neurotransmitter is termed *cholinergic* (from acetylcholine).

TABLE 4-1 EFFECTS OF THE AUTONOMIC NERVOUS SYSTEM (ANS) ON EFFECTOR ORGANS

Organ	Aspect	PANS	Receptor	SANS
Eye	Lens (ciliary muscle)	Contraction (near vision)	β_2	Relaxation (distant vision)
	Iris	Contraction miosis	α_1	Contraction
				Radial muscle mydriasis
CVS	Heart force (inotropic)		β_1, β_2	Increases force
	Heart, SA node rate (chronotropic)	Decreases heart rate	β_1, β_2	Increases heart rate
Blood vessels, smooth muscles	Coronary		$\alpha_1, \beta_1, \beta_2$	Constriction (α), dilation (β)
	Skin/mucosa		α_1, α_2	Constriction
	Skeletal muscle	Dilation	α_1	Constriction
			β_2	Dilation
	Abdominal viscera		α_1	Constriction
			β_2	Dilation
	Salivary glands	Dilation	α_1, β_2	Constriction
Lungs	Bronchial smooth muscle	Contraction	β_2	Relaxation
	Secretions bronchial, nasopharyngeal		α_1, β_1	Secretion increase/decrease
Gastrointestinal tract/ genitourinary tract	Motility/tone	Contracts, increases	$\alpha_1, \alpha_2, \beta_1, \beta_2$	Relaxes
Stomach, intestine, bladder	Sphincters	Relaxation	α_1	Contraction
	Secretions from gastrointestinal tract	Stimulation	α_2	Inhibition
	Secretion from salivary glands	Increase profuse and watery	α	Viscous thick
	Uterus		α_1, β_2	Relaxation
Endocrine	Pancreas, acini	Secretion	α_1	Decreases secretions
	Pancreas, islet cells		α_2	Decreases secretions
	Adrenal medulla	Secretion epinephrine/ norepinephrine		
Skin	Sweat	Secretion, generalized		Secretion, local
	Pilomotor muscles		α_1	Contraction
Liver	Glycogen synthesis		α_1	Glycogenolysis
			β_2	Gluconeogenesis
Other	Adipose tissue		$\alpha_2, \beta_1, \beta_2$	Lipolysis
	Male sex organs	Erection	α_1	Ejaculation
	Skeletal muscle		β_2	Contraction

CVS, Cardiovascular system; *PANS,* parasympathetic autonomic nervous system; *SA,* sinoatrial; *SANS,* sympathetic autonomic nervous system.

TABLE 4-2 TYPES OF CHOLINERGIC RECEPTORS

Receptor Site	Location	Neurotransmitter	Stimulating Agent	Blocking Agent
Muscarinic	B	Acetylcholine	Muscarine	Atropine
Nicotinic	C	Acetylcholine	Nicotine	Hexamethonium
Somatic-skeletal muscle	D	Acetylcholine	Nicotine	*d*-Tubocurarine (curare)

B, Muscarinic cholinergic; *C,* nicotinic cholinergic; *D,* cholinergic somatic.

- A drug that acts at the location where NE is the neurotransmitter released is termed *adrenergic* (taken from the early trade name of epinephrine, Adrenalin).
- A drug that acts at the location where the PANS acts has the prefix *parasympatho-*.
- A drug that acts at the location where the SANS acts has the prefix *sympatho-*.
- A drug that acts at the location where a division of the ANS acts and produces the same effect as the neurotransmitter has

the suffix *-mimetic* (as in mime, acts like). It can also be referred to as an agonist (see Chapter 2).
- A drug that acts at the location where a division of the ANS acts and blocks the action of the neurotransmitter has the suffix *-lytic* or *-blocker*. It can also be referred to as an antagonist (see Chapter 2).

Using this nomenclature, the four groups of ANS drugs can be abbreviated as P+ (cholinergics, parasympathomimetics), P− (anticholinergics, parasympatholytics, or cholinergic-blockers),

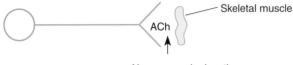

FIGURE 4-3

The neuromuscular junction of skeletal muscle releases acetylcholine.

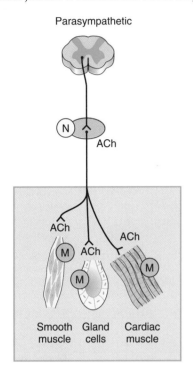

FIGURE 4-4

The parasympathetic autonomic nervous system (PANS). *ACh,* Acetylcholine; *M,* muscarinic receptors; *N,* nicotinic receptors. (From McKenry L, Tessier E, Hogan MA: *Mosby's pharmacology in nursing,* ed 22, St Louis, 2006, Mosby.)

S+ (sympathomimetics, adrenergics), and S− (adrenergic blockers, sympathetic blockers, sympatholytics).

PARASYMPATHETIC AUTONOMIC NERVOUS SYSTEM

Acetylcholine has been identified as the principal mediator in the PANS. When an action potential travels along the nerve, it causes the release of the stored acetylcholine from the synaptic storage vesicles, and if sufficient acetylcholine is released, it will initiate a response in the postsynaptic tissue. If the postsynaptic tissue is a postganglionic nerve, depolarization with generation of an action potential occurs in that neuron. In the postganglionic parasympathetic fibers, the postsynaptic tissue is an effector organ and the response will be the same as that of the neurotransmitter. The action of the released acetylcholine is terminated by hydrolysis by acetylcholinesterase to yield the inactive metabolites choline and acetic acid (or acetate) (Figure 4-7).

> Three acetylcholine (ACh) receptors:
> 1. Parasympathetic autonomic nervous system (PANS)
> 2. Ganglionic
> 3. Neuromuscular junction

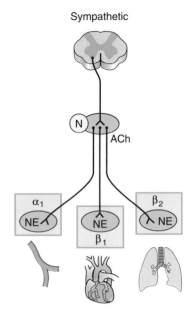

FIGURE 4-5

Sympathetic autonomic nervous system (SANS). *ACh,* Acetylcholine; *N,* nicotinic receptors; *NE,* norepinephrine. (From McKenry L, Tessier E, Hogan MA: *Mosby's pharmacology in nursing,* ed 22, St Louis, 2006, Mosby.)

Some of the postsynaptic tissues respond to acetylcholine because of an interaction between acetylcholine and these tissues. To be an effective mediator, acetylcholine must fit both physically and chemically at the receptor. It has been shown that atropine (A-troe-peen) can block the action of acetylcholine at the postganglionic endings in the PANS but not at the neuromuscular junction. In contrast, curare blocks the response of skeletal muscle to acetylcholine but does not block its effect on tissues such as the salivary gland. Hexamethonium blocks the action of acetylcholine at the ganglia. From these observations, one can infer that there are differences among receptors that have acetylcholine as a neurotransmitter—subtypes of acetylcholine-innervated receptors that are located in anatomically different synapses. Other factors, such as the amount of acetylcholine released, the size of the synaptic cleft, and the tissue penetration of a drug, may also account for differences in the response of the receptor to drugs at each acetylcholine-mediated junction.

Cholinergic (Parasympathomimetic) Agents

Depending on their mechanism of action (Table 4-3) the cholinergic (parasympathomimetic) agents are classified as direct acting (acts on receptor) or indirect acting (causes release of neurotransmitter). The direct-acting agents (Figure 4-8) include the choline derivatives and pilocarpine. The choline derivatives include both acetylcholine and other, more stable choline derivatives. These derivatives of acetylcholine possess activity similar to PANS stimulation but have a longer duration of action and are more selective.

The indirect-acting (see Figure 4-8) parasympathomimetic agents or cholinesterase inhibitors act by inhibiting the enzyme cholinesterase.

When the enzyme that normally destroys acetylcholine is inhibited, the concentration of acetylcholine builds up (it is not being destroyed), resulting in PANS stimulation.

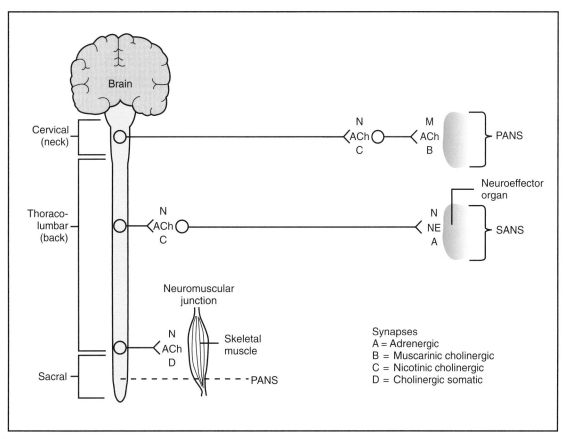

FIGURE 4-6
Parasympathetic autonomic nervous system *(PANS)*, sympathetic autonomic nervous system *(SANS)*, and neuromuscular junction.

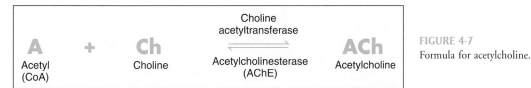

FIGURE 4-7
Formula for acetylcholine.

TABLE 4-3   CHOLINERGIC (PARASYMPATHOMIMETIC) AGENTS

Type	Classification	Drug Name	Therapeutic Use
Direct acting	Choline esters	Bethanechol (Urecholine)	Urinary retention not due to urinary tract obstruction
	Other	Pilocarpine (Isopto Carpine)	Glaucoma
	Other	Pilocarpine (Salagen)	Xerostomia
Indirect acting	Reversible agents	Physostigmine (Antilirium)	Some drug overdoses
		Neostigmine (Prostigmin)	Myasthenia gravis, reversible nondepolarizing muscle relaxants
		Pyridostigmine (Mestinon)	
	Irreversible organophosphates	Malathion, parathion	Agricultural insecticides
		Sarin (GB)	No known therapeutic uses
		Tabun	

◆ PHARMACOLOGIC EFFECTS

Cardiovascular Effects. The cardiovascular effects associated with the cholinergic agents are the result of both direct and indirect actions. The direct effect on the heart produces a negative chronotropic and negative inotropic action. A decrease in cardiac output is associated with these agents.

The cholinergic agents' effects on the smooth muscles around the blood vessels result in relaxation and vasodilation, producing a decrease in total peripheral resistance. The indirect effect of these agents is an increase in heart rate and cardiac output. Because the direct and indirect effects of these agents on the heart rate and cardiac output are opposite, the resulting effect will depend on the concentration of the drug present. Generally, there is bradycardia and a decrease in blood pressure and cardiac output.

Gastrointestinal Effects. The cholinergic agents excite the smooth muscle of the gastrointestinal tract, producing an increase in activity, motility, and secretion.

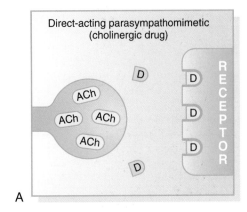
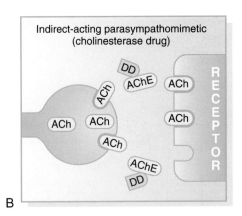

FIGURE 4-8

A, Direct-acting parasympathomimetic (cholinergic drugs). Cholinergic drugs resemble acetylcholine and act directly on the receptor. **B,** Indirect-acting parasympathomimetic (cholinesterase inhibitors). Cholinesterase inhibitors inactivate the enzyme acetylcholinesterase (cholinesterase), thus permitting acetylcholine to react to the receptor. *ACh,* Acetylcholine; *AChE,* acetylcholinesterase, or cholinesterase; *D,* cholinergic drug; *DD,* cholinesterase inhibitor (anticholinesterase). (From Kee JL, Hayes ER, McCuiston LE: *Pharmacology: a nursing process approach,* ed 6, St Louis, 2009, Saunders.)

Effects on the Eye. The cholinergic agents produce miosis and cause cycloplegia. Cycloplegia is a paralysis of the ciliary muscles of the eye that results in the loss of visual accommodation. Because intraocular pressure is also decreased, these agents are useful in the treatment of glaucoma.

ADVERSE REACTIONS

The adverse reactions that are associated with the administration of the cholinergic agents are essentially extensions of their pharmacologic effects. When large doses of these agents are ingested, the resultant toxic effects are described by the acronym SLUD: *s*alivation, *l*acrimation, *u*rination, and *d*efecation. With even larger doses, neuromuscular paralysis can occur as a result of the effect on the neuromuscular junction. CNS effects, such as confusion, can be seen if toxic doses are administered.

The treatment of an overdose of cholinesterase inhibitors, such as the insecticides or organophosphates (parathion), includes a combination of pralidoxime (pra-li-DOX-eem) (2-PAM, Protopam) and atropine. Pralidoxime regenerates the irreversibly bound acetylcholine receptor sites that are bound by the inhibitors (knocks them off like a prizefighter), and atropine blocks (competitively) the muscarinic effects of the excess acetylcholine present.

CONTRAINDICATIONS

The relative contraindications to or cautions with the use of the cholinergic agents stem from these agents' pharmacologic effects and adverse reactions. They include the following:

- *Bronchial asthma:* Cholinergic agents may cause bronchospasms or precipitate an asthmatic attack.
- *Hyperthyroidism:* Hyperthyroidism may cause an increased risk of atrial fibrillation.
- *Gastrointestinal tract or urinary tract obstruction:* If either the gastrointestinal tract or the urinary tract is obstructed and a cholinergic agent is given, an increase in secretions and motility could cause pressure and the system could "back up."
- *Severe cardiac disease:* The reflex tachycardia that can result from administering cholinergic agents may exacerbate a severe cardiac condition.
- *Myasthenia gravis treated with neostigmine:* Patients with myasthenia gravis should not be given irreversible cholin-

esterase inhibitors because neostigmine occupies the enzyme and the irreversible agent would not function.
- *Peptic ulcer:* Cholinergic agents stimulate gastric acid secretion and increase gastric motility. This action could exacerbate an ulcer.

USES

The direct-acting agents are used primarily in the treatment of glaucoma, a condition in which the intraocular pressure is elevated. Occasionally, they are used to treat myasthenia gravis, a disease resulting in muscle weakness from an autoimmune reaction that reduces the effect of acetylcholine on the voluntary muscles. The urinary retention that occurs after surgery is also treated with the choline esters (see Table 4-3).

Pilocarpine (pye-loe-KAR-peen) (Salagen), a naturally occurring cholinergic agent, is used in the treatment of xerostomia, but its success may be limited because of the myriad of potential side effects. Common side effects from pilocarpine include perspiration (sweating), nausea, rhinitis, chills, and flushing. Pilocarpine is available in 5-mg tablets. The usual dose of pilocarpine is 5 mg three times a day (tid). This can be obtained by giving one 5-mg tablet tid [three times a day]). Pilocarpine is also available as ophthalmic solution in strengths ranging from 0.5% to 10%. It is used topically in the eye to treat glaucoma. Several strengths (e.g., 2%) are available as generic preparations.

The indirect-acting cholinergic agents, the cholinesterase inhibitors, are divided into groups based on the degree of reversibility with which they are bound to the enzyme. Edrophonium is rapidly reversible, whereas physostigmine and neostigmine are slowly reversible. These agents are used to treat glaucoma and myasthenia gravis.

Physostigmine (fi-zoe-STIG-meen) (Antilirium) has been used to treat reactions caused by several different kinds of drugs. Acute toxicity from the anticholinergic agents (e.g., atropine) and other agents that have anticholinergic action (e.g., the phenothiazines, tricyclic antidepressants, and antihistamines) has been treated with physostigmine.

The cholinesterase inhibitors developed for use as insecticides and chemical warfare agents are essentially irreversible and are called the *irreversible cholinesterase inhibitors.* Members of this group include parathion, malathion, and sarin (used on a subway in Japan to poison riders).

Anticholinergic (Parasympatholytic) Agents

The anticholinergic agents prevent the action of acetylcholine at the postganglionic parasympathetic endings. The release of acetylcholine is not prevented, but the receptor site is competitively blocked by the anticholinergics (Figure 4-9). Thus the anticholinergic drugs block the action of acetylcholine on smooth muscles (e.g., intestines), glandular tissue (e.g., salivary glands), and the heart. These agents are called *antimuscarinic agents* because they block the muscarinic receptors and not the nicotinic receptors.

◆ PHARMACOLOGIC EFFECTS

Central Nervous System Effects. Depending on the dose administered, the anticholinergics can produce CNS stimulation or depression. For example, usual therapeutic doses of scopolamine more often cause sedation, whereas atropine in high doses can cause stimulation. Atropine and scopolamine are tertiary agents,

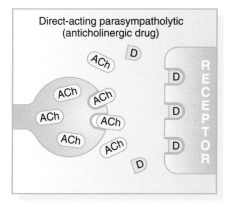

FIGURE 4-9
Anticholinergic response. The anticholinergic drug occupies the receptor sites, blocking acetylcholine. *ACh,* Acetylcholine; *D,* anticholinergic drug. (From Kee JL, Hayes ER, McCuiston LE: *Pharmacology: a nursing process approach,* ed 6, St Louis, 2009, Saunders.)

and propantheline (proe-PAN-the-leen) (Pro-Banthine) and glycopyrrolate (Robinul) are quaternary agents (Figure 4-10). Because of their water solubility, quaternary agents do not penetrate the CNS well. The tertiary agents are lipid soluble, and they can easily penetrate the brain. The quaternary agents have fewer CNS adverse reactions because they are less likely to enter the brain.

Effects on Exocrine Glands. The anticholinergics affect the exocrine glands by reducing the flow and the volume of their secretions. These glands are located in the respiratory, gastrointestinal, and genitourinary tracts. This effect is used therapeutically in dentistry to decrease salivation and create a dry field for certain dental procedures such as obtaining a difficult impression.

Effects on Smooth Muscle. Anticholinergics relax the smooth muscle in the respiratory and gastrointestinal tracts. Ipratropium is an anticholinergic inhaler used to treat asthma. The effect of anticholinergics on gastrointestinal motility has given rise to the name spasmolytic agents. If these drugs are used repeatedly, constipation can result. By delaying gastric emptying and by decreasing esophageal and gastric motility, the anticholinergics may exacerbate the condition. The smooth muscle in the respiratory tract is relaxed by the anticholinergic agents, causing bronchial dilation. This effect is used to treat asthma.

Effects on the Eye. The parasympatholytics have two effects on the eye, mydriasis and cycloplegia. Cycloplegia refers to paralysis of the ciliary muscles of the eye that results in the loss of visual accommodation. The effects of cycloplegia and mydriasis are useful to prepare the eye for ophthalmologic examinations. For eye examinations, mydriasis dilates the pupil so that the retina can be examined, and cycloplegia allows for proper measurements to make glasses. These effects occur when the drug is given topically or systemically.

Cardiovascular Effects. With large therapeutic doses, the anticholinergic agents can produce vagal blockade, resulting in tachycardia. This effect has been used therapeutically to prevent cardiac slowing during general anesthesia. With small doses, bradycardia predominates. This variable response in the heart rate occurs because heart rate is a function of both

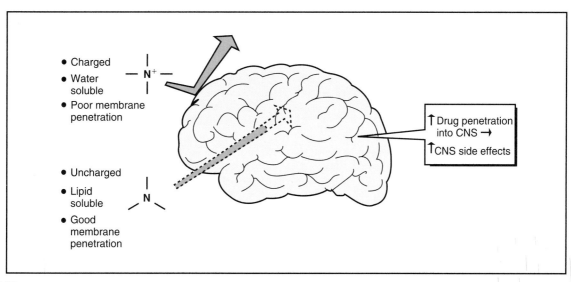

FIGURE 4-10
Anticholinergics, brain penetration. Quaternary amines are charged and hydrophilic (water soluble), so they cannot easily penetrate the brain. Tertiary amines are uncharged and lipophilic (lipid soluble), so they easily penetrate the brain. *CNS,* Central nervous system.

direct (increased heart rate) and indirect (decreased heart rate) effects.

ADVERSE REACTIONS

Salivation
Lacrimation
Urination
Defecation

The adverse reactions associated with the anticholinergics are essentially extensions of their pharmacologic effects. These can include xerostomia (see Appendix E for a discussion of drugs that cause xerostomia and a discussion of artificial salivas), blurred vision, photophobia, tachycardia, fever, and urinary and gastrointestinal stasis. Hyperpyrexia (elevated temperature) and hot, dry, flushed skin caused by a lack of sweating are also seen. Hyperpyrexia is treated symptomatically.

Anticholinergic toxicity can cause signs of CNS excitation including delirium, hallucinations, convulsions, and respiratory depression.

CONTRAINDICATIONS

Specific contraindications or cautions to the use of the anticholinergic agents include the following.

Glaucoma. Anticholinergics are the only ANS drug group that can cause an acute rise in intraocular pressure in patients with narrow-angle glaucoma (angle closure). Glaucoma is divided into narrow-angle (5% of glaucoma cases) and open-angle glaucoma (95% of glaucoma cases); cases of narrow-angle glaucoma are uncommon. Anticholinergic drugs can precipitate an acute attack in unrecognized cases of this rare condition. If narrow-angle glaucoma is diagnosed, emergency ophthalmic surgery must be performed to relieve the eye pressure. In contrast, the patient with open-angle glaucoma who is currently receiving treatment with eyedrops (many types) can be given a few doses of anticholinergic agents with impunity.

Prostatic Hypertrophy. Because the anticholinergic agents can exacerbate urinary retention, older men with prostatic hypertrophy (many men older than 50 years) who already have difficulty urinating should not be given these drugs. Acute urinary retention that may require catheterization can occur.

Intestinal or Urinary Obstruction or Retention. Constipation or acute urinary retention can be precipitated by the use of these agents in susceptible patients. Constipation can be exacerbated, especially in patients with chronic constipation. (One should not give them an opioid [narcotic] for pain control.)

Cardiovascular Disease. Because anticholinergic agents have the ability to block the vagus nerve, resulting in tachycardia, patients with cardiovascular disease should be given these agents cautiously.

USES

Table 4-4 provides examples of anticholinergic (parasympatholytic) agents, as well as their usual oral doses and routes of administration.

Preoperative Medication. The anticholinergic agents are used preoperatively for two reasons. First, they inhibit the secretions of saliva and bronchial mucus that can be stimulated by general anesthesia. Second, they have the ability to block the vagal slowing of the heart that results from general anesthesia.

Treatment of Gastrointestinal Disorders. Many types of gastrointestinal disorders associated with increased motility or acid secretion have been treated with anticholinergic agents. For example, patients with gastric ulcers are sometimes treated with

TABLE 4-4 EXAMPLES OF ANTICHOLINERGIC (PARASYMPATHOLYTIC) AGENTS

Category	Agent	PO Dose (mg)*	Route of Administration
Tertiary			
Natural alkaloids	Atropine	0.4	PO, P, ophth, topical
	Scopolamine (hyoscine) (Maldemar) (Transderm-Scop)	0.4	P, ophth, transdermal
Synthetic esters	Dicyclomine (Bentyl)	10, 20; 10 mg/5 ml (syrup)	PO, P
Quaternary			
Esters	Ipratropium (Atrovent)	—	Inhalation
	Propantheline (Pro-Banthine)	7.5, 15	PO

ophth, Ophthalmic; *P*, parenteral (injection); *PO*, oral.
*Usual oral dose (mg).

the anticholinergic agents, although there is little proof of their effectiveness. Both nonspecific diarrhea and hypermotility of the colon have also been treated with these agents. In the doses used, it is difficult to prove that the anticholinergic agents are effective for these purposes.

Ophthalmologic Examination. Because of the ability of anticholinergic agents to cause mydriasis and cycloplegia, they are commonly used topically before examinations of the eye. Producing mydriasis allows the full visualization of the retina. Cycloplegia is useful to relax the lens so that the proper prescription for eyeglasses may be determined.

Reduction of Parkinson-Like Movements. Before the advent of levodopa, anticholinergic agents were commonly used to reduce the tremors and rigidity associated with Parkinson's disease. Patients treated with these agents predictably experienced the side effects of dry mouth and blurred vision. At present, anticholinergic agents are only occasionally used in combination with levodopa for the treatment of Parkinson's disease.

The phenothiazines, used to treat psychoses, can produce extrapyramidal (Parkinson-like) side effects (see Chapter 17). These include abnormal mouth and tongue movements, rigidity, tremor, and restlessness. Anticholinergic agents, such as trihexyphenidyl (trye-hex-ee-FEN-I-dill) (Artane) and benztropine (BENZ-troe-peen) (Cogentin), are often administered concurrently with the phenothiazines to reduce rigidity and tremor.

Motion Sickness. Scopolamine, because of its CNS depressant action, is used to treat motion sickness. Transdermal scopolamine is applied behind the ear to prevent motion sickness before boating trips.

DRUG INTERACTIONS

The most important drug interaction associated with the anticholinergic agents is an additive anticholinergic effect. Other agents that have anticholinergic effects, such as the phenothiazines, antihistamines, and tricyclic antidepressants, can be additive with the parasympatholytics. Mixing more than one drug group possessing anticholinergic effects can lead to symptoms of anticholinergic toxicity, including urinary retention, blurred vision, acute glaucoma, and even paralytic ileus. Dental office personnel must pay careful attention to the medications the patient is taking to rule out excessive anticholinergic effects.

Nicotinic Agonists and Antagonists

Nicotine, which is present in cigarettes, is so toxic that one drop on the skin is rapidly fatal. In low doses, it produces stimulation because of depolarization. At high doses, it produces paralysis of the ganglia, resulting in respiratory paralysis. Peripherally, it increases blood pressure and heart rate and increases gastrointestinal motility and secretions. Nicotine constricts the blood vessels and reduces blood flow to the extremities. Nicotine is addicting, and withdrawal can occur. It is used as an insecticide.

SYMPATHETIC AUTONOMIC NERVOUS SYSTEM

The major neurotransmitters in the SANS include NE and epinephrine. They are synthesized in the neural tissues and stored in synaptic vesicles. NE is the major neurotransmitter released at the terminal nerve endings of the SANS. With stimulation, epinephrine is released from the adrenal medulla and distributed throughout the body via the blood. Dopamine receptors are important in the brain and splanchnic and renal vasculature. There are currently several dopamine receptor subtypes (D_1 to D_5). They are divided into two groups: one group is D_1 and D_5 and the other group is D_2, D_3, and D_4. Each of these receptor subtypes may be further divided into A and B, for example, D_{1A} and D_{1B}.

The term *catecholamine* is made up of two terms that relate to their structure. *Catechol* refers to 1,2-dihydroxybenzene. *Amine* refers to the chemical structure NH_2. NE, epinephrine, and dopamine are endogenous sympathetic neurotransmitters that are catecholamines. Isoproterenol (Isuprel) is an exogenous catecholamine. This term is used to refer to the epinephrine contained in a lidocaine with epinephrine solution.

The adrenergic drugs can be classified by their mechanism of action (Figure 4-11) as follows:

*   *Direct acting:* Epinephrine, NE, and isoproterenol produce their effects directly on the receptor site by stimulating the receptor.
*   *Indirect acting:* These agents, such as amphetamine, release endogenous NE, which then produces a response. Depletion

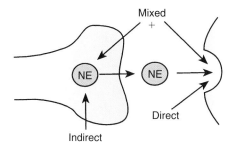

FIGURE 4-11
Sympathetic autonomic nervous system (SANS): direct-, mixed-, and indirect-acting adrenergic agents. *NE,* Norepinephrine.

of the endogenous NE with reserpine diminishes the response to these agents.

*   *Mixed acting:* These agents, such as ephedrine, can either stimulate the receptor directly or release endogenous NE to cause a response.

NE's action is terminated primarily by reuptake into the presynaptic nerve terminal by an amine-specific pump. The NE taken up in this manner is stored for reuse. In addition, two enzyme systems, monoamine oxidase (MAO) and catechol-*O*-methyltransferase (COMT), are involved in the metabolism of a portion of both epinephrine and NE.

Sympathetic Autonomic Nervous System Receptors

As early as 1948, the existence of at least two types of adrenergic receptors, termed *alpha* (α) and *beta* (β), was recognized. The activation of α-receptors causes a different response than the activation of β-receptors. More subreceptor types are now known.

♦ α-RECEPTORS

The stimulation of the α-receptors results in smooth-muscle excitation or contraction, which then causes vasoconstriction. Because α-receptors are located in the skin and skeletal muscle, vasoconstriction of the skin and skeletal muscle follows stimulation. Drugs that block the action of neurotransmitters on the α-receptors are referred to as α-adrenergic blocking agents.

♦ β-RECEPTORS

There are at least two types of β-receptors, $β_1$ and $β_2$. $β_1$-Receptor excitation causes stimulation of the heart muscle, resulting in a positive chronotropic effect (increased rate) and a positive inotropic effect (increased strength). The $β_1$-receptor controls the heart (one can remember the receptor that controls the heart by remembering that humans have only one heart) (Figure 4-12). Other actions thought to be associated primarily with $β_1$-receptor stimulation include metabolic effects on glycogen formation.

The stimulation of the $β_2$-receptors results in smooth-muscle relaxation. Because the blood vessels of the skeletal muscle are innervated by $β_2$-receptors, stimulation causes vasodilation. Relaxation of the smooth muscles of the bronchioles, also containing $β_2$-receptors, results in bronchodilation. $β_2$-Receptor stimulation produces bronchodilation in the lungs (one can remember the receptor that controls the lungs by remembering that humans have two lungs) (see Figure 4-12). Drugs with this effect have been used in the treatment of asthma. The type of receptor found in a given tissue determines the effect adrenergic agents will produce on that tissue (see Table 4-1).

Agents that block β-receptor effects are called β-adrenergic blocking agents. Some (e.g., propranolol) are nonspecific, blocking both $β_1$-receptors and $β_2$-receptors, whereas others are more selective, blocking primarily $β_2$-receptors.

Adrenergic (Sympathomimetic) Agents

Adrenergic agents play an important part in the treatment of anaphylaxis and asthma and are added to local anesthetic solutions (vasoconstrictors) to prolong their action. Table 4-5 lists some adrenergic agents.

◆ PHARMACOLOGIC EFFECTS

When discussing the pharmacologic effects associated with the adrenergic drugs, it is important to note the proportion of α-receptor and β-receptor activity each possesses. For example, epinephrine has both α-receptor and β-receptor activity, NE

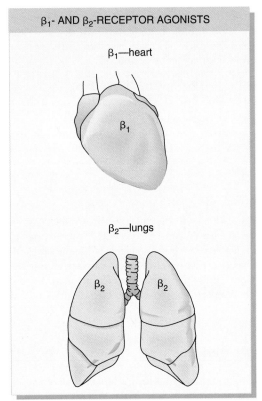

β₁- AND β₂-RECEPTOR AGONISTS

β₁—heart

β₁

β₂—lungs

β₂   β₂

FIGURE 4-12
β-Receptors: β₁ and β₂.

and phenylephrine stimulate primarily α-receptors, and isoproterenol acts mainly on β-receptors. Although the effects of these agents depend on their ability to stimulate various receptors, the general actions of the adrenergic agents are discussed with specific reference to α-receptor or β-receptor effects as applicable.

Central Nervous System Effects. The sympathomimetic agents, such as amphetamine, produce CNS excitation, or alertness. With higher doses, anxiety, apprehension, restlessness, and even tremors can occur.

Cardiovascular Effects

Heart. The general effect of the sympathomimetics, such as epinephrine, on the heart is to increase its force and strength of contraction. The final effect on blood pressure is a combination of the direct and the indirect effects. NE, primarily an α-agonist, produces vasoconstriction that increases peripheral resistance, resulting in an increase in blood pressure. With an increase in blood pressure, the vagal reflex decreases the heart rate. Epinephrine, an α- and β-agonist, constricts the α-receptors and dilates the β-receptors. This produces a widening of the pulse pressure (systolic blood pressure–diastolic blood pressure) with an increase in systolic and a decrease in diastolic blood pressures. Isoproterenol, primarily a β-agonist, produces vasodilation (lowers peripheral resistance) that triggers an increase in heart rate (vagal reflex).

Vessels. The vascular responses observed with the sympathomimetics depend on the location of the vessels and whether they are innervated by α-receptors, β-receptors, or both. Agents with α-receptor effects will produce vasoconstriction primarily in the skin and mucosa (innervated with α-receptor fibers), whereas agents with β-receptor effects will produce vasodilation of the skeletal muscle (innervated with β-receptor fibers). The resultant effect on the total peripheral resistance is an increase with an α-receptor agent and a reduction with a β-receptor agent.

Blood Pressure. The sympathomimetic effect on the blood pressure is generally an increase. With epinephrine,

TABLE 4-5   EXAMPLES OF ADRENERGIC RECEPTOR AGONISTS (SYMPATHOMIMETIC ADRENERGIC AGONISTS)

Type	Drug	Receptors	Indications
Endogenous catecholamines	Epinephrine (Adrenalin) (Primatene) (EpiPen)	α/β	Anaphylaxis, asthma
	Norepinephrine (Levophed)	α/β	Hypotension
α₁-Selective	Phenylephrine (Neo-Synephrine)	α₁	Hypotension, nasal congestion
	Tetrahydrozoline (Tyzine, Visine)	α	Conjunctivitis, rhinitis
	Oxymetazoline (Afrin, Neo-Synephrine 12 hour, OcuClear)	α	Conjunctivitis, nasal congestion
α₂-Selective	Clonidine (Catapres)	α₂	Hypertension
	Methyldopa (Aldomet)	α	Hypertension
β-Nonselective	Isoproterenol (Isuprel)	β	Heart block, bronchospasm
β₁-Selective	Dobutamine (Dobutrex)	β₁ > β₂	Cardiac decompensation
β₂-Selective	Albuterol (Proventil, Ventolin)	β₂ > β₁	Asthma
	Metaproterenol (Alupent)	β₂ > β₁	Asthma
Miscellaneous indirect-acting	Amphetamine	CNS/α/β	ADHD, narcolepsy
	Dextroamphetamine (Dexedrine)	CNS/α/β	ADHD, narcolepsy
	Amphetamine aspartate, sulfate, saccharate, and sulfate (Adderall)	CNS/α/β	ADHD, narcolepsy
	Methamphetamine (Desoxyn)	CNS/α/β	ADHD, obesity
	Methylphenidate (Ritalin)	CNS/α/β	ADHD
	Ephedrine	α/β	Methamphetamine precursor
	Pseudoephedrine (Sudafed)	α/β	Nasal congestion

ADHD, Attention-deficit hyperactivity disorder; *CNS,* central nervous system.

which has both α-receptor–stimulating and β-receptor–stimulating properties, there is a rise in systolic pressure and a decrease in diastolic pressure. With NE, there is a rise in both systolic and diastolic pressures. With isoproterenol, there is little change in systolic pressure, but a decrease in diastolic pressure occurs.

Effects on the Eye. The sympathomimetic agents have at least two effects on the eye: a decrease in intraocular pressure, which makes them useful in the treatment of glaucoma, and mydriasis.

Effects on the Respiratory System. These agents cause a relaxation of the bronchiole smooth muscle because of their β-adrenergic effect. This has made them useful in the treatment of asthma and anaphylaxis.

Metabolic Effects. The hyperglycemia resulting from β-receptor stimulation can be explained on the basis of increased glycogenolysis and decreased insulin release. Fatty acid mobilization, lipolysis, and gluconeogenesis are stimulated, and the basal metabolic rate is increased.

Effects on the Salivary Glands. The mucus-secreting cells of the submaxillary glands and sublingual glands are stimulated by the sympathomimetic agents to release a small amount of thick, viscous saliva. Because the parotid gland has no sympathetic innervation (only parasympathetic) and the sympathomimetics produce vasoconstriction, the flow of saliva is often reduced, resulting in xerostomia.

◆ ADVERSE REACTIONS

The adverse reactions associated with the adrenergic drugs are extensions of their pharmacologic effects. Anxiety and tremors may occur, and the patient may have palpitations. Serious arrhythmias can result. Agents with an α-adrenergic action can also cause a dramatic rise in blood pressure. The sympathomimetic agents should be used with caution in patients with angina, hypertension, or hyperthyroidism.

◆ CONTRAINDICATIONS

These drugs should not be used in persons with uncontrolled hypertension, angina, or hyperthyroidism. These drugs stimulate α- and β-receptors in the heart and as such would further increase blood pressure and heart rate in persons with already increased blood pressure and heart rates. This could lead to arrhythmias or a myocardial infarction.

◆ USES

Vasoconstriction

Prolonged Action. The sympathomimetic agents are used in dentistry primarily because of their vasoconstrictive action on the blood vessels. Agents with an α-effect (vasoconstriction) are often added to local anesthetic solutions. These vasoconstrictors prolong the action of the local anesthetics and reduce their potential for systemic toxicity.

Hemostasis. The adrenergic agents have been used in dentistry to produce hemostasis. Epinephrine can be applied topically or infiltrated locally around the bleeding area. Epinephrine-containing retraction cords, used to stop bleeding and to retract the gingiva before taking an impression, can produce problems such as systemic toxicity. Epinephrine is quickly absorbed after topical application if the tissue is injured. The total amount of epinephrine given by all routes must be noted to prevent an overdose.

Decongestion. Sympathomimetic agents are often incorporated into nose drops or sprays (see Table 4-5) to treat nasal congestion. These agents provide symptomatic relief by constricting the vessels and reducing the swelling of the mucous membranes of the nose. Within a short time, the congestion can return; this is a condition called *rebound congestion*. With repeated local use, systemic absorption can cause problems even greater than rebound congestion. Systemic decongestants or topical intranasal steroids are now preferred.

Cardiac Effects

Treatment of Shock. The value of the adrenergic agents in the treatment of shock is controversial. These drugs will elevate a lowered blood pressure, but correcting the cause of shock is more important. Some agents with both α-effects and β-effects (e.g., epinephrine) are used.

Treatment of Cardiac Arrest. The sympathomimetic agents, especially epinephrine, are used to treat cardiac arrest.

Bronchodilation. The use of the sympathomimetic agents in the treatment of respiratory disease stems from their action as bronchodilators. Patients with asthma or emphysema are often treated with adrenergic agents to provide bronchodilation. In the treatment of anaphylaxis, when bronchoconstriction is predominant, epinephrine is the drug of choice.

Central Nervous System Stimulation. Amphetamine-like agents have been used and abused as "diet pills." They are indicated for the treatment of attention deficit disorder (ADD) and narcolepsy.

Adrenergic agonists with some specificity for CNS stimulation are used for both legitimate and illegitimate purposes.

Methylphenidate (meth-ill-FEN-I-date) (Ritalin) and dextroamphetamine (dex-troe-am-FET-a-meen) (Dexedrine) are adrenergic agents used to treat ADD in both children and adults. These agents, given to hyperactive children and adults, reduce impulsivity and increase attention span. Some children with ADD will exhibit excessive motor activity—turn around in the chair, stand up from the chair, grab dental instruments, squirt water, and ask about everything. Side effects exhibited with this use include insomnia and anorexia. ADD has also been known as *attention deficit hyperactivity disorder* (ADHD) and *minimal brain dysfunction* (MBD), and children with the disorder have been referred to as *hyperkinetic* children.

Diethylpropion (dye-eth-il-PROE-pee-on) (Tenuate) is an adrenergic drug that is used as a "diet pill." Uses for weight loss, to produce euphoria, and for "staying awake" are not legitimate medical uses for adrenergic agents. Truck drivers have used these agents to keep themselves awake for long hours. Hallucinations and psychosis make these truck drivers dangerous.

Narcolepsy, a disease in which spontaneous deep sleep can occur at any time, is treated with the sympathomimetic amines. Tolerance to the effect does not seem to occur.

◆ SPECIFIC ADRENERGIC AGENTS

Epinephrine. The drug of choice for acute asthmatic attacks and anaphylaxis, epinephrine (Epi) (ep-i-NEF-rin) (Adrenalin), may be administered by both the intravenous and subcutaneous routes. It is also used in patients with cardiac arrest. It is added to local anesthetic solutions to delay absorption and reduce systemic toxicity (see Chapter 9). Epinephrine should be stored in amber-colored containers and placed out of the reach of sunlight because light causes deterioration. As it deteriorates, epinephrine first turns pink, then brown, and finally precipitates. Solutions of epinephrine with any discoloration or precipitate should be discarded immediately. (One should check the expiration date, too.)

Phenylephrine. Phenylephrine (fen-ill-EF-rin) (Neo-Synephrine) causes primarily α-receptor stimulation, which produces vasoconstriction in the cutaneous vessels. This leads to an increase in total peripheral resistance and systolic and diastolic pressures. A reflex vagal bradycardia also results. Phenylephrine is used as a mydriatic and in nose sprays (Neo-Synephrine) or drops to relieve congestion.

Levonordefrin. Levonordefrin (lee-voe-nor-DEF-rin) (Neo-Cobefrin), a derivative of NE, is a vasoconstrictor often added to local anesthetic solutions. Although claims made for this drug include less CNS excitation and cardiac stimulation, the dose required to produce vasoconstriction equal to that caused by epinephrine is higher. Therefore it is difficult to distinguish levonordefrin's effects from those of other vasoconstrictors. Its effects resemble those of α-receptor stimulation.

Ephedrine and Pseudoephedrine. In contrast to the catecholamines, ephedrine and pseudoephedrine (soo-doe-e-FED-rin) (Sudafed) are effective when taken orally and have a longer duration of action. They have both α- and β-receptor activity. Their mechanism of action is mixed, that is, they have both direct and indirect action. Ephedrine is often used in combination with other agents for patients with asthma as nonprescription remedies. Pseudoephedrine is also present in OTC products designed for the treatment of the common cold or allergies such as pseudoephedrine (Sudafed). The newest use of these agents is to "cook" them to produce methamphetamine, which is used illicitly. Because of this, their availability has been restricted. Ephedrine, in any form (herbal or chemical), is no longer available in dietary supplements. Its use, as such, is illegal in the United States. Pseudoephedrine is now kept "behind the counter" with a pharmacist. Those wishing to purchase pseudoephedrine must be older than 18 and need to go to the pharmacist to purchase it. In most states, the patient must sign a log. There is also a limit as to how much a person can purchase each month.

Dopamine. Dopamine (DOE-pa-meen) (Intropin) is a neurotransmitter in parts of the CNS. It is both an α-agonist and a β-agonist and is used primarily in the treatment of shock. It is a precursor of NE and epinephrine synthesis, as shown in Figure 4-13. Dopamine first acts on the β-receptors of the heart, producing a positive chronotropic and inotropic effect. In higher doses, it stimulates the α-receptors, producing vasoconstriction. However, it exerts an unusual vasodilating effect in certain vessels and produces an increase in blood flow to the renal, splanchnic, cerebral, and coronary vessels. Ventricular arrhythmias and hypotension can occur.

Dipivefrin. Dipivefrin (dye-PIV-e-frin) (Propine) and epinephrine are sympathomimetic ophthalmics that are used to treat glaucoma. They decrease the production of aqueous humor (β-receptor effect), increase its outflow (β-effect), and produce mydriasis (primarily α-effect). Dipivefrin, a prodrug, is metabolized in vivo to epinephrine. It may produce fewer side effects than epinephrine because it penetrates into the eye better and is used to treat chronic open-angle glaucoma.

Adrenergic Blocking Agents

Adrenergic blocking agents can block all the adrenergic receptors (α- and β-blockers), just the α-receptors (α-blockers), just the

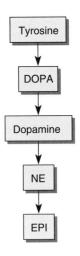

FIGURE 4-13
Synthesis of epinephrine from tyrosine, including the intermediate steps involving dopamine. *DOPA,* 3, 4 dihydrophenylalanine; *EPI,* epinephrine; *NE,* norepinephrine.

TABLE 4-6 EXAMPLES OF ADRENERGIC RECEPTOR ANTAGONISTS (SYMPATHOLYTICS, ADRENERGIC BLOCKERS)

Receptor	Examples
α-Adrenergic Receptor Antagonists	
α	Phentolamine (Regitine)
$\alpha_1 > \alpha_2$	Phenoxybenzamine (Dibenzyline)
$\alpha_1 >>> \alpha_2$	Prazosin (Minipress)
α_2	Yohimbine
α Partial agonist and antagonist	Ergot
β-Adrenergic Receptor Antagonists (L = low, I = intermediate, H = high ISA)	
Nonspecific (nonselective) β	Propranolol (Inderal)
Specific (selective) $\beta_1 > \beta_2$	Acebutolol (Sectral)
	Atenolol (Tenormin)
α- and β-Adrenergic Antagonists	
α, β	Labetalol (Normodyne, Trandate)

ISA, Intrinsic sympathetic activity.

β-receptors (β-blockers), or just α_1-receptors (α_1-blockers), α_2-receptors (α_2-blockers), β_1-receptors (β_1-blockers), or β_2-receptors (β_2-blockers) (Table 4-6).

◆ α-ADRENERGIC BLOCKING AGENTS

The α-adrenergic blocking agents competitively inhibit the vasoconstricting effects (α-receptor effects) of the adrenergic agents. This reduces the sympathetic tone in the blood vessels, producing a decrease in the total peripheral resistance. The resulting decrease in blood pressure stimulates the vagus, thereby producing a reflex tachycardia. Patients who are pretreated with α-blocking agents and given epinephrine exhibit a predominance of β-effects (vasodilation), which lowers blood pressure. This effect is termed epinephrine reversal because the blood pressure goes down instead of going up. The α-adrenergic blockers also block the mydriasis that these agents normally cause.

The agents phenoxybenzamine (fen-ox-ee-BEN-za-meen) (Dibenzyline) and phentolamine (fen-TOLE-a-meen) (Regitine) are α-blockers. They are used in the treatment of peripheral vascular disease in which vascular spasm is a common feature (e.g., Raynaud's syndrome) and in the diagnosis and treatment of pheochromocytoma, a catecholamine-secreting tumor of the adrenal medulla.

Other examples of α_1-adrenergic blocking agents are tolazoline (toe-LAZ-a-zeen) (Priscoline), prazosin (PRA-zoe-sin) (Minipress), terazosin (ter-AY-zoe-sin) (Hytrin), and doxazosin (dox-AY-zoe-sin) (Cardura), which are competitive blockers of the α-receptor. They are effective in the treatment of hypertension and are discussed in Chapter 15. These agents are also indicated in the management of Raynaud's vasospasm and in the treatment of benign prostatic hypertrophy (to increase ease of urination).

β-ADRENERGIC BLOCKING AGENTS

The β-blocking drugs competitively block the β-receptors in the adrenergic nervous system. Their generic names end in *olol*, so they can be easily recognized. Because β-receptor stimulation produces vasodilation, bronchodilation, and tachycardia, β-blockers would block these effects, producing bradycardia and in asthmatics, possible bronchoconstriction. Their exact effect is determined by the tone in the sympathetic nervous system. The β-blockers may be either nonspecific (nonselective), such as propranolol (proe-PRAN-oh-lole) (Inderal), or specific (selective) such as atenolol (a-TEN-oh-lole) (Tenormin). The specific β-blockers have more activity on the heart and blood vessels (β-receptors) than on the lungs (β-receptors). This specificity, or selectivity, produces fewer side effects. The selective β-blockers also have a lower chance of causing drug interactions.

Propranolol (Inderal) is a β-blocker that depresses the heart (negative chronotropic and inotropic effect), produces bronchoconstriction, and can cause hypoglycemia. It is used in the treatment of arrhythmias (for its quinidine-like effect), angina, hypertension, and migraine headache prophylaxis. Diseases in which tachycardia occurs, such as hyperthyroidism and pheochromocytoma, can be symptomatically treated with propranolol. The β-blockers are discussed in Chapter 15.

α- AND β-BLOCKING AGENTS

Labetalol (la-BET-a-lole) (Normodyne, Trandate) has both α- and β-blocking action. Because the β-blockers are designated using the suffix *-olol*, this α- and β-blocker uses the suffix *-alol*. It is a selective α-blocker and nonselective β-blocker. It is indicated for the treatment of hypertension and produces a fall in blood pressure without reflex tachycardia.

Neuromuscular Blocking Drugs

The neuromuscular blocking drugs are agents that affect transmission between the motor nerve endings and the nicotinic receptors on the skeletal muscle. These blocking agents act either as antagonists (nondepolarizing) or as agonists (depolarizing).

NONDEPOLARIZING (COMPETITIVE) BLOCKERS

Indigenous people living along the Amazon have used poison arrows when hunting animals. The poison is the neuromuscular blocking drug curare, or *d*-tubocurarine. This nondepolarizing blocker combines with the nicotinic receptor and blocks the action of acetylcholine. The depolarization of the membrane is inhibited and muscle contraction is blocked. These competitive blockers can be overcome by the administration of cholinesterase inhibitors such as neostigmine. Current examples include vecuronium and pancuronium.

Paralysis of the small facial muscles is followed by paralysis of the fingers, limbs, extremities, and trunk. The function of the muscles involved in respiration is lost, beginning with the intercostal muscles. The last function lost is the most primitive diaphragmatic breathing. Nature has planned that loss of function is in the order of least important to most important (the diaphragm). The duration of action of these drugs range between 20 minutes and 2 hours, depending on the dose.

DEPOLARIZING AGENTS

Depolarizing agents, such as succinylcholine (suk-sin-ill-KOE-leen), attach to the nicotinic receptor and like acetylcholine, result in depolarization. The constant stimulation of the receptor causes the sodium channel to open, producing depolarization (phase I). Transient fasciculations of the muscles result. With time, the receptor cannot transmit any further impulses and repolarization occurs as the sodium channel closes (phase II). A flaccid paralysis is produced by resistance to depolarization.

Succinylcholine produces muscle fasciculations followed by paralysis. The paralysis lasts only a few minutes because succinylcholine is broken down by plasma cholinesterase.

Succinylcholine can produce cardiac arrhythmias, hyperkalemia, and increased intraocular pressure. When it is used in general anesthesia in conjunction with halothane, succinylcholine precipitates malignant hyperthermia in susceptible patients (heredity). The drug of choice for malignant hyperthermia is dantrolene (Dantrium). Sometimes a small dose of curare is administered before the administration of succinylcholine to block the fasciculations of the succinylcholine. This reduces postoperative muscle pain.

DENTAL HYGIENE CONSIDERATIONS

Cholinergic Drugs
- Dental hygienists need to encourage patients to use good oral hygiene to help with the effects of increased salivation from cholinergic drugs.
- The dental hygienist should raise a patient into the sitting position slowly and have the patient rise slowly from the dental chair to help minimize the hypotensive effects from cholinergic drugs.

Anticholinergic Drugs
Xerostomia
- Xerostomia can be minimized with meticulous oral hygiene, including brushing and flossing.
- Patients should also drink plenty of water and keep a glass of water by their bedside at night.
- Patients should avoid prescription and nonprescription mouth rinses that contain alcohol because alcohol can exacerbate dry mouth.
- Caffeinated beverages can also exacerbate dry mouth.
- Fruit juices and sodas contain sugar, which can put the patient at increased risk for caries.
- Have the patient chew tart, sugarless gum or suck on tart, sugarless candy to help minimize dry mouth.

DENTAL HYGIENE CONSIDERATIONS—cont'd

Tachycardia

- Always check the patient's pulse and blood pressure, especially before a procedure that may require epinephrine.

Sedation

- Caution should be used if another sedating drug, such as an opioid analgesic, is necessary.
- The patient should have someone drive him or her to and from the appointment.
- The patient should avoid any activity that requires thought or concentration.

Adrenergic Agonists
Tachycardia

- The patient's blood pressure and pulse rate should be checked at each visit, especially if epinephrine or levonordefrin is required.
- Patients with uncontrolled hypertension or uncontrolled hyperthyroidism should not receive these drugs.

Central Nervous System Excitation and Tremors

- These effects can be exacerbated in a patient with existing CNS health issues or with hyperthyroidism.
- Both can be avoided or minimized with detailed medication/health histories and lower doses of a vasoconstrictor.

Drug Interactions

- Many over-the-counter (OTC) cough and cold products contain adrenergic agonists, which can interact with vasoconstrictors that can lead to increased blood pressure.
- Check the patient's blood pressure and pulse rate.
- This can be avoided by carefully questioning the patient about his or her OTC drug use.

Oral β-Adrenergic Agonists

- These drugs have the ability to increase blood pressure and heart rate, especially in combination with a vasoconstrictor.
- This can be avoided or minimized by measuring the patient's blood pressure and pulse rate before administering a vasoconstrictor.
- Ask specific questions about the patient's medications and health.

CLINICAL SKILLS ASSESSMENT

1. Explain the difference in mechanism of action between the direct-acting and indirect-acting cholinergic agents.
2. Describe the pharmacologic effects of the cholinergic agents on the heart, gastrointestinal tract, and eye.
3. State two major uses of the cholinergic agents.
4. Describe a unique dental use for pilocarpine.
5. Describe the pharmacologic effects of the anticholinergic agents on the exocrine glands, smooth muscle, and eye.
6. List the adverse reactions associated with the anticholinergic agents.
7. State the contraindications and cautions to the use of anticholinergic agents and explain their relationship to the pharmacologic effects of these agents.
8. State the major therapeutic uses of the anticholinergics.
9. State the pharmacologic effect of the adrenergic agents on the eye, bronchioles, and salivary glands.
10. State the therapeutic uses of the adrenergic agents, especially the uses these agents have in dentistry.
11. Explain the limits to the accepted medical uses of the amphetamine-like agents. Explain why ephedrine tablets are bought by the case by some individuals.
12. Name the pharmacologic class to which atenolol (Tenormin) belongs. Describe the effects that make β-blockers useful in the treatment of arrhythmias, angina, and hypertension.
13. Differentiate between "selective" and "nonselective" β-blockers. Name a difference important to the dental health team (drug interaction).

⊖volve ─────────────────────────────

Please visit http://evolve.elsevier.com/Haveles/pharmacology for review questions and additional practice and reference materials.

5 Nonopioid (Nonnarcotic) Analgesics

CHAPTER OUTLINE

PAIN
CLASSIFICATION
SALICYLATES
    Acetylsalicylic Acid
    Other Salicylates
NONSTEROIDAL ANTIINFLAMMATORY
    DRUGS
    Chemical Classification
    Mechanism of Action
    Pharmacokinetics
    Pharmacologic Effects
    Adverse Reactions
    Drug Interactions
    Contraindications and Cautions
    Therapeutic Uses
    Specific Nonsteroidal Antiinflammatory
        Drugs
ACETAMINOPHEN
    Pharmacokinetics
    Pharmacologic Effects
    Adverse Reactions
    Drug Interactions
    Uses
    Dose and Preparations
DRUGS USED TO TREAT GOUT
    Colchicine
    Allopurinol
    Probenecid

LEARNING OBJECTIVES

1. Describe pain and its purpose and main components.
2. Discuss the chemistry and pharmacokinetics, pharmacologic effects, adverse reactions, toxicity, drug interactions, and uses of aspirin.
3. Define the term *nonsteroidal antiinflammatory drug* and discuss the chemistry, pharmacokinetics, pharmacologic effects, adverse reactions, toxicity, drug interactions, and uses of these drugs.
4. Discuss the properties, pharmacologic effects, drug interactions, and uses of acetaminophen.
5. Explain the disease known as *gout* and summarize the drugs used to treat it.

Pain control is of great importance in dental practice. Pain often brings the patient to the dental office. Conversely, pain can be the factor that keeps the patient from seeking dental care at the appropriate time. Thus dental treatment is often rendered on inflamed, hypersensitive tissues of a patient who suffers from mental fatigue after enduring pain for a length of time.

The dental health care provider must be able to recognize and evaluate a patient's need for medication to control pain. Because pain is such a complex phenomenon, the entire patient must be considered before the type of medication that may be needed is determined.

PAIN

The sensation of pain is the means by which the body is made urgently aware of the presence of tissue damage. Pain represents a protective reflex for self-preservation. Just as the hand is quickly removed from a hot object, a painful dental abscess brings the patient to the dental office seeking professional assistance for its resolution. Pain is a diagnostic symptom of an underlying pathologic condition. Although the relief of pain is an immediate objective, only by treatment of the underlying cause is the ultimate resolution achieved.

The two components of pain are perception and reaction. Perception is the physical component of pain and involves the message of pain that is carried through the nerves eventually to the cortex. Reaction is the psychological component of pain and involves the patient's emotional response to the pain. Although individuals are surprisingly uniform in their perception of pain, they vary greatly in their reaction to it. A decrease in the pain threshold (a greater reaction to pain) has been said to be associated with emotional instability, anxiety, fatigue, youth, certain nationalities, women, and fear and apprehension. The pain threshold is raised by sleep, sympathy, activities, and analgesics (Figure 5-1). As a result, analgesic therapy must be selected for the individual. A level of discomfort that may not require drug treatment in one person may demand extreme therapy in another. Although some patients undergoing routine exodontia require no postoperative medication, even the strongest analgesics will not completely control postoperative extraction pain in other persons.

49

CLASSIFICATION

The analgesic agents can be divided into two groups, the nonopioids, also called the *nonnarcotic, peripheral, mild,* and *antipyretic analgesics,* and the opioids, also called the *narcotic, central,* or *strong analgesics* (Figure 5-2).

An important difference between the nonopioid and the opioid analgesics (narcotic analgesics) is their sites of action.

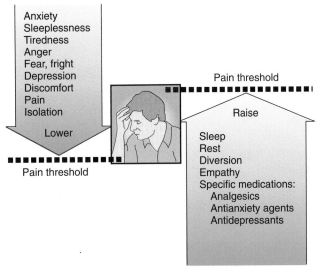

FIGURE 5-1
Factors that alter the pain threshold. Sleep raises the threshold, and fear lowers it. (From McKenry L et al: *Mosby's pharmacology in nursing,* ed 22, St Louis, 2006, Mosby.)

Nonopioid analgesics act primarily at the peripheral nerve endings, although their antipyretic effect is mediated centrally. Opioids act primarily within the central nervous system (CNS).

Another difference between the opioids and the nonopioid analgesic agents is their mechanism of action. The action of the nonopioid analgesic agents is related to their ability to inhibit prostaglandin synthesis (Figure 5-3). The opioids affect the response to pain by depressing the CNS (the reaction). The side effect profiles of the two groups also differ.

The nonopioids can be divided into the salicylates (aspirin-like group), acetaminophen, and the nonsteroidal antiinflammatory drugs (NSAIDs) (Box 5-1). Aspirin, a member of the salicylates, is discussed first.

SALICYLATES

Since antiquity, extracts of willow bark containing salicin have been used to reduce fever. Over the years, many other salicylates (sa-LI-si-lates) have been synthesized, but aspirin is the most useful salicylate for analgesia. Box 5-2 lists some analgesic and some topical salicylates. Because aspirin is the prototype salicylate, it is discussed.

Acetylsalicylic Acid

♦ CHEMISTRY

Acetylsalicylic acid (aspirin, ASA) is broken down into acetic acid (HA) and salicylic acid (SA) (Figure 5-4). Acetic acid imparts the characteristic vinegar odor to a bottle of aspirin. Therefore the degree of breakdown of aspirin can be roughly determined by smelling a bottle of aspirin tablets. (If one thinks

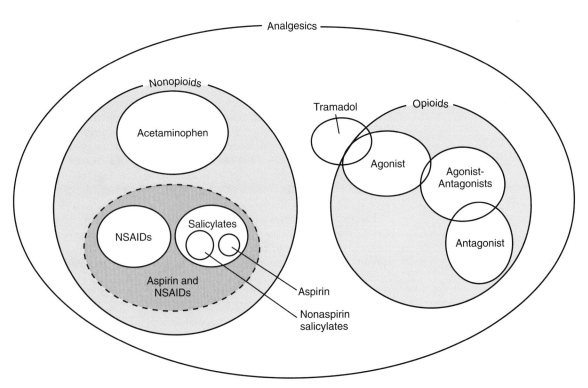

FIGURE 5-2
Categories of analgesics.

"phew" when opening an aspirin bottle, it is time to purchase a new bottle.) In addition, salicylic acid is a strong keratolytic agent (used to remove plantar warts from the bottom of feet) and may cause additional adverse gastrointestinal effects if degraded aspirin is administered orally.

♦ MECHANISM OF ACTION

The mechanism of aspirin's analgesic, antipyretic, antiinflammatory, and antiplatelet effects is related to its ability to inhibit prostaglandin synthesis. Aspirin inhibits the enzyme cyclo-oxygenase (COX, prostaglandin synthase) by acetylating serine, which results in inhibition of the production of prostaglandins. Figure 5-5 shows the synthesis of the prostaglandins and leuko-

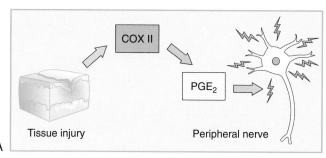
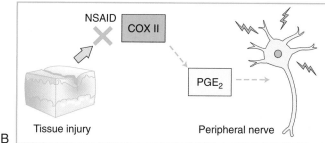

FIGURE 5-3
Model for nociceptive pain. **A,** Tissue injury triggers cyclo-oxygenase II (COX II) in peripheral tissue to convert arachidonic acid to prostaglandin E_2 (PGE_2), resulting in stimulation of the nociceptor in peripheral nerve to send a signal for pain to the central nervous system. **B,** Nonsteroidal antiinflammatory drug (NSAID) interfering with COX II–mediated prostaglandin synthesis. (From McKenry L et al: *Mosby's pharmacology in nursing,* ed 22, St Louis, 2006, Mosby.)

BOX 5-1 SELECTED NONOPIOID ANALGESICS

Salicylates
Aspirin
Choline salicylate
Diflunisal
Magnesium salicylate
Salsalate

NSAIDs
Etodolac
Ibuprofen
Ketoprofen
Naproxen

Nonsalicylates/Nonnarcotics
Acetaminophen

NSAIDs, Nonsteroidal antiinflammatory drugs.

BOX 5-2 SALICYLATES

Oral
Aspirin
Choline salicylate (Arthropan)
Diflunisal (Dolobid)
Magnesium salicylate (Doan's)
Salsalate (Disalcid)
Sodium salicylate combination (Trilisate)

Topical
Methyl salicylate, oil of wintergreen (toxic PO) (Icy Hot, Ben-Gay)
Salicylic acid (Compound W, DuoFilm)
Trolamine salicylate (Myoflex)

PO, By mouth.

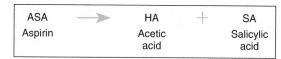

FIGURE 5-4
Formula for acetylsalicylic acid.

trienes from arachidonic acid. Prostaglandins, which are lipids that are synthesized locally by inflammatory stimuli, can sensitize the pain receptors to substances such as bradykinin. Therefore a reduction in prostaglandins results in a reduction in pain. Because aspirin blocks the synthesis of prostaglandins, it is more effective if given before the painful stimuli are experienced. Because of this mechanism, aspirin is more effective against "throbbing" pain (caused by inflammation and common in dentistry) than against "stabbing" pain (direct effect on nerve endings).

♦ PHARMACOKINETICS

Aspirin is rapidly and almost completely absorbed from the stomach and small intestine, producing its peak effect on an empty stomach in 30 minutes (90 minutes for salicylate). The buffered tablet reaches its peak in about 20 minutes (salicylate). Before a tablet of aspirin can be absorbed, it must be dispersed and dissolved. Addition of a buffer to the tablet facilitates this process. This is borne out by the somewhat quicker peak of action and higher blood levels attained with buffered aspirin preparations. Buffered aspirin has a higher proportion of the aspirin in the ionized form, which should make absorption slower, but this is offset by the increase in the rate of dissolution, which is facilitated. This difference in absorption has not been shown to translate into a clinically significant quicker effect.

Aspirin may be administered rectally as suppositories if vomiting is present. Because this route is more erratic and unpredictable, it should only be used when the oral route is not feasible. An aspirin tablet should never be applied topically to the oral mucosa to treat a toothache. A painful ulceration can occur. Any benefit from this practice would come from inadvertent swallowing of the aspirin or local damage to nerve endings.

Aspirin is widely distributed into most body tissues and fluids. It is poorly bound to plasma proteins. It is hydrolyzed to salicylate in the mucosa of the gastrointestinal tract and on first pass through the liver. The half-life of unhydrolyzed aspirin is about 15 minutes. The half-life of hydrolyzed aspirin is dose-dependent. With small doses, the half-life is 2 to 3 hours; with

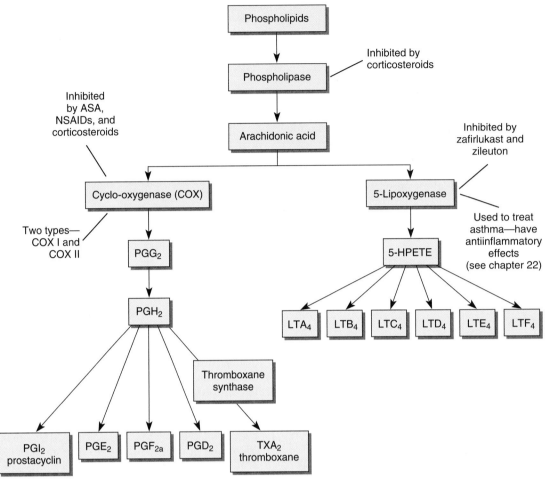

FIGURE 5-5
Synthesis of prostaglandins and leukotrienes and site of action of aspirin and nonsteroidal antiinflammatory drugs (NSAIDs) that interfere with prostaglandin synthesis.

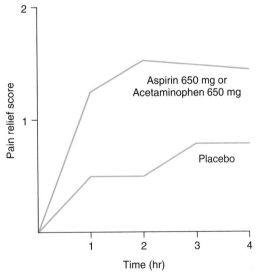

FIGURE 5-6
Analgesic efficacy over time of aspirin versus placebo.

higher doses, a half-life of 15 to 30 hours can be attained. The half-life varies with the dose because a constant amount rather than a constant percentage of the drug is metabolized per hour. This type of metabolism is called *zero-order kinetics* (see Chapter 2).

♦ PHARMACOLOGIC EFFECTS

Analgesic Effect. Aspirin's analgesic effect has been repeatedly demonstrated in many clinical trials. In fact, new drugs are often compared in analgesic strength to aspirin. Aspirin typically relieves mild-to-moderate pain such as a headache or toothache. For more intense pain, the agents or stronger opioids are required because the analgesic potency of aspirin is weaker than the other agents mentioned. Because of its easy accessibility and long history of use, aspirin's worth as an analgesic is often unrecognized by the lay public. Figure 5-6 shows the analgesic efficacy of aspirin over time as compared to placebo.

Antipyretic Effect. The ability of aspirin to reduce fever (antipyretic effect) results from its inhibition of prostaglandin synthesis in the hypothalamus. Hypothalamic prostaglandin synthesis is caused by elevated blood levels of leukocyte pyrogens induced by inflammation. Increased hypothalamic prostaglandin levels produce increased body temperature. Therefore the inhibition of hypothalamic prostaglandin synthesis results

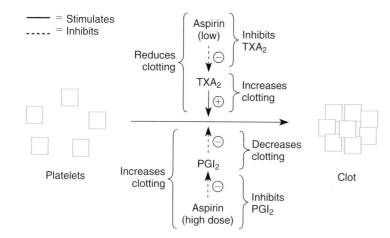

───── = Stimulates
----- = Inhibits

FIGURE 5-7
The effects and mechanism of action of aspirin, thromboxane, and prostacyclin synthesis.

in a return to more normal body temperature. Aspirin reduces fever by inducing peripheral vasodilation and sweating. Although it reduces an elevated temperature, it has no effect on normal body temperature. In fact, in toxic doses it produces hyperthermia (see the section on Adverse Reactions).

Antiinflammatory Effect. Aspirin's antiinflammatory effect is derived from its ability to inhibit prostaglandin synthesis. The prostaglandins are potent vasodilating agents that also increase capillary permeability. Therefore aspirin causes decreased erythema and swelling of the inflamed area. This antiinflammatory action is useful in dental patients because inflammation is a significant part of most dental pain. Patients with arthritis may be given large doses of aspirin to provide symptomatic relief of pain and inflammation in the joints.

Uricosuric Effect. Although large doses (greater than 3 gm/day) of aspirin can produce a uricosuric effect, small doses (less than 1 gm/day) produce uric acid retention. Aspirin can also counteract the uricosuric effect of probenecid (proe-BEN-e-sid) (Benemid), which is used to treat gout. Aspirin is no longer used as a uricosuric agent because more effective agents are available to treat gout.

Antiplatelet Effect. Aspirin irreversibly binds to platelets. Its antiplatelet effect has been shown to be clinically effective for secondary myocardial infarction prevention in adults, the primary prevention of coronary artery disease, and the treatment of an ischemic event or the prevention of a further ischemic event. The effect of aspirin on platelets depends on the dose taken. Aspirin has (±) an effect on two substances involved in blood clotting: thromboxane A_2 and prostacyclin. Depending on the dose, aspirin can inhibit either prostacyclin (inhibits aggregation) or thromboxane A_2 (stimulates aggregation). Figure 5-7 demonstrates that inhibition of thromboxane A_2 would prevent clotting because thromboxane A_2 promotes clotting. Further studies are needed to determine aspirin's usefulness and dose in preventing clotting events in different patient populations. Low-dose aspirin has been shown to be effective for prevention of myocardial infarction, and it is now recommended for both men and women older than the age of 50 years. Other recommendations include taking an aspirin if a heart attack is suspected. Aspirin's effects by dose are illustrated in Figure 5-8.

◆ ADVERSE REACTIONS

In sufficiently high doses, aspirin can produce a variety of undesirable effects. Some of aspirin's side effects can be minimized

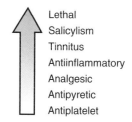

Lethal
Salicylism
Tinnitus
Antiinflammatory
Analgesic
Antipyretic
Antiplatelet

FIGURE 5-8
Pharmacologic effects and adverse reactions of aspirin from low to high doses.

but not eliminated. Precautions and contraindications for the administration of aspirin are listed in Table 5-1.

Gastrointestinal Effects. Aspirin's most frequent side effect is related to the gastrointestinal tract. It may be simple dyspepsia, nausea, vomiting, or gastric bleeding. These adverse effects result from direct gastric irritation and inhibition of prostaglandins. Because prostaglandins are responsible for inhibition of gastric acid secretion and stimulation of the cytoprotective mucus in the stomach, aspirin counteracts these effects. In high doses, aspirin's stimulation of the chemoreceptor trigger zone in the CNS can also produce nausea and vomiting. Salicylates may exacerbate preexisting ulcers, gastritis, or hiatal hernia.

> Gastric effects are common.

Bleeding. At usual therapeutic doses, aspirin irreversibly interferes with the clotting mechanism by reducing platelet adhesiveness caused by interfering with adenosine diphosphate (ADP) release. The bleeding time is prolonged, and each platelet is affected until new platelets are formed (4 to 7 days). Replacement of all of the affected platelets is not required to produce normal clotting. After about 20% of the platelets have been replaced with newly formed platelets, clotting will return to normal by about 36 hours. Therefore with lower doses of aspirin, 1.5 days should elapse to obtain normal clotting. With large doses of aspirin, the half-life is prolonged. Aspirin inhibits the production of prothrombin, resulting in hypoprothrombinemia. Three other mechanisms—the local irritant effects on the stomach, the decrease in platelet stickiness, and the loss of protective mucosa—magnify adverse effects on the stomach. Salicylate-induced gastric bleeding is painless. With a small loss of blood, aspirin does not produce significant bleeding. Salicylates may exacerbate preexisting conditions such as ulcers, gastritis,

TABLE 5-1   PRECAUTIONS AND CONTRAINDICATIONS FOR THE ADMINISTRATION OF ASPIRIN

Disease or Condition	Drug Used	Comments
Myocardial infarction, atrial fibrillation, valve replacement	Warfarin (Coumadin)	Increases anticoagulant effect of warfarin
Peptic ulcer (heartburn), GERD	H$_2$-blockers (e.g., cimetidine)	Gastric irritant effect
Gout	Probenecid (Benemid)	Antagonizes uricosuric effect of probenecid
Arthritis, cancer, psoriasis	MTX	Increases toxicity of methotrexate
Rheumatic fever, arthritis	Large doses of aspirin	Do not add more aspirin if patient is taking large doses already
Hemophilia	Factor VIII	Gastric bleeding
Hypoprothrombinemia		Bleeding
Vitamin K deficiency, alcoholism		Bleeding
G6PD deficiency		Hemolysis
Diabetes	Oral hypoglycemics	Hypoglycemia

GERD, Gastroesophageal reflux disease; MTX, methotrexate; G6PD, glucose-6-phosphate dehydrogenase.

hiatal hernia, or gastrointestinal esophageal reflux disease (GERD).

Reye's Syndrome. In children and adolescents with either chickenpox or influenza, the use of aspirin has been epidemiologically associated with Reye's (pronounced rize) syndrome. In place of aspirin, acetaminophen is used in pediatrics for both its analgesic and antipyretic action. Reye's syndrome is associated with hepatotoxicity and encephalopathy, commonly fatal.

Hepatic and Renal Effects. Rarely, aspirin can produce hepatotoxicity. Renal papillary necrosis and interstitial nephritis leading to dialysis is associated with certain analgesic use. It may be caused by the concomitant administration of aspirin and acetaminophen.

Pregnancy and Nursing Considerations. Although animal studies have shown that aspirin can produce birth defects, human studies have demonstrated only a slight positive correlation between chronic aspirin ingestion and congenital abnormalities. With aspirin abuse, increased risk of stillbirth, neonatal death, and decreased birth weight occur. With near-term, high-dose administration of aspirin, gestation can be prolonged, parturition delayed, and risk of hemorrhage increased in the newborn and mother. Even premature closure of the patent ductus arteriosus (hole in fetal heart) has been reported. Although salicylates are excreted in the breast milk, usual occasional therapeutic doses of aspirin do not present a problem for the healthy nursing infant.

Hypersensitivity (Allergy). The incidence of true aspirin allergy is less than 1% (0.2% to 0.4%).

> True aspirin allergy is uncommon.

Many patients with "allergy to aspirin" in their charts, on questioning, actually have stomach problems rather than a true allergy. In the patient's chart, it is important to differentiate aspirin's adverse reactions from its hypersensitivity reactions. Adequate questioning of patients who "claim" to be allergic to aspirin is needed because patients with true aspirin hypersensitivity cannot be given any of the NSAIDs because of some cross-hypersensitivity. Allergic reactions can vary from rash, wheezing, urticaria, and angioneurotic edema to anaphylactic shock. When a true aspirin allergy exists, any aspirin-containing products or NSAIDs should be avoided.

Persons with asthma are more likely to have a hypersensitivity reaction to aspirin, with the incidence ranging from 5% to 15%. The aspirin hypersensitivity triad: *aspirin hypersensitivity, asthma,* and *nasal polyps* often occur together. This reaction is thought to be the result of the shunting of the products of arachidonic acid from the production of prostaglandins to the leukotrienes and is thought to be a potential mechanism for this hypersensitivity. These patients exhibit cross-hypersensitivity between aspirin and other agents, including the NSAIDs, and they should not be given any NSAIDs.

♦ TOXICITY

An overdose of aspirin can produce harmful effects and even death.

Symptoms. When the blood level of salicylates reaches a certain level, a toxic reaction, referred to as salicylism, occurs. It is characterized by tinnitus (ringing in the ears), headache, nausea, vomiting, dizziness, and dimness of vision. Hyperthermia and electrolyte imbalance can also occur. With higher levels, stimulation of respiration leads to hyperventilation, which produces respiratory alkalosis. Compensatory alkalosis results in renal loss of bicarbonate, sodium, and potassium. Both respiratory and metabolic acidosis ensue. The cause of death from aspirin poisoning is usually acidosis and electrolyte imbalance.

Prevention. Children are the primary victims of accidental poisoning. The lethal dose of aspirin

> Toxicity prevention involves child-proof containers.

for a child is 4 gm, and the lethal dose of aspirin for an adult is 10 to 30 gm. Education of the parents regarding the potential for poisoning and proper storage and childproof containers for over-the-counter (OTC) aspirin have significantly reduced accidental poisonings in children.

Treatment. Treatment of aspirin poisoning includes removing excess drug in the stomach by inducing emesis or administering activated charcoal to absorb the aspirin. Other symptoms are treated symptomatically. For example, hyperthermia is treated with cooling baths or "blankets," acidosis with sodium bicarbonate, hypokalemia with potassium, and hypoglycemia with intravenous (IV) glucose. Box 5-3 lists the patient instructions for aspirin.

BOX 5-3 PATIENT INSTRUCTIONS FOR USE OF ASPIRIN
• Take with a full glass of water. • Take with food, milk, or an antacid to minimize gastrointestinal irritation. • Do not use NSAIDs concurrently. • Do not take OTC analgesics with aspirin. • Do not give to children under the age of 18 because of the risk for Reye's syndrome. • Aspirin use can prolong bleeding time. • If the pain does not subside within a few days, call the dentist.

NSAIDs, Nonsteroidal antiinflammatory drugs; *OTC,* over the counter.

◆ DRUG INTERACTIONS

The drug interactions of aspirin are listed in Table 5-1. Some of the more notable are briefly discussed in the following:

* *Warfarin:* The drug interaction between aspirin and warfarin can result in bleeding. Warfarin (WAR-far-in), an oral anticoagulant, is highly protein bound to plasma protein–binding sites. If aspirin is administered to a patient taking warfarin, it can displace the warfarin from its binding sites, increasing its anticoagulant effect. In addition, aspirin affects both platelets and the gastrointestinal tract. Bleeding and hemorrhage may result from these interactions.
* *Probenecid:* Aspirin interferes with probenecid's (proe-BEN-e-sid) uricosuric effect. Aspirin has been reported to precipitate an acute attack of gout. One should avoid using aspirin in patients taking probenecid.
* *Methotrexate:* Methotrexate (meth-oh-TREX-ate) (MTX) is an antineoplastic drug used to treat certain kinds of cancer and autoimmune diseases (arthritis, psoriasis). Aspirin can displace MTX from its protein-binding sites and can also interfere with its clearance. This results in an increased serum concentration and MTX toxicity such as bone marrow depression.
* *Sulfonylureas:* Higher doses of salicylates (more than 2 gm) may produce a hypoglycemic effect. One proposed mechanism involves the displacement of the sulfonylureas from their plasma protein–binding sites by aspirin. This hypoglycemia effect can also be observed with insulin.
* *Antihypertensives:* Aspirin reduces the antihypertensive effect of many hypertensives including angiotensin-converting enzyme (ACE) inhibitors, β-blockers, and thiazide and loop diuretics. This requires several doses of aspirin over a few days. Aspirin's effect on the renal function, resulting in water and sodium retention, may contribute to this effect.

◆ USES

One use of aspirin is to provide analgesia for mild-to-moderate pain. It is the analgesic against which new analgesics are measured for efficacy. Its antipyretic effect is useful in the control of fever but should be avoided in children (Reye's syndrome). Its antiinflammatory action is used in the treatment of inflammatory conditions such as rheumatic fever and arthritis. Because of its effect on platelet aggregation (inhibition), aspirin is used to prevent unwanted clotting (in patients older than 50 years or with previous myocardial infarction). In some patients, the incidence of myocardial infarction has decreased, but the overall mortality remained the same.

◆ DOSE AND PREPARATIONS

The usual adult dose of aspirin for the treatment of pain or fever is 325 to 650 mg every 4 hours. The dose for arthritis is between 3 and 6 gm/day. For prevention of myocardial infarction, the dose is 75 to 325 mg/day. The dose for children is 10 to 15 mg/kg every 4 to 6 hours (maximum 3.6 gm/24 hr) (see Table 5-9).

Many types of preparations containing aspirin are available by prescription and OTC (Table 5-2). Some of these types are as follows.

Regular Aspirin. A single-entity form of aspirin includes the commonly used 325-mg (5-gr) tablet and the 81-mg flavored children's tablet. Many brand and generic products are available in all strengths.

Enteric-Coated Aspirin. Aspirin can be formulated with a coating that dissolves in the intestine rather than in the stomach. The advantage of enteric-coated aspirin is that gastric symptoms are reduced. The disadvantage is that these products can give erratic absorption and unreliable blood levels. The onset of action is too long to make them useful for acute dental pain. They have limited use in treatment of chronic arthritis when gastric irritation is a problem. They can be used when daily aspirin is used for clot prevention.

Combinations

With Buffer. Although claimed to produce fewer gastrointestinal side effects, buffered tableted preparations have never been shown to do so. They are absorbed at a slightly quicker rate. The liquid buffered preparations do produce less gastrointestinal irritation, but they contain sodium, which is relatively contraindicated in high blood pressure.

With Another Analgesic. Aspirin can be combined with an opioid analgesic or acetaminophen. Caffeine is part of this combination. Mixing aspirin with an opioid can allow a decrease in the amount of the opioid in the product and therefore reduce its side effects.

With Sedatives. Adding a sedative to aspirin can make it more effective if anxiety is a substantial component of the pain. Prescribing a separate antianxiety agent would give the prescriber more control and is preferred.

With Caffeine. Caffeine potentiates the analgesic effect of aspirin and other analgesics. The addition of 130 mg of caffeine is equivalent to increasing the dose of the analgesic by one third or more. Most proprietary preparations contain about one-half this much caffeine. (However, one can always take two tablets of most analgesics.)

Other Salicylates

◆ COMMON AGENTS

Sodium, choline, magnesium salicylate and salicylamide, and salsalate are other salicylates. These agents claim to have fewer gastrointestinal side effects, but this claim has little documentation. Their efficacy as analgesic agents and the appropriate doses for analgesia must be determined. Two advantages of these agents are that they are thought to have no effect on platelets and no cross-hypersensitivity with aspirin. Magnesium is contraindicated in renal disease, and sodium is contraindicated in cardiovascular disease. Salicylamide is a weak analgesic. Salsalate is made up of the combination of two salicylic acids.

TABLE 5-2 SELECTED OVER-THE-COUNTER (OTC) ASPIRIN-CONTAINING PRODUCTS

| | ASPIRIN | | INGREDIENTS | |
Type of Aspirin	Selected Brand Names	Amount of Aspirin (mg)	Other	Approximate Amount (mg)
Regular	Bayer	500, 325	None	
	Empirin	325		
	St. Joseph	81	None	
	Bayer, low dose	81	None	
Enteric coated	Ecotrin	500, 325	None	
	Ecotrin, low dose	81	None	
Buffered tablets	Bufferin	325	Buffered with calcium carbonate, magnesium oxide, and magnesium carbonate	Each tablet contains 65 mg of calcium and 50 mg of magnesium
	Bufferin Extra Strength	500	Buffered with calcium carbonate, magnesium oxide, and magnesium carbonate	Each tablet contains 90 mg of calcium and 70 mg of magnesium
	Ascriptin	325	Magnesium-aluminum hydroxide	150
Effervescent tablets	Alka-Seltzer Flu effervescent	500	Chlorpheniramine Dextromethorphan	2 mg (chlorpheniramine); 15 mg (dextromethorphan)
Combinations	Excedrin tablets	250	Caffeine Acetaminophen	65 250
	Anacin	400	Caffeine	32
	Fiorinal*	325	Butalbital Caffeine	50 40

*By prescription only.

◆ DIFLUNISAL

Diflunisal (dye-FLOO-ni-sal) (Dolobid) is a salicylate classified as an NSAID. Its peak action occurs 2 to 3 hours after ingestion, and its half-life is 8 to 12 hours in the normal patient. It is as effective as the other NSAIDs in the treatment of pain. Like other NSAIDs, diflunisal can be administered before a dental procedure to delay the onset of postsurgical pain. Because of its long half-life, it is dosed only two or three times daily. The general comments relating to the NSAIDs also apply to diflunisal. Its antipyretic effect is not clinically useful.

NONSTEROIDAL ANTIINFLAMMATORY DRUGS

NSAIDs have important applications in dentistry. Their mechanism of action and many of their pharmacologic effects and adverse reactions resemble those of aspirin. Many authors agree that the NSAIDs are the most useful drug group for the treatment of dental pain. The availability of OTC NSAIDs gives the dental health care worker several products that can be recommended for purchase. Whether a prescription should be written for an NSAID or an OTC NSAID recommended depends on appraisal of the patient's attitudes.

Chemical Classification

NSAIDs are divided into several chemical derivatives: the propionic acids, acetic acids, fenamates, pyrazolones, oxicams, and others. Table 5-3 lists the NSAIDs by chemical classification, pharmacokinetic parameters, analgesic dose, and dosing interval. Most members of the propionic acid derivative group, along

with mefenamic acid and diflunisal, are approved for the management of pain.

Mechanism of Action

Like aspirin, NSAIDs inhibit the enzyme COX (prostaglandin synthase), resulting in a reduction in the formation of prostaglandin precursors and thromboxanes from arachidonic acid (see Figure 5-4). Many of the actions and the adverse reactions of the NSAIDs result from their inhibition of prostaglandin synthesis.

Pharmacokinetics

Most NSAIDs peak in about 1 to 2 hours (see Table 5-3). The effect of food on absorption of the NSAIDs approved to treat pain is to reduce the rate but not the extent of absorption of ibuprofen, the naproxens, and diflunisal. There is no effect on absorption of the NSAIDs with oral antacids, except for diflunisal (antacids reduce absorption). They are metabolized in the liver and excreted by the kidney. The half-lives of the individual agents are listed in Table 5-3. Biliary or fecal excretion occurs with the fenamates, piroxicam, sulindac, and tolmetin.

Pharmacologic Effects

Alcoholics should avoid acetaminophen.

The analgesic, antipyretic, and antiinflammatory actions of the NSAIDs result from the same mechanism as aspirin inhibition of prostaglandin synthesis by inhibiting COX. NSAIDs are useful for treating dysmenorrhea (painful menstruation) because an excess of prostaglandins in the uterine wall produces painful contractions. In the treatment of gout, the action of the NSAIDs is related to their analgesic and

TABLE 5-3   NONSELECTIVE NONSTEROIDAL ANTIINFLAMMATORY DRUGS, PEAK, HALF-LIFE, AND ANALGESIC AND MAXIMUM DOSE

Drug Name	Action	Peak (hr)	Half-Life (hr)	Analgesic Dose (mg) and Interval q (hr)	Maximum Daily Dose (mg)
Propionic Acid Derivatives					
Ibuprofen[a] (Motrin, Advil)		1-2	1.8-2.5	400 q4-6	3200
Flurbiprofen[b] (Ansaid PO, Ocufen-Ophth)[c]		1.5	5.7	50 q4-6	300
Fenoprofen (Nalfon)		1-2	2-3	200 q4-6	3200
Naproxen (Naprosyn)		2-4	12-15	500 stat; 250 q6-8	1500
Naproxen sodium[d] (Anaprox)		1-2	12-13	550 stat; 275 q6-8	1375
Ketoprofen (Orudis)[e]	I	0.5-2	2-4	25-50 q6-8	300
Ketoprofen (Oruvail)	SR	None	2-4	[f]	300
Oxaprozin (Daypro)		3-5	42-50	1200 mg/24 hr	1800
Acetic Acid Derivatives					
Indomethacin (Indocin)	I	1-2	4.5	25 mg q8-12	200
Indomethacin SR (Indocin SR)	SR	2-4	4.5-6	75 mg q12-24	150
Sulindac (Clinoril)[g]		2-4	(8-16)[h]	150-200 mg q12	400
Tolmetin (Tolectin)		0.5-1	1-1.5	400 mg q8	2000
Diclofenac (Cataflam)	I	1	1-3	50 q6-8	200
Diclofenac (Voltaren)	SR	2-3	1-2	[f]	225
Etodolac (Lodine)	I	1-2	7.3	200-400 q6-8	1200
Etodolac (Lodine-XL)	SR	None	7.3	400-1000 mg/24 hr	1200
Ketorolac (Toradol)[i]		0.5-1	2.4-8.6	10 q4-6 (PO) 60 mg as a single dose or 30 mg q6	40 (PO) 120 (IM)
Nonacidic Agent					
Nabumetone[j] (Relafen)		3-6	(22.5-30)[k]	1000 mg/24 hr	2000
Fenamic Acid Derivatives					
Meclofenamate (Meclomen)		0.5-1	2-3	50 q4-6	400
Mefenamic acid[b] (Ponstel)		2-4	2-4	500 stat; 250 q6	1000
Salicylates					
Diflunisal (Dolobid)[l]		2-3	8-12	1000 stat; 500 q8-12	1500
Oxicams					
Piroxicam (Feldene)[m]		3-5	30-86	20 mg/24 hr	20
Meloxicam (MOBIC)		5-10	15-20	7.5 mg/24 hr	15

OTC, Over the counter; *I,* immediate action; *IM,* intramuscular; *PO,* by mouth; *SR,* sustained-release action.
[a]OTC as Ibuprofen, Motrin-IB, Haltran, Medipren.
[b]Therapy not usually to exceed 1 week.
[c]Ophthalmic solution to prevent inhibition of intraoperative miosis.
[d]OTC as Aleve.
[e]OTC as Orudis-KT.
[f]Not approved for use as simple analgesic.
[g]Prodrug converted in liver to active sulfide metabolite.
[h]Half-life of metabolite.
[i]For short-term (<5 days) treatment following the use of the parenteral form.
[j]Prodrug converted to active metabolite.
[k]Half-life with chronic use in parentheses ( ).
[l]Salicylate.
[m]qd dosing for arthritis, very long acting.

antiinflammatory actions but is independent of their effect on serum uric acid.

Adverse Reactions

◆ GASTROINTESTINAL EFFECTS

Gastrointestinal irritation, pain, and bleeding problems leading to tarry stools can occur with all NSAIDs. The prostaglandins stimulate the production of cytoprotective mucus that protects the stomach against gastric acid secretion. Prostaglandin inhibitors, such as NSAIDs, can interfere with the normal protective mechanisms in the stomach and increase acid secretion, causing symptoms or even an ulceration or perforation. A prostaglandin, misoprostol (mye-soe-PROST-ole) or prostaglandin E$_2$ (Cytotec, PGE$_2$), is available to prevent NSAID-induced ulcers.

◆ CENTRAL NERVOUS SYSTEM EFFECTS

The dose-dependent CNS side effects include sedation, dizziness, confusion, mental depression, headache, vertigo, and convulsions. Because of the CNS effects of the NSAIDs, patients taking them should be cautioned about driving an automobile. These agents are not addicting, tolerance does not develop, and no withdrawal syndrome can be induced.

◆ BLOOD CLOTTING

The NSAIDs reversibly inhibit platelet aggregation because they inhibit thromboxane A$_2$ production. In contrast to aspirin, their effect remains only as long as the drug is present in the blood: 1 day for ibuprofen, 4 days for naproxen, and 2 weeks for oxaprozin.

◆ RENAL EFFECTS

Renal effects of the NSAIDs include renal failure, cystitis, and an increased incidence of urinary tract infections. The NSAIDs have little effect on the patient with normal kidney function; however, with renal disease, decreases in both renal blood flow and glomerular filtration rate can occur. NSAIDs have precipitated renal insufficiency. With decreased renal function, peripheral edema with fluid retention has been noted.

◆ OTHER EFFECTS

Other adverse effects associated with the NSAIDs are muscle weakness, ringing in the ears, hepatitis, hematologic problems, and blurred vision.

◆ ORAL EFFECTS

Oral manifestations reported include ulcerative stomatitis, gingival ulcerations, and dry mouth.

◆ HYPERSENSITIVITY REACTIONS

Like aspirin, the NSAIDs can induce a wide range of hypersensitivity reactions, including hives or itching, angioneurotic edema, chills and fever, Stevens-Johnson syndrome, exfoliative dermatitis, and epidermal necrolysis. Anaphylactoid reactions including bronchospasm (wheezing) have been reported.

◆ PREGNANCY AND NURSING CONSIDERATIONS

| Contraindicated in pregnancy. |

Like aspirin, the NSAIDs given late in pregnancy can prolong gestation, delay parturition, and produce dystocia or premature closure of the ductus arteriosus. The uterine prosta-glandins are responsible for parturition and closure of the ductus arteriosus. Fenoprofen, ibuprofen, and naproxen have not been shown to be teratogenic in animal studies (Food and Drug Administration [FDA] pregnancy category B). Diflunisal, tolmetin, and mefenamic acid have been shown to be teratogenic in animals (FDA pregnancy category C).

Ibuprofen has not been detected in breast milk, whereas fenoprofen and mefenamic acid are present in small quantities. Small amounts of both naproxen (1% of serum) and diflunisal (5% of serum) are excreted in breast milk. Ibuprofen is the drug of choice for treating a nursing woman.

Drug Interactions

The drug interactions of the NSAIDs are summarized in Table 5-4. Interactions continue to be under investigation for their clinical significance and presence with each NSAID. Lithium toxicity has been produced in those patients taking lithium for bipolar affective disorders. NSAIDs may increase the effect of digoxin, a drug used for congestive heart failure. Digoxin's narrow therapeutic index is one reason for caution. NSAIDs have been shown to reduce the effect of agents used as antihypertensives such as diuretics, ACE inhibitors, and β-blockers. Probenecid can increase the serum levels of the NSAIDs. NSAIDs can increase the toxicity of cyclosporin and MTX. Before patients are given NSAIDs, the drug interactions should be checked.

Contraindications and Cautions

The contraindications and cautions for using an NSAID (Table 5-5) are related to their adverse reactions. Patients with asthma, cardiovascular or renal diseases with fluid retention, coagulopathies, peptic ulcer, and ulcerative colitis should be given NSAIDs cautiously, if at all.

Patients also at higher risk for adverse reactions include those with renal function impairment or a history of previous hypersensitivity to aspirin or other NSAIDs and geriatric patients who are more prone to adverse hepatic or renal reactions. Box 5-4 lists the patient instructions for NSAIDs.

Therapeutic Uses

◆ MEDICAL

Depending on the specific NSAID and the clinical trials that have been conducted, medical use of NSAIDs may include many conditions. Osteoarthritis, rheumatoid arthritis, gouty

TABLE 5-4	SELECTED DRUG INTERACTIONS OF THE NONSTEROIDAL ANTIINFLAMMATORY DRUGS
Drug	**Potential Outcome**
Lithium	Increased effect of lithium
MTX	Increased effect of MTX leads to bone marrow toxicity
Diuretics	Reduced antihypertensive effect
ACE inhibitors	Reduced antihypertensive effect
β-Blockers	Reduced antihypertensive effect
Digoxin	Increased digoxin effect

ACE, Angiotensin-converting enzyme; *MTX,* methotrexate.

TABLE 5-5   CONTRAINDICATIONS AND CAUTIONS TO USE OF ASPIRIN AND NONSTEROIDAL ANTIINFLAMMATORY DRUGS

Drugs	Disease	Comments
Aspirin: Small doses	Prevent clotting, heart disease	May use NSAIDs, continue aspirin
Aspirin: High doses	Rheumatic fever	Aspirin lowers blood level of NSAIDs
Lithium	Bipolar (manic) disorder	NSAIDs reduce lithium clearance; potential lithium toxicity
H_2-blockers Proton pump inhibitors	Peptic ulcer, gastroesophageal reflux disease	Gastric bleeding, esophagitis
MTX	Rheumatoid arthritis, psoriasis, cancer	Potentiates MTX toxicity, bone marrow suppression*
Vitamin K deficiency	Alcoholism, liver disease	Bleeding
Warfarin	Myocardial infarction, atrial fibrillation, prosthetic heart valve	Aspirin contraindicated; bleeding; use NSAIDs with caution; increases anticoagulant effect of warfarin
Factor VIII	Hemophilia	Gastric bleeding
Probenecid*	Gout	Probenecid inhibits excretion of NSAIDs
Colchicine	Gout	More GI adverse reactions
Allopurinol	Gout	No contraindications
None	Pregnancy	Use should be avoided during pregnancy, especially during the third trimester
None	G6PD deficiency	Hemolysis
None	Hypoprothrombinemia	Bleeding

NSAIDs, Nonsteroidal antiinflammatory drugs; *MTX,* methotrexate; *GI,* gastrointestinal; *G6PD,* glucose-6-phosphate dehydrogenase.
*Once-a-week dosing as for autoimmune diseases can be used with caution.

BOX 5-4   PATIENT INSTRUCTIONS FOR USE OF NONSTEROIDAL ANTIINFLAMMATORY DRUGS

- Take with a full glass of water.
- Take with food to minimize gastrointestinal irritation.
- Use caution with driving because of possible drowsiness or dizziness.
- Do not use aspirin concurrently.
- If pain does not subside within a few days, call the dentist.
- Do not take OTC analgesics with prescription NSAIDs.

OTC, Over the counter; *NSAIDs,* nonsteroidal antiinflammatory drugs.

arthritis, fever, dysmenorrhea, and pain are indications for the NSAIDs. Accepted unlabeled indications for which NSAIDs are often prescribed include bursitis and tendonitis.

◆ **DENTAL**

NSAIDs are useful in the management of dental pain. Many studies that have compared the analgesic efficacy of the NSAIDs with that of the opioid analgesics find that they are equivalent in many clinical situations. For example, usual analgesic doses of NSAIDs have been shown to be as effective as 650 mg of aspirin or acetaminophen plus 60 mg of codeine and even as effective as the intermediate-strength opioid combinations (oxycodone plus aspirin or acetaminophen). In usual prescription doses, NSAIDs can be shown to be statistically significantly better than codeine alone, aspirin, acetaminophen, or placebo. It is difficult to understand why the dental use of the NSAIDs has decreased. All NSAIDs are equally efficacious at equianalgesic doses. Figure 5-9 shows the pain relief over time of several commonly used analgesics. Their relative effectiveness is discussed in the following paragraphs.

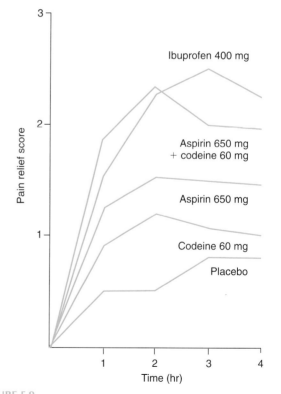

FIGURE 5-9

Time-effect curves for placebo, codeine, aspirin, aspirin plus codeine, and ibuprofen. The mean pain relief scores are plotted against time in hours. (From Cooper SA et al: Analgesic efficacy of an ibuprofen-codeine combination, *Pharmacotherapy* 2:162, 1982.)

Specific Nonsteroidal Antiinflammatory Drugs

♦ IBUPROFEN

Ibuprofen (eye-byoo-PRO-fen) (Advil, Motrin), the oldest member of the NSAIDs, has the most clinical experience. It is rapidly absorbed orally, and food decreases its rate but not its extent of absorption; antacids have no effect. The half-life is about 2 hours. Its onset of action is about half an hour, and its duration of action is 4 to 6 hours. It undergoes hepatic metabolism and is excreted by the kidney. It is an effective analgesic and has been studied in many dental situations. Ibuprofen is the drug of choice for treatment of dental pain when an NSAID is indicated. Only in rare cases or if new information becomes available are other NSAIDs indicated. When a longer-acting agent is desired for patient convenience, the naproxens can be used.

Clinical trials in dental pain management testify to ibuprofen's effectiveness. A dose of 400 mg of ibuprofen is usually more effective than 650 mg of aspirin, 600 mg of acetaminophen, and both aspirin and acetaminophen when combined with 60 mg of codeine (see Figure 5-9). A shallow dose-response curve for ibuprofen has been demonstrated, with some finding no difference between the 200- and 300-mg doses and others finding no difference between the 400- and 800-mg doses. The 200-mg (OTC) dose of ibuprofen has been shown to be as effective as two 325-mg doses of acetaminophen or aspirin. The 400- to 600-mg doses produce about the same degree of effectiveness, but the higher doses produce a longer duration of action (drug level stays above an analgesic dose longer because the blood level is higher).

The usual analgesic dose of ibuprofen is 400 to 800 mg every 4 to 6 hours (maximum dose: 3.2 gm/day). The higher range of dose may produce more antiinflammatory effects. Most studies can easily demonstrate that 400 mg of ibuprofen is better than any usual therapeutic doses of codeine.

Ibuprofen is available OTC in 200-mg tablets and by prescription in 400-, 600-, and 800-mg tablets. Side effects, such as CNS effects, are dose dependent, so they occur more often at the higher end of the dose range. Ibuprofen is also available OTC in suspension form for pediatric use and is often used as an antipyretic.

♦ NAPROXEN AND NAPROXEN SODIUM

| Longer acting |

Naproxen (na-PROX-en) (Naprosyn) and naproxen sodium (Anaprox) are propionic acid NSAIDs that have slightly longer half-lives than ibuprofen and can be dosed on an 8- to 12-hour schedule. They should also be given with a loading dose (see Table 5-3). Their pharmacologic effects, adverse reactions, and efficacy are similar to those of ibuprofen. In addition to tablets, this product is available in suspension form. Figure 5-10 shows data for a patient taking lithium who begins taking naproxen. One should note that lithium levels rise when naproxen is given because it inhibits lithium clearance.

♦ OTHER NONSTEROIDAL ANTIINFLAMMATORY DRUGS

Other NSAIDs (see Table 5-3), such as fenoprofen, ketorolac, or diflunisal (discussed previously), may be used for patients who do not respond to either ibuprofen or naproxen sodium. Certain patients need an agent with which they are not familiar. "Shoppers" looking for scheduled drugs respond better to an

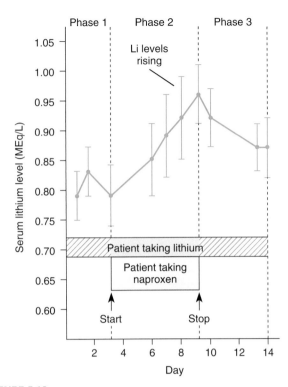

FIGURE 5-10
Change in serum lithium levels in patients given naproxen (N = 7). Results are expressed as mean ± standard error.

unknown drug's name. Prescribing one of the new NSAIDs whose name has not yet become familiar may be effective.

Ketorolac (kee-TOE-role-ak) (Toradol) is a newer NSAID. The use of this agent increased because it was being heavily advertised to dental professionals. It is equivalent in efficacy to the other NSAIDs; however, unlike other NSAIDs, it is available parenterally. One should make sure that before a new agent is prescribed it has some documented clinical advantage.

Ketorolac is an NSAID indicated for the short-term (up to 5 days) management of moderately severe acute pain that requires analgesia at the opioid level. It is contraindicated as a prophylactic analgesic before any major surgery when hemostasis is critical because of the increased risk of bleeding. Oral ketorolac is indicated only as continuation therapy to IV or intramuscular (IM) ketorolac (must use injectable before prescribing the tablets).

♦ CYCLO-OXYGENASE II SPECIFIC AGENTS

All of the currently available NSAIDs inhibit both COX I and COX II. COX I is a widely distributed constitutive (present at all times) enzyme responsible for the adverse reactions of the NSAIDs such as stomach problems, reduced renal function, fluid retention, and reduced platelet adhesiveness. COX II is an inducible enzyme that is synthesized only when inflammation occurs.

COX II–specific inhibitors selectively decrease the inflammatory effects of COX II, while leaving the protective effects of COX I largely in place, leading to fewer adverse reactions than the older, nonselective NSAIDs. Celecoxib (Celebrex), a COX II–specific inhibitor, is indicated for arthritis. Drugs, such as celecoxib, were thought to offer an advantage over nonselective NSAIDs because they were believed to be less irritating to the

TABLE 5-6 CYCLO-OXYGENASE (COX) RECEPTORS: COX I AND COX II

COX Receptors	Enzyme	Effects	Examples
COX I-II	Both		Ibuprofen Naproxen Meclofenamate
COX I-specific	Constitutive, always present, wide distribution	Side effects seen in renal blood flow, fluid and electrolytes, stomach mucosal integrity, vasomotor tone, uterus	Indomethacin Sulindac
COX II-specific COX II >> I	Inducible; expression variable	Antiinflammatory	Celecoxib (Celebrex)

stomach. However, they have significantly higher incidences of serious gastrointestinal adverse effects. Clinically, they are equivalent to nonselective NSAIDs. Rofecoxib (Vioxx) and valdecoxib (Bextra) were removed from the U.S. market in 2005 as a result of a high incidence of cardiovascular events (heart attacks) associated with these two drugs. Celecoxib remains on the market but must be used in the lowest dose possible. Because these drugs offer no therapeutic advantage over nonselective NSAIDs they have no real use in dentistry. Table 5-6 lists some NSAIDs grouped by COX inhibition.

ACETAMINOPHEN

Acetaminophen (a-seet-a-MEE-noe-fen) (paracetamol, N-acetyl p-aminophenol; Tylenol; APAP) is the only member of the p-aminophenols currently available for clinical use. Acetanilid, the parent compound, was introduced in 1886 and rapidly shown to be too toxic. Phenacetin, removed from the market in 1983, was more toxic than acetaminophen. Acetaminophen is used as an analgesic and antipyretic in children and in adults when aspirin is contraindicated.

Pharmacokinetics

Acetaminophen is rapidly and completely absorbed from the gastrointestinal tract, achieving a peak plasma level in 1 to 3 hours. After therapeutic doses, it is excreted with a half-life of 1 to 4 hours. Acetaminophen is metabolized by the liver microsomal enzymes to the glucuronide conjugate, the sulfuric acid conjugate, and cysteine. When large doses are ingested, an intermediate metabolite is produced that is thought to be hepatotoxic and possibly nephrotoxic. Acetaminophen and aspirin are equally efficacious (kills the same degree of pain) and equally potent (same dose in milligrams needed for effect) as analgesics and antipyretics.

Pharmacologic Effects

The analgesic and antipyretic effects of acetaminophen are approximately the same potency (on a milligram for milligram basis) as aspirin (see Figure 5-6). This means that acetaminophen and aspirin are equally efficacious, and because virtually the same doses are used for each agent, they are equally potent. However, acetaminophen does not possess any clinically significant antiinflammatory effect. Therefore it is less useful in the treatment of arthritis or any other type of inflammatory pain. Differences in degree of prostaglandin synthesis inhibition at different sites may account for this difference in action.

Therapeutic doses of acetaminophen have no effect on the cardiovascular or respiratory system. In contrast to aspirin, acetaminophen does not produce gastric bleeding or affect platelet adhesiveness or uric acid excretion.

Adverse Reactions

The principal toxic effects of acetaminophen are hepatic necrosis and nephrotoxicity.

◆ HEPATIC EFFECTS

The toxic metabolite of acetaminophen that contributes to hepatic necrosis is N-acetyl-p-benzoquinonamine. Hepatic necrosis may occur in adults after the acute ingestion of a single dose of 20 to 25 gm of acetaminophen; 25 gm or more is potentially fatal. More often than not, children experience more cases of accidental overdose with acetaminophen. This occurs because the wrong dose form is used (e.g., infant drops are given to older children or adult doses are given to children). Infant drops are concentrated, and doses for toddlers to 11-year-old children are not the same as doses for infants. Parents may give the infant liquid to the older child and pour it in the measuring cup, not realizing that they have overdosed their child. Also, normal doses over extended periods of time can lead to toxicity. Symptoms during the first 2 days after intoxication are minor. Nausea, vomiting, anorexia, and abdominal pain may occur. Liver injury becomes manifest on the second to third day, with alterations in plasma enzyme levels (elevated transaminase and lactic hydrogenase), elevated bilirubin levels, and prolongation of prothrombin time. Hepatotoxicity may progress to encephalopathy, coma, and death. If the patient recovers, no residual hepatic abnormalities persist. Patients with hepatic disease, such as those with a history of hepatitis, should avoid acetaminophen.

Most recently, the Food and Drug Administration (FDA) has recommended tighter dose controls and warnings with acetaminophen use in the hopes of preventing even more cases of accidental liver toxicity. The FDA advisory committee is recommending that persons receive no more than 650 milligrams (2 regular strength tablets) at any one time. Doses of 1000 mg four times per day can, after only 1 or 2 days, lead to liver toxicity. This would include decreasing the amount of acetaminophen that is often used in combination with opioid analgesics.

Alcohol stimulates the oxidizing enzymes that metabolize acetaminophen to its toxic metabolite. Depending on the amount of alcoholic beverages ingested, the maximum dose of acetaminophen varies. The normal maximum dose of acetaminophen (4 gm) may be used in patients who usually do not drink. The dose should be restricted to 2 gm if a patient is a moderate drinker (less than three alcohol beverages daily). Alcoholics or

TABLE 5-7	MAXIMUM ACETAMINOPHEN (APAP) DOSE RELATED TO ALCOHOL USE	
Chronic Alcohol Consumed	**Maximum Daily Dose of APAP (gm)**
None	4 for a short period; 2.6 for chronic use
Moderate drinking (fewer than three drinks per day)	2
Alcoholic and three or more drinks per day	None

APAP, N-Acetyl-*p*-aminophenol (acetaminophen).

patients who normally ingest three or more alcohol beverages daily should avoid acetaminophen completely (Table 5-7).

◆ TREATMENT OF TOXICITY

The treatment of overdose toxicity should begin with gastric lavage if a drug has recently been ingested. The administration of activated charcoal and magnesium or sodium sulfate solution should follow. The administration of sulfhydryl groups in the form of oral *N*-acetylcysteine reduces or even prevents liver damage if given soon enough after ingestion.

◆ NEPHROTOXICITY

Nephrotoxicity has been associated with long-term consumption. The primary lesion appears to be a papillary necrosis with secondary interstitial nephritis. Although no single agent can be identified, prolonged consumption of analgesics can lead to kidney disease. Because analgesics are used in dental practice on a short-term basis, the possibility of nephrotoxicity does not present a significant problem in dental therapy. Concurrent chronic use of the combination of acetaminophen and aspirin or NSAIDs increases the risk of analgesic nephropathy, renal papillary necrosis, end-stage renal disease, and cancer of the kidney or urinary bladder.

Drug Interactions

Acetaminophen is remarkably free of drug interactions at its usual therapeutic doses. The hepatotoxicity of acetaminophen can be potentiated by administration of agents that induce hepatic microsomal enzymes such as barbiturates, carbamazepine, phenytoin, and rifampin. Chronic large doses of alcohol can increase the toxicity of acetaminophen.

Uses

Acetaminophen is used as an analgesic and antipyretic. It is especially useful in patients who have aspirin hypersensitivity or in whom aspirin-induced gastric irritation would present a problem. In young children, its use as an antipyretic has replaced aspirin because of aspirin's association with Reye's syndrome. It is not known to what degree the long-term use of therapeutic doses of acetaminophen might produce renal lesions. It has a greater propensity for producing hepatic necrosis when a large acute dose (overdose) is ingested. Box 5-5 lists the patient instructions for acetaminophen.

Dose and Preparations

Acetaminophen is available in many combinations and elixirs (Tylenol, Tempra). The usual adult dose is 325 to 650 mg every

BOX 5-5	PATIENT INSTRUCTIONS FOR USE OF ACETAMINOPHEN

- Follow the specific directions regarding dose of acetaminophen.
- Do not increase the dose or take more than is recommended in a 24-hour period because of the risk of liver toxicity.
- Give children the correct dose form and dose because of the risk of liver toxicity.
- If the pain does not subside within 24 hours, call the dentist.

TABLE 5-8	ACETAMINOPHEN DOSING CHART (mg)		
Weight (lb)	**Age (yr)**	**mg**	**Liquid/Elixir*** **160 mg/5 ml (no. tsp)**
24	<2	Consult	Consult
25-35	2-3	160	1
36-47	4-5	240	1.5
48-59	6-8	320	2
60-71	9-10	400	2.5
72-95	11	480	3

Obtain the child's weight in pounds; check weight column and determine applicable row; read the dose (mg) column to determine dose; identify preparation parent has or will purchase; determine the volume or number of tablets needed for the dose and product.
*CAUTION: Preparations with different concentrations available, number of teaspoonfuls only for this concentration; infants' concentrated drops use much less volume.

TABLE 5-9	ANALGESIC DOSING BY mg/lb	
Drug	**Dose in mg/lb**
Acetaminophen	5
Aspirin	5
Ibuprofen	5
Naproxen	2.5

4 to 6 hours or 1000 mg three to four times a day. Not more than 4 gm in 24 hours should be ingested by adults. However, the FDA is recommending that not more than 650 mg every 4 to 6 hours three to four times a day be given. Various elixirs, drops, and chewable tablets that are convenient for administration to children are available. The concentration of the elixir is 120 mg/5 ml (1 teaspoonful) or 160 mg/5 ml; the drops contain 60 mg/0.6 ml. Acetaminophen should not be administered to children younger than 3 years or for more than 10 days except on a prescriber's advice. The dosing of acetaminophen in children can be determined using Table 5-8. Table 5-9 provides the doses of acetaminophen, aspirin, ibuprofen, and naproxen on a milligram per pound basis.

DRUGS USED TO TREAT GOUT

Gout is an inherited disease occurring primarily in men, with an onset that usually involves one joint, often the big toe or knee. Both hyperuricemia and urate crystals, or tophi, may be found in the joints or other tissues. The excess uric acid may be the result of excessive production or reduced excretion of uric acid (two types of gout). The disease responds to colchicine.

Both the NSAIDs and colchicine are used to treat acute attacks of gout. Other agents, such as probenecid and allopurinol (al-oh-PURE-i-nole), are available to prevent gout. These are briefly mentioned here, although they are not analgesics per se.

Colchicine

Colchicine (KOL-chi-seen) has only one indication: the treatment of an acute attack of gout. It is so specific in its action on gouty attacks that it is sometimes used to diagnose the disease. Colchicine is taken hourly at the onset of the attack or until side effects, such as nausea and vomiting, are intolerable. Its mechanism is complex, but it appears to inhibit the chemotactic property of leukocytosis and interfere with the inflammatory response to urate crystals. Colchicine possesses many side effects, but gastrointestinal toxicity, including nausea, vomiting, and diarrhea, occurs often (up to 80%). Bone marrow depression and hypersensitivity have also been reported.

Allopurinol

Allopurinol (Zyloprim) is a xanthine oxidase inhibitor that inhibits the synthesis of uric acid. It is used to prevent excessive uric acid from forming. It is also used in patients receiving either chemotherapy or irradiation for malignancy because the death of many cells causes a release of large amounts of uric acid precursors. The side effects associated with allopurinol include hepatotoxicity of a hypersensitivity type. If a pruritic rash should occur, the drug should be promptly discontinued because fatalities have been reported. This drug is not indicated for asymptomatic hyperuricemia.

Probenecid

The other approach to prevention of gout is to increase the excretion of uric acid by the administration of a uricosuric agent such as probenecid (Benemid) (see Figure 5-7). Probenecid, by blocking the tubular reabsorption of filtered urate, prevents new tophi and mobilizes those present. Increasing frequency or severity of acute gouty attacks is an indication for uricosuric administration.

Gastrointestinal side effects and hypersensitivity may occur with probenecid use. Headaches and sore gums have also been reported. Concurrent administration of aspirin can interfere with the uricosuric action of probenecid. Diabetic tests using the copper sulfate urine test (Clinitest) may have false-positive results. Occasionally, probenecid and colchicine are combined, with the colchicine preventing acute attacks and the probenecid enhancing the excretion of uric acid. Probably a more rational approach is to administer each drug separately as needed. Maintenance of adequate urinary output (at least 2 L) is important to minimize the precipitation of uric acid in the urinary tract.

Probenecid increases the level of the NSAIDs and penicillin. In the latter case, this effect can be used therapeutically (see discussion of penicillin in Chapter 7). For prevention of acute gout, either probenecid or allopurinol can be used. Acute gout normally is treated with NSAIDs and colchicine.

For mild-to-moderate pain, the drug of choice is either acetaminophen or aspirin in adults. Aspirin provides an antiinflammatory effect but is contraindicated in children and adolescents.

If both aspirin and acetaminophen provide inadequate pain relief, then ibuprofen can be used. Its analgesic efficacy parallels that of many products combining nonopioids with opioids such as aspirin with codeine (Empirin #3).

DENTAL HYGIENE CONSIDERATIONS

1. If nonopioid analgesics are necessary, the dental hygienist should conduct a thorough medication/health history in order to determine if any contraindications or drug interactions exist.
2. Information regarding salicylates, NSAIDS, and acetaminophen should include warnings to not exceed the manufacturer's recommended daily dose over a 24-hour time period.
3. The dental hygienist should encourage patients to check the OTC labels for any overlapping ingredients. Oftentimes, these products contain ibuprofen, aspirin, acetaminophen, or any combination of the three with antihistamines and decongestants.
4. The dental hygienist should also be aware of the fact that many opioid analgesics are combined with nonopioid analgesics. Remind patients to not supplement with OTC analgesics if a combination nonopioid/opioid analgesic is prescribed.
5. Warnings of significant side effects associated with OTC nonopioid analgesics (such as bleeding) should be given to the patient along with instructions to call the dental practice if an adverse reaction occurs.
6. NSAIDs should be avoided in persons with asthma.
7. If patients complain of gastrointestinal adverse effects, then they may require a semisupine chair position during dental treatment.
8. Review the information in Boxes 5-3, 5-4, and 5-5.

CLINICAL SKILLS ASSESSMENT

1. What is the rationale for using acetaminophen in a patient with an ulcer?
2. What dose and duration of therapy should be recommended for an adult male patient?
3. What are the adverse reactions of acetaminophen?
4. Are nephrotoxicity and hepatotoxicity only associated with toxic doses of acetaminophen?
5. How can acetaminophen toxicity be avoided?
6. What would increase the risk of developing nephrotoxicity with acetaminophen?
7. What are the pharmacologic effects of acetaminophen?
8. Compare and contrast acetaminophen to aspirin in terms of pharmacologic and therapeutic effects.
9. Are there any possible interactions with acetaminophen? If so, what are they and how can they be avoided?
10. What should be said to a patient during a counseling session on acetaminophen?
11. What is the role of aspirin in the prevention of heart attacks and stroke?
12. Are there any dental concerns associated with one baby aspirin each day?
13. Should a patient taking high blood pressure medication take a drug like ibuprofen? Why or why not?
14. Compare and contrast the OTC NSAIDs.
15. When would a prescription NSAID be appropriate?

16. Are there interactions between NSAIDs and antihypertensive drugs?

17. The dentist recommends a short course of OTC ibuprofen. What should a patient be told about this drug?

18. Can aspirin be used in children under the age of 18? Why or why not?

19. Why is it important to use the correct dose form of acetaminophen in children?

⊖volve ——————————————————————

Please visit http://evolve.elsevier.com/Haveles/pharmacology for review questions and additional practice and reference materials.

6 Opioid (Narcotic) Analgesics and Antagonists

LEARNING OBJECTIVES

1. Explain the classification, mechanism of action, and pharmacokinetics of opioids.
2. List and describe the pharmacologic effects and potential adverse reactions of opioids.
3. Discuss the addiction potential of opioids, including treatment.
4. Name and explain the analgesic actions of the most common opioid agonists.
5. Discuss the actions of and provide examples of the mixed opioids.
6. Summarize the mechanism of action of tramadol.
7. Apply the use of opioids to dentistry.

The opioid analgesics are often used to manage dental pain in patients in whom nonsteroidal antiinflammatory drugs (NSAIDs) are contraindicated. The dental hygienist and the dentist should be aware of the opioid groups, side effects, relative potency, and proper place in the management of dental pain.

HISTORY

Opium is the dried juice from the unripe seed capsules of the opium poppy. As early as 4000 BC, many cultures had recognized the euphoric effect of the poppy plant. In the early 1800s, morphine and codeine were isolated from opium. Until about 1920, patent medicines (medicines whose efficacy and safety were questionable) containing opium were promoted for numerous uses. When these agents, used orally, became unlawful, narcotic (opioid) abuse by injection began and has continued until the present.

TERMINOLOGY

The terms used to refer to this drug group have changed over the years. *Narcotics,* the original name for this group of drugs, is derived from the Greek word that means "stupor." At first, the term *narcotics* was used to refer to drugs that are derivatives of opium poppy. Drugs in different pharmacologic classes with central nervous system (CNS) depressant effects also began to be lumped into the narcotic group because they caused stupor. This designation then became confusing because the drugs in it had different properties. *Opiates* was the next term that was used. It refers to drugs that are derived from the substances in the opioid poppy. Other chemical agents that produced opiate effects but did not have a structure like the opiates were synthesized but were not opiate-like. To be more inclusive, the term *opioids* was then used to include not only the former opiates but also other structurally different agents, their antagonists, and the receptors stimulated by the opioids. The old term *narcotic* is still used in older publications or by older practitioners.

CLASSIFICATION

The clinically useful opioids may be divided in several different ways. One way to divide these agents is by their mechanism of action at the receptor sites: agonists, mixed opioids, and antagonists. Table 6-1 shows the classifications.

The opioids may also be classified by their chemical structure (Box 6-1). Structural classification is useful when the patient has a history of an allergy. Agents with the most similar chemical structure are more likely to be cross-allergenic; conversely, those with very different structures are much less likely to exhibit cross-allergenicity. The chemical structure groups include morphine/codeine, methadone, morphinan, meperidine, and others. The largest group is the morphine/codeine group, which includes codeine. A patient with a true allergy to codeine should not be given an analgesic in that group.

Opioids may be classified by their efficacy (Table 6-2). Efficacy classification assists in selection of the proper opioid based on the amount of pain relief needed. The amount of pain experienced is usually related to the individual patient and his or her reaction to the dental procedure and the specific dental procedure being performed. Although "bigger" procedures may elicit

BOX 6-1	OPIOID ANALGESIC AGENTS BY STRUCTURE GROUP
Morphine and Codeine	
Hydromorphone (Dilaudid)	
Hydrocodone (in Vicodin)	
Dihydrocodeine (in Synalgos-DC)	
Oxycodone (in Percodan, Percocet, Tylox)	
Methadone	
Methadone (Dolophine)	
Propoxyphene (Darvon)	
Morphinan	
Butorphanol (Stadol)	
Pentazocine (in Talwin-NX)	
Meperidine	
Meperidine (Demerol)	
Fentanyl (Sublimaze)	
Diphenoxylate (in Lomotil)	
Loperamide (Imodium) OTC	
Other	
Buprenorphine (Buprenex)	

TABLE 6-1	CLASSIFICATION OF THE OPIOIDS BY RECEPTOR ACTION	
Group	Subgroup	Example
Opioid agonists		Morphine, codeine
Mixed opioids	Agonist antagonists	Pentazocine
	Partial agonists	Buprenorphine
Antagonists		Naloxone

TABLE 6-2 SELECTED OPIOID ANALGESICS BY EFFICACY, DOSING INTERVAL, USUAL DOSES, AND SCHEDULE				
Drug Name	Dosing Interval (hr)	Usual Dose (mg)*	Comments	Schedules for Controlled Substances
Strongest				
Morphine	4-6	IM: 10	Standard agent; prototype	II
Methadone (Dolophine)	4-6†	IM: 10 PO: 10	Used PO for "methadone maintenance"	II
Meperidine (Demerol)	3-4	IM: 100 PO: 50	Abused by professionals	II
Hydromorphone (Dilaudid)	4-6	PO: 2	Most potent on a mg-for-mg basis	II
Intermediate				
Oxycodone (in Percodan, Percocet, Tylox, Roxiprin, Roxicet)	4-6	PO: 5	Popular with addicts "shopping" for opioids	II
Pentazocine (in Talwin NX)	4-6	PO: 50	Has antagonist properties	IV
Weakest				
Hydrocodone (in Vicodin, Lortab, Lorcet)	4-6	PO: 5		III
Codeine (in Tylenol #3, Empirin #3)	4-6	PO: 30	#2 = 15 mg; #3 = 30 mg; #4 = 60 mg	III
Dihydrocodeine (in Synalgos-DC)	4-6	PO: 30	16 mg per dose	III
Propoxyphene (in Darvocet-N 100)	4-6	PO: 65 (HCI) or 100 (N)	65 mg HCl = 100 mg napsylate	IV

HCI, Hydrochloride; *IM*, intramuscular; *N*, napsylate; *PO*, by mouth.
*Average dose.
†Dosing interval in methadone maintenance 24 hours.

more pain, the characteristics of the patient play a more important role.

MECHANISM OF ACTION

The opioids bind to receptors located in both the CNS and the spinal cord, producing an altered perception of reaction to pain. Receptors that mediate specific pharmacologic effects and adverse reactions are stimulated to varying degrees by individual opioids.

> Important receptors include μ, κ, and δ.

The discovery of three groups of endogenous substances with opioid-like action, the enkephalins, endorphins, and dynorphins, has helped explain the presence of these receptors. These naturally occurring peptides possess analgesic action and have addiction potential. They probably function as neurotransmitters, but their exact function has not been elucidated. They may be involved in the analgesic action of a placebo and the enhancement of well-being that occurs with running (an increase in β-endorphins).

Table 6-3 describes the pharmacologic effects of selected opioid receptors and the effect of some opioids on these receptors. Opioids may be complete agonists, partial agonists, agonist-antagonists, or antagonists. The three opioid receptors that have been characterized in more detail and that are stimulated by the opioids are the mu (μ), kappa (κ), and delta (δ) receptors. Differences in affinity for and action of different opioids in tolerance to pain might even be the result of variations in the endogenous levels of the neurotransmitters. Differences in affinity for and action of different opioids at these and other specific receptors explain some of the distinctions among the different opioids' adverse reactions. For example, stimulation of μ-receptors produce analgesia. The k-receptor is responsible for dysphoria. Pentazocine, a κ-receptor agonist, produces dysphoria; morphine has no effect on the κ-receptor and produces less dysphoria than pentazocine. Naloxone is an antagonist at the three receptor sites (Figure 6-1). More opioid receptors are sure to be identified and characterized. As more subreceptor types are elucidated, it will be possible to further separate beneficial (analgesic) effects of the opioids from their side effects (e.g., respiratory depression, constipation, or drug dependence).

PHARMACOKINETICS

> First-pass metabolism reduces bioavailability.

ADME, which is an acronym of the first letters of each component of drug handling, refers to absorption, distribution, metabolism, and excretion:

TABLE 6-3   OPIOID RECEPTORS, EFFECTS, AND STIMULATION BY VARIOUS OPIOIDS

	μ (mu)		δ (delta)	Sigma (σ)	Epsilon (ε)	κ (kappa)
Effects	Supraspinal analgesia, sedation, miosis (pruritus)	Spinal analgesia, respiratory depression, euphoria, physical dependence, constipation	?Analgesia (?emotion, seizures)	Autonomic stimulation, dysphoria, hallucinations, nightmares, anxiety, ?antianalgesic	Analgesia	Analgesia (1 = spinal, 3 = supraspinal), sedation, miosis (?micturition, diuresis), ?dysphoria
	μ1	μ2	δ1	δ2	κ1	κ2	κ3
Endogenous Opioids						
Enkephalins	Ag		Ag			
β-Endorphins	Ag		Ag			
Dynorphin	wk Ag				Ag	
Opioid Agonists						
Morphine	Ag		wk Ag		wk Ag	
Codeine	wk Ag		wk Ag			
Fentanyl	Ag		Ag		Ag	
Mixed Opioids						
Pentazocine	wk Ant, pAg				Ag	
Buprenorphine	pAg				Ant	
Butorphanol	wk pAg				Ag	
Nalbuphine	Ant				Ag	
Dezocine	pAnt				Ag	
Opioid Antagonists						
Naloxone	Ant		wk Ant		Ant	
Nalmefene	Ant		?Ant		?Ant	
Naltrexone	Ant		?Ant		?Ant	

Ag, Agonist; *Ant,* competitive antagonist; *pAg,* partial agonist; *pAnt,* partial antagonist;; *wk,* weak; *?,* unknown.

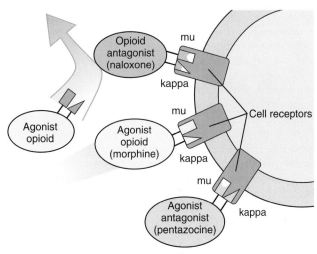

FIGURE 6-1
Receptor actions of opioids. (From McKenry L, Tessier E, Hogan MA: *Mosby's pharmacology in nursing,* ed 22, St Louis, 2006, Mosby.)

- *Absorption:* Most opioid analgesic agents are absorbed well when taken orally; absorption occurs from the lungs and from the nasal and oral mucosa. Absorption occurs through the mucous membranes of the nose and the intact skin. A nasal spray for one opioid, butorphanol (Stadol NS), is available. Absorption through the skin is used to advantage with transdermal patches of fentanyl (Duragesic).
- *Distribution:* After absorption, the opioids undergo variable first-pass metabolism in the liver or intestinal cell wall, which reduces their bioavailability. The oral-to-parenteral ratio determines the difference in bioavailability between an opioid administered orally and one given parenterally. For example, the ratio is 0.2 to 0.3 for morphine, 0.25 to 0.7 for meperidine, and 0.4 to 0.7 for codeine. Therefore about two-thirds of codeine administered orally reaches the systemic circulation, whereas only about one-fourth of morphine does. The opioids are bound to plasma proteins to varying degrees (morphine 35%, meperidine 60%). The opioids are also distributed to the fetus in pregnant women, accounting for the respiratory depression produced in the fetus when the mother is given opioids near term.
- *Metabolism:* The major route of metabolism for the opioids is conjugation with glucuronic acid in the liver. Given orally, most opioids have a similar duration of action for analgesia—4 to 6 hours.
- *Excretion:* Metabolized opioids are excreted by glomerular filtration as their metabolites. The metabolites and the unchanged drug are excreted in the urine.

The dosing interval and usual dose of some opioids are listed in Table 6-2. In general, their onset is within 1 hour and their duration necessitates dosing every 4 to 6 hours.

PHARMACOLOGIC EFFECTS

Although the pharmacologic effects and adverse reactions of the opioids are closely related, they are discussed separately. A pharmacologic effect may also be an adverse reaction, depending on the clinical use of the agent. In general, the severity of the side effects is proportional to the agent's efficacy (strength).

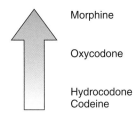

Morphine

Oxycodone

Hydrocodone
Codeine

FIGURE 6-2
Comparing strengths of opioids. Opioids vary in efficacy (maximal effect attained) from codeine (low) to morphine (high).

Analgesia

| Efficacy is variable among opioids. |

The opioid analgesics provide varying degrees of analgesia, depending on the strength of the agent. Figure 6-2 shows the relative analgesic efficacy of selected opioids. Morphine is the opioid agonist by which other opioids are measured. The strongest opioids can reduce even the most severe pain; the weaker agents mixed with nonopioids are equivalent to the NSAIDs in their ability to relieve pain; and the analgesic potency of the weakest agent (codeine) is low (see Table 6-2).

Codeine raises the pain threshold and affects the cerebral cortex to depress the reaction to pain. Both m-receptors and k-receptors are involved in producing analgesia. The opioids alter the patient's reaction to painful stimuli, possibly by altering the release of certain central neurotransmitters.

Sedation and Euphoria

In the usual therapeutic doses, the opioid analgesics generally produce sedation by k-receptor stimulation. This may potentiate their analgesic effect and relieve anxiety. This effect is additive with other CNS depressants such as alcohol. With larger doses, or if the pain is suddenly removed, euphoria can result. CNS excitation rarely occurs.

Cough Suppression

The opioids exert their antitussive action by depressing the cough center, located in the medulla. The dose that produces the antitussive effect is much lower than that required for analgesia, so the least potent agents are effective (e.g., codeine). Related compounds, such as dextromethorphan, are often used as antitussives.

Gastrointestinal Effects

The opioids increase the smooth muscle tone of the intestinal tract and markedly decrease its propulsive contractions and motility. This effect has made opioids useful in the symptomatic treatment of diarrhea. Opioid-like agents without analgesic properties, such as diphenoxylate (in Lomotil), are used to treat diarrhea.

ADVERSE REACTIONS

Unlike many other drugs, the adverse reactions of the opioids are not related to a direct damaging effect on hepatic, renal, or hematologic tissues but instead are an extension of their pharmacologic effects. Like the pharmacologic effects, the adverse reactions of the opioid analgesics are proportional to their anal-

TABLE 6-4   CONTRAINDICATIONS AND CAUTIONS TO THE USE OF OPIOIDS

Condition	Comment
Alcoholic or addict	Greater potential for abuse
Head injury	Can increase intracranial pressure
Chronic pain	Addiction potential limits (e.g., TMD) duration
Respiratory disease	Respiratory depression can occur
Pregnancy	Respiratory depression near term (fetus)
Nursing	No problem: watch infant
Nausea	Additive nausea
Constipation	Exacerbates or produces constipation

TMD, Temporomandibular disease.

gesic strength. Table 6-4 lists contraindications and cautions for the use of opioids.

Respiratory Depression

Not a problem with usual doses in normal patients.

The opioid analgesic agonists depress the respiratory center in a dose-related manner. This is usually the cause of death with an overdose. The depression is related to a decrease in the sensitivity of the brainstem to carbon dioxide. Both the rate and depth of breathing are reduced. In elderly or debilitated patients, the usual therapeutic dose of morphine can produce a significant decrease in pulmonary ventilation. Reduced ventilation produces vasodilation, which results in an increase in intracranial pressure. Opioids should not be used in patients with head injuries. Opioids may also mask CNS diagnostic symptoms. Patients with hyperthyroidism are more tolerant of the depression, whereas patients with hypothyroidism are more sensitive.

Nausea and Emesis

Analgesic doses of opioid analgesics often produce nausea and vomiting. This is the result of their direct stimulation of the chemoreceptor trigger zone (CTZ), located in the medulla. This side effect is reduced if the patient does not ambulate. Administration of repeated, regular doses of an opioid can prevent vomiting by depressing the vomiting center (VC), another area in the CNS distinct from the CTZ.

Constipation

The opioids produce constipation by causing a tonic contraction of the gastrointestinal tract. Small doses of even weak opioids often have this effect, and their duration outlasts their analgesic effect. Even with continued administration, tolerance does not develop to this effect.

Miosis

The opioid analgesics cause miosis, an important sign (pinpoint pupils) in diagnosing an opioid overdose or identifying an addict. Tolerance does not develop to this effect.

Urinary Retention

The opioids increase the smooth muscle tone in the urinary tract, thereby causing urinary retention. They also produce an antidiuretic effect by stimulating the release of antidiuretic hormone (ADH) from the pituitary gland. This reaction may pose a problem in patients with prostatic hypertrophy.

Central Nervous System Effects

Occasionally, opioids may produce CNS stimulation, exhibited by anxiety, restlessness, or nervousness. Dysphoria can also occur from the opioids.

Cardiovascular Effects

The opioids may depress the vasomotor center and stimulate the vagus nerve. With high doses, postural hypotension, bradycardia, and even syncope may result.

Biliary Tract Constriction

In high doses, the opioids may constrict the biliary duct, resulting in biliary colic (pain associated with gallstones). This effect is important in patients passing gallstones who are being treated with opioids.

Histamine Release

Because the opioids can stimulate the release of histamine, itching and urticaria can result from their administration. This effect can occur at the site of intramuscular injection or at remote sites (e.g., itchy nose).

Pregnancy and Nursing Considerations

Opioids have not been shown to be teratogenic, although they may prolong labor or depress fetal respiration if given near term. Infants born to mothers using high-dose opioids, such as an addict, can have marked depressed respiration and experience withdrawal symptoms. The amount of opioid excreted in the mother's milk when therapeutic doses are given to the mother would pose no problem to the normal infant. Morphine and codeine are classified as Food and Drug Administration (FDA) pregnancy category C. Acetaminophen is a pregnancy category B drug. Caution is urged because acetaminophen is often combined with opioid analgesics.

Addiction

The degree of addiction potential of opioids is proportional to their analgesic strength. This fact limits the usefulness of the strongest of these agents. Because the duration of use in dentistry is usually short, addiction does not often pose a problem for the dentist. NSAIDs should be used to control dental pain in the addict. An addict will develop tolerance to the effects of the opioids, except for miosis and constipation. The rate of development of tolerance is related to the strength of the opioid and its frequency of use.

◆ OVERDOSE

The major symptom of opioid overdose is respiratory depression. In addition to pinpoint pupils and coma, this symptom is characteristic of opioid overdose. Opioid overdose is treated with an antagonist, naloxone, discussed later in this chapter.

◆ WITHDRAWAL

After abruptly discontinuing the opioids, a withdrawal syndrome occurs. The symptoms include yawning, lacrimation, perspiration, rhinorrhea, gooseflesh ("cold turkey"), irritability, nausea, vomiting, tachycardia, tremors, and chills. The name *cold turkey* comes from the symptom of piloerection (like when a person is cold); this reaction reminded addicts of the way a turkey looks (little bumps).

♦ IDENTIFICATION OF AN ADDICT

"Shoppers" are addicts who try to find a physician or dentist who will prescribe their drug of choice. There have even been organized groups of shoppers headed by an individual. The members of the groups are directed to physicians and dentists with complaints whose symptoms are taught to them. Prescriptions for controlled substances that are given to these "patients" are returned to the leader, and the "patients" are paid for their time. New dentist offices are often targets for "shopping." If a prescription for a controlled substance is obtained, more addicts will be contacting the office. This is not the type of "practice builder" that any dental office needs. Dental practitioners should become suspicious if any of the following shopper symptoms are present in a patient:

- Requests a certain drug and says it is better; he or she may stumble over the name
- Claims many allergies and says lots of pain medications do not work
- Cancels dental appointments because he or she claims to be going out of town on business
- Experiences pain for days after scaling and root planing
- Moves from dental office to dental office because "others do not understand"
- Claims a "low pain threshold"
- Needs refills several days after a dental procedure without complications

♦ TREATMENT

> Methadone maintenance is one method.

The following four general methods are used for treating opioid addiction:
1. One method involves substituting the equivalent amount of an oral opioid (usually methadone) for the injectable form that the addict had been using (e.g., heroin) and then gradually withdrawing that oral form.
2. Another method involves going cold turkey by abruptly withdrawing the opioid and using adjunctive medication to alleviate the symptoms of withdrawal, such as phenothiazines, clonidine, or benzodiazepines.
3. A third method involves maintaining a patient on high doses of methadone, termed *methadone maintenance*. With this method, the patient takes supervised large oral doses of methadone on a daily basis. Because the patient develops a tolerance for the effects of the opioids, a block is produced that prevents heroin-like agents from producing the "rush" feeling after injecting.
4. The last method involves administering an orally effective, long-acting antagonist, naltrexone (Trexan). Naltrexone blocks the action of usual doses of opioid administered illicitly. No treatment for opioid addiction is successful in all patients.

Allergic Reactions

> True opioid allergy is uncommon.

The most common type of true allergic reactions to the opioids is dermatologic in nature, including skin rashes and urticaria. Reports of gastrointestinal side effects are often reported as allergies but are side effects of the opioids. Contact dermatitis can occur with topical exposure. These allergic reactions have to be differentiated from the symptoms related to the histamine-releasing properties of the opioids. If a patient gives a history of a true allergic reaction to an opioid, an opioid from a different chemical class should be chosen (see Box 6-1). Figure 6-3 shows choices of analgesics for the patient allergic to codeine. Some brands of opioid analgesic combinations are formulated with sodium bisulfite. In patients with sulfite hypersensitivity, reference sources should be consulted to determine which brand contains sulfites.

Drug Interactions

Some of the drug interactions of the opioids are listed in Table 6-5. The most common outcome is sedation.

The respiratory depression produced by the opioids is additive with that produced by other CNS depressants. Alcohol or sedative-hypnotic agents can potentiate the opioids' respiratory depressant effect. When promethazine or hydroxyzine (antihistamines) is added to an opioid regimen, the opioid dose should be reduced.

All opioids can interact with the monoamine oxidase inhibitors (MAOI), a group of drugs used to treat depression. CNS excitation, hypertension, and hypotension have been reported. The accumulation of a metabolite of meperidine, normeperidine, may be responsible for the increased effect of meperidine in the presence of the antipsychotic agents such as chlorpromazine.

SPECIFIC OPIOIDS

Opioid Agonists

The analgesic action of the most commonly used opioids (agonists) is related to their action on the μ-receptors and κ-receptors (see morphine in Table 6-3). These agonist opioids are discussed first.

♦ MORPHINE

Morphine (more-FEEN) is considered to be the prototype opioid agonist against which other opioids are measured. An equivalent number of milligrams of each opioid is compared with 10 mg of morphine. Morphine is used parenterally to control postoperative pain in hospitalized patients. It is also used orally, primarily in the treatment of terminal illnesses. Sustained-release morphine tablets are the most commonly used form of morphine for outpatient use in the terminally ill. Few, if any, sustained-release analgesics are useful in dentistry because the patient needs immediate relief not future relief. The usual oral dosing interval and route of administration are listed in Table 6-2.

♦ OXYCODONE

Oxycodone (ox-i-KOE-done) is used alone or combined with either aspirin (in Percodan) or acetaminophen (in Percocet and Tylox) (Table 6-6) to provide relief of moderate-to-severe pain. Combining an opioid with a nonopioid analgesic produces an additive analgesic effect with fewer adverse reactions. Oxycodone retains about two-thirds of its action when given orally. It bridges the gap between codeine and morphine in terms of strength of analgesic action.

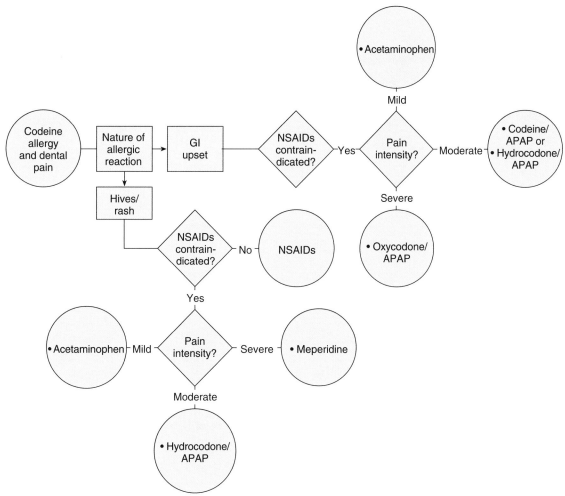

FIGURE 6-3

Codeine allergy decision tree. Use this decision tree to choose an analgesic for patients with a history of codeine allergy. *APAP,* Acetaminophen; *NSAIDs,* nonsteroidal antiinflammatory drugs; *NX,* naloxone.

TABLE 6-5	DRUG INTERACTIONS OF THE OPIOIDS	
	Medical Drug	**Potential Outcome**
General opioids	Alcohol	Additive CNS depression
	Barbiturates	
Specific Opioids		
Propoxyphene	Carbamazepine	Carbamazepine toxicity
Meperidine	Barbiturates	↑Toxicity of meperidine
	Chlorpromazine, neuroleptics	↓BP →CNS depression
	MAOIs	Severe reactions, excitation, rigidity, ↑BP
Methadone	Barbiturates	↓Methadone levels
	Phenytoin	↓Methadone levels; withdrawal
	Rifampin	

BP, Blood pressure; *CNS,* central nervous system; *MAOIs,* monoamine oxidase inhibitors.

♦ HYDROCODONE

There are many combinations of hydrocodone (hye-droe-KOE-done) and acetaminophen, including the original, which contains 5 mg of hydrocodone and 500 mg of acetaminophen (5/500). Various combinations of the two ingredients, hydroco-done and acetaminophen, include ranges of 2.5 to 10 mg of hydrocodone and 500 to 750 mg of acetaminophen. The companies offering brand name combinations seem to manufacture new combinations to thwart the development of generic equivalents. The original product combination (hydrocodone 5 mg and acetaminophen 500 mg) is recommended for the majority of dental patients with pain. To change the dose of this drug combination, the number of tablets per dose can be altered (from one-half to two tablets). This strength is available generically and is inexpensive. As with any opioid product containing acetaminophen, the total dose of acetaminophen should not exceed 4 gm (see Chapter 5). Upper limits for the total daily dose per day must not be exceeded. With combination products, the maximum daily dose (for a person who does not drink) is six tablets for products containing 650 mg and five tablets for those with 750 mg per dose form.

♦ CODEINE

Codeine (KOE-deen) is the most commonly used opioid in dentistry, and it is combined with acetaminophen (Tylenol #3) for oral administration. Other constituents, including caffeine and aluminum/magnesium hydroxides (antacid), are often included in these analgesic combinations. Codeine has a relatively weak analgesic action compared with morphine, hydromorphone, hydrocodone, or even oxycodone. Some commonly

TABLE 6-6   CONSTITUENTS OF COMMON OPIOID ANALGESIC PRODUCTS

Trade Name	Opioid	Efficacy (+ to ++++)	Other Ingredients (mg)
Propoxyphene (Darvon) compound-65	Propoxyphene HCl (65)	+	Aspirin (389) Caffeine (32.4)
Darvocet* N-100	Propoxyphene napsylate (100)	+	Acetaminophen (650)
Tylenol #1-4†	Codeine #1 (7.5) #3 (30) #2 (15) #4 (60)	++	Acetaminophen (300) Sodium metabisulfite (trade name); generic also available
Tylenol with codeine elixir	Codeine (12 mg/5 ml)	++	Alcohol (7%) Sucrose
Phenaphen #2-4	Codeine (15, 30, 60)	++	Acetaminophen (325)
Empirin #2-4	Codeine (15, 30, 60)	++	Aspirin (325)
Fiorinal #3	Codeine (30)	++	Aspirin (325) Butalbital (50) Caffeine (40)
Fioricet with codeine	Codeine (30)	++	Acetaminophen (325) Butalbital (50) Caffeine (40)
Talwin NX†	Pentazocine (50)	+++	Naloxone (0.5)
Vicodin, Lortab, Lorcet	Hydrocodone (5-10)	++	Acetaminophen (500-700)
Vicoprofen	Hydrocodone (7.5)	++	Ibuprofen (200)
Percodan, Roxiprin, Endodan†	Oxycodone (~5)	+++	Aspirin (325)
Percocet, Roxicet, Endocet, Oxycocet	Oxycodone (5)	+++	Acetaminophen (325)
Tylox	Oxycodone (5)	+++	Acetaminophen (500)
OxyContin‡	Oxycodone (10, 20, 40, 80)	+++	None
Oxycodone liquid	Oxycodone 20 mg/ml, 5 mg/5 ml	+++	
Demerol	Meperidine (50, 100)	+++	None
Demerol APAP	Meperidine (50, 100)	+++	Acetaminophen (300)
Mepergan Fortis	Meperidine (50)	+++	Promethazine (25)
Dilaudid	Hydromorphone (1, 2, 3, 4, 8)	++++	None

APAP, Acetaminophen.
*Suffix of "-cet" shows drug contains acetaminophen.
†Most commonly prescribed.
‡Sustained-release product; not for acute pain.

used analgesic combinations are listed in Table 6-6. Evidence for hydrocodone's efficacy being more than that of codeine is lacking because hydrocodone was previously used (and therefore tested) as an antitussive.

The amount of codeine in combination products is designated by #2 (15 mg; ¼ gr), #3 (30 mg; ½ gr), and #4 (60 mg; 1 gr). Generally, doses greater than 30 to 60 mg of codeine are poorly tolerated by the patient (too much nausea). In pain studies, it is difficult to show that 30 mg of codeine is any better than a placebo, and 60 mg of codeine has an analgesic strength about the same as 650 mg of aspirin, 650 mg of acetaminophen, or 200 mg of ibuprofen. Because of codeine's weak analgesic efficacy, prescription doses of NSAIDs often produce better results in the management of dental pain. When codeine is combined with nonopioid analgesics, there is additive analgesic activity. In the combination products, lower doses of each analgesic may be used and there is a potential for a reduction in adverse reactions.

◆ PROPOXYPHENE

> Popularity is unrelated to analgesic efficacy.

An opioid that is synthetic and is chemically similar to methadone is propoxyphene (proe-POX-i-feen), which is in Darvocet N-100. Its analgesic efficacy has been questioned (see Table 6-6), and it is certainly no more efficacious than two tablets of aspirin or acetaminophen. It is available combined with aspirin and caffeine or acetaminophen, which adds to its puny efficacy. Its adverse effects include nausea, vomiting, dizziness, and physical dependence. These adverse effects are significantly higher and more dangerous in the elderly. Also, its active metabolite is cardiotoxic. Hundreds of deaths have been associated with its overdose, often in combination with alcohol. With the availability of other agents, it is difficult to justify the use of propoxyphene. However, propoxyphene is very commonly prescribed in medicine. The reason for this is that it acts as the bridge (in the provider's perception) when "waffling" on whether to give an opioid. (There must be lots of "wafflers.")

◆ MEPERIDINE

Meperidine (me-PAIR-i-deen) (Demerol) is intended for the acute management of moderate-to-severe pain. It requires 100 mg to equal about 10 mg of morphine. However, its use has resulted in inadequate pain control and adverse effects for many patients over the years. Morphine, hydromorphone, or oxycodone should be used in its place. The drug interactions between meperidine and both the MAOIs and phenothiazines must be considered before using meperidine. Meperidine is a poor choice for oral use because it has a high first-pass effect, a short duration of action, and more drug interactions. It may be useful as an ingredient in an anxiolytic "medley" given as an oral preoperative. Although occasionally used in outpatient dentistry, it has little if any use.

◆ HYDROMORPHONE

An orally effective opioid, hydromorphone (hye-droe-MORE-fone) (Dilaudid) is reserved for the management of severe pain. It is more potent than morphine and better absorbed orally, but it tends to produce similar adverse reactions. Its use in dentistry should be limited to rare situations, limited numbers, and careful monitoring. It is a favorite of the addict because of its strength (see Table 6-6).

◆ METHADONE

Methadone (METH-e-done) (Dolophine) is used primarily in the treatment of opioid addicts. It is used either to withdraw the patient gradually or for methadone maintenance. Because it has a longer duration of action, withdrawal from methadone is easier than from heroin. However, because it is an opioid analgesic the risk for dependence still exists. Lately, methadone has been used as an analgesic in the treatment of chronic pain because it can be dosed less frequently than short-acting opioids such as morphine or hydrocodone. It also has a long half-life, good bioavailability, and it is cost-effective. The downside to methadone use is the risk of death and life-threatening changes in breathing and heart rates. These incidences have been reported in persons newly starting methadone or in persons switching to methadone after using stronger opioid analgesics. As a result, only low doses should be prescribed for pain.

◆ FENTANYL FAMILY

Fentanyl (FEN-ta-nil) (Duragesic, Sublimaze), sufentanil (sue-FEN-ta-nil) (Sufenta), and alfentanil (al-FEN-ta-nil) (Alfenta) are short-acting parenterally administered agonist opioid analgesics that are used perioperatively or during general anesthesia. They provide analgesia during and immediately after general anesthesia. Fentanyl is used in combination with droperidol (droe-PER-i-dol) (Inapsine) to induce or supplement general or regional anesthesia and to produce general anesthesia. Postoperative ventilation and observation are needed when these agents are used. Fentanyl is also available as a patch (Fentanyl [Duragesic] Transdermal System) for application to the skin every 3 days. The patches provide constant pain relief for the terminally ill. Sometimes, oral morphine is used concomitantly as needed to control "breakthrough" pain.

Mixed Opioids

Mixed opioids include the agonist-antagonist opioid analgesics and the partial agonists. The only mixed opioid available for oral use is the agonist-antagonist pentazocine. Butorphanol (Stadol), available as a nasal spray, is also in this group. This group is ripe for research to develop opioids with adequate analgesic potency and fewer side effects, such as respiratory depression and addiction potential, than the agonist opioids. At present, their place in dental therapeutics is unclear.

◆ AGONIST-ANTAGONIST OPIOIDS

The only agonist-antagonist opioid available in oral form is pentazocine (pen-TAZ-oh-seen) (Talwin). It produces CNS effects not unlike the opioid agonists, including analgesia, sedation, and respiratory depression. The type of analgesia it produces is somewhat different from that produced by the agonist opioids. This may be the result of its agonist action at the κ-receptors and δ-receptors and its antagonist action at the μ-receptor. (References differ in attributing the dysphoric and psychomimetic adverse reactions—some say δ, and others say σ.)

The adverse reactions of pentazocine include sedation, dizziness, nausea, vomiting, and headache. Opioid-like effects on the gastrointestinal tract occur with pentazocine. Psychomimetic effects, including nightmares, hallucinations, and dysphoria, have been reported. With high doses, respiratory depression can occur. Unlike the agonist opioids, increasing the dose of pentazocine does not result in a commensurate increase in respiratory depression, that is, respiratory depression is nonlinear. Unlike the opioid agonists, pentazocine can increase both the blood pressure and heart rate. This may be related to its catecholamine-releasing properties.

The drug of choice to treat pentazocine overdose is naloxone. With abuse, repeated injections in the same location can result in severe sclerosis, fibrosis, and ulceration. Because pentazocine was initially thought not to have abuse potential, many pentazocine abusers have been produced. A popular mixture termed "Ts and Blues" is a combination of pentazocine (Talwin) and pyribenzamine (blue-colored tablet), an antihistamine. Because of its weak antagonist property, it may precipitate withdrawal in the addict.

Pentazocine is available as tablets containing 50 mg of pentazocine and 0.5 mg of naloxone, a pure opioid antagonist (Talwin-NX). Naloxone, a Schedule IV opioid, was added to pentazocine to reduce its addiction potential. How does it do this? First, naloxone, a pure antagonist, is effective parenterally but not orally because it is inactivated. Second, if the tablet is taken by the intended oral route, the naloxone will not affect its analgesic potency because it is rapidly inactivated when taken orally. Third, if the contents of the tablet are injected parenterally, the active naloxone will counteract the action of pentazocine, reducing its positive effects. This combination tablet has resulted in a tablet that is more difficult to abuse and whose street value was cut in half. (One cannot say that drug addicts do not know their pharmacology.)

Parenterally available agonist-antagonists include dezocine (DEZ-oh-seen) (Dalgan), nalbuphine (NAL-byoo-feen) (Nubain), and butorphanol (byoo-TOR-fa-nol) (Stadol). Dezocine has agonist action at the κ-receptor and antagonist action at the μ-receptor. Its analgesic strength is comparable to morphine at usual therapeutic doses. Like pentazocine, these other agonist-antagonists demonstrate nonlinear respiratory depression. Sedation, nausea, vomiting, xerostomia, and headache are side effects of these drugs. These agents produce fewer psychomimetic effects than pentazocine but more than the agonists.

When originally marketed, these agonist-antagonists were said to have much less addiction potential or even none at all. They were not placed on any narcotic schedule by the Drug Enforcement Administration (DEA). Butorphanol, available as a nasal spray, has been marketed for some time. Because of the nature of the patient use of this agent in clinical practice, most pharmacists consider this product to be "addicting." The current literature and clinical practice has determined that these agents do in fact have addiction potential. If they are added to the list, it will not be surprising.

◆ PARTIAL AGONISTS

The first and only available partial agonist is buprenorphine (byoo-pre-NOR-feen) (Buprenex, Subutex). It is a partial m-receptor agonist but has no d-receptor action. In abstinent morphine-dependent patients, buprenorphine suppresses withdrawal; in stabilized opioid-dependent patients, it precipitates withdrawal. Its abuse potential appears to be moderate, and it is classified as a Schedule III drug. It is available for oral and parenteral use.

◆ OPIOID ANTAGONISTS

Naloxone reverses opioid overdose.

Naloxone. Naloxone (nal-OX-zone) (Narcan) is an essentially pure opioid antagonist that is active parenterally. It antagonizes the μ-receptors, κ-receptors, and δ-receptors. When given alone, it produces few pharmacologic effects in the usual therapeutic doses. Naloxone is the drug of choice for treating agonist or mixed opioid overdoses. It will reverse opioid-induced respiratory depression. If another agent, such as a barbiturate, is responsible for the depression, naloxone does not add to the respiratory depression. If administered to an addict who has taken an overdose of an opioid, small doses must be carefully titrated or opioid withdrawal may be produced. It also serves as a useful tool in research to determine the role of the opioid receptors in hypnosis, acupuncture, and the placebo effect.

Naloxone is given intravenously or intramuscularly with an average adult dose of 2 mg and a range of doses between 0.4 and 10 mg. Doses should be repeated if the duration of action of the opioid is longer than that of naloxone.

Effects should occur within 1 to 2 minutes. Doses may be repeated at 2- to 3-minute intervals. If no response occurs after 10 mg is administered, the diagnosis of opioid overdose must be questioned. If any opioid is used in the dental office, the dental office emergency kit should contain naloxone.

Nalmefene reverses opioid overdose.

Nalmefene. Nalmefene (NAL-me-feen) (Revex) is another parenteral opioid antagonist used to reverse opioid overdose.

Naltrexone is used to prevent opioid and alcohol use in addicts.

Naltrexone. A long-acting, orally effective opioid antagonist, naltrexone (nal-TREKS-zone) (ReVia, Vivitrol) is indicated for the maintenance of the opioid-free state in detoxified, formerly opioid-dependent patients. It should not be administered until the patient has remained opioid free for at least 1 week and has had a negative naloxone challenge. It is also used in the management of alcohol abstinence. Its adverse reactions include insomnia, nervousness, headache, abdominal cramping, nausea, vomiting, and arthralgia. Acute hepatitis and liver failure have been associated with naltrexone. It is administered daily or in some instances three times weekly. Patients on naltrexone should not be given opioid analgesic agents for management of dental pain.

Tramadol

Analgesic efficacy unimpressive; lack of addiction potential questionable.

Tramadol (Ultram) is a unique analgesic with an interesting mechanism of action. It has μ-opioid agonist action and inhibits the reuptake of norepinephrine and serotonin (modifies the ascending pain pathways). It has some but not all properties of an opioid (like codeine and hydrocodone) because of its μ-agonist activity and it does not affect the other two opioid receptors the κ-receptors and δ-receptors. Tramadol's other mechanism involves the inhibition of reuptake of norepinephrine and serotonin, similar to the mechanism of the antidepressants.

Adverse reactions of tramadol include CNS effects such as dizziness, somnolence, headache, and stimulation. Gastrointestinal tract side effects include nausea, diarrhea, constipation, and vomiting. Palpitations, diaphoresis, and seizures have been reported in patients taking tramadol. One should watch for signs of addiction (currently this drug is not scheduled).

Tramadol use is associated with physical dependency and withdrawal symptoms. Tramadol causes typical opiate withdrawal symptoms and atypical symptoms including anxiety, palpitations, and anguish.

Tramadol's analgesic efficacy is difficult to assess because most studies are unpublished and therefore cannot be judged; studies comparing tramadol with nonsteroidal agents or stronger opioids have not been done. Tramadol efficacy is stated in Table 6-7.

The usual adult dose is 50 to 100 mg every 4 to 6 hours, not to exceed 400 mg/day. Because of its weak analgesic activity and its high cost compared with established analgesics, its use is difficult to justify.

DENTAL USE OF OPIOIDS

The advent of the NSAIDs has produced a change in the use of the opioids in dental practice. Most dental pain can be better managed by the use of NSAIDs. In the patient in whom NSAIDs are contraindicated, the dentist has a wide range of opioids from

TABLE 6-7   RELATIVE EFFICACY OF TRAMADOL (ULTRAM)

Tramadol Dose (mg)	Compared with Codeine (mg)	Comparison with Combinations
50	= 60	<#2 ASA/#3 codeine (total = 650/60)
75		≥APAP/propoxyphene 650/100
100	>60	<#2 ASA/#3 codeine (total = 650/60)
150	>60	≥APAP/propoxyphene 650/100
5 times a day		
50		= #1 tablet acetaminophen 300/codeine 30 mg
		= #1 tablet of aspirin 300/codeine 30 mg

APAP, Acetaminophen; *ASA*, aspirin.

BOX 6-2   PATIENT INSTRUCTIONS FOR USE OF OPIOID ANALGESICS

- Take with a full glass of water.
- Take with food to minimize gastrointestinal irritation.
- Use caution with driving because of the likelihood of dizziness and drowsiness.
- Avoid any situations that require thought or concentration because of the likelihood of sedation.
- These drugs can cause xerostomia. Drink plenty of water and avoid caffeinated beverages, juices, and sodas.

which to choose. By beginning with codeine or hydrocodone combinations and progressing to oxycodone combinations, almost all dental pain can be managed. Only in rare cases and for very short periods (1 to 2 days) should stronger opioids be prescribed for outpatient dental pain. Box 6-2 lists the patient instructions for opioid analgesics.

Patients with chronic pain should be managed with nonopioid therapies and referred to appropriate specialists, depending on the nature of their chronic pain. In the treatment of chronic pain, opioids are not indicated. New patients with a complaint of pain should be seen in the dental office, and definitive treatment rendered. Opioid prescriptions should be given only for small amounts without refills and only if the patient has dental treatment performed. If dental pain persists, the patient should be seen in the dental office for evaluation and local treatment. If the patient demands opioids repeatedly, the patient should be referred to a pain clinic for evaluation. Temporomandibular disease (TMD), formerly called temporomandibular joint (TMJ) disease, often produces chronic pain. When pain becomes chronic, the mechanisms producing the pain differ from that of acute pain. Treatment of TMD should include NSAIDs and possibly muscle relaxants and tricyclic antidepressants.

DENTAL HYGIENE CONSIDERATIONS

1. If opioid analgesics are necessary, the dental hygienist should conduct a thorough medication/health history of the patient to determine if any contraindications or drug interactions exist.
2. The dental hygienist should be aware that many opioid analgesics are combined with nonopioid analgesics. Remind patients to not supplement with OTC analgesics if a combination nonopioid/opioid analgesic is prescribed.
3. The most common side effect associated with opioid analgesics is sedation. Other sedating drugs should be avoided or used with caution if the drug is essential.
4. Patients should avoid anything that requires thought or concentration while taking the opioid analgesic.
5. If patients complain of gastrointestinal adverse effects, they may require a semisupine chair position during dental treatment.
6. The dental hygienist should be aware of the signs of opioid addiction and how to identify an addict.
7. Consult Box 6-2 for patient instructions regarding opioid analgesics.

CLINICAL SKILLS ASSESSMENT

1. What are some red flags associated with opioid addiction?
2. Is any one opioid more addicting than another? If so, what is this based on?
3. Is there a need for concern with opioid addiction for patients taking these drugs to treat or manage dental pain? Why or why not?
4. What is hydrocodone and how effective is it in treating or managing dental pain?
5. Compare and contrast hydrocodone with ibuprofen.
6. What are the adverse reactions associated with hydrocodone?
7. Are there drug interactions with hydrocodone?
8. What are the dental concerns associated with hydrocodone?
9. What should patients be told about this medication?
10. Can tramadol be used instead of hydrocodone?

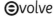

Please visit http://evolve.elsevier.com/Haveles/pharmacology for review questions and additional practice and reference materials.

7 Antiinfective Agents

LEARNING OBJECTIVES

1. Outline the history and basic principles of infection and its relevance to dentistry.
2. Summarize the principal indications for the use of antimicrobial agents.
3. Name and describe the major adverse reactions and disadvantages associated with the use of antiinfective agents.
4. Discuss penicillin, macrolides, tetracyclines, cephalosporins—their chemical makeup, properties, mechanisms of action, uses, and potential adverse reactions—and name several specific types.
5. Name and describe several other types of antibiotics and antiinfectives.
6. Discuss the use of antiinfective agents in dentistry.
7. Describe the drugs used to treat tuberculosis and the difficulties this disease presents.
8. Summarize the concept and practice of antibiotic prophylaxis in dentistry.

Antiinfective agents play an important role in dentistry because infection, after pain management, is the dental problem for which drugs are most often prescribed. As the knowledge about the etiology of dental diseases is continually increasing and the involvement of microorganisms becoming better understood, dental health care workers continue to better understand the proper place of antibiotics and their effect on microorganisms. Another important piece of the puzzle of infection is the immunologic response of the host. This puzzle piece has not yet led to therapeutic intervention strategies.

Dental infections can be divided into several types as follows:

- *Caries:* Caries, produced by *Streptococcus mutans,* is the first important dental infection of the newly erupting teeth of the young patient. At present, traditional antiinfective agents have not been useful for this problem in the general population. The treatments of choice involve the use of fluoridated water, local physical removal of bacterial plaque from teeth on a regular basis (good oral hygiene, dental prophylaxis), and appropriately placed sealants.

- *Periodontal disease:* In the adult patient, the dental health care team's biggest dental problem is periodontal disease. With an increase in knowledge about antiinfective agents, dental teams will be better able to understand and properly administer new treatments for this disease such as tetracycline fibers. Because it is now known that microorganisms, such as *Actinobacillus actinomycetemcomitans,* black-pigmented bacteroides, motile rods, and spirochetes, are involved in periodontal disease, development of a more rational approach to treatment of periodontal disease may be possible. Table 7-1 lists the common organisms that are involved in periodontal infections and the sensitivity or resistance to the antibiotics tested. Treatments that use localized methods of drug delivery (e.g., tetracycline fibers) hold promise for the future management of periodontal disease.

- *Localized dental infections:* Most localized dental infections are extensions that arise from either periodontic- or endodontic-related sources. For most localized dental infections, if adequate drainage can be obtained, antiinfective agents are not indicated unless the patient is immunocompromised (Box 7-1). In the

TABLE 7-1   PERIODONTAL MICROBES, THEIR PRESENCE, AND IN VITRO SUSCEPTIBILITY TO CERTAIN ANTIMICROBIAL AGENTS (BY MINIMUM INHIBITORY CONCENTRATION)

Organisms	LJP	AP	R	PEN	AMX	TET	DOX	CLN	MET	CIP
Aggregatibacter actinomycetemcomitans	+	+	+	1-16	1-16	2-8	6	R	32	<1
Porphyromonas gingivalis	—	+	+	<1	ND	2	1	<1	4	<1-2
Prevotella intermedia	+	+	+	5	ND	6	3	<1	2	<1
Eikenella corrodens	+	+	+	8-9	8	3-32	6	R	R	<1
Fusobacterium spp.	+	+	+	2-5	2	2	2	<1	1	3
Campylobacter rectus (Wolinella recta)	—	+	+	1	1	2	1	1	2	R

Data from Slots J, Rams TE: Antibiotics in periodontal therapy: advantages and disadvantages, *J Clin Periodontol* 17:479, 1990.

+, Elevated proportions of bacteria; —, regular proportions or not detected or studied; *AMX,* amoxicillin; *AP,* adult periodontitis; *CIP,* ciprofloxacin; *CLN,* clindamycin; *DOX,* doxycycline; *LJP,* localized juvenile periodontitis; *MET,* metronidazole; *MIC,* minimal inhibitory concentrations for 90% of strains (μg/m), except penicillin G, which is U/ml; *ND,* not determined; *PEN,* penicillin G; *R,* "refractory" adult periodontitis; *TET,* tetracycline.

BOX 7-1   DISEASES, CONDITIONS, AND DRUGS THAT DECREASE RESISTANCE TO INFECTION

Diseases/Conditions	Drugs
Addison's disease	Immunosuppressive drugs such as:
AIDS-related complex	Azathioprine (Imuran)
HIV	Cyclophosphamide (Cytoxan)
Alcoholism	Cyclosporin (Sandimmune)
Blood dyscrasias	Methotrexate (Rheumatrex)
Cancer	Glucocorticosteroids
Cirrhosis of the liver	
Diabetes mellitus	
Down syndrome	
Immunoglobulin deficiency	
Leukemia	
Malnutrition	
Splenectomy	

AIDS, Acquired immunodeficiency syndrome; *HIV,* human immunodeficiency virus.

---

occasional situation in which antibiotics are indicated, the antibiotic of choice is determined by the organisms likely to be present.

- *Systemic infections:* Systemic dental infections can be identified because they produce systemic symptoms such as fever, malaise, and tachycardia. Lesions associated with infections producing these types of symptoms should be drained, but if this is not possible, antibiotics should be given. The duration of therapy should include the number of days for the signs and symptoms to be totally gone plus 2 or 3 days. If the dental infection has systemic symptoms, the use of antiinfective agents is indicated and may even be critical.

DENTAL INFECTION "EVOLUTION"

Dental infections often follow similar pathways of evolution from their beginning to their end. In the beginning, the organisms responsible for a dental infection are primarily gram-positive cocci, such as *Streptococcus viridans,* or α-hemolytic streptococci. After a short time, the gram-positive infection begins to include a variety of both gram-positive and gram-negative anaerobic organisms, such as *Peptostreptococcus (Peptococcus)* and *Bacteroides* (*Porphyromonas* and *Prevotella* species). At this point, the infection is termed a *mixed* infection. Over time, the proportion of organisms that are anaerobic increases. With additional time and no treatment, the infection progresses until it consists of predominantly anaerobic flora. At this point, the anaerobic organisms coalesce into an abscess, often visible on radiograph (x-ray).

The choice of antibiotics for a dental patient's infection depends on where it is in its evolution. If the infection is just beginning, the organisms most likely to be present are gram-positive cocci. Penicillin is the drug of choice, unless the patient has a penicillin allergy. Amoxicillin is most often used because it is less irritating to the stomach and can be taken with food or milk. In patients allergic to penicillin, alternatives might include erythromycin or clindamycin. When the infection is at the mixed stage, agents effective against either gram-positive organisms or anaerobic organisms may be successful. Treating gram-positive organisms is easier, and the drug of choice is penicillin/amoxicillin or with a penicillin allergy, a macrolide antibiotic. For anaerobic organisms, metronidazole is effective. By eradicating one group of organisms, the balance between the two types of organisms is altered and the body can then resolve the infection. Clindamycin affects both gram-positive cocci and gram-positive and -negative anaerobes. Historically, oral surgeons have been comfortable using clindamycin, but other dentists have avoided it because of the association with pseudomembranous colitis (bloody diarrhea).

To treat a dental infection, it is critical to know what organism(s) are likely to be involved and the sensitivity of those organisms to antibiotics. Decisions are based on the likelihood of certain infections and their sensitivities.

HISTORY

In 1932, Gerhard Domagk of Germany observed that Prontosil protected mice against infection by streptococcal bacteria. This milestone in medical history led to the development of the sulfonamides and marked the beginning of systemic antimicrobial therapy.

In 1940, Chain and Florey of England observed that interest had been focused on the sulfonamides and that other possibilities, notably those connected with naturally occurring substances, should be considered.

In 1928, Fleming of England observed that a mold, *Penicillium notatum,* produced a substance that inhibited the growth of certain bacteria. He named this substance "penicillin" and suggested that it might be useful for application to infected wounds. In their classic paper, Chain and coworkers reported the low toxicity and systemic antibacterial effectiveness of penicillin. The excitement that began with the sulfonamides was transferred to the penicillins. As each new antibiotic is marketed, this excitement is transferred to the newest antibiotic developed. For years, scientists have been concerned about the indiscriminate use of antibiotics. Recent developments, such as totally resistant strains of bacteria, have made this concern even more important.

DEFINITIONS

A discussion of individual antimicrobial agents is preceded by definitions of the following terms:

- *Antiinfective agents:* Substances that act against or destroy infections.
- *Antibacterial agents:* Substances that destroy or suppress the growth or multiplication of bacteria.
- *Antibiotic agents:* Chemical substances produced by microorganisms that have the capacity, in dilute solutions, to destroy or suppress the growth or multiplication of organisms or prevent their action. The difference among the terms *antibiotic, antiinfective,* and *antibacterial* is that antibiotics are produced by microorganisms, whereas the other agents may be developed in a chemistry laboratory (not from a living organism). *Antibacterial* refers to a substance from any source that inhibits or kills bacteria. The term *antiinfective* refers to a substance from any source that inhibits or kills organisms that can produce infection, such as bacteria, protozoa, viruses, and so forth. This difference is largely ignored in general conversation, and antiinfectives are often referred to as "antibiotics."
- *Antimicrobial agents:* Substances that destroy or suppress the growth or multiplication of microorganisms.
- *Antifungal agents:* Substances that destroy or suppress the growth or multiplication of fungi.
- *Antiviral agents:* Substances that destroy or suppress the growth or multiplication of viruses.
   The following are definitions of commonly used terms:
- *Bactericidal:* The ability to kill bacteria. This effect is irreversible, that is, if the bacteria are removed from the drug, they do not live.
- *Bacteriostatic:* The ability to inhibit or retard the multiplication or growth of bacteria. This is a reversible process because if the bacteria are removed from the agent, they are able to grow and multiply. Whether an antibacterial agent is labeled bactericidal or bacteriostatic depends on variables such as the dose used or the organism being treated. Box 7-2 lists the

BOX 7-2 CLASSIFICATION OF ANTIINFECTIVE AGENTS: BACTERICIDAL OR BACTERIOSTATIC	
Bactericidal	**Bacteriostatic**
Aminoglycosides	Chloramphenicol
Bacitracin	Clindamycin*
Cephalosporins	Macrolides*
Metronidazole	Spectinomycin
Macrolides*	Sulfonamides
Penicillins	Tetracyclines
Polymyxin	Trimethoprim
Quinolones	
Rifampin	
Vancomycin	

*May be bactericidal against some organisms at higher blood levels.

most common antimicrobial agents and classifies them as bacteriostatic or bactericidal.

- *Blood (serum) level:* Concentration of the antiinfective agent present in the blood or serum. The importance of the serum level is that certain levels of an antibiotic are required to produce an effect on various types of organisms. For an antibiotic to be effective, the dose given must produce this concentration in the blood.
- *Infection:* Infection is not only an invasion of the body by pathogenic microorganisms but also a reaction of the tissues to their presence. The presence of a pathogen does not constitute "invasion." In fact, many potential oral pathogens are part of the normal floral in the mouth, but they only cause infection if their relative numbers rise.
- *Minimum inhibitory concentration (MIC):* Lowest concentration needed to inhibit visible growth of an organism on media after 18 to 24 hours of incubation. This in vitro test is more reliable and quantitative than the disk tests.
- *Spectrum:* Range of activity of a drug. The spectrum of activity of an antibacterial agent may be narrow, intermediate, or broad. A narrow-spectrum agent acts primarily against a smaller group of bacteria such as gram-positive cocci, gram-negative rods, gram-positive or gram-negative anaerobes, or viruses.
- *Superinfection, suprainfection:* Infection caused by the proliferation of microorganisms different from those causing the original infection. When antiinfectives disturb the normal flora of the body, the emergence of organisms unaffected by or resistant to the antibiotic used can occur. Superinfection is more often caused by broad-spectrum antibiotics such as tetracycline and increases when taken for a longer period. In this case, a reduction in the number of gram-positive and gram-negative bacteria allows the overgrowth of the fungus, *Candida albicans.* The pathogenic organisms emerging in a superinfection generally are more difficult to eradicate than the original organism and are more likely to exhibit resistance. The fact that the practitioner can cause and eliminate infections emphasizes the importance of determining a definite need before these drugs are used. (Dental practitioners should stamp out, or at least reduce, health care–acquired infections.)
- *Synergism:* Synergism occurs when the combination of two antibiotics produces more effect than would be expected

if their individual effects were added (in other words, 1 + 1 > 2). Combinations of antibiotics that are bactericidal are generally synergistic. Combinations of those that are bacteriostatic are merely additive (1 + 1 = 2).

- *Antagonism:* Antagonism occurs when a combination of two agents produces less effect than either agent alone (see Box 7-2).

INFECTION

The factors that determine the likelihood of a microorganism causing an infection are the following:
- Disease-producing power of the microorganism (virulence)
- Number of organisms present (inoculum)
- Resistance of the host (immunologic response): Host resistance should be considered as having both local and systemic components. Systemically, both drugs (steroids and antineoplastic agents) and diseases (acquired immunodeficiency syndrome [AIDS] and insulin-dependent diabetes mellitus [IDDM]) may reduce a patient's immunity (see Box 7-1) and increase the chance of an infection. Sleep deprivation and anxiety can also reduce a patient's immunologic response to infection.

CULTURE AND SENSITIVITY

Ideally, all infections requiring antimicrobial therapy would be cultured, and sensitivity tests would be performed. Culturing involves growing the bacteria from a sample of infective exudate, and sensitivity testing involves exposing the organism to certain test antibiotics and determining whether the organism is sensitive or resistant. Today, in part at least because of the inappropriate use of antiinfective agents, organisms are more quickly becoming resistant to antibiotics.

Culture and sensitivity is the only way to be sure that a drug will kill or inhibit the growth of the infecting microorganisms in a patient-specific infection. In practice, this is often difficult. In dentistry, the need for anaerobic culturing makes obtaining a sample and culturing it more difficult. Another problem is that many dental infections are often of mixed origin so that the results of the cultures are difficult to interpret. In cases of a serious infection, an infection in a compromised patient, or an infection that is not responding to treatment, it is imperative that a culture be taken.

Culture

When a culture is taken, proper collection materials (tubes or vials with the correct media) and methods must be used to obtain reliable results. Dental professionals need to communicate to the laboratory personnel the nature of the appropriate cultures to be taken. The laboratory personnel should perform a Gram stain so that they may report all of the bacteria that are present in high numbers. Both obligate and facultative anaerobes should be preserved.

Depending on the site, the collection method varies. Examples of methods include the following: for an abscess, aspiration with a needle; for a draining lesion, a swab from an anaerobic pack; and for endodontic treatment, properly handled absorbent

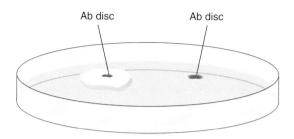

FIGURE 7-1
Culture and sensitivity. Antibiotic *(Ab)* disc with zone around it shows sensitivity.

points. Collection methods should be adapted to keep the anaerobes alive. For the periodontal pocket, the sterile paper point or the explorer can be used to sample the pocket.

Care must be taken not to contaminate the sample with supragingival plaque, which has a different microbial constitution. In at-risk patients, a culture should be taken before antibiotics are administered because antibiotics can alter the nature of the microbes so that identification is more difficult. Infections in problem sites and in problem patients should be cultured.

Sensitivity

After the organism is identified, it is grown on culture medium (Figure 7-1). Observing whether the organisms are sensitive or resistant to certain test antibiotics assists in determining which antibiotic to use in difficult infections. One to 2 days are required before the results of this test are available. Although therapy can start before this time, it may be changed after the results are available. If clinical response has been adequate, often the original antibiotic is continued despite sensitivity results.

RESISTANCE

Resistance (related to antibiotics) is the natural or acquired ability of an organism to be immune to or to resist the effects of an antiinfective agent. Natural resistance occurs when an organism has always been resistant to an antimicrobial agent because of the bacteria's normal properties such as lipid structures in the cell wall. Acquired resistance occurs when an organism that was previously sensitive to an antimicrobial agent develops resistance. This can occur by natural selection of a spontaneous mutation ("survival of the fittest"). An increase in the use of an antibiotic in a given population (e.g., a hospital) increases the proportion of resistant organisms in that population. Conversely, a decrease in the use of an antibiotic decreases the proportion of organisms resistant to that antibiotic in that given population. Another method by which resistance develops is by the transfer of deoxyribonucleic acid (DNA) genetic material from one organism to another via transduction, transformation, or bacterial conjugation. The first organism, which is resistant to one or more antibiotics, transfers its genetic material to a second organism. The second organism, which was not previously resistant, thus becomes resistant to the same antibiotic as the first organism without ever having been exposed to that antibiotic. This transfer of genetic material from one organism to another may occur among very different microorganisms, including transfer from a nonpathogenic bacteria to a pathogenic bacteria. The three most common mechanisms of acquired resistance are a decrease in bacterial permeability, the production of bacterial enzymes, and an alteration in the target site.

INDICATIONS FOR ANTIMICROBIAL AGENTS

Considerable controversy exists regarding the need for antimicrobial agents in various situations. The two categories of indications are prophylactic and therapeutic.

Therapeutic Indications

Although there is no simple rule to determine whether antimicrobial therapy is needed in dentistry, many infections do not require it. Most patients without immune function deficiencies, in whom drainage can be obtained, need no antibiotics to manage their dental infections. (Patients with acne are not prescribed an antibiotic every time a pimple is pinched.) Table 7-2 lists the indications for treatment of dental infections and the antibiotics of choice and their alternatives. If local resistance patterns vary from those found in the table, antibiotic choice should be based on that information. However, before a decision is made, there are several factors that must be considered.

◆ PATIENT

The best defense against a pathogen is the host response. A properly functioning defense mechanism is of primary importance. When this defense is lacking, the need for antimicrobial agents is more pressing.

◆ INFECTION

The virulence and invasiveness of the microorganism are important in deciding the acuteness, severity, and spreading tendency of an infection. An acute, severe, rapidly spreading infection should generally be treated with antimicrobial agents, whereas a mild, localized infection in which drainage can be established need not be treated. If the periodontal pocket (site) remains active despite repeated root planing, then the use of antibiotics to alter the flora may be considered.

When antimicrobial agents are to be used in the treatment of dental infections, the organisms likely to produce the infection and their susceptibility to antimicrobial agents must be considered. Table 7-2 lists the antimicrobials of choice for various dental situations (when culture and sensitivity tests are unavailable) and alternatives if the drug of choice cannot be used. When two antimicrobial agents have approximately the same therapeutic effect and their cost to the patient is very different, the cost of therapy is another consideration.

To answer the question as to whether an antibiotic is effective in a certain dental infection, one needs many patients with similar infections in which half are given active antibiotics and half are given a placebo. This study would help to define the proper use of antibiotics in dental infections. This slow testing has begun, using antibiotics in periodontal situations, but there is still much to discover.

TABLE 7-2 ANTIMICROBIAL USE IN DENTISTRY*

Infection Situation	Drug(s) of Choice	Alternative Drug(s)
Periodontal Disease		
Acute necrotizing ulcerative gingivitis†	Penicillin VK Amoxicillin	Metronidazole Tetracycline
Abscess (perio)	Penicillin VK	Tetracycline
LJP	Doxycycline Tetracycline	Amoxicillin + metronidazole Augmentin (amoxicillin + clavulanate)
Adult periodontitis†	Not usually treated with drugs	Clindamycin
RAP	Doxycycline Tetracycline Metronidazole	Amoxicillin + metronidazole
Oral Infections		
Soft tissue infections (abscess, cellulitis, postsurgical, pericoronitis)	Penicillin VK Amoxicillin	Doxycycline Clindamycin Cephalosporin Tetracycline
Osteomyelitis	Penicillin VK Amoxicillin	Clindamycin Cephalosporin
Mixed Infections Insensitive To Penicillin		
Aerobes	Amoxicillin	Cephalosporin Sulfonamides Tetracycline
Anaerobes and chronic infections	Metronidazole Clindamycin	Cephalosporin Augmentin Tetracycline Metronidazole + penicillin
Prophylaxis for Infective Endocarditis		
Prosthetic heart valve‡	No penicillin allergy: Amoxicillin§	Penicillin allergy: Clarithromycin Azithromycin Clindamycin
Patient with LJP	Doxycycline for 3 weeks followed by usual regimen (see above)	

LJP, Localized juvenile periodontitis; *RAP,* rapid advancing periodontitis.
*Clinical conditions may alter drug therapy.
†No antimicrobial agents are usually required for these conditions.
‡See Table 7-4.
§See Table 7-3.

Prophylactic Indications

Few situations arise for which a definite indication for prophylactic antibiotic coverage exists. One clear-cut use of antibiotics for prophylaxis before a dental procedure (recommended by the American Heart Association and the American Dental Association) is a history of infective endocarditis, presence of a heart valve prosthesis, or congenital heart disease. The most current guidelines regarding antibiotic prophylaxis are discussed in detail at the end of this chapter.

GENERAL ADVERSE REACTIONS AND DISADVANTAGES ASSOCIATED WITH ANTIINFECTIVE AGENTS

Superinfection (Suprainfection)

All antiinfective agents can produce an overgrowth of an organism that is different from the original infecting organism and resistant to the agent being used. The wider the spectrum of the antiinfective agent and the longer the agent is administered, the greater the chance of superinfection occurring. This side effect can be minimized by use of the most specific antiinfective agent, the shortest effective course of therapy, and adequate doses.

Allergic Reactions

All antiinfective agents, just like all drugs, have the potential to produce a variety of allergic reactions, ranging from a mild rash to fatal anaphylaxis. Some antiinfective agents, such as the penicillins and the cephalosporins, are more allergenic than other agents. Many antiinfective agents, such as erythromycin and clindamycin, have a low allergenic potential.

Drug Interactions

Antiinfective agents can interact with oral contraceptives, oral anticoagulants, and other antiinfectives (a bacteriostatic agent interferes with a bactericidal agent).

◆ ORAL CONTRACEPTIVES

Some antibiotics have been found to decrease oral contraceptive efficacy by increasing their clearance from the body. This drug interaction, although unlikely, should be discussed with the patient whenever a patient using oral contraceptives receives a prescription for an antibiotic. Of those antibiotics used in dentistry, ampicillin and the tetracyclines are the most likely to produce this effect. In certain patients, additional birth control measures should be used during antibiotic administration.

◆ ORAL ANTICOAGULANTS

Antiinfective agents can potentiate the effect of oral anticoagulants. Oral anticoagulants are vitamin K inhibitors, so interfering with the production of vitamin K could increase the anticoagulant effect. Bacterial flora in the intestine produce most of the vitamin K in human bodies. Antiinfective agents (e.g., tetracycline) reduce the bacterial flora that produce vitamin K. With the vitamin K reduced, the oral anticoagulant's effect is increased. Erythromycin inhibits the enzymes that metabolize warfarin, leading to an increase in warfarin levels. Prolongation of the international normalized ratio (INR) leading to bleeding or hemorrhage may result. INR should be monitored more closely in patients on antiinfective therapy. Antiinfective agents interact to varying degrees depending on the antibiotic.

◆ OTHER ANTIINFECTIVES

Antibiotics that act at the same receptor may compete for that receptor and should not be given together (e.g., erythromycin and clindamycin). An antibiotic that has bacteriostatic properties stops the bacteria from growing, thereby inhibiting the action of a bactericidal agent (requires growing and actively dividing cells to work). Except in a few unusual, nondental cases, one antibiotic should be chosen and used alone.

Gastrointestinal Complaints

All antiinfective drugs can produce a variety of gastrointestinal complaints. The complaints include stomach pain, increased motility, and diarrhea. The incidence varies greatly, depending on the particular agent used, the dose of that agent, and whether the patient takes the drug with food. Erythromycin has the highest incidence of gastrointestinal complaints of any of the antibiotics. More serious gastrointestinal complaints, such as pseudomembranous colitis, which has been historically linked with clindamycin, are now known to occur not only with a wide variety of antiinfective agents (cephalosporins, amoxicillin) but also in the absence of any antimicrobial agents.

Pregnancy Considerations

The antimicrobial agents that can be used during pregnancy to treat infections are limited. Although the risk-to-benefit ratio must be considered whenever pregnant women are given any medications, penicillin and erythromycin have not been associated with teratogenicity and are often used. The use of clindamycin is probably also acceptable, but before any antibiotics are used in the pregnant dental patient, the patient's obstetrician should be contacted (this procedure also helps prevent medical-legal problems). Metronidazole is not usually used during pregnancy, but exceptions exist. The tetracyclines are contraindicated during pregnancy because of their effect on developing teeth and skeleton.

Dose Forms

Adult dose forms of antibiotics are commonly tablets and capsules. Children's dose forms, including liquid and chewable antibiotic dose forms, contain sugar as their sweetening agent. After the dentition has erupted, the dental health care worker should encourage the parent or child to brush the child's teeth after the use of these agents. The chewable tablets can stick to the teeth, especially in the pits. Long-term administration of antibiotics could increase the child's caries rate.

Cost

Cost is an important factor in choosing an antibiotic for a patient. If the perfect antibiotic is chosen and prescribed but the patient does not purchase the medication because it is too expensive, then poor results are likely. The best inexpensive antibiotic that can be taken will be more effective than an expensive one that cannot be purchased. Figure 7-2 compares the cost of various antiinfective agents.

PENICILLINS

The penicillins (pen-i-SILL-ins) can be divided into four major groups (see Table 7-3). The first group contains penicillin G and V, the second group is composed of the penicillinase-resistant penicillins, the third group contains amoxicillin, and the fourth group consists of extended-spectrum penicillins. Because the penicillins have many properties in common, their similarities are discussed first. In dentistry, the first and third groups are commonly used.

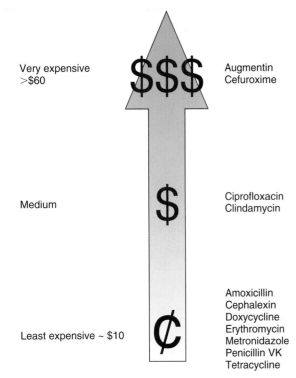

Very expensive
>$60

$$$

Augmentin
Cefuroxime

Medium

$

Ciprofloxacin
Clindamycin

Least expensive ~ $10

¢

Amoxicillin
Cephalexin
Doxycycline
Erythromycin
Metronidazole
Penicillin VK
Tetracycline

FIGURE 7-2
Relative cost of dentally useful antibiotic agents.

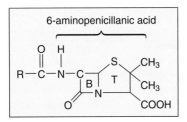

FIGURE 7-3
β-Lactam ring.

Source and Chemistry

The mold *Penicillium notatum* and related species produce the naturally occurring penicillins. The semisynthetic penicillins are produced by chemically altering the naturally produced penicillins. The penicillin structure includes a β-lactam ring fused to a five-member, S-containing thiazolidine ring. Neither of these rings has much antimicrobial action alone. Active penicillins are produced by adding different functional groups to position 6. Cleaving these functional groups from their two-ring structure results in a loss of antimicrobial activity. When the β-lactam ring is broken, such as in the presence of penicillinase, the antimicrobial activity of the compound is lost (Figure 7-3).

The addition of organic groups at the R position confers antibacterial activity to the compounds formed from 6-aminopenicillanic acid. These R groups create the various penicillins that were originally designated with letters, for example, penicillin G and penicillin V. The penicillins can be inactivated by any reaction that removes the R group or in the case of penicillinase, breaks the β-lactam ring *(B)*. Salts of the penicillins are

made by reactions at the thiazolidine *(T)* carboxyl (–COOH) group.

Although many naturally occurring penicillins have been produced, only penicillin G (Na+/K+ penicillin) is of use today. The various semisynthetic penicillins are formed by substituting other groups at the R position.

Pharmacokinetics

Penicillin tubular secretion in the kidney; half life = ½ hour

Penicillin can be administered either orally or parenterally but should not be applied topically because its allergenicity is greatest by that route. When penicillin is administered orally, the amount absorbed depends on the type of penicillin. The percentage can vary from 0% to more than 90% (see Table 7-3). When the percentage absorbed is too low, as with methicillin, the penicillin is available only for injection. Penicillin V is better absorbed orally than penicillin G, so penicillin V is used for administration of oral penicillin.

The oral route provides the advantages of convenience and less likelihood of a life-threatening allergic reaction. The disadvantages of using the oral rather than the parenteral route are that the blood levels rise slower, the blood levels are less predictable because of variable absorption or lack of patient compliance (biggest problem), and some penicillins are degraded by gastric acid. The highest blood levels are obtained if the patient takes the penicillin orally at least 1 hour before or 2 hours after meals, but penicillin V and amoxicillin can be taken without regard to meals.

After absorption, penicillin is distributed throughout the body, with the exception of cerebrospinal fluid, bone, and abscesses. This includes the tissue, saliva, and kidneys. Penicillin crosses the placenta and appears in breast milk.

Penicillin is metabolized by hydrolysis in the liver and undergoes tubular secretion in the kidney. The elimination half-life for both penicillin G and penicillin V is about 0.5 hour. In five half-lives, about 2.5 hours, these penicillins are virtually eliminated from the body.

Mechanism of Action

Penicillin is a very potent bactericidal agent that attaches to penicillin-binding proteins (PBPs) on the bacterial cell membrane. The PBPs are enzymes that are involved in the synthesis of the cell wall and the maintenance of the cell's structural integrity. Penicillin acts as the structural analog of acyl-D-alanyl-D-alanine, inhibiting the formation of cross-linkages (transpeptidases). This destroys cell wall integrity and leads to lysis. The penicillins are more effective against rapidly growing organisms. Table 7-3 summarizes the types, routes of ingestion, and other properties of the types of penicillins.

Spectrum

Penicillin G and V's narrow spectrum of activity includes gram-positive cocci, such as *Staphylococcus aureus, Staphylococcus pneumoniae, Streptococcus pyogenes, Streptococcus viridans,* and certain gram-negative cocci, such as *Neisseria gonorrhoeae* (produces gonorrhea) and *N. meningitidis.* Penicillin is also effective against spirochetes and anaerobes such as *Actinomyces, Peptococcus, Peptostreptococcus, Bacteroides, Corynebacterium,* and *Clostridium* species. The spectrum of action of the penicillins matches the microbes responsible for many periodontal conditions. The other penicillins have a somewhat different spectrum that is discussed in each section.

The antibacterial activity of penicillin is standardized in international units (IU). One international unit has the activity of 0.6 mg of the master standard of sodium penicillin G, so 1 mg of pure sodium penicillin G equals 1667 IU. About 400,000 IU of penicillin V is equivalent to 250 mg. Penicillin G is usually measured in international units, whereas other penicillins are expressed in milligrams.

Resistance

Resistance to penicillin can occur by several different mechanisms. Penicillinase-producing staphylococci are resistant because their enzymes destroy some penicillins. These penicillinases inactivate the penicillin moiety by cleaving the β-lactam ring.

In hospital environments, more than 95% of the population of staphylococci are penicillinase-producing organisms. Clavulanic acid serves as an inhibitor, which allows the use of amoxicillin to treat penicillinase-producing organisms. Certain bacteria have an outer cell membrane that prevents penicillin from reaching the PBPs.

Although most oral strains of *S. viridans* are sensitive to penicillin, an increasing number of strains are becoming resistant. The amount of bacterial resistance is proportional to the clinical use of the antibiotic; frequent use leads to increased resistance (and vice versa).

Adverse Reactions

The untoward reactions to the penicillins can be divided into toxic reactions and allergic or hypersensitivity reactions. The penicillins are the most common cause of drug allergies.

◆ TOXICITY

Because penicillin's toxicity is almost nonexistent, large doses have been tolerated without adverse effects. For this reason, there is a large margin of safety when penicillin is administered. With massive intravenous (IV) doses, direct central nervous system (CNS) irritation can result in convulsions. Large doses of penicillin G have been associated with renal damage manifested as fever, eosinophilia, rashes, albuminuria, and a rise in blood urea nitrogen (BUN). Hemolytic anemia and bone marrow depression have also been produced by penicillin. The penicillinase-resistant penicillins are significantly more toxic than penicillin G. Gastrointestinal irritation can manifest itself as nausea with or without vomiting. The irritation caused by injection of penicillin can produce sterile abscesses if given intramuscularly or thrombophlebitis if given intravenously.

◆ ALLERGY AND HYPERSENSITIVITY

Allergic reactions to penicillin always should be considered when penicillin is prescribed. Some studies indicate that 5% to 10% of patients receiving penicillin will have a reaction. Allergic reactions to oral penicillin are less common than with parenteral penicillin. Anaphylactic reactions are more frequent in patients pretreated with β-blockers and subsequently given oral penicil-

TABLE 7-3	PENICILLINS					
Drug Name	Routes	Penicillinase Resistant	Acid Stable	Absorbed Orally (%)	Protein Bound (%)
Penicillin G and V					
Penicillin G (Pentids)	PO, IM, IV	No	No	15-30	60
Penicillin G procaine (Crysticillin)	IM	No	No	—	60
Penicillin G benzathine (Bicillin L-A)	IM	No	No	—	60
Penicillin V (Pen-Vee K, V-Cillin K)	PO	No	Yes	60-75	75-80
Penicillinase Resistant					
Methicillin (Staphcillin)	IM, IV	Yes	No	0	30-45
Nafcillin (Unipen, Nafcil)	IM, IV	Yes	Yes	10-15	90
Oxacillin (Prostaphlin, Bactocill)	PO, IM, IV	Yes	Yes	20-30	95
Ampicillins					
Ampicillin (Polycillin, Omnipen)	PO, IM, IV	No	Yes	30-40	20
Amoxicillin (Amoxil, Larotid)	PO	No	Yes	75-90	20
Amoxicillin + clavulanate (Augmentin)	PO	Yes	Yes	Very good	20
Extended Spectrum					
Carbenicillin indanyl (Geocillin)	PO	No	Yes	80	50
Carbenicillin (Geopen, Pyopen)	IM, IV	No			50
Ticarcillin (Ticar)	IM, IV	No			45
Piperacillin (Pipracil)	IM, IV	No			16

PO, By mouth; *IM*, intramuscular; *IV*, intravenous.
Bold type indicates drugs most used in dentistry.

lin. Anaphylactic reactions in these patients have been reported to be difficult to treat.

The following are types of allergic reactions associated with the penicillins:

- *Anaphylactic reactions:* Anaphylactic shock, an acute allergic reaction, occurs within minutes after the administration of penicillin and presents the most serious danger to patients. It is characterized by smooth muscle contraction (e.g., bronchoconstriction), capillary dilation (shock), and urticaria caused by the release of histamine and bradykinin. If treatment does not begin immediately, death can result. The treatment of anaphylaxis is the immediate administration of parenteral epinephrine.

- *Rash:* All types of skin rashes have been reported in association with the administration of penicillin. This type of reaction accounts for 80% to 90% of allergic reactions to the penicillins. These rashes are usually mild and self-limiting but can occasionally be severe. Even contact dermatitis has occurred as a result of topical exposure, for example, while preparing an injectable solution (type IV).

- *Delayed serum sickness:* Serum sickness is manifested as fever, skin rash, and eosinophilia or severely as arthritis, purpura, **lymphadenopathy**, splenomegaly, mental changes, an abnormal **electrocardiogram**, and edema. It usually takes at least 6 days to develop and can occur during treatment or up to 2 weeks after treatment has ceased.

- *Oral lesions:* Delayed reactions to penicillin can exhibit themselves in the oral cavity. These include severe stomatitis, furred tongue, black tongue, acute glossitis, and cheilosis. These oral lesions can occur most commonly with topical application but have been reported from other routes.

- *Other reactions:* Interstitial nephritis, hemolytic anemia, and eosinophilia are types of allergic reactions occasionally reported during penicillin therapy.

When reactions to penicillin occur, the consequences are often serious. It is estimated that an anaphylactic reaction occurs in up to 0.05% of penicillin-treated patients, with a mortality of 5% to 10%. It is estimated that 100 to 300 deaths occur annually in the United States because of an allergic reaction to penicillin. Although the chance of a serious allergic reaction to penicillin is greater after parenteral administration, anaphylactic shock and death after oral use have also been reported. Patients who have a history of any allergy are more likely to be allergic to penicillin.

Allergic reactions to penicillin of any type may be followed by more serious allergic reactions on subsequent exposure. Any history of an allergic reaction to penicillin contraindicates its use, and another antibiotic should be substituted. However, a negative history does not guarantee the lack of a penicillin allergy. If a penicillin is prescribed and any question of a reaction remains, one should make sure that, after the first dose is taken, the patient is somewhere where help can be summoned if necessary.

Uses

Penicillin is an important antibiotic in medical and dental practice. Its use in dentistry results from its bactericidal potency, lack of toxicity, and spectrum of action, which includes many oral flora. It is often used for the treatment of dental infections. Table 7-2 demonstrates the dental infections for which penicillin is the drug of choice if patients are not allergic

to it. Amoxicillin, a close penicillin relative, is also used for specific prophylactic indications. It is the agent of choice for the prophylaxis of infective endocarditis in nonallergic patients who have a history of rheumatic heart disease or valve damage (see the discussion on antibiotic prophylaxis of infective endocarditis at the end of this chapter). Penicillin's effectiveness in the treatment of dental infections is explained by its effectiveness against many aerobic and anaerobic bacteria.

Specific Penicillins

◆ PENICILLIN G

Penicillin G, the prototype penicillin, is available as sodium, potassium, procaine, or benzathine salts. These salts differ in their onset and duration of action and the plasma levels attained. Figure 7-4 compares the blood levels attained by the IV administration of the potassium salt and the intramuscular (IM) administration of the potassium, procaine, and benzathine salts. One should note that the potassium salt given intravenously produces the most rapid and highest blood level, whereas the benzathine salt given intramuscularly produces the lowest and most sustained blood level. The potassium and procaine salts, given intramuscularly, produce intermediate blood levels and durations of action. The penicillin's duration of action is inversely proportional to the solubility of the penicillin form: the least soluble is the longest acting.

The sodium salts of penicillin should be avoided in patients with a limited sodium intake such as cardiovascular patients. Renal patients should not be given potassium salts, which can result in hyperkalemia. Patients may be allergic to the procaine moiety in procaine penicillin G. Both procaine and benzathine penicillins are suspensions given intramuscularly, from which the penicillin is slowly released.

◆ PENICILLIN V

Penicillin V has a spectrum of action very similar to that of penicillin G. The potassium salt of penicillin V (K penicillin V or penicillin VK) is more soluble than the free acid and therefore is better absorbed when taken orally. Table 7-2 lists some situations in which penicillin is the drug of first choice if the patient is not allergic to it. The usual adult dose is 500 mg four times a day (qid) for treatment of an infection for a minimum of 5 days and preferably 7 to 10 days.

◆ PENICILLINASE-RESISTANT PENICILLINS

Penicillinase-resistant penicillins should be reserved for use against only penicillinase-producing staphylococci. Compared with penicillin G, the penicillinase-resistant penicillins are less effective against penicillin G–sensitive organisms. They also produce more side effects such as gastrointestinal discomfort, bone marrow depression, and abnormal renal and hepatic function. Patients allergic to penicillin are also allergic to the penicillinase-resistant penicillins.

Because cloxacillin and dicloxacillin are better absorbed than the other penicillinase-resistant penicillins, they are the drugs of choice.

◆ AMPICILLINS

Ampicillin (am-pi-SILL-in) and amoxicillin (a-mox-i-SILL-in) are most often used in medicine. These penicillinase-susceptible penicillins have a spectrum of action that includes gram-positive

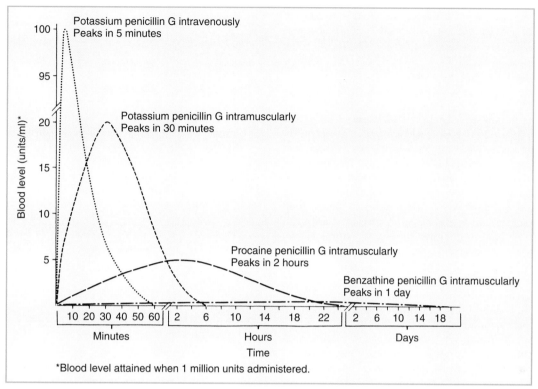

FIGURE 7-4
Comparative blood levels of penicillin G salts.

cocci, *Haemophilus influenzae,* and enterococci such as *Escherichia coli, Proteus mirabilis,* and *Salmonella* and *Shigella* species.

Amoxicillin, a relative of ampicillin, is most often used to treat infections because it produces higher blood levels, is better absorbed, requires less frequent dosing (three times daily versus four times daily for penicillin VK or ampicillin), and its absorption is not impaired by food. Amoxicillin is the drug of choice for prophylaxis for bacterial endocarditis before a dental procedure. Amoxicillin is used to treat upper respiratory tract infections *(H. influenzae),* urinary tract infection *(E. coli),* and meningitis *(H. influenzae).* Otitis media in children is often treated with amoxicillin. Amoxicillin is also available mixed with clavulanic acid, a β-lactamase inhibitor (Augmentin). Clavulanic acid combines with and inhibits the β-lactamases produced by bacteria. Therefore the amoxicillin is protected from enzymatic inactivation. This combination can be used with penicillin-producing organisms. It has had some use in the management of certain periodontal conditions (see Table 7-2).

Both ampicillin and amoxicillin can produce a variety of allergic reactions. Ampicillin is much more likely to produce rashes than other penicillins. Most agree that the ampicillin rash is not of an allergic or immunologic nature. This unusual ampicillin-related rash is much more common in patients with mononucleosis (almost 100%) or those taking allopurinol. Cross-allergenicity between penicillin VK, amoxicillin, and ampicillin is complete (omitting the "weird" ampicillin rash).

♦ EXTENDED-SPECTRUM PENICILLINS

Carbenicillin (kar-ben-i-SILL-in) has a wider spectrum of action than penicillin G, with special activity against *Pseudomonas aeruginosa* and some strains of *Proteus.* It is not penicillinase resistant and is available parenterally to treat systemic infections.

Drug	Food	Metabolism/ Excretion	Dose
TABLE 7-4 MACROLIDES			
Erythromycin			
Base (E-Mycin, Ery-Tab, ERYC, PCE, various)	MT	Hepatic, in bile	250-500 mg q6h
Stearate (Erythrocin)	MT	Hepatic, in bile	250-500 mg q6h
Estolate (Ilosone)	OK	Hepatic, in bile	250-500 mg q6h
Ethyl succinate (EES)	OK	Hepatic, in bile	400-800 mg q6h
Azithromycin (Zithromax)	MT	Unchanged in bile	500 mg stat, then 250 mg qd
Clarithromycin (Biaxin)	OK	Metabolized to active; renal	500 mg bid

bid, Twice a day; *MT,* take on an empty stomach (1 hour before or 2 hours after eating); *OK,* may take without regard to meals; *qd,* daily.

MACROLIDES

The macrolide antibiotics consist of erythromycin, clarithromycin, and azithromycin (Table 7-4).

Erythromycin

♦ MECHANISM AND SPECTRUM

Erythromycin is usually bacteriostatic and interferes with protein synthesis by inhibiting the enzyme peptidyl transferase at the 50S ribosomal subunit. Its spectrum of action closely resembles that of penicillin against gram-positive bacteria. It is also the drug of choice for *Bordetella, Legionella,* and *Actinomyces* organisms, *Mycoplasma pneumoniae, Entamoeba histolytica,* some *Chlamydia* species, and diphtheria. It is also indicated for streptococcal and staphylococcal infections.

◆ PHARMACOKINETICS

Erythromycin is administered orally as tablets and capsules, oral suspensions in IV and IM forms, and in topical preparations. Because erythromycin is broken down in the gastric fluid, it is formulated as an enteric-coated tablet, capsule, or insoluble ester to reduce degradation by stomach acid. It should be administered 2 hours before or 2 hours after meals (see Table 7-4). The peak blood level varies between 1 and 6 hours. Although food reduces the absorption of erythromycin, it may be necessary to administer it with food to minimize its adverse gastrointestinal effects. Its half-life is 2 hours.

◆ ADVERSE REACTIONS

With usual therapeutic doses of erythromycin, side effects other than gastrointestinal are usually minimal. Allergic reactions to erythromycin are uncommon.

Gastrointestinal Effects. The side effects most often associated with erythromycin administration are gastrointestinal and include stomatitis, abdominal cramps, nausea, vomiting, and diarrhea. These effects occur more often in four times daily versus twice daily dosing and with higher (2 gm/day) versus lower (1 gm/day) doses. In one study, at least one gastrointestinal side effect occurred in an average of about 50% of patients, with about 20% discontinuing their medication because of side effects.

Cholestatic Jaundice. Cholestatic jaundice has been reported primarily with the estolate form but has also been reported with the ethylsuccinate form. Erythromycin base has not been associated with this reaction. Symptoms include nausea, vomiting, and abdominal cramps followed by jaundice and elevated liver enzyme levels. Patients with a history of hepatitis should be given erythromycin base or stearate. The mechanism of this adverse effect is believed to be a hypersensitivity reaction.

◆ DRUG INTERACTIONS

Erythromycin can increase the serum concentrations of theophylline, digoxin, triazolam, warfarin, carbamazepine, and cyclosporine. This effect may produce toxicity, depending on the doses of each drug. The mechanism by which erythromycin produces these drug interactions may involve inhibition of hepatic metabolism of these drugs. Table 7-5 lists some drug interactions of the macrolides.

◆ USES

Because erythromycin is active against essentially the same aerobic microorganisms as penicillin, it is the drug of first choice against these infections in penicillin-allergic patients. Erythromycin is not effective against the anaerobic *Bacteroides* species implicated in many dental infections.

Azithromycin and Clarithromycin

Both azithromycin (ay-ZITH-roe-my-sin) (Zithromax, Z-Pak) and clarithromycin (klare-ITH-roe-my-sin) (Biaxin) are newer macrolide antibiotics like erythromycin. They inhibit RNA-dependent protein synthesis by binding to the 50S ribosomal subunit They have activity against aerobic gram-positive cocci, such as *Staphylococcus* and *Streptococcus* organisms, and gram-negative aerobes. In contrast to erythromycin, azithromycin and clarithromycin have variable action against some anaerobes. They are bacteriostatic and can be taken without regard to meals.

The incidence of adverse reactions is lower with azithromycin and clarithromycin as compared to erythromycin. Adverse reactions relate to the gastrointestinal tract, including dyspepsia, diarrhea, nausea, and abdominal pain. Azithromycin has been reported to elevate liver function tests (LFTs) and should be used with caution in patients with hepatic impairment. Clarithromycin can produce an abnormal or metallic taste.

Several drug interactions can occur with both agents because of their reduction in the metabolism of certain drugs metabolized in the liver. Azithromycin can increase the levels of astemizole, loratadine, carbamazepine, digoxin, and triazolam but does not affect either warfarin or theophylline. The peak of azithromycin is reduced by cations, such as magnesium and aluminum, but the total drug absorbed is not affected. Clarithromycin increases the levels of drugs metabolized in liver such as theophylline, carbamazepine, digoxin, omeprazole, and astemizole. Like the other macrolides, clarithromycin inhibits the cytochrome P (CYP)-450 liver microsomal enzymes.

Azithromycin and clarithromycin are indicated as alternative antibiotics in the treatment of common orofacial infections caused by aerobic gram-positive cocci and susceptible anaerobes. The dose for azithromycin consists of 5 days of therapy: first day, 250 mg twice a day (bid), and then 250 mg/day for 4 more days; for clarithromycin, the dose is 500 mg bid for 7 to 10 days. When amoxicillin and clindamycin cannot be used for the prophylaxis of endocarditis and prosthetic joint infections, these macrolides can be used as alternative antibiotics. The dose for prevention of bacterial endocarditis or joint prosthesis is 500 mg 1 hour before the dental procedure.

TABLE 7-5   ERYTHROMYCIN DRUG INTERACTIONS

Drug Interacting	Mechanism	Management
Antibiotics (clindamycin, penicillin)	Interferes with action of other antibiotics	Choose one antibiotic for both purposes; stop one while administering the other
Carbamazepine (Tegretol)	Increased serum levels of carbamazepine	Monitor
OC, BCP	Decreased effectiveness of OC	Use alternative method of birth control (e.g., condoms) until end of that cycle (rest of the month)
Warfarin (Coumadin)	Increased warfarin effect	Bleeding increased
Theophylline (Theo-Dur, Slo-bid)	Increased theophylline toxicity	OK to give 2 doses

OC, Oral contraceptives; *BCP,* birth control pills.

TETRACYCLINES

The tetracyclines (te-tra-SYE-kleens) are broad-spectrum antibiotics affecting a wide range of microorganisms (Table 7-6). Their adverse effects on developing teeth are well known.

The first tetracycline was isolated from a *Streptomyces* strain in 1948. Since then, other tetracyclines have been derived from different species of *Streptomyces,* and the rest have been produced semisynthetically. The tetracyclines are closely related chemically and clinically.

Pharmacokinetics

The tetracyclines are most commonly given by mouth (PO). Absorption after oral administration varies but is fairly rapid. There is wide tissue distribution, and tetracyclines are secreted in the saliva and in the milk of lactating mothers (one-half plasma concentration). Tetracyclines are concentrated by the liver and excreted into the intestines via the bile. Enterohepatic circulation prolongs the action of the tetracyclines after they have been discontinued. The tetracyclines are also stored in the dentine and enamel of unerupted teeth and are concentrated in the gingival crevicular fluid. The long-acting agents are concentrated to at least four times serum levels.

The various tetracyclines differ clinically in their duration of action, percent absorbed when taken orally, half-lives, and mechanism of elimination. Doxycycline is excreted in the feces, whereas tetracycline is eliminated essentially unchanged by glomerular filtration and minocycline is metabolized in the liver and excreted in the urine. Both doxycycline and minocycline may be given safely to patients with renal dysfunction. All tetracyclines cross the placenta and enter the fetal circulation.

Spectrum

The tetracyclines are bacteriostatic and interfere with the synthesis of bacterial protein by binding at the 30S subunit of bacterial ribosomes. As broad-spectrum antibiotics, they are effective against a wide variety of gram-positive and gram-negative bacteria (both aerobes and anaerobes), Rickettsia, spirochetes *(Treponema pallidum),* some protozoa *(Entamoeba histolytica),* and *Chlamydia* and *Mycoplasma* organisms.

Bacterial resistance to the tetracyclines develops slowly in a stepwise fashion. Cross-resistance among tetracyclines is prob-

ably complete. This resistance is caused by a decreased uptake of the tetracycline by the organism. In the study of sensitivity of organisms isolated from dental infections, one-fifth to three-fifths of *S. viridans* and one-fifth to two-fifths of *S. aureus* were found to be resistant to tetracycline. The advantage of penicillin over tetracycline in these aerobic gram-positive infections is clear.

Adverse Reactions

Although most adverse reactions to the tetracyclines occur infrequently, gastrointestinal distress is not uncommon.

◆ GASTROINTESTINAL EFFECTS

The gastrointestinal adverse effects include anorexia, nausea, vomiting, diarrhea, gastroenteritis, glossitis, stomatitis, xerostomia, and superinfection (moniliasis). The side effects are largely related to local irritation from alteration of the oral, gastric, and enteric flora.

If diarrhea occurs in a patient receiving tetracycline, the possibility of infectious enteritis, such as staphylococcal enterocolitis, intestinal candidiasis, and pseudomembranous colitis (secondary to *Clostridium difficile* overgrowth), must be ruled out. Some patients taking tetracyclines have developed a yellowish-brown discoloration of the tongue. This can occur with either topical or systemic administration. Patients with ill-fitting dentures are likely to have candidiasis (moniliasis) caused by superinfection associated with the areas of the oral mucosa tissue where breakdown has occurred.

◆ EFFECTS ON TEETH AND BONES

Tetracyclines are incorporated into calcifying structures. If they are used during the period of enamel calcification, they can produce permanent discoloration of the teeth and enamel hypoplasia (see Plate 15). Consequently, they should not be used during the last half of pregnancy or in children younger than 9 years. Tetracycline will affect the primary teeth if given to the mother during the last half of pregnancy or to the infant during the first 4 to 6 months of life. If tetracycline is administered between 2 months and 7 or 8 years of age, the permanent teeth will be affected. The mechanism involves the deposition of tetracycline in the enamel of the forming teeth. These stains are permanent and darken with age and exposure to light. They begin as a yellow fluorescence and progress with time to brown.

TABLE 7-6   ORAL AND TOPICAL TETRACYCLINES

Drug Name/Form	Serum Protein Binding (%)	Normal Serum t½ (hr)	Usual Oral Adult Dosage	Lipid Solubility
Tetracycline* (Sumycin)	20-65	6-10	250-500 mg q6h	Intermediate
Fibers (Actisite)†			12.7 mg/fiber	
Doxycycline caps (Vibramycin)‡	60-90	14-25	50 mg q12h or 100 mg q24h	High
Caps (Periostat)‡,§			20 mg bid	
Gels (Atridox)†				
Minocycline (Minocin)‡,¶	55-75	11-20	100 mg q12h	High

bid, Twice a day.
*Avoid concomitant administration with food or divalent or trivalent cations.
†Used topically in sulcus.
‡May be taken with food or milk but not high concentration of divalent or trivalent cations.
§Systemic very low doses; effect because of collagenase, not antibacterial action.
¶Vestibular side effects, blue oral lesions.

This process is accelerated by exposure to light. The permanent discoloration ranges from light gray to yellow to tan. With large doses of tetracyclines, a decrease in the growth rate of bones has been demonstrated in the fetus and infants.

Minocycline can cause black pigmentation of mandibular and maxillary alveolar bone and the hard palate. When viewed through the mucosa, the pigment appears bluish. Other cases of oral pigmentation have been said to involve the crowns of the permanent teeth (half of incisal surface) and the gingival mucosa. The incidence of this oral pigmentation in adults is 10% after 1 year and 20% after 4 years of therapy. With discontinuation of minocycline, the pigmentation becomes less intense but is usually not completely reversible.

♦ HEPATOTOXICITY

The incidence of liver damage increases with the IV use of tetracyclines. Deaths have occurred, especially in pregnant women. Renal impairment leads to accumulation of tetracycline and may increase the likelihood of hepatic damage.

♦ NEPHROTOXICITY

Toxic renal effects with characteristic disorders of renal tubular function, producing Fanconi's syndrome, have been reported after the use of old (degraded) tetracycline. Old or outdated tetracycline should be discarded to prevent future use. Because the nephrotoxic effect of the tetracyclines is additive with that of other drugs, tetracyclines should not be used concomitantly with other nephrotoxic drugs.

♦ HEMATOLOGIC EFFECTS

Although uncommon, the hematologic changes hemolytic anemia, leukocytosis, and thrombocytopenic purpura have been reported after tetracycline therapy.

♦ SUPERINFECTION

With superinfection, resistant organisms multiply and may cause disease. One common situation, especially prevalent in the compromised host, is an overgrowth of *C. albicans.* Oral or vaginal candidiasis can result from the administration of oral tetracycline.

♦ PHOTOSENSITIVITY

Patients taking tetracyclines who are exposed to the sunlight sometimes react with an exaggerated sunburn. Although the incidence seems to vary with the different tetracyclines, patients receiving a prescription for a tetracycline should be told to use a sunscreen before exposure to the sun.

♦ OTHER EFFECTS

Minocycline (min-oh-SYE-kleen) has been associated with CNS side effects, including lightheadedness, dizziness, and vertigo. Patients who will be driving a car should be warned about this reaction.

♦ ALLERGY

Anaphylactic and various dermatologic reactions to the tetracyclines have occasionally occurred, but the overall allergenicity of these drugs is low. Glossitis and cheilosis have also been attributed to a hypersensitive reaction to tetracycline. A patient who is allergic to one tetracycline is almost certain to be allergic to all tetracyclines.

Drug Interactions

♦ CATIONS

Divalent (Ca^{+2}, Mg^{+2}, Fe^{+2}, Zn^{+2}) and trivalent (Al^{+3}) cations reduce the intestinal absorption of tetracyclines by forming nonabsorbable chelates of tetracycline with, for example, calcium. Dairy products containing calcium, antacids (Ca^{+2}, Mg^{+2}, Al^{+3}), and mineral supplements (iron, calcium, zinc, or fortified foods) should not be taken within 2 hours of ingesting tetracycline. Reasonable quantities of dairy products can be taken with doxycycline and minocycline because there is less interference with absorption, but concomitant administration with antacids or mineral supplements should be avoided.

♦ ENHANCED EFFECT OF OTHER DRUGS

Tetracycline enhances the effect of the oral sulfonylureas, which has the potential to result in hypoglycemia. The effects of digoxin, lithium, and theophylline may also be enhanced, which leads to toxicity from these agents with narrow therapeutic indices. Furosemide's toxicity may also be increased by tetracycline.

♦ REDUCED DOXYCYCLINE EFFECT

The barbiturates and phenytoin can reduce the action of doxycycline. The mechanism is stimulation of hepatic microsomal enzymes so that doxycycline is metabolized more rapidly.

♦ GENERAL ANTIBIOTIC INTERACTIONS

Like all the antibiotics, tetracyclines may reduce the effectiveness of oral contraceptives or increase the effectiveness of oral anticoagulants. Also, in most instances, mixing tetracyclines with another antibiotic results in antagonism, especially if the other antibiotic is bactericidal.

Uses

Tetracyclines, including both tetracycline and doxycycline, have extensive medical and dental use.

♦ MEDICAL

Although active against a wide variety of microorganisms, tetracyclines are rarely the drug of choice for a specific infection. Occasionally, they are alternative drugs to treat chlamydial and rickettsial infections. They are used to treat acne (topically and systemically), pulmonary infections in patients with chronic obstructive pulmonary disease (COPD), and traveler's diarrhea. Tetracyclines should not be used for prophylaxis against infective endocarditis except in one unusual situation in dentistry, which is discussed in the next section.

♦ DENTAL

Tetracyclines are not indicated as the drug of choice or the alternative drug of choice for dental infections unrelated to periodontal disease. They are often used for certain periodontal conditions. Conventional treatment with local measures should have failed before tetracycline therapy is initiated. A potential advantage of the tetracyclines in treatment of certain periodontal situations relates to their ability to concentrate in the gingival crevicular fluid. Because long-acting tetracyclines are concentrated to a greater extent in the gingival fluid and they require once-daily dosing, they may have some advantage over tetracycline itself. The ideal tetracycline therapy would be delivered directly to the gingival crevice, thereby greatly reducing the systemic dose. A variety of plastic strips, hollow fibers, or collars to deliver the tetracycline directly to the sulcus are being used but continue to be evaluated.

CLINDAMYCIN

Clindamycin (klin-da-MYE-sin) (Cleocin) is a bacteriostatic antibiotic effective primarily against gram-positive organisms and anaerobic *Bacteroides* species. Clindamycin is produced by adding a −Cl group to lincomycin, which is elaborated by *Streptomyces lincolnensis,* found in a soil sample taken near Lincoln, Nebraska. Clindamycin is structurally unrelated to any other antimicrobial agent other than lincomycin, which is not used.

Pharmacokinetics

Clindamycin may be administered orally, topically, intramuscularly, intravenously, or vaginally. Oral clindamycin is well absorbed, and food does not interfere with its absorption. It reaches its peak concentration in 45 minutes with a half-life of about 2.5 hours. Clindamycin is distributed throughout most body tissues, including bone, but not to the cerebrospinal fluid. Concentration in the bone can approximate that in the plasma. It crosses the placental barrier, and it is more than 90% bound to plasma proteins. Only about 10% of the active drug is eliminated in the urine. The majority of clindamycin is excreted as inactive metabolites in the urine and feces (via the bile).

Spectrum

The antibacterial spectrum of clindamycin includes many gram-positive organisms and some gram-negative organisms. The antibacterial action results from interference with bacterial protein synthesis. Clindamycin is bacteriostatic in most cases, although occasionally it can be bactericidal at higher blood levels.

Similar to erythromycin, clindamycin's activity includes *S. pyogenes* and *S. viridans,* pneumococci, and *S. aureus.* In contrast to erythromycin, clindamycin is very active against several anaerobes, including *Bacteroides fragilis* and *Bacteroides melaninogenicus, Fusobacterium* species, *Peptostreptococcus* (anaerobic streptococci) and *Peptococcus* species, and *Actinomyces israelii.*

Bacterial resistance to clindamycin develops in a slow, stepwise manner. It occurs by mutations in the bacterial ribosomes that result in a decrease in affinity and binding capacity of these drugs. Cross-resistance between clindamycin and erythromycin is often noted. An antagonistic relationship has been observed between clindamycin and erythromycin because of competition for the same binding site (50S subunit) on the bacteria.

Adverse Reactions

♦ GASTROINTESTINAL EFFECTS

Pseudomembranous colitis (PMC) possible but not common.

The most commonly observed side effects of clindamycin are gastrointestinal, including diarrhea, nausea, vomiting, enterocolitis, and abdominal cramps. Glossitis and stomatitis have also been reported with these agents. The incidence of diarrhea with clindamycin is approximately 10%.

The development of pseudomembranous colitis (PMC), also known as *antibiotic-associated colitis (AAC),* has been a more serious consequence associated with clindamycin. It is characterized by severe, persistent diarrhea and the passage of blood and mucus. This colitis, which can be fatal, is caused by a toxin produced by the bacterium *Clostridium difficile.* It is associated not only with clindamycin but also with other antibiotics such as tetracycline, ampicillin, and the cephalosporins. Treatment of colitis includes discontinuation of the drug, vancomycin or cholestyramine administered orally, and fluid and electrolyte replacement. Systemically administered corticosteroids have sometimes proved helpful. Opioid-like agents, such as diphenoxylate and atropine (Lomotil), may exacerbate the condition and should not be used. PMC may occur during treatment, several weeks after cessation of antibiotic therapy, or without any antibiotic use.

♦ SUPERINFECTION

As with other antibiotics, superinfection by *C. albicans* is sometimes associated with the use of clindamycin.

♦ OTHER EFFECTS

Adverse reactions affecting the formed elements in the blood include neutropenia, thrombocytopenia, and agranulocytosis. Abnormal LFTs and renal dysfunction have been noted.

♦ ALLERGY

Morbilliform skin rashes occasionally occur in patients given clindamycin. Oral allergic manifestations include glossitis and stomatitis. More severe allergic reactions include urticaria, angioneurotic edema, erythema multiforme, serum sickness, and anaphylaxis.

Uses

Although clindamycin is effective against many gram-positive organisms, other agents are available that are at least as effective as clindamycin and do not usually cause PMC. The indications for treatment with clindamycin are limited to a number of infections caused by anaerobic organisms, especially *Bacteroides* species and some staphylococcal infections, when the patient is allergic to penicillin.

Many oral infections have been shown to contain a predominance of anaerobic organisms. Many of these anaerobes, such as *Bacteroides oralis, Peptostreptococcus, Fusobacterium,* and *Veillonella* species and clostridia, are sensitive to oral penicillin V. Clindamycin is the drug of choice for some *Bacteroides* species and other anaerobes, endocarditis prophylaxis with penicillin allergy, and some pelvic infections.

Mixed gram-positive and gram-negative anaerobic infections may be treated with clindamycin. The use of clindamycin when anaerobic osteomyelitis is suspected is indicated if the organism is susceptible. It is important to emphasize that clindamycin should be used only when specifically indicated, not indiscriminately, and the patient should be warned of the potential for PMC and informed about its symptoms (bloody diarrhea mixed with mucus). The dose of clindamycin is 150 to 300 mg q6h (qid).

METRONIDAZOLE

Metronidazole (me-troe-NI-da-zole) (Flagyl) is an antiinfective that is a synthetic nitroimidazole with trichomonacidal *(Trichomonas vaginalis)*, amebicidal (*Entamoeba histolytica* species), and bactericidal action. It has exceptional action against most obligate anaerobes such as *Bacteroides* species. As with all antibiotics, resistance to this agent is increasing. It freely enters cells and is reduced into unknown polar compounds that do not contain the nitro group. This short-lived product is cytotoxic, but it causes DNA to lose its cyclic structure and inhibits nucleic acid synthesis, leading to death of the organisms. It affects cells whether they are or are not dividing.

In addition to its antiinfective effects, metronidazole also has antiinflammatory effects. It affects neutrophil motility, lymphocyte action, and cell-mediated immunity. What therapeutic purpose these actions might serve is yet to be identified.

Pharmacokinetics

Taken orally, metronidazole is well absorbed, with a peak level occurring between 1 and 2 hours after administration. Between 60% and 80% of a dose is excreted in the urine. Metabolites account for about 20% of the dose. Its half-life averages 8 hours, but with alcoholic liver disease it averages 18 hours. It is less than 20% protein bound. Metronidazole is somewhat concentrated in the gingival crevicular fluid, producing concentrations that are bactericidal to pathogenic periodontal organisms. Metronidazole is distributed into the cerebrospinal fluid, saliva, and breast milk in levels approximating that of the serum.

Spectrum

Metronidazole is bactericidal and penetrates all bacterial cells. The spectrum of action of metronidazole includes the protozoa *T. vaginalis* and *E. histolytica*. Metronidazole is active against obligate anaerobic bacteria such as *Bacteroides, Fusobacterium, Veillonella, Treponema, Clostridium, Peptococcus, Campylobacter,* and *Peptostreptococcus* organisms. The increased use of antibiotics is resulting in a continuing rise in the incidence of resistance. One should compare the spectrum of action of metronidazole with the bacteria responsible for periodontal conditions and the concentration effective against those bacteria to minimize resistance.

Adverse Reactions

◆ GASTROINTESTINAL EFFECTS

Stomach distress is common.

Metronidazole's most common adverse reactions involve the gastrointestinal tract. This side effect occurs in 12% of patients taking metronidazole. It includes nausea, anorexia, diarrhea, and vomiting. Epigastric distress and abdominal cramping have also been reported.

◆ CENTRAL NERVOUS SYSTEM EFFECTS

Headache, dizziness, vertigo, and ataxia have been reported. Confusion, depression, weakness, insomnia, and serious convulsive seizures are rarely associated with metronidazole use.

◆ RENAL TOXICITY

Cystitis, polyuria, dysuria, and incontinence can occur with metronidazole. Rarely, darkening of the urine as a result of a metabolite has been reported.

◆ ORAL EFFECTS

Xerostomia, unpleasant metallic taste

Another effect that has been reported is a dry mouth. Often, an unpleasant or sharp metallic taste has been reported. Altered taste of alcohol has been noted. Glossitis, stomatitis, and a black-furred tongue are side effects the dental health care worker might observe. These side effects may be related to monilial overgrowth. Appendix E discusses xerostomia in more detail.

◆ OTHER EFFECTS

Transient neutropenia in humans and carcinogenicity, mutagenicity, and tumorigenicity in lower life forms have been reported. Metronidazole is in Food and Drug Administration (FDA) pregnancy category B because administration to pregnant mice caused fetal toxicity. Administration of metronidazole for dental infections during pregnancy is contraindicated. Nursing mothers should not be given metronidazole unless milk is expressed and discarded beginning when the metronidazole is taken and continuing for 48 hours after discontinuing the drug.

Drug Interactions

No alcohol with metronidazole

When alcohol is ingested with metronidazole, a disulfiram-like reaction can occur. Disulfiram (Antabuse) is a drug used to treat persons with alcohol problems (see Chapter 25). Symptoms include nausea, abdominal cramps, flushing, vomiting, or headache. Alcohol should be avoided during metronidazole administration and for 1 day after therapy has ceased. Products, such as mouthwashes or elixirs, that contain alcohol should not be used during this period.

Metronidazole can potentiate the effect of warfarin. The combination of metronidazole and disulfiram has led to confusion and should be avoided. Drugs that stimulate liver microsomal enzymes, such as phenobarbital and phenytoin, can reduce the plasma levels of metronidazole. Before metronidazole is administered to patients, the possibility of a drug interaction should be checked.

Uses

Metronidazole is used for the treatment of infections caused by susceptible organisms in both medical and dental conditions. It has special usefulness because of its anaerobic spectrum.

◆ MEDICAL

The medical uses of metronidazole include treatment of trichomoniasis, giardiasis, amebiasis, and susceptible anaerobic bacterial infections. It is effective against serious anaerobic infections of the abdomen, skeleton, and female genital tract. Endocarditis and lower respiratory tract infections caused by *Bacteroides* species are treated with metronidazole. It is available as oral tablets and capsules; vaginal cream and gel for vaginal infections; topical cream, gel, and lotions for the treatment of rosacea; and IV solution for anaerobic infections.

◆ DENTAL

Because of its anaerobic efficacy, metronidazole is useful in the treatment of many periodontal infections. One notable exception is that it has no action against *A. actinomycetemcomitans.* One advantage of metronidazole is that when prescribed generically it is inexpensive (see Figure 7-3).

CEPHALOSPORINS

"Expensive cousins" to the penicillins

The cephalosporin (sef-a-loe-SPOR-in) group of antibiotics is structurally related to the penicillins. Cephalosporins are active against a wide variety of both gram-positive and gram-negative organisms. The oral cephalosporin products, listed in Box 7-3, are divided into first-, second-, third-, and fourth-generation agents. Most third-generation cephalosporins are available for parenteral use. The orally active cephalosporins are discussed.

The source of the original cephalosporins was *Cephalosporium acremonium,* which was isolated from a sewer outlet near Sardinia in Italy. Because cephalosporins are true antibiotics, they were originally produced by organisms. Those available for oral use are relatively acid stable and highly resistant to penicillinase, but they are destroyed by cephalosporinase, an enzyme elaborated by some microorganisms.

Pharmacokinetics

The cephalosporins can be administered orally, intramuscularly, or intravenously. The agents that cannot be used orally are too poorly absorbed to provide adequate blood levels. The cephalosporins used orally are well absorbed. They are bound between 10% and 65% to the plasma proteins (see Box 7-3). After absorption, they are widely distributed throughout the tissues. Like penicillin, the cephalosporins are excreted by glomerular filtration and tubular secretion into the urine. Their half-lives vary between 50 and 240 minutes.

BOX 7-3   ORAL CEPHALOSPORINS
First-Generation
Cephalexin (Keflex)
Cephradine (Velosef, Anspor)
Cefadroxil (Duricef, Ultracef)
Second-Generation
Cefaclor (Ceclor, Raniclor)
Cefuroxime (Ceftin, Kefurox, Zinacef)
Cefprozil (Cefzil)
Third-Generation
Cefixime (Suprax)
Cefpodoxime proxetil (Vantin)
Cefdinir (Omnicef)
Carbacephem Relative
Loracarbef (Lorabid)

Spectrum

The cephalosporins, which are bactericidal, are active against most gram-positive cocci, penicillinase-producing staphylococci, and some gram-negative bacteria. They inhibit most *Salmonella* and *Klebsiella* organisms, some paracolon strains, and *E. coli. Serratia* and *Enterobacter* species, *H. influenzae,* indole-positive *Proteus,* methicillin-resistant staphylococci, and most *Pseudomonas* strains are unaffected. The generation of the cephalosporin (first, second, or third) designates the width of antimicrobial action; the first-generation width is narrower (gram-positive, few gram-negative) than the second-generation width (gram-positive, more gram-negative and anaerobes), and the third-generation agents (gram-positive weaker, many gram-negative and anaerobes) have the broadest spectrum of action.

Mechanism of Action

The mechanism of action of the cephalosporins is like that of the penicillins: inhibition of cell wall synthesis. They bind to enzymes in the cell membrane involved in cell wall synthesis. The cephalosporin acts as an analog of acyl-D-alanyl-D-alanine to produce a deficiency in the cell walls, leading to lysis. They are more effective against rapidly growing organisms (which explains the potential drug interaction between bacteriostatic and bactericidal antibiotics).

Adverse Reactions

In general, the cephalosporins have a low incidence of adverse reactions (excluding allergic reactions) and are well tolerated. They have more adverse reactions than penicillin VK. The following adverse reactions may occur.

◆ GASTROINTESTINAL EFFECTS

The most common adverse reaction associated with the cephalosporins is gastrointestinal, including diarrhea, nausea, vomiting, abdominal pain, anorexia, dyspepsia, and stomatitis.

◆ NEPHROTOXICITY

Evidence suggests that the cephalosporins may produce nephrotoxic effects under certain conditions. Although some have suggested that this is a toxic reaction, it may be an allergic reaction.

◆ SUPERINFECTION

As with all antibiotics, especially those with a broader spectrum of action, superinfection has been reported. Resistant gram-negative organisms are often the culprits.

◆ LOCAL REACTION

As with penicillin, the irritating nature of the cephalosporins can produce localized pain, induration, and swelling when given intramuscularly and abscess and thrombophlebitis when given intravenously.

◆ HEMOSTASIS AND DISULFIRAM-LIKE REACTION

Certain parenteral cephalosporins can impair hemostasis or produce a disulfiram-like reaction. Dental health care workers do not use parenteral cephalosporins, and therefore this side effect is of no concern to dentistry.

♦ ALLERGY

Various types of hypersensitivity reactions have been reported in approximately 5% of patients receiving cephalosporins. These reactions include fever, eosinophilia, serum sickness, rashes, and anaphylaxis. Large doses often produce a direct positive Coombs' reaction (immune mechanism is attacking the patient's own red blood cells). This can lead to a significant degree of hemolysis.

The cephalosporins and penicillin have similar structures; some cross-hypersensitivity can occur. Clinically, the incidence of hypersensitivity reactions to the cephalosporins is higher in patients with a history of penicillin allergy. The degree of cross-hypersensitivity reported is about 10%. Cephalosporins are often given to patients with a history of penicillin allergy, especially if the reaction was mild and in the distant past.

Uses

The cephalosporin antibiotics are indicated for the treatment of gram-positive organisms. The cephalosporins are indicated for infections that are sensitive to these agents but resistant to penicillin. They are especially useful in certain infections caused by gram-negative organisms such as *Klebsiella*. Their dental use includes prophylaxis for patients with "at-risk" joints who are undergoing dental procedures likely to produce bleeding. They are also used to treat infections with sensitive organisms when other agents are ineffective or cannot be used.

RATIONAL USE OF ANTIINFECTIVE AGENTS IN DENTISTRY

Figure 7-5 shows the progression of most dental infections. The early phase, stage 1, is primarily gram-positive organisms; the mixed stage, stage 2, has both aerobes and anaerobes; and the last stage, stage 3, is exclusively anaerobes. If incision and drainage is possible, most dental infections in patients with normal immunity, whether the infection is in stage 1, 2, or 3, do not need antiinfective agents.

Stage 1

Acute abscess and cellulitis are primarily the result of gram-positive organisms. The drug of choice in patients without a penicillin allergy is penicillin V 500 mg q6h for 5 to 7 days (actually the patient must take the antibiotic every day as long as symptoms persist plus 2 or 3 days). For those with an allergy

to penicillin, erythromycin ethylsuccinate or clindamycin may be used (see Appendix D for a flowchart).

Stage 2

During stage 2, the infection is mixed. This can be handled by attacking either the gram-positive organisms or the anaerobes. The gram-positive organisms can be managed with the same drugs as in stage 1. To attack the anaerobes, an antiinfective with good anaerobic coverage is needed. The two antibiotics with the most anaerobic coverage are clindamycin and metronidazole. Penicillin V also has anaerobic coverage. If drainage can be established, antiinfective agents are not indicated in the immunocompetent patient.

Stage 3

In stage 3, the organisms have coalesced into one area and are almost solely anaerobic. Most often incision and drainage is sufficient. In fact, this sometimes happens spontaneously and the patient is "cured" (in his or her mind because he or she does not have pain). If chronic infection persists or if the patient is immunocompromised, use of an antibiotic with anaerobic coverage is warranted.

When a prescribed antiinfective is not effective, there may be several reasons for this outcome. If an antibiotic failure occurs, the patient must be reevaluated taking into account the following reasons why an antibiotic may be ineffective:

- **Patient compliance:** The patient may not be taking the antibiotic.
  - *Did not get the prescription filled:* Was the patient informed about the benefit that the medicine would have? Was the patient informed about the risk of not taking the medicine? Consequences?
  - *Tried and failed to get the prescription filled:* There was a long wait at the pharmacy. The children have to be picked up from school. The checkbook was forgotten. When the patient was told the price of the prescription, he or she was not able to pay for it. The patient was told that antibiotics can interfere with the effectiveness of birth control pills and she did not want to get pregnant.
  - *Got prescription filled but … :* The patient noticed that the tablets "smelled bad" or were "hard to swallow" or "decided to take an herbal product."
  - *Did not complete prescription:* Patients state that they "began to feel better," "forgot to take some pills," "took

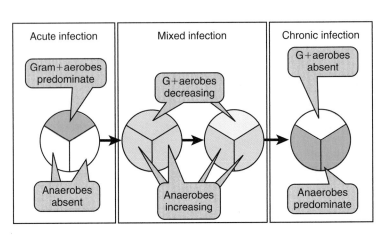

FIGURE 7-5
Mix of organisms present in dental infections over time from early to late.

a few but then quit," "saved them for the next time I have a toothache," and so on.

- **Ineffective antibiotic:** The antibiotic chosen may not be effective against the organism producing the infection. If antibiotics do not spawn a response after 2 or 3 days, consideration should be given to changing the antibiotic (check compliance first).
- **Poor debridement:** Dead tissue, purulent exudate, or foreign bodies were not completely removed from the site of infection.
- **Resistant organism:** The antibiotic may not be effective because the organism is resistant to the antibiotic chosen. Knowledge about the resistance patterns in the dental area is important to consider before prescribing an antibiotic.
- **Concentration did not reach the site of the infection:** There are several mechanisms by which an adequate concentration of the antibiotic does not reach the site of the infection. Lack of penetration may occur because of decreased vascularity, an isolated location or "walled off" area, or a drug interaction inactivating the antibiotic before absorption. Microvascular disease, often seen in diabetics, further reduces the blood flow and the amount of antibiotic sent to the area.
- **Host defenses inadequate:** The ability of the host's immune system to fight the infection is very important in ridding the body of the infection.

ANTIMICROBIAL AGENTS FOR NONDENTAL USE

Vancomycin

Used intravenous (IV) for systemic effect; used by mouth (PO) for local effect

Vancomycin (van-koe-MYE-sin) (Vancocin) is an antibiotic elaborated by *Streptomyces orientalis,* an actinomycete found in soil samples from India and Indonesia. It is unrelated to any other antibiotic currently marketed. Because it has very poor gastrointestinal absorption and it causes irritation when used intramuscularly, it is usually administered only intravenously for a systemic effect. When given PO, it is being used to eradicate organisms within the gastrointestinal tract.

◆ SPECTRUM

Vancomycin is bactericidal and has a narrow spectrum of activity against many gram-positive cocci, including both staphylococci and streptococci. It acts by inhibition of bacterial cell wall synthesis. In the past, resistance did not develop readily, but recently vancomycin-resistant organisms have appeared. When resistance was uncommon, vancomycin was rarely used. After resistance to other organisms increased, the use of vancomycin increased. This led, predictably, to an increase in resistance to vancomycin. Cross-resistance with other antibiotics is not believed to occur because it has a different structure from other antibiotics.

◆ ADVERSE REACTIONS

Except when vancomycin is given in large doses, significant toxic reactions are infrequent. With oral use, nausea, vomiting, and a bitter taste may be experienced. With IV use, an erythematous rash on the face and upper body has been reported (red man syndrome). Hypotension accompanied by flushing, chills, and drug fever are also associated with vancomycin.

Aminoglycosides

As the name implies, the *aminoglycoside* (a-mee-noe-GLYE-koe-side) antibiotics are made up of amino sugars in glycosidic linkage. In 1943, a strain of *Streptomyces griseus* was isolated that elaborated streptomycin. Further strains of *Streptomyces* species furnished neomycin, kanamycin, tobramycin, and amikacin, and *Micromonospora* organisms produced gentamicin and netilmicin. They are bactericidal and appear to inhibit protein synthesis and to act directly on the 30S subunit of the ribosome. The aminoglycosides are as follows:
- Neomycin (Neo-Fradin, Neo-Rx)
- Gentamicin (Garamycin)
- Tobramycin (AKTob, TOBI, Tobrex)
- Amikacin (Amikin)

◆ PHARMACOKINETICS

Because aminoglycosides are poorly absorbed after oral administration, they must be administered intramuscularly or intravenously for a systemic effect. Aminoglycosides are used orally for their local effect within the intestines. Before gastrointestinal surgery, aminoglycosides reduce the intestinal bacterial flora.

◆ SPECTRUM

The aminoglycosides are bactericidal and have a broad antibacterial spectrum. They are used primarily to treat aerobic gram-negative infections when other agents are ineffective. They have little action against gram-positive anaerobic or facultative bacteria.

◆ ADVERSE REACTIONS

The adverse reactions of the aminoglycoside antibiotics seriously limit their use in clinical practice. Their major adverse effects include the following.

Ototoxicity. The aminoglycosides are toxic to the eighth cranial nerve, which can lead to auditory and vestibular (in ear) disturbances, or ototoxicity. Patients may have difficulty maintaining equilibrium and can develop vertigo. Hearing impairment and deafness, which can be permanent, have resulted from the administration of these agents. This side effect is more common in patients with renal failure because the drug accumulates in the body. Elderly patients are also more susceptible.

Nephrotoxicity. The aminoglycosides can cause kidney damage by concentrating in the renal cortex. The blood levels and total amount of drug given correlate with the incidence of nephrotoxicity.

◆ USES

The aminoglycosides are indicated for the treatment of hospitalized patients with serious gram-negative infections. Topical aminoglycosides are used to treat certain eye infections and skin infections.

Chloramphenicol

Chloramphenicol (klor-am-FEN-i-kole) (Chloromycetin), a broad-spectrum, bacteriostatic antibiotic, inhibits bacterial protein synthesis by acting primarily on the 50S ribosomal unit. It is active against a large number of gram-positive and gram-negative organisms, *Rickettsiae*, and some *Chlamydia* organisms. It is particularly active against *Salmonella typhi*.

Chloramphenicol has fallen into disuse primarily because of its serious adverse effects, which include fatal blood dyscrasias such as aplastic anemia, agranulocytosis, hypoplastic anemia, and thrombocytopenia. Chloramphenicol can produce bone marrow suppression with pancytopenia. Although the incidence is low (1:40,000), this condition is often fatal. Chloramphenicol has no use in dentistry.

Sulfonamides

Sulfonamides were the first antibiotics that went on to pave the way for the antibiotic revolution.

◆ MECHANISM OF ACTION

p-Aminobenzoic acid (PABA) analog inhibits synthesis of folic acid.

The structural similarity between the sulfonamide agents and *p*-aminobenzoic acid (PABA) is the basis for most of their antibacterial activity. Unlike humans, many bacteria are unable to use preformed folic acid, which is essential for their growth. They must synthesize folic acid from PABA. Because of their structural similarity to PABA, the sulfonamides competitively inhibit dihydropteroate synthetase, the bacterial enzyme that incorporates PABA into dihydrofolic acid, an immediate precursor of folic acid (Figure 7-6). Drugs that are metabolized to PABA (e.g., ester local anesthetics) could theoretically interfere with the action of the sulfonamides.

◆ SPECTRUM

The sulfonamides are bacteriostatic against many gram-positive and some gram-negative bacteria. They are often used in medicine to treat acute otitis media in children *(H. influenzae)*, acute exacerbations of chronic bronchitis in adults *(S. pneumoniae)*, and urinary tract infections *(Klebsiella* and *Enterobacter* organisms and *E. coli)*. They are ineffective against *S. viridans* but are active against some *Chlamydia* organisms. Sulfonamides are also used for prophylaxis of *Pneumocystis carinii* pneumonitis and for traveler's diarrhea caused by enterotoxigenic *E. coli* or *Cyclospora* organisms.

The readily absorbed sulfonamides are used for their systemic effects and are distributed throughout the body. Some poorly

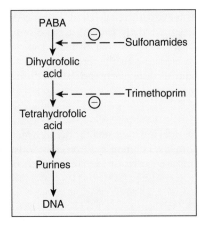

FIGURE 7-6

Location of action of sulfonamides and trimethoprim. They inhibit the synthesis of folic acid at two different locations. *PABA, p*-Aminobenzoic acid.

soluble sulfonamides, when given orally, act locally in the treatment of ulcerative colitis or before surgical procedures on the bowel.

◆ ADVERSE REACTIONS

Drink plenty of water.

The most common adverse reaction to the sulfonamides is an allergic skin reaction. Patients with an allergy to "sulfa" drugs may exhibit some cross-hypersensitivity with thiazide diuretics and the sulfonylureas (used orally to treat diabetes). There is no cross-hypersensitivity between sulfa drugs and sulfites, sulfates, or sulfur.

The allergic reactions may manifest as rash, urticaria, pruritus, fever, a fatal exfoliative dermatitis, or periarteritis nodosa (serious blood vessel disease in which small- and medium-sized arteries become swollen and damaged). Other cutaneous allergic reactions include erythema nodosum, erythema multiforme, Stevens-Johnson syndrome, and epidermal necrolysis.

Other relatively common side effects include nausea, vomiting, abdominal discomfort, headache, and dizziness. Liver damage, depressed renal function, blood dyscrasias (agranulocytosis, thrombocytopenia, aplastic and hemolytic anemia), and precipitation of lupus erythematosus are seen less often.

Patients with human immunodeficiency virus (HIV) are much more likely to exhibit adverse effects (65%), such as rash, fever, or leukopenia, and to discontinue therapy. In patients with HIV, the sulfisoxazole-trimethoprim combination is used prophylactically to prevent *P. carinii* pneumonia.

The possibility of renal crystallization (crystalluria) must always be kept in mind with the sulfonamides. The earlier sulfonamides had low solubility in the urine, and there was danger of crystallization in the kidney. The new sulfonamides are more soluble and therefore less likely to precipitate in the kidney. This is the reason patients taking sulfonamides are encouraged to drink plenty of water.

◆ USES

These agents have no use in dentistry.

Sulfamethoxazole-Trimethoprim

Trimethoprim (trye-METH-oh-prim), an antibacterial and antimalarial agent, and sulfamethoxazole (sul-fa-meth-OX-a-zole), a sulfonamide, are commonly used in combination (co-trimoxazole, SMX-TMP, Bactrim, or Septra). Because sulfamethoxazole (SMX) inhibits the incorporation of PABA into folic acid and trimethoprim (TMP) inhibits the reduction of dihydrofolate to tetrahydrofolate (see Figure 7-6), this combination inhibits two separate steps in the essential metabolic pathway of the bacteria, thus delaying resistance and leading to a synergistic effect.

SMX-TMP (Bactrim, Septra) is bacteriostatic against a wide variety of gram-positive bacteria and some gram-negative bacteria. Its adverse effects are similar to those of the sulfonamides. Approximately 75% of the adverse reactions associated with this combination involve skin disorders.

SMX-TMP is indicated in the treatment of selected urinary tract infections and selected respiratory and gastrointestinal infections. It is used extensively to treat acute otitis media in children, which is often caused by *H. influenzae*. A combination of erythromycin and sulfisoxazole (Pediazole) is also used to treat otitis media in children. SMX-TMP is used prophylactically to prevent *P. carinii* pneumonia in patients with AIDS, *Serratia* sepsis, and systemic *Salmonella* (ampicillin-resistant) and *Shigella* infections. SMX-TMP has no documented use in dentistry, but pediatric patients coming to the dental office may be taking it prophylactically for prevention of chronic ear infections.

Nitrofurantoin

Nitrofurantoin (nye-troe-fyoor-AN-toyn) (Macrodantin) possesses a wide antibacterial spectrum including both gram-positive and gram-negative bacteria. It is bacteriostatic against many common urinary tract pathogens, including *E. coli*. Many strains of *Klebsiella* and *Enterobacter* and all strains of *P. aeruginosa* are resistant. The most common adverse reactions are nausea, vomiting, and diarrhea, but taking the drug with food decreases these effects. Nitrofurantoin can also cause a brownish discoloration of urine. Many hypersensitivity reactions are associated with nitrofurantoin. Nitrofurantoin is used in the treatment or prophylaxis of certain urinary tract infections.

Quinolones (Fluoroquinolones)

Orally effective and active versus *Pseudomonas* organisms

A group of orally effective antibacterial agents, called the *quinolones* (KWIN-a-lones), are chemically related to nalidixic (nal-i-DIX-ik) acid (NegGram). The number of agents in this group of drugs has risen exponentially. This group may have potential use in dentistry because of their spectrum of action. As with all antibiotics, their overuse produces resistance. They are bactericidal against most gram-negative organisms and many gram-positive organisms. They are the first orally active agents against certain *Pseudomonas* species. There is no cross-resistance with other antimicrobial agents.

The mechanism of action of the quinolones is unique and involves antagonism of the A subunit of DNA gyrase, which is an enzyme involved in DNA synthesis. The interference with DNA gyrase results in cell death and resistance is not transferred from a resistant bacteria to an unexposed bacteria. Examples of the fluoroquinolones are listed in Box 7-4. The discussion concentrates on ciprofloxacin (sip-roe-FLOKS-a-sin) (Cipro), a prototype of the quinolones.

♦ PHARMACOKINETICS

Ciprofloxacin is well absorbed orally and is eliminated with a half-life of 4 hours. Both antacids and probenecid interfere with ciprofloxacin's absorption and serum concentration. Patients should be well hydrated to prevent any possibility of crystalluria (drink water while taking).

♦ SPECTRUM

Ciprofloxacin is bactericidal against a wide range of gram-negative organisms, including *Klebsiella* and *Enterobacter* species,

BOX 7-4   EXAMPLES OF FLUOROQUINOLONES
Ciprofloxacin (Cipro)
Enoxacin (Penetrex)
Levofloxacin (Levaquin)
Lomefloxacin (Maxaquin)
Norfloxacin (Noroxin)
Ofloxacin (Floxin)
Sparfloxacin (Zagam)
Trovafloxacin (Trovan)

E. coli, P. aeruginosa, and gram-positive organisms such as *S. aureus*. Its special spectrum is against *Pseudomonas* organisms. Unlike other antiinfective agents, an additive action may result when ciprofloxacin is combined with other antimicrobial agents. The emergence of organisms resistant to the fluoroquinolones and the cross-resistance among the fluoroquinolones is increasing. Use of fluoroquinolones in chickens may be partially responsible for increasing resistance.

Ofloxacin (o-FLOKS-a-sin) (Floxin) is the quinolone with activity against organisms present in dental infections. When the spectrums of ciprofloxacin and ofloxacin are compared, ofloxacin's spectrum of action most closely parallels the spectrum of microbes found in dental infections. After consulting many sources for information about the spectrum of action of the fluoroquinolones, the conclusion reached is that intraspecies variation is at least as great as interspecies variation. In other words, spectrum of action is difficult to predict and depends on which sample of microorganisms is tested. Because of this action, ciprofloxacin or other quinolones may be used in dentistry in the future.

♦ ADVERSE REACTIONS

Gastrointestinal Effects. Nausea, diarrhea, vomiting, painful oral mucosa, bad taste, and oral candidiasis have been reported. Pseudomembranous colitis has been seen in patients taking quinolones.

Central Nervous System Effects. CNS adverse reactions include headache, restlessness, lightheadedness, and insomnia. CNS stimulation has been noted.

Hypersensitivity. Rash, pruritus, urticaria, hyperpigmentation, and edema of the lips have been noted. Fluoroquinolones are associated with photosensitivity reactions when the patient is exposed to the sun. The patient should be advised to use sunscreen or wear clothes that cover the whole body. A few anaphylactic reactions have been reported.

Other Effects. Disturbed vision, joint pain, renal problems, and palpitations have rarely been reported. An unusual reaction affecting the Achilles tendon has become fairly common in patients taking quinolones. These agents can produce tendonitis or tendon rupture in the Achilles tendon, so exercise should be limited. Hepatotoxicity has rarely been attributed to the quinolones.

Pregnancy and Nursing Considerations. Ciprofloxacin is contraindicated in the pregnant or nursing woman.

♦ USES

Ciprofloxacin is indicated for lower respiratory tract, skin, bone and joint, and urinary tract infections caused by susceptible organisms. Because of the spectrum of the quinolones, future use may include dental periodontal disease. In summary, the new quinolones have an advantage over other antimicrobial agents because of their unique mechanism of action, making the development and transfer of resistance more difficult. Their gram-negative spectrum coupled with their oral efficacy and bactericidal action makes these agents a welcome addition to the antimicrobial armamentarium. Many more members of this group of agents currently have been released, and more wait in the wings. Overuse of these agents has already begun, and it is hoped that they do not become much less useful as a result of overprescribing.

ANTITUBERCULOSIS AGENTS

The treatment of tuberculosis (TB), a disease caused by the acid-fast bacterium *Mycobacterium tuberculosis,* is difficult for several reasons.

- First, patients with TB often have inadequate defense mechanisms (e.g., AIDS).
- Second, tubercle bacilli develop resistant strains easily and possess unusual metabolic characteristics, including long periods of inactivity (they become dormant) when they are resistant to treatment.
- Third, most of the drugs available are not bactericidal and because of their toxicity often cannot be used in sufficient doses.
- Finally, people using antituberculosis agents often do not take them as prescribed.

For these reasons, the development of multidrug-resistant TB (MDR TB) has continued to increase because of its spread in patients with HIV, the homeless, and in other countries. (On an airline flight, a patient with active TB has been reported to have infected several other passengers. The latest report of the spread of TB infection occurred in a fast-food line.) The newest development in the worldwide problem with TB is the practice of manufacturing and selling drugs used for treatment of TB containing only a fraction of the labeled amount (counterfeit tablets).

Treatment of TB relies almost entirely on chemotherapy (Table 7-7). Because of the problem of resistance, at least three drugs are administered concurrently in all active cases. Isoniazid (INH), rifampin, and pyrazinamide are combined for the treatment of pulmonary TB. INH and rifampin are continued every day for 9 to 12 months. Pyrazinamide is continued for 2 months. With susceptible organisms, a patient, if compliant, usually becomes noninfective within 2 to 3 weeks. This compliance presents a problem because patients often stop taking their medication before the designated time.

The Centers for Disease Control and Prevention (CDC) recommends that the following patients receive INH because they are at risk of developing TB: close contacts of recently diagnosed patients, patients with a positive skin test and radiographic findings consistent with nonprogressive TB, patients whose skin test has become positive (converted), and immunosuppressed patients. If patients have been vaccinated against TB (with Bacillus Calmette-Guérin [BCG]), skin tests (purified protein derivative [PPD]) will always be positive, and chest x-rays are required for screening. Because many people have TB, it is not unlikely that a TB-positive person may come in and request treatment. If a person with active TB seeks oral health care, contact that person's physician and delay health care until the disease is no longer in the active state.

Isoniazid

Isoniazid (eye-soe-NYE-a-zid) (Laniazid), or INH, is bactericidal only against actively growing tubercle bacilli. The mechanism of action may relate to inhibition of mycolic acid synthesis resulting in disruption of the bacterial cell wall. "Resting" bacilli exposed to the drug are able to resume normal growth when the drug is removed. Within a few weeks after beginning therapy, resistant strains develop.

◆ PHARMACOKINETICS

INH is readily absorbed from the gastrointestinal tract and is distributed throughout the body. Its metabolism varies by race. Most Eskimos and Japanese are fast acetylators, whereas whites and blacks in the United States are split 50-50 between fast and slow acetylators. The ability to acetylate rapidly is inherited as an autosomal dominant trait. Whether this ability to metabolize INH rapidly is related to the chance of developing INH-induced

TABLE 7-7   ANTITUBERCULOSIS AGENTS

Drug Name	Dose	Side Effects	Comments
Isoniazid (INH, Laniazid)	300 mg/day; 900 mg 2 × wk	Hepatitis (acetaminophen, alcohol exacerbates); peripheral neuropathy, give pyridoxine (vitamin B_6); CNS toxicity; GI	Alone for conversion or prophylaxis; combined with other TB drugs for treatment
Rifampin (Rifadin, Rimactane) Rifapentine (Priftin)*	600 mg/day	GI (nausea, vomiting, anorexia, pseudomembranous colitis); rash; kidney (hematuria, pyuria, or proteinuria); hepatitis (alcohol exacerbates); CNS (mood changes, fatigue); blood dyscrasias	Reddish-orange to reddish-brown discoloration of urine, feces, saliva, sputum, sweat, and tears (discolor contact lenses permanently); induces enzymes
PZA	50-70 mg/kg 2 × wk	Hepatotoxicity; nausea, vomiting; hyperuricemia (gouty attack)	Used with ciprofloxacin for MDR TB
Rifater		Isoniazid + rifampin + PZA	
Ethambutol (Myambutol)	15 mg/kg/day	Retrobulbar optic neuritis (eye examination for visual fields and acuity and red-green discrimination); peripheral neuritis; gouty arthritis; GI symptoms; CNS (confusion)	
Streptomycin	15 mg/kg/day; max 1 g	Ototoxicity (vertigo), nephrotoxicity	Given by IM injection; dose adjusted per renal function

TB, Tuberculosis; *CNS,* central nervous system; *GI,* gastrointestinal; *IM,* intramuscular; *INH,* isonicotinyl hydrazine; *MDR TB,* multidrug-resistant tuberculosis; *PZA,* pyrazinamide.
*Cyclopentyl rifamycin.

hepatitis is unknown. The half-life for fast acetylators is 1.5 hours and for slow acetylators is 3 hours.

◆ ADVERSE REACTIONS

The incidence of all adverse reactions to INH is approximately 5%. The most common adverse reaction, occurring in about 20% of patients, involves the nervous system, which may be a result of INH causing vitamin B_6 depletion. Peripheral and optic neuritis, muscle twitching, toxic encephalopathy, insomnia, restlessness, sedation, incoordination, convulsions, and even psychoses have been reported. These neurotoxic symptoms can be prevented by coadministration of pyridoxine (vitamin B_6).

The other major adverse effect associated with INH is hepatotoxicity. Approximately 1% of patients taking INH exhibit clinical hepatitis and up to 10% develop abnormal laboratory values. Some cases of hepatitis have been fatal. The risk for developing this adverse effect is age related: it rarely occurs in patients younger than 20 years, whereas 2.5% of patients older than 50 develop hepatitis. This differential in incidence of hepatitis by age may modify the treatment plan for an individual patient. Other side effects include hematologic effects, gastrointestinal effects, dryness of the mouth, and a lupuslike reaction or rheumatic syndrome with arthralgia. Urinary retention and gynecomastia have been noted in males. Hypersensitivity reactions, including rashes, hepatitis, lymphadenopathy, and fever, are occasionally reported. The choice of whether to use INH depends on many factors such as patient age, presence of renal or hepatic deficiency, history of seizures, gastrointestinal disturbances, alcoholism, or history of neurotoxicity.

INH is both an inhibitor and an inducer of cytochrome P-450 2E isoenzymes. The benzodiazepines that are oxidized in the liver, such as diazepam and midazolam, may have an increased effect in patients taking INH. Foods (e.g., cheese and fish) and drugs that are contraindicated with monoamine oxidase (MAO) inhibitors may also react with INH.

◆ USES

INH is used alone for prophylaxis or for converters (patients with a change in their TB test results). It is used in combination with other antituberculosis agents. The usual adult dose is 300 mg daily.

Rifampin

Rifampin (RIF-am-pin) (Rifadin, Rimactane) is a semisynthetic derivative of rifamycin, an antibiotic produced by *Streptomyces mediterranei.* Its mechanism of action involves inhibition of DNA-dependent ribonucleic acid (RNA) polymerase, which then suppresses the initiation of chain formation. It is active against *M. tuberculosis* and many gram-positive and some gram-negative bacteria. Rifampin's spectrum also includes *S. aureus, N. meningitidis, H. influenzae,* and *Legionella* species. In TB, resistance quickly develops to rifampin administered alone in a one-step process as a result of a change in the RNA polymerase. Administering rifampin with other antituberculosis agents reduces the development of resistance.

◆ PHARMACOKINETICS

Rifampin is absorbed from the gastrointestinal tract and eliminated in the bile, where enterohepatic circulation occurs. Its half-life is 1.5 to 5 hours and is increased in hepatic disease but unaltered by renal disease. The half-life is reduced by INH

coadministration because of enzyme induction. By blocking the hepatic uptake of rifampin, probenecid increases the concentration of rifampin in the serum.

◆ ADVERSE REACTIONS

The most common adverse reactions are gastrointestinal, including anorexia, stomach distress, nausea, vomiting, abdominal cramps, and diarrhea. Occasionally, rashes, thrombocytopenia, nephritis, and impairment of liver function are seen. A flulike reaction can occur with infrequent administration. Rifampin gives a red-orange color to body fluids, including tears (affecting contact lenses), urine, feces, saliva, and sweat.

◆ USES

Rifampin is used in combination with other agents for treatment of TB. The adult dose is 600 mg daily. It is used to treat meningococcal carriers prophylactically and children exposed to *H. influenzae* meningitis.

Pyrazinamide

Pyrazinamide (peer-a-ZIN-a-mide) (PZA), a relative of nicotinamide, is well absorbed and widely distributed throughout the body. It is hepatotoxic and can produce rash, hyperuricemia, and gastrointestinal disturbances. The CDC currently recommends PZA for use during the first 2 months with INH and rifampin to treat TB. PZA, which used to be a tertiary drug, now plays a much more important role than it had in the past. One treatment regimen includes the use of INH and rifampin every day for 9 to 12 months. PZA is continued for 2 months (Figure 7-7).

If a patient is compliant and the organisms susceptible, he or she usually becomes noninfective within 2 to 3 weeks to 2 to 3 months. A negative sputum sample is required to ensure that the patient is noninfective.

Ethambutol

Ethambutol (e-THAM-byoo-tole) (Myambutol) is a synthetic tuberculostatic agent effective against *M. tuberculosis.* Resistance among tubercle bacilli develops very rapidly when this drug is used alone.

The most important side effect is optic neuritis, resulting in a decrease in visual acuity and loss of ability to perceive red and green. Periodic ophthalmologic examinations are recommended. Other side effects include rash, joint pain, gastrointestinal upset, malaise, headache, and dizziness. This drug is used when other antituberculosis agents cannot be used or resistance is encountered.

TOPICAL ANTIBIOTICS

In general, the use of topical antibiotics is discouraged. Systemic administration is superior in most cases. If an agent is used topically, it should be one that cannot be used systemically. One old and one newer product are mentioned briefly.

Neomycin, Polymyxin, and Bacitracin

The combination of an aminoglycoside, neomycin (nee-oh-MYE-sin), and two polypeptide antibiotics, polymyxin (pol-i-MIX-in) and bacitracin (bass-i-TRAY-sin), is available in ointment form (Neosporin, triple antibiotic ointment).

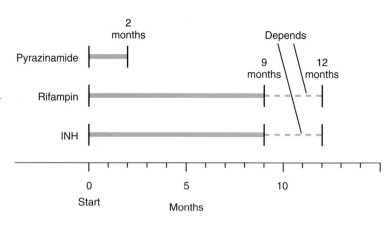

FIGURE 7-7
Treatment and time course of tuberculosis with a minimum of three drugs used. Depending on the recommended regimen, treatment with rifampin and isoniazid (INH) may last between 9 and 12 months.

Neomycin affects gram-negative organisms, and polymyxin and bacitracin affect gram-positive organisms. This combination product is used topically on scratches; if the wound is infected, systemic antibiotics are indicated.

Mupirocin

Mupirocin (myoo-PEER-oh-sin) (Bactroban) is a topical antibacterial produced by *Pseudomonas fluorescens.* Mupirocin inhibits protein synthesis by binding to bacterial isoleucyl transfer-RNA synthetase. It shows no cross-resistance with other antibiotics. It is active versus certain *Streptococcus* and *Staphylococcus* organisms and is indicated for the topical treatment of impetigo. Local itching and stinging have been reported. Mupirocin is as effective as the usual systemic treatments (penicillinase-resistant penicillins) and has fewer side effects.

In dentistry, mupirocin can be used to treat the bacterial infection with streptococci or staphylococci that are occasionally present with angular cheilitis (chronic inflammatory condition at the corners of the mouth). The secondary infection can be determined by its clinical presentation. Because angular cheilitis most commonly is a fungal infection, topical antifungal agents should be used first.

ANTIBIOTIC PROPHYLAXIS USED IN DENTISTRY

Infective endocarditis is caused by an infection of the heart valves or endocardium with an organism. Infective endocarditis often begins with sterile vegetative cardiac lesions consisting of amalgamations of platelets, fibrin, and bacteria. When bacteria are introduced into the bloodstream, they may infect the damaged valves. Infective endocarditis can also occur in patients without predisposing cardiac factors. The difficult question, to which there is currently no proved answer, is this: "Which factors will be predictive in identifying patients in whom appropriate antibiotics will prevent infective endocarditis when specific dental procedures are performed?"

Prevention of Infective Endocarditis

- Dental
- Cardiac
- Drug

Prophylaxis for infective endocarditis is based on the concept (which may not be true) that giving certain antibiotics to certain patients before certain procedures can prevent these patients from developing infective

endocarditis. In March 2007, the journal *Circulation* published the most current guidelines from the American Heart Association (AHA) for antibiotic prophylaxis before dental procedures to prevent infective endocarditis. The newest guidelines recommend that only those people who are at highest risk for bad outcomes from infective endocarditis receive short-term preventive antibiotics before select, common, and routine dental procedures.

According to the AHA, these newest guidelines are based on a comprehensive review of published studies that suggest that infective endocarditis is more likely to occur from bacteria entering the bloodstream as a result of daily activities than from a dental procedure. There was also no compelling evidence in the medical and dental literature that antibiotic prophylaxis before a dental procedure would prevent infective endocarditis in those at risk for developing it. Also, the antibiotics used to prevent infective endocarditis carry risks, including adverse effects, risk of fatal allergic reactions, and the possibility of bacterial resistance.

For every situation in which it may be appropriate to use prophylactic antibiotics, the following factors should be considered:
- The specific dental procedure being performed
- The cardiac and medical condition of the patient
- Risk for bad outcomes from infective endocarditis
- The drug and the dose that may be needed

The updated guidelines also emphasize that maintaining optimal oral health and practicing daily oral hygiene are more important in reducing the risk for infective endocarditis than taking an antibiotic before a dental procedure.

◆ DENTAL PROCEDURES

When dental treatment is rendered (including periodontal probing), organisms are more likely to enter the blood supply, producing bacteremia. Bacteremia is also produced when eating potato chips, brushing teeth, or chewing wax. The organisms can then produce infective endocarditis.

To determine whether prophylactic antibiotic coverage is needed before a dental procedure, see the infective endocarditis decision tree in Appendix D. According to the 2007 guidelines from the AHA regarding prophylactic antibiotic coverage, one should ask the following:
- Does the cardiac/medical condition warrant prophylaxis? Is the patient at highest risk for bad outcomes from infective endocarditis?

BOX **7-5** DENTAL PROCEDURES FOR WHICH ENDOCARDITIS PROPHYLAXIS IS REASONABLE FOR PATIENTS WITH SPECIFIC CARDIAC CONDITIONS

Prophylaxis Is Considered Reasonable

All dental procedures that involve manipulation of gingival tissue or the periapical region of the teeth or perforation of the oral mucosa

No Prophylaxis Is Necessary

- Routine anesthetic injections through noninfected tissues
- Oral radiographs
- Placement of removable prosthodontic or orthodontic appliances
- Adjustment of orthodontic appliances
- Placement of orthodontic brackets
- Shedding of deciduous teeth
- Bleeding from trauma to the lips or oral mucosa

From Wilson W, Taubert KA, Gewitz M et al: Prevention of infective endocarditis: guidelines from the American Heart Association, *Circulation* 116:1736, 2007.

BOX **7-6** CARDIAC CONDITIONS ASSOCIATED WITH THE HIGHEST RISK OF ADVERSE OUTCOMES FROM ENDOCARDITIS

Prophylaxis Reasonable

- Prosthetic cardiac valve
- Previous infective endocarditis
- Congenital heart disease (CHD):
  - Unrepaired cyanotic CHD, including palliative shunts and conduits
  - Completely repaired congenital heart defect with prosthetic material or device, whether placed by surgery or by catheter intervention, during the first 6 months after the procedure
  - Repaired CHD with residual defects at the site or adjacent to the site of a prosthetic patch or device (which inhibits endothelialization)
  - Cardiac transplant recipients who develop cardiac valvulopathy

No Prophylaxis Necessary

- With the exception of the cardiac conditions listed above, antibiotic prophylaxis is no longer recommended for any other form of CHD.
- Mitral valve prolapse
- Rheumatic heart disease
- Bicuspid valve disease
- Calcified aortic stenosis
- Congenital heart conditions:
  - Ventricular septal defect
  - Atrial septal defect
  - Hypertrophic cardiomyopathy

From Wilson W, Taubert KA, Gewitz M et al: Prevention of infective endocarditis: guidelines from the American Heart Association, *Circulation* 116:1736, 2007.

- Will the dental procedure to be performed involve manipulation of gingival tissue or the periapical region of the teeth or perforation of the oral mucosa?

Only if both of these questions are answered in the affirmative would prophylaxis be indicated.

Depending on the dental procedure being performed, patients may or may not need prophylactic antibiotic coverage. Box 7-5 divides dental procedures into those procedures that involve manipulation of the gingival mucosa or the periapical region of the teeth or perforation of the oral mucosa and those that do not require prophylaxis. Clinical judgment will determine the need either for or against antibiotic coverage for each patient.

◆ CARDIAC CONDITIONS

Patients with cardiac conditions can be divided into groups based on the cardiac condition (Box 7-6). The first group contains patients at highest risk for developing infective endocarditis (e.g., prosthetic cardiac valve, previous infective endocarditis) and who suffer the worst outcomes. Oral antibiotic prophylaxis is required for these patients if the dental procedure warrants it. The second cardiac group includes those conditions that do not require prophylactic antibiotic coverage (e.g., coronary bypass surgery after 6 months). Several new additions to this group include mitral valve prolapse and rheumatic heart disease. Although these people still have a lifelong risk of infective endocarditis, they have a much higher risk from a random blood-borne bacterial infection from day-to-day activities than from a dental or medical procedure. These changes were made based on the most current recommended guidelines from the AHA for preventing infective endocarditis.

◆ ANTIBIOTIC REGIMENS FOR DENTAL PROCEDURES

Table 7-8 lists the antibiotic regimens for prophylaxis of endocarditis before dental procedures. These situations include treating those patients with no allergies and those patients allergic to penicillin antibiotics or ampicillin.

When a patient's physician is contacted concerning the patient, the current medical condition of the patient should be explored. Based on the patient's medical status and the current recommendations, the dental health care worker determines

whether antibiotics are indicated. Explain to the medical provider that the choice of therapy will be determined based on the patient's medical condition and the dental treatment being rendered. An agreement between the dentist and medical provider should be reached, but the dentist should not agree to practice outside the recommendation. This will minimize suggestions of inappropriate antibiotics or regimens. When no recommendations exist and the literature is contradictory, the choice should be based on a consensus between the dental health care worker and the patient's physician. If the patient is at highest risk for bad outcomes from infective endocarditis, then the usual regimens should be administered before providing dental treatment.

Prosthetic Joint Prophylaxis

Both the American Dental Association (ADA) and the American Academy of Orthopaedic Surgeons (AAOS) continue to recommend that all patients receive antibiotic prophylaxis before certain dental procedures during the first 2 years after total joint replacement (Box 7-7). Like other preprocedure prophylaxis situations, the joint condition, the dental procedures, and the appropriate drugs must be considered.

Appendix D provides a flowchart to determine when prophylaxis is needed in a patient with a joint prosthesis. Box 7-5 may be consulted to determine which dental procedures require antibiotic prophylaxis.

Whether the use of antibiotics is indicated after the patient is 2 years postreplacement surgery should be determined by those involved most closely with the patient's condition. The ADA and the AAOS recommend that antibiotic

TABLE 7-8	PROPHYLACTIC ANTIBIOTIC DRUG REGIMENS FOR DENTAL PROCEDURES					
		ORAL DOSE (1 HOUR BEFORE PROCEDURE)		PARENTERAL DOSE (SINGLE DOSE ADMINISTERED 30 MINUTES PRIOR TO PROCEDURE)		
Situation	Drug	Adult (mg)	Child (mg/kg)	Adult (mg)	Child (mg/kg)
No allergies to penicillin or amoxicillin (oral)	Amoxicillin	2000	50		
Unable to take oral medications and no penicillins or ampicillin allergies	Ampicillin (IM/IV) or			2000	50
	Cefazolin (IM/IV) or			1000	50
	Ceftriaxone (IM/IV)			1000	50
Allergic to penicillins or ampicillin and can take oral medications	Cephalexin*† or	2000	50		
	Clindamycin or	600	20		
	Azithromycin or	500	15		
	Clarithromycin	500	15		
Allergic to penicillins or ampicillin and can not take oral medication	Cefazolin† (IM/IV) or			1000	50
	Ceftriaxone† (IM/IV) or			1000	50
	Clindamycin (IM/IV)			600	20

IM, Intramuscular; *IV*, intravenous.
*Or other first- or second-generation cephalosporins in equivalent adult or pediatric doses.
†Cephalosporins should not be used in individuals with a history of anaphylaxis, angioedema, or urticaria with penicillins or ampicillin.
Modified from Wilson W et al: Prevention of infective endocarditis; guidelines from the American Heart Association, *Circulation* 116:1736, 2007.

BOX 7-7   INCREASED RISK FACTORS IN PATIENTS WITH TOTAL JOINT REPLACEMENT

Antibiotic prophylaxis is recommended for the first 2 years after total joint replacement surgery in **all** patients. Antibiotic prophylaxis is usually necessary after 2 years in the following groups of individuals:
- Immunocompromised or immunosuppressed individuals, including those with the following:
  - Rheumatoid arthritis or systemic lupus erythematosus
  - Drug- or radiation-induced immunosuppression
- Individuals with comorbidities such as the following*:
  - Previous prosthetic joint infections
  - Malnourishment
  - Hemophilia
  - HIV infection
  - Type 1 diabetes
  - Malignancy

From American Dental Association, American Academy of Orthopaedic Surgeons: Advisory statement: antibiotic prophylaxis for dental patients with total joint replacements, *J Am Dent Assoc* 134(7):895, 2003. Copyright © 2003 American Dental Association. All rights reserved. Adapted 2009 with permission.
Based on Ching et al, Brause, Murray et al, Poss et al, Jacobson et al, Johnson and Bannister, Jacobson et al (1986), and Berbari et al (see Bibliography).
HIV, Human immunodeficiency virus.
*This list is not all inclusive.

prophylaxis before dental procedures, greater than 2 years after joint replacement, be reserved for those people that are immunocompromised or have certain comorbid conditions (see Box 7-7). Appendix D includes a decision tree on total joint replacement.

Noncardiac Medical Conditions

Patients with noncardiac medical conditions may also require prophylactic antibiotic coverage before dental procedures, but lack of agreement among practitioners for these situations causes confusion. For some conditions in this group, there is consensus that antibiotics are indicated or that antibiotics are not indicated. For other conditions there is little consensus. One should consult with the most current guidelines established by the AHA to determine if antibiotic prophylaxis is necessary.

BIBLIOGRAPHY

American Dental Association, American Academy of Orthopaedic Surgeons: Advisory statement: Antibiotic prophylaxis for dental patients with total joint replacements, *J Am Dent Assoc* 134:895, 2003.

Berbari EF, Hanssen AD, Duffy MC, et al: Risk factors for prosthetic joint infection: case-control study, *Clin Infect Dis* 27:1247, 1998.

Brause BD: Infections associated with prosthetic joints, *J Antimicrob Chemother* 23:676, 1989.

Ching DW, Gould IM, Rennie JA, et al: Prevention of late haematogenous infection in major prosthetic joints, *J Antimicrob Chemother* 23:676, 1989.

Fitzgerald RH, Jacobson JJ, Luck JV, et al: Antibiotic prophylaxis for dental patients with total joint replacements, *J Am Dent Assoc* 128(7):1004, 1997.

Garvin J: Antibiotic prophylaxis: making sense of new AHA guidelines, *ADA News* June 2007. Available at: www.ada.org/prof/resources/pub/adanews/adanewsarticle.asp?articleid=2567. Accessed September 20, 2007.

Hersh EV: Adverse drug interactions in dental practice: interactions involving antibiotics, *J Am Dent Assoc* 130(2):236, 1999.

Jacobson JJ, Millard HD, Plezia R, et al: Dental treatment and late prosthetic joint infections, *Oral Surg Oral Med Oral Pathol* 61:413, 1986.

Jacobson JJ, Patel B, Asher G, et al: Oral *Staphylococcus* in elderly subjects with rheumatoid arthritis, *J Am Geriatr Soc* 45:1-5, 1997.

Johnson DP, Bannister GG: The outcome of infected arthroplasty of the knee, *J Bone Joint Surg Br* 68(2):289, 1986.

Murray RP, Bourne MH, Fitzgerald RH Jr: Metachronous infection in patients who have had more than one total joint arthroplasty, *J Bone Joint Surg Am* 73(10):1469, 1991.

Poss R, Thornhill TS, Ewald FC, et al: Factors influencing the incidence and outcome of infection following total joint arthroplasty, *Clin Orthop* 182:117, 1984.

Wilson W, Taubert KA, Gewitz M, et al: Prevention of infective endocarditis: guidelines from the American Heart Association, *Circulation* 116:1736, 2007.

DENTAL HYGIENE CONSIDERATIONS

1. Establish a clear indication for antiinfective therapy.
2. Determine the patient's health status.
3. Select the appropriate antibiotic. Choose the antibiotic with the most narrow spectrum and lowest toxicity.
4. Establish a dose regimen, duration of therapy, and route of administration. Review this with the patient.
5. Remind the patient that antibiotics should be taken on an empty stomach and with a full glass of water.
5. Counsel the patient about the side effects, potential allergic reaction, drug interactions, and food interactions associated with the prescribed antibiotic therapy.
6. Advise the patient to notify the dentist if adverse effects develop.
7. Advise the patient to stop taking the drug and seek medical help if he or she begins to experience an allergic reaction with the antibiotic.
8. Explain the importance of taking the antibiotic as prescribed and completing the full course of therapy.
9. Monitor for compliance with antibiotic prophylaxis.

CLINICAL SKILLS ASSESSMENT

1. Under what conditions is antibiotic prophylaxis necessary?
2. Should antibiotic prophylaxis be given to a patient with prosthetic joint before dental procedures? Describe the factors, if any, that would influence the decision.
3. What antibiotic dose and dosing regimen should be used?
4. What should a patient be told about an antibiotic?
5. What are the adverse reactions associated with penicillin? What should a patient be told about them?
6. What are some reasons that a patient might be noncompliant with medication?
7. A patient has called and complained of nausea, itching, and a rash after taking a prescription for penicillin. What is happening to this patient?
8. What should the patient do?
9. Is nausea caused by an allergic reaction or is it a side effect of penicillin?
10. Can a patient allergic to penicillin receive other types of penicillin antibiotics?
11. What is the role of tetracycline antibiotics in the treatment of periodontitis?
12. What are the different dose forms available and how do they differ from one another?
13. What are the adverse reactions associated with tetracycline, and what should a patient be told about them?
14. Who is tetracycline contraindicated in and why?
15. What is the role of metronidazole in dentistry, and what are its adverse effects? Are there any drug/food interactions?
16. Compare and contrast antituberculosis drugs in terms of mechanism of action and adverse effects.
17. What are the dental concerns associated with tuberculosis and when is it okay to treat a person with tuberculosis?

evolve

8 Antifungal and Antiviral Agents

LEARNING OBJECTIVES

1. Name several types of antifungal agents and discuss their indications in dentistry and potential adverse reactions.
2. Discuss the treatment of herpes simplex.
3. Describe the various drugs and drug combinations used to treat acquired immunodeficiency syndrome.

The antibiotics and antiinfectives discussed in Chapter 7 are effective against a certain spectrum of organisms: bacteria, protozoa, rickettsia, trichomonads, amoebas, and spirochetes. These agents are not effective against either fungal or viral infections. This chapter discusses treatment and management of fungal and viral infections commonly encountered in the dental office: the fungus *Candida albicans* (candidiasis or thrush) and the herpes simplex virus. The viral infection, acquired immunodeficiency syndrome (AIDS), and the different types of hepatitis (A, B, C, D, Ex) are discussed with reference to factors that might affect dental treatment. Other fungal and viral infections that are common in the population are briefly mentioned.

ANTIFUNGAL AGENTS

Candida albicans: most common oral fungus

Although fungal infections are not often encountered in dental practice, when they are present, they are often difficult to treat. Unlike bacterial infections, fungal infections are more insidious. Fungal infections are more likely to occur in patients who are immunocompromised, and these infections can become chronic. Fungal infections can be divided into those that affect primarily the skin or mucosa (mucocutaneous) and those that affect the whole body (systemic). The dental health care worker usually treats skin or mucosal lesions, most commonly within the mouth. These mucosal lesions may be treated with a topical or systemic antifungal agent.

Although there are different groups of fungi, two common groups are candida-like and tinea. Dental health care workers manage mucocutaneous candidal infections, primarily caused by *C. albicans,* with nystatin, clotrimazole, ketoconazole, or fluconazole (Table 8-1). Infections with tinea affect the skin and produce athlete's foot, "jock itch," and ringworm. Both over-the-counter (OTC) and prescription products are used to manage these conditions topically (Table 8-2).

Mucocutaneous candidal infections commonly occur in the vaginal canal. If the patient can recognize the symptoms (by having had a previous infection), an antifungal OTC product can be purchased and used.

Systemic mycoses produced by fungi include aspergillosis, blastomycosis, coccidioidomycosis, cryptococcosis, histoplasmosis, mucormycosis, and paracoccidioidomycosis. Chromomycosis, mycetoma, and sporotrichosis may progress to deep mycotic infections. These serious infections are medical management situations beyond the scope of this chapter. Figure 8-1 provides comparative acquisition.

TABLE 8-1   DENTALLY USEFUL ANTIFUNGAL AGENTS FOR ORAL CANDIDIASIS

Drug Name	Dentally Useful Dose Forms	Comments	Dose	Dose (gm)
Nystatin (Mycostatin, Nilstat, others)	Aqueous suspension, vaginal tablets, cream, ointment, pastilles	Side effects uncommon	*Suspension:* 5 ml qid *Vaginal tab:* 1 qid *Pastilles:* one 4-5 times/day	2.5* (50%) 1.2†
Clotrimazole (Mycelex)	Troches (lozenges)	Nausea	*Troches:* Dissolve 1-5 times/day	0.9‡ (90%)
Ketoconazole (Nizoral)	Oral tablets (200 mg), cream	Hepatoxicity, anaphylaxis, teratogenic, drug interactions	*Tablet:* 1 or 2 tablets daily *Cream:* apply once or twice daily	N/A N/A
Fluconazole (Diflucan)	Oral tablets (50, 100, 150, 200 mg)		200 mg first day; then 100 mg daily	N/A

N/A, Not available; *qid,* four times a day.
*Sucrose.
†0.4 gm sucrose + 0.8 gm glucose.
‡Glucose.

TABLE 8-2   TOPICAL ANTIFUNGAL AGENTS

Drug Name	Route	Spectrum
OTC		
Undecylenic acid (Desenex, Cruex)	Powder, ointment, cream, liquid, foam, soap	Tinea
Tolnaftate (Tinactin, Aftate)	Cream, powder, liquid, solution, aerosol, gel	Tinea
Miconazole (Fungoid, Micatin, Monistat-Derm)	Cream, powder, spray, tincture	*Candida*
Clotrimazole (Lotrimin, Mycelex)	Cream, solution	*Candida*
Butoconazole (Femstat)	Cream	*Candida*
Sulconazole (Exelderm)	Cream, solution	Tinea
Triacetin (Enzactin)	Cream, ointment	
Haloprogin (Halotex)	Cream, solution	*Trichophyton,* tinea
Rx		
Terbinafine (Lamisil)	Cream, solution	*Candida, Trichophyton*
Butenafine (Mentax)	Cream	Tinea
Naftifine (Naftin)	Cream, gel	Tinea
Ciclopirox (Loprox, Penlac)	Lotion, solution (nail lacquer)	*Candida,* tinea
Econazole (Spectazole)	Cream	*Candida,* tinea
Ketoconazole (Nizoral)	Cream, shampoo	*Candida,* tinea

OTC, Over-the-counter; *Rx,* prescription.

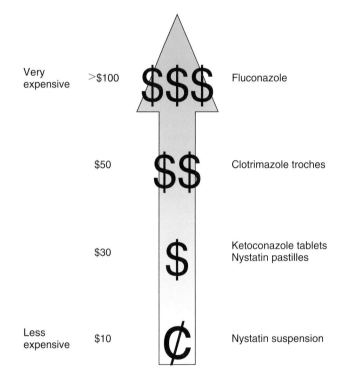

FIGURE 8-1
Relative cost of antifungal prescriptions.

Nystatin

Nystatin (nye-STAT-in) (Mycostatin, Nilstat) is a prescription antifungal agent that is produced by *Streptomyces noursei.* Its mechanism of action involves binding to sterols in the fungal cell membrane. This produces an increase in membrane permeability and allows leakage of potassium and other essential cellular constituents. Because bacteria do not contain sterols in their cell membranes, nystatin is not active against these organisms.

Nystatin is not absorbed from the mucous membranes or through intact skin; taken orally, it is poorly absorbed from the gastrointestinal tract. In usual therapeutic doses, blood levels are not detectable. When administered orally, it is not absorbed but is excreted unchanged in the feces. Nystatin is fungicidal and fungistatic against a variety of yeasts and fungi. In vitro, nystatin inhibits *C. albicans* and some other species of *Candida.*

The adverse reactions associated with nystatin are minor and infrequent. Applied topically or taken orally (through the gastrointestinal tract), there is little if any absorption. When higher doses have been used, nausea, vomiting, and diarrhea have occasionally occurred. Rarely, hypersensitivity reactions have been reported.

Nystatin is used for both the treatment and the prevention of oral candidiasis in susceptible cases. Although *C. albicans* is a frequent inhabitant of the oral cavity, only under unusual conditions does it produce disease. Often, patients affected are immunocompromised.

For the treatment of oral candidiasis, nystatin is available (see Table 8-1) in the form of an aqueous suspension (100,000 U/ml) containing 50% sucrose. The directions to the patient are to swish, swirl, and spit or swallow 5 ml (1 tsp) four times daily. The suspension should remain in the mouth 2 minutes for the best effect. For infants and small children with thrush, half of a dropperful (2.5 ml) is placed in each side of the mouth and rubbed into the recesses of the mouth and on the lesions. If swallowed, diabetics using this suspension must take the sugar content into account (2.5 gm sucrose per tsp) when planning their meals and insulin use.

Nystatin pastilles are licorice-flavored, are rubbery, and also contain sugar. Informal feedback has indicated that patients with xerostomia might not find this dose form acceptable. The advantage of this preparation is that it takes 15 minutes for the lozenge to dissolve in the mouth, thus bathing lesions in the antifungal agent for a longer period. It is allowed to dissolve in the mouth four times daily. The dental health care worker must discuss patients' oral health habits, especially when patients are chronically ingesting these cariogenic agents.

Nystatin is available in vaginal tablets for use in vaginal infections. Occasionally, these vaginal tablets can be used orally. They are dissolved in the mouth four times daily. The advantages of the vaginal tablet used as a lozenge are that the drug remains in contact with the infected oral mucosa longer than it does when in the suspension form and it contains no sugar. The disadvantage is that it is not flavored for oral use.

Patients should be instructed to use the nystatin product for 10 to 14 days, depending on the severity of the infection, or for 48 hours after the symptoms have subsided and cultures have returned negative. Cultures are typically not performed. Some patients, especially if immunocompromised, may require long-term prophylactic antifungal agents to control candidiasis.

Imidazoles

Imidazoles useful in dentistry include clotrimazole, miconazole, and ketoconazole.

♦ CLOTRIMAZOLE

Clotrimazole (kloe-TRIM-a-zole) (Mycelex) is a synthetic antifungal agent available in the form of a slowly dissolving, sugar-containing lozenge for oral use. It is also available as an OTC cream for topical application to the skin or vaginal canal.

Clotrimazole's mechanism of action involves alteration of cell membrane permeability. It binds with the phospholipids in the cell membrane of the fungus. As a result of the alteration in permeability, the cell membrane loses its function and the cellular constituents are lost.

Clotrimazole troches:
1 box = 70 lozenges

Clotrimazole oral lozenges dissolve in approximately 15 to 30 minutes. Patients with xerostomia may have difficulty dissolving this product. Saliva concentrations that are sufficient to inhibit most *Candida* species are maintained in the mouth for about 3 hours. The drug is bound to the oral mucosa,

from which it is slowly released. The amount of clotrimazole absorbed systemically by this route is unknown, but some absorption occurs. Each lozenge also contains 0.9 gm of glucose. The spectrum of action of clotrimazole is primarily against the *Candida* species.

The most common adverse reactions associated with clotrimazole involve the gastrointestinal tract, including abdominal pain, diarrhea, and nausea. Clotrimazole has been reported to produce elevated liver enzyme (aspartate aminotransferase) levels in approximately 15% of patients.

Systemic clotrimazole has been assigned to Food and Drug Administration (FDA) pregnancy category C. Very high doses have been embryotoxic in rats and mice. High doses have caused impaired mating and a decrease in both the number and survival of the young. No teratogenic effects have been found in several other species tested. No carcinogenicity has been demonstrated in rats.

Clotrimazole is indicated for the local treatment of oropharyngeal candidiasis. Patients should be instructed to dissolve the lozenge in the mouth slowly, like a cough drop, to minimize gastrointestinal discomfort. They should also be told to take all of the medication prescribed to minimize relapse. The usual adult dosage is 1 lozenge (10 mg) five times daily for 10 to 14 days (or longer for immunosuppressed patients) or for 48 hours after the symptoms have cleared. Some clinicians advocate dissolving one 100-mg clotrimazole (Mycelex) vaginal tablet four times daily in the oral cavity, like a lozenge or troche. The advantages of the vaginal tablet used as a lozenge are that the drug remains in contact with the infected oral mucosa longer than it does when in the suspension form and it contains no sugar. The disadvantage is that it is not flavored for oral use.

♦ KETOCONAZOLE

Ketoconazole (kee-toe-KON-a-zole) (Nizoral), another imidazole used in dentistry, alters cellular membranes and interferes with intracellular enzymes. By interfering with the synthesis of ergosterol, a cellular component of fungi, membrane permeability is altered and purine transport inhibited. The imidazoles inhibit the C-14 demethylation of lanosterol, an ergosterol precursor. It also inhibits sex steroid biosynthesis, including testosterone, perhaps by blocking several P-450 enzyme steps.

Systemic imidazole
ketoconazole

Pharmacokinetics. For the adequate systemic absorption of ketoconazole, an acidic environment is required. Patients with achlorhydria should take ketoconazole with hydrochloride acid (use straw to minimize damage to teeth). Medications that interfere with the normal production of stomach acid, such as H_2-blockers or H_2-receptor antagonists (H_2-RA) and proton pump inhibitors, reduce the absorption of ketoconazole. If ketoconazole must be taken with drugs that reduce the stomach acid, the ketoconazole should be taken as long a time as possible before or after the acid-reducing drug. All imidazole antifungal agents require an acidic environment for optimal absorption. With the exception of the cerebrospinal fluid (CSF), it is well distributed in humans. It crosses the placenta and is excreted in breast milk. The peak serum concentration occurs between 1 and 4 hours after administration. Ketoconazole is metabolized in the liver, and approximately 13% is excreted by the kidney, with a half-life between 2 and 8 hours. Because of the small contribution of the kidney to the excretion of ketoconazole, patients with renal impairment do not generally require a reduction in their dose. Because the primary route of excretion for ketoconazole is biliary, patients with hepatic impairment may require a lower dose.

Spectrum. Ketoconazole is effective against a wide variety of fungal infections. It is indicated in many systemic fungal infections, including blastomycosis, candidiasis, coccidioidomycosis, and histoplasmosis. Although effective against organisms causing tinea, it is not the drug of choice unless traditional agents have failed.

Adverse Reactions

Gastrointestinal Effects. The most frequent adverse reactions (3% to 10%) associated with ketoconazole are nausea and vomiting, which can be minimized by taking ketoconazole with food.

Hepatotoxicity. The most serious adverse reaction associated with ketoconazole is hepatotoxicity. Its incidence is at least 1 : 10,000. It is usually reversible on discontinuation of the drug, but occasionally it has been fatal. It is thought to be an idiosyncratic reaction that can happen at any time. With extended use, the patient should have periodic liver function tests (LFTs). Patients taking other hepatotoxic agents, those with liver disease (e.g., alcoholic hepatitis), or those on prolonged therapy should be watched closely because they may be more susceptible to this hepatotoxicity.

Ketoconazole, in higher doses, inhibits the secretion of the corticosteroids and lowers the serum levels of testosterone. In men, this effect can produce gynecomastia and impotence. This adverse effect is specific to ketoconazole.

Other Effects. Other adverse reactions reported include headache, dizziness, drowsiness, photophobia, skin rash or pruritus, and insomnia. Fever, chills, dyspnea, tinnitus, arthralgias, and thrombocytopenia have occurred in a few patients. When ketoconazole is applied topically, irritation, pruritus, and stinging are the most commonly reported side effects.

Pregnancy and Nursing Considerations. Animal studies have shown that ketoconazole is teratogenic. The FDA pregnancy category for ketoconazole is C. Because ketoconazole is excreted in breast milk, the risk-to-benefit ratio must be considered before it is used in the nursing mother.

Drug Interactions. Ketoconazole has many drug interactions that have been reported in the literature. Because an acidic environment is required for dissolution and absorption of ketoconazole, agents that alter the amount of stomach acid could theoretically reduce the absorption of ketoconazole (H₂-RA, H⁺-pump inhibitors, anticholinergic agents, and antacids). At least 2 hours should elapse between the ingestion of these agents and ketoconazole's administration.

Ketoconazole inhibits the cytochrome P (CYP)-450 3A4 hepatic microsomal isoenzyme, which can produce drug interactions with many other drugs also metabolized by this isoenzyme. Ketoconazole can increase the blood levels of cyclosporine, warfarin, corticosteroids, phenytoin, digoxin, lovastatin, and simvastatin, to name a few.

Isoniazid, phenytoin, and theophylline can decrease ketoconazole serum levels. Ketoconazole should not be used with rifampin because rifampin renders its blood level undetectable. Ketoconazole may decrease the effect of oral contraceptives; an alternative method of birth control should be suggested. Ketoconazole may produce a disulfiram-like reaction or enhance hepatotoxicity with alcohol.

Uses

Dental. Ketoconazole is indicated in the treatment and management of mucocutaneous and oropharyngeal candidiasis (oral thrush). It can be used prophylactically in chronic mucocutaneous candidiasis. Because of its adverse reaction profile, ketoconazole should be used only after topical antifungal agents have been ineffective or if there is reason to believe that they will be ineffective.

Medical. Ketoconazole is indicated in the treatment of candidiasis, histoplasmosis, and paracoccidioidomycosis. It is also used to treat certain recalcitrant cutaneous dermatophytoses such as tinea corporis, tinea cruris, tinea versicolor, and seborrheic dermatitis.

Dose. The usual adult dose of ketoconazole for the treatment of *Candida* species is 200 to 400 mg orally (PO) daily (qd). It should be used for at least 2 weeks, and 6 to 12 months may be required for chronic mucocutaneous candidiasis. Maintenance therapy may be necessary for certain patients. Ketoconazole is available for topical administration in a 2% aqueous vehicle (cream) for tinea or candidal infections. It is applied once or twice daily for at least 2 weeks. Ketoconazole (Nizoral) shampoo is used twice weekly to treat dandruff, a condition caused by the fungus.

♦ OTHER IMIDAZOLES

Other imidazoles, such as fluconazole (floo-KON-a-zole) (Diflucan), an oral triazole antifungal agent, are used to treat certain fungal infections. Fluconazole prevents the synthesis of ergosterol in the fungal cell membranes by inhibiting fungal CYP-450 enzymes. Phospholipids and unsaturated fatty acids accumulate in the fungal cells.

Fluconazole is indicated for treatment of oropharyngeal and esophageal candidiasis and serious systemic candidal infections. One tablet of fluconazole is now indicated to treat vaginal candidiasis. Fluconazole is used prophylactically against candidiasis in immunocompromised patients or for the treatment of candidal infections that do not respond to other agents.

Itraconazole (it-ra-KON-a-zole) (Sporanox), another systemic imidazole, is used for blastomycosis, histoplasmosis, and aspergillosis. It is the first antifungal agent to be effective in the treatment of onychomycosis of the toenail or fingernail (pulse therapy is used, i.e., on-off-on-off).

Other Antifungal Agents

♦ AMPHOTERICIN B

Used for serious systemic fungal infections

An important agent in the treatment of many serious systemic fungal infections is amphotericin B (am-foe-TER-i-sin) (Fungizone). Because of its side effects, it has earned the nickname "amphoterrible." It must be administered parenterally because it is poorly absorbed from the intestinal tract.

Amphotericin is produced by *Streptomyces nodosus*. It binds to the sterols in the fungus cell membrane, altering membrane permeability and allowing the loss of potassium and small molecules from the cells.

The spectrum of amphotericin includes many fungi, such as certain strains of *Aspergillus, Paracoccidioides, Coccidioides, Cryptococcus, Histoplasma, Mucor,* and *Candida* organisms. It is also effective against the protozoa *Leishmania*.

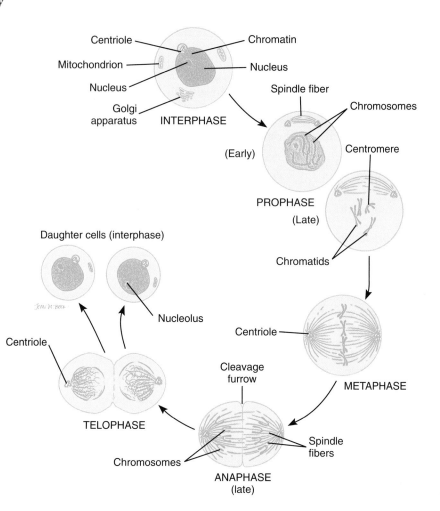

FIGURE 8-2

The process of mitosis. Note the mitotic spindle structure formed during cell division. The drug griseofulvin disrupts this structure and arrests cell division to produce its antifungal action. (From Thibodeau GA, Patton KT: *Structure & function of the body,* ed 13, St Louis, 2008, Mosby.)

The adverse reactions associated with amphotericin are wide ranging and potentially serious, but it is often the only effective treatment for certain serious systemic fungal infections. Most patients experience hypokalemia, headache, chills (50%), fever, malaise, muscle and joint pain, gastric complaints, and nephrotoxicity (80%). Amphotericin has many potentially serious drug interactions.

Topical amphotericin has produced burning, itching, and in rare cases an allergic contact dermatitis. It is available as a 3% cream or ointment. The parenteral forms of amphotericin include liposomal and cholesteryl forms.

♦ GRISEOFULVIN

Commonly used for tinea capitis (ringworm of scalp)

Griseofulvin (gri-see-oh-FUL-vin) (Fulvicin P/G, Grisactin Ultra, Gris-PEG) is an antibiotic produced by *Penicillium griseofulvum.* Its antifungal action is produced by disrupting the cell's mitotic spindle structure and arresting cell division in metaphase (Figure 8-2). Unlike many drugs, griseofulvin's absorption is enhanced by taking it with a fatty meal. It is tightly bound and preferentially deposited in diseased keratin precursors (hair, nails, and skin). Its spectrum includes tinea (e.g., ringworm), *Trichophyton, Microsporum,* and *Epidermophyton* species but does not include *Candida* organisms.

The adverse reactions of griseofulvin include headache, gastrointestinal complaints, and overgrowth of *Candida* organisms in the oral cavity (thrush). Hypersensitivity reactions include urticaria, photosensitivity, and lupuslike reactions. The possibility of some cross-sensitivity with penicillins should be considered because the organism that makes griseofulvin is in a family related to penicillin. Depression of hematopoietic functions and carcinogenicity in animals have been demonstrated. It can also produce a disulfiram-like reaction.

Griseofulvin is indicated in the treatment of susceptible infections of the skin, hair, and nails. Because the drug is deposited only in the growing tissues, the duration of treatment depends on the time it takes for the affected area to completely grow out, which may be from 2 weeks to 8 months. Although there is no known use in dentistry, the side effects of griseofulvin, hematopoietic suppression and oral candida infection, must be considered when a dental patient is taking this drug.

ANTIVIRAL AGENTS

The search for drugs useful in the treatment of viral infections has posed the greatest problem of all infectious organisms. This is because viruses are obligate intracellular organisms that require cooperation from their host's cells. Therefore to kill the virus, often the host's cell must also be harmed. The herpes virus, because of the location of the lesions around the oral cavity or in some cases on the dentist's or hygienist's finger (herpetic whitlow), has been of the most interest to the dental health care

TABLE 8-3 ANTIVIRAL AGENTS, EXCLUDING HUMAN IMMUNODEFICIENCY VIRUS DRUGS

Drug Name	Route(s)	Indication(s)	Comments
Acyclovir (Zovirax)	PO, topical, IV	Primary and recurrent herpes in immunocompromised patients	*Local:* burning *Oral:* nausea, CNS effects
Penciclovir (Denavir)	Topical	Oral herpes simplex labialis (cold sores)	
Docosanol (Abreva)	Topical	Oral herpes simplex labialis	Available without a prescription (OTC)
Vidarabine (Ara-A, Vira-A)	IV, ophthalmic ointment	Herpes encephalitis, keratoconjunctivitis, recurrent epithelial keratitis	
Idoxuridine (IDU, Herplex, Stoxil)	Ophthalmic ointment, solution	Herpes simplex keratitis	Irritation, pruritus, edema, inflammation
Ganciclovir (Cytovene)	IV, IM, SC, PO	CMV retinitis (AIDS): CMV disease prevention (transplant)	Granulocytopenia
Ribavirin (Virazole, Rebetol, Copegus)	Aerosol, PO	Infants with severe RSV	Very costly, difficult to administer, requires special machine
Amantadine (Symmetrel)	PO	Prophylaxis of influenza A virus	Also used to treat parkinsonism

AIDS, Acquired immunodeficiency syndrome; *CMV,* cytomegalovirus; *CNS,* central nervous system; *IM,* intramuscular; *IV,* intravenous; *OTC,* over-the-counter; *PO,* orally; *RSV,* respiratory syncytial virus; *SC,* subcutaneous.

worker. Now, with the symptoms of AIDS being seen clinically in the mouth, the treatment of this virus takes on more importance. Table 8-3 lists some antiviral agents along with their routes of administration and indications. Figure 8-3 separates the antivirals into related groups.

Herpes Simplex

Herpes viruses are associated with "cold sores," and dental practitioners are asked for "something to help." Most antiviral agents are either purine or pyrimidine analogs that inhibit DNA synthesis (Figure 8-4 and Color Plates 1 and 2).

◆ ACYCLOVIR

Acyclovir: activated by herpes enzymes

Acyclovir (ay-SYE-kloe-veer) (Zovirax) is a purine nucleoside that works by inhibiting deoxyribonucleic acid (DNA) replication. It is much less toxic to normal uninfected cells because it is preferentially taken up by infected cells. In the host's cells, acyclovir is only minimally phosphorylated. This explains its excellent adverse reaction profile.

Pharmacokinetics. When acyclovir is taken orally, between 15% and 30% is absorbed. Peak concentrations occur within about 2 hours. Food does not affect the drug's absorption. Acyclovir is distributed widely throughout the body. Approximately 10% of a dose of acyclovir is metabolized in the liver.

Spectrum. The antiviral action of acyclovir includes various herpesviruses, including herpes simplex types 1 and 2 (HSV-1 and HSV-2), varicella-zoster, Epstein-Barr, *Herpesvirus simiae* (B virus), and cytomegalovirus. Several mechanisms of resistance to acyclovir have been found.

Adverse Reactions. The type and extent of the adverse reactions experienced depend on the route of administration of acyclovir.

Topical Administration. When administered topically, acyclovir produces burning, stinging, or mild pain in about one-third of patients. Itching and skin rash have also been reported.

Oral Administration. One of the most common adverse effects associated with oral acyclovir is headache (13%). Other central nervous system (CNS) effects include vertigo, dizziness, fatigue,

insomnia, irritability, and mental depression. Oral acyclovir also commonly produces gastrointestinal adverse reactions, including nausea, vomiting, and diarrhea. Anorexia and a funny taste in the mouth have also been reported rarely. Other side effects associated with oral acyclovir include acne, accelerated hair loss, arthralgia, fever, menstrual abnormalities, sore throat, lymphadenopathy, thrombophlebitis, edema, muscle cramps, leg pain, and palpitation.

Parenteral Administration. With parenteral administration, local reactions at the injection site are the most common side effects reported; these include irritation, erythema, pain, and phlebitis. Because acyclovir can precipitate in the renal tubules, it can occasionally affect the blood urea nitrogen or serum creatine levels. Symptoms of encephalopathy, including lethargy, obtundation, tremors, confusion, hallucination, agitation, seizures, and coma, have been reported in about 1% of patients given parenteral acyclovir.

Uses

Topical. The indications for topical acyclovir include initial herpes genitalis and limited non–life-threatening initial and recurrent mucocutaneous herpes simplex (HSV-1 and HSV-2) in immunocompromised patients. Topical acyclovir has not been effective in the treatment of recurrent herpes genitalis or herpes labialis infections in nonimmunocompromised patients. It does produce a limited shortening in the duration of viral shedding in males by a few hours. It does not prevent the transmission of infection, and it does not prevent recurrence. Although available literature does not support the use of topical acyclovir for management of herpes labialis in dentistry, it is used extensively. No acyclovir products are approved for the treatment of recurrent herpes labialis in the immunocompetent patient.

Oral. The oral form of acyclovir is indicated in the treatment of initial herpes genitalis and management of recurrent herpes genitalis infections in both immunocompromised and nonimmunocompromised patients. It is effective in the prophylaxis of recurrent herpes genitalis infections in both patient groups. It is not indicated for the suppression of recurrent herpes genitalis in patients with mild infections. In the treatment of herpes labialis,

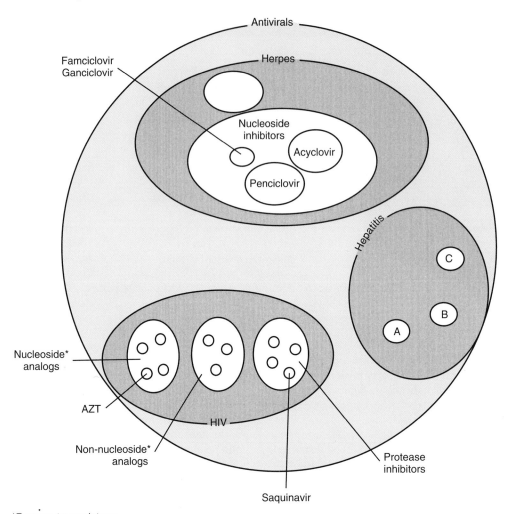

FIGURE 8-3
Related groups of antiviral agents.

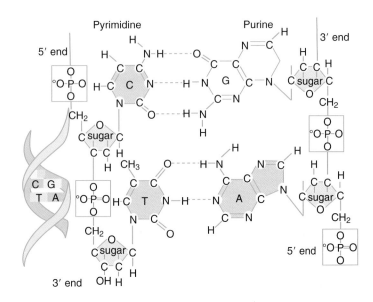

FIGURE 8-4
Purine and pyrimidine base of DNA.

oral acyclovir has shown unimpressive results. Even with hundreds of patients in some studies, only a small difference in a few measured parameters is seen. Higher doses may prove to be effective.

Injectable. The parenteral form of acyclovir is used for severe initial herpes genitalis infections in the nonimmunocompromised patient. It is also indicated for the treatment of initial and recurrent mucocutaneous herpes simplex infections in the immunocompromised patient. Other uses include herpes zoster and varicella-zoster treatment.

Dose. The usual oral adult dosage of acyclovir for the treatment of initial genital herpes is 200 mg every 4 hours (q4h) while the patient is awake five times daily for 10 days. Treatment should be started as soon as the prodromal stage is noticed. The prophylactic dosage for recurrent episodes is 400 mg twice a day (bid) not to exceed 12 months. Some patients may need up to 200 mg five times daily. For intermittent therapy of recurrent episodes, the dose is 200 mg q4h five times a day for 5 days. This is the common dose that has been studied in herpes labialis. Acyclovir has not been shown to effectively treat herpes labialis in topical, tablet, or capsule forms. The slight decrease in crusting or pain does not warrant its use. A larger dose is used in the treatment of herpes zoster (shingles) or chickenpox. It does not prevent the postherpetic neuralgia produced by shingles.

♦ DOCOSANOL 10%

Docosanol 10% (Abreva), available topically and without a prescription, has been shown to decrease healing time by about a half day in patients with recurrent orolabial herpes when started within 12 hours of the appearance of prodromal symptoms. The advantage of docosanol 10% is that it is available without a prescription.

♦ PENCICLOVIR

Penciclovir (pen-CY-klo-veer) (Denavir), available topically, has been shown to reduce both the duration of the lesion and the pain of the lesions on the lips and face associated with both primary and recurrent herpes simplex. The advantages of penciclovir over acyclovir are that it can achieve a higher concentration within the cell and that the drug remains in the cells longer.

♦ FAMCICLOVIR

Famciclovir (fam-CY-klo-veer) and valacyclovir (val-a-CY-klo-veer) are prodrugs converted to penciclovir and acyclovir, respectively, as they pass through the intestinal wall. They are indicated in the treatment of recurrent episodes of genital herpes. They have not been studied for use in herpes labialis. Organisms that have resistance to acyclovir often have cross-resistance with these other agents. Famciclovir and valacyclovir are indicated for acute localized varicella-zoster infections. Intravenous ganciclovir is indicated for serious cytomegalovirus retinitis in immunocompromised patients.

Acquired Immunodeficiency Syndrome

AIDS is the disease produced by infection with the retrovirus human immunodeficiency virus (HIV). Antiretroviral agents are used in combinations called "cocktails" to manage AIDS. Nucleoside reverse transcriptase inhibitors, nonnucleoside reverse transcriptase inhibitors, and protease inhibitors are the groups discussed in this chapter. Table 8-4 lists examples of drugs used to treat HIV. Opportunistic infections often occur in patients

TABLE 8-4   EXAMPLES OF DRUGS USED TO TREAT HUMAN IMMUNODEFICIENCY VIRUS (HIV)

Drug Class	Drug Name
Nucleoside analogs	Didanosine (ddI) (Videx)
	Lamivudine (3TC) (Epivir)
	Stavudine (d4T) (Zerit)
	Zalcitabine (ddC) (Hivid)
	Zidovudine (AZT, ZVD) (Retrovir)
Nonnucleoside analogs	Delavirdine (Rescriptor)
	Nevirapine (NVP) (Viramune)
Protease inhibitors	Indinavir (Crixivan)
	Nelfinavir (Viracept)
	Ritonavir (Norvir)
	Saquinavir (Invirase, Fortovase)

TABLE 8-5   OPPORTUNISTIC INFECTIONS IN PATIENTS WITH HUMAN IMMUNODEFICIENCY VIRUS (HIV) AND DRUGS OF CHOICE

Organism	Effect	Treatment
Cryptococcus neoformans	Meningitis	Amphotericin B
Candida	Esophagitis	Clotrimazole, ketoconazole
Pneumocystis carinii	Pneumonia	TMP-SMZ, pentamidine
CMV	Lungs, pneumonitis	Ganciclovir
Mycobacterium tuberculosis	Lungs	INH + rifampin + pyrazinamide
Toxoplasma gondii	Encephalitis	Pyrimethamine-sulfadiazine

CMV, Cytomegalovirus; INH, isoniazid; TMP-SMZ, trimethoprim-sulfamethoxazole.

with AIDS, so they may be taking various antiinfective agents to prevent diseases such as tuberculosis, *Pneumocystis carinii* pneumonia, herpes infections, and candidiasis (Table 8-5).

♦ NUCLEOSIDE REVERSE TRANSCRIPTASE INHIBITORS

Zidovudine (zye-DOE-vue-deen) (AZT, Retrovir), a thymidine analog, is converted into zidovudine triphosphate by cellular enzymes. This AZT derivative is then integrated into DNA polymerase (reverse transcriptase) so that synthesis of viral DNA is terminated. The reverse transcriptase of HIV is 100 times more susceptible to inhibition than are normal human cells. The nucleoside antiretroviral agents block viral replication and conversion into a form that can get into an uninfected host cell. It has no effect on cells already containing HIV. AZT is well absorbed orally, metabolized by the liver, and excreted by the kidneys with a half-life of about 1 hour. It is distributed to most body tissue, including CSF. AZT inhibits HIV synthesis and reduces the morbidity and mortality from AIDS and AIDS-related complex. Opportunistic infections are reduced in both number and frequency.

The toxicity of AZT is related to bone marrow depression, which can lead to anemia, granulocytopenia, and thrombocytopenia. Transfusions are often required. CNS effects include headache, agitation, and insomnia. Nausea occurs in almost half the patients. A causal relationship to AZT has not been established, but oral manifestations reported include altered sense of taste, edema of the tongue, bleeding gums, and mouth ulcers. Adverse reactions sometimes limit treatment with AZT.

Acetaminophen, indomethacin, and aspirin can inhibit AZT's metabolism and potentiate the toxicity of both drugs. Other nonsteroidal antiinflammatory agents have not been implicated, but current literature should be consulted. A higher incidence of granulocytopenia was reported when acetaminophen was used with AZT.

◆ NONNUCLEOSIDE REVERSE TRANSCRIPTASE INHIBITORS

Nevirapine (ne-VYE-ra-peen) (VP, Viramune), a nonnucleoside reverse transcriptase inhibitor, is specific for HIV-1. HIV-2 is different from HIV-1 in that it is only transmitted from a woman to her child while it is in the womb. This particular form of the virus appears to be centralized in western Africa. HIV-1 is transmitted via sexual intercourse, sharing of bodily fluids, and intravenous substance abuse, and during pregnancy and childbirth. These agents inhibit the same enzymes as the nucleoside analogs, but they do not require bioactivation. Adverse reactions include CNS effects (headache, drowsiness), rash, gastrointestinal effects (diarrhea, nausea), and elevated LFTs. When these agents are used alone, resistance to them develops quickly. This group is combined with the nucleoside analogs and the protease inhibitors.

◆ PROTEASE INHIBITORS

Saquinavir (sa-KWIN-a-veer) (Invirase), a protease inhibitor, prevents the cleavage of viral protein precursors needed to generate functional structural proteins in and modulation of reverse transcriptase activity, preventing the maturation of HIV-infected cells. The difference between the protease inhibitors and the other two groups is that the protease inhibitors can interfere with the action of the HIV-infected cells. Its adverse reactions include rash, hyperglycemia, and paresthesias. Gastrointestinal adverse reactions include pain, diarrhea, and vomiting. Oral adverse reactions involve buccal mucosal ulceration. Ketoconazole significantly increases the levels of saquinavir. Patients taking saquinavir should take it 2 hours after a full meal and avoid sunlight. Although adverse reactions can occur, they are generally less serious than with the older agents. The discovery of the protease inhibitors has made a substantial difference in both the mortality and morbidity of AIDS patients.

◆ COMBINATIONS

In the management of HIV and AIDS, drugs are combined to produce an improved effect. The combinations of drugs, called "cocktails," used to manage HIV or AIDS are changing constantly. Rapid changes in retroviral drug therapy make it impossible to predict what specific agents will be used in a few years. Within each group, the agents chosen are often the newest agents, which have quickly been brought to the market. Because the drugs that patients with AIDS will be taking will be the newest agents, it is important to obtain information about these drugs before planning dental treatment. Normally, patients with HIV will be taking three drugs: a nucleoside, a nonnucleoside reverse transcriptase inhibitor, and a protease inhibitor. An example of this combination is lamivudine, nevirapine, and saquinavir.

Other Antiviral Agents

◆ AMANTADINE

Amantadine (a-MAN-ta-deen) (Symmetrel) inhibits the penetration of the adsorbed virus into the host's cells or inhibits the uncoating of the influenza A viruses. Its common side effects include nausea, dizziness, lightheadedness, and insomnia. It can be used prophylactically for prevention of an influenza A viral infection or for treatment to reduce the symptoms of the infection. It is used in institutional patients (e.g., nursing homes) to prevent the spread of infection during outbreaks. It also has antiparkinsonian action. A new relative of amantadine with similar action is rimantadine (Flumadine). Resistance to both drugs is widespread, and as a result, the use of both drugs is limited.

◆ INTERFERONS

The interferons (in-ter-FEER-ons) are a large group of endogenous proteins that have antiviral, cytotoxic, and immunomodulating action. Recombinant DNA technology now produces interferons. The FDA has approved several interferons currently classified as alfa* (α), beta (β), and gamma (γ) for certain indications, but they are used for other, unapproved indications. Many more are available that have not been marketed; for example, there are 16 known subtypes of α-interferons. The types of interferons available and their indications are listed in Table 8-6. All currently available interferons are parenteral. The most common uses of the interferons are for the treatment of hepatitis C and multiple sclerosis.

Interferons are used parenterally, and injection site reactions, such as necrosis, can occur. The interferons interact with cells through cell surface receptors. Activation of these receptors produces the following effects: induction of gene transcription, inhibition of cellular growth, alteration of the state of cellular

TABLE 8-6   INTERFERONS

Interferon Type	Trade Name	Indications, Selected
Alfa-2a	Roferon-A	Hairy cell leukemia, chronic hepatitis B or C
Peginterferon alfa-2a With ribavirin	Pegasys Copegus	Hepatitis B or C
Alfa-2b	Intron-A	Hairy cell leukemia, chronic non-A, non-B/C hepatitis AIDS-related Kaposi's sarcoma, acute hepatitis, chronic hepatitis B
Peginterferon alfa-2b Plus ribavirin	PEG-Intron Rebetol	Chronic hepatitis C
Alfa-n3	Alferon N	Condyloma acuminatum
Beta-1a	Avonex	Multiple sclerosis, relapsing
Beta-1b	Betaseron	Multiple sclerosis, relapsing

AIDS, Acquired immunodeficiency syndrome.

---

*Spanish spelling is used for global consistency.

differentiation, and interference with oncogene expression. Other effects include altering cell surface antigen expression, increasing phagocytic activity of macrophages, and augmenting the cytotoxicity of lymphocytes. With so many actions, it is no wonder that these agents are being explored for other indications.

Adverse reactions vary, depending on the interferon, but some can be serious and even require discontinuation of the drug. A flulike syndrome, consisting of myalgias, fatigue, headache, and arthralgia, occurs in many patients. Other side effects include CNS effects (fatigue, fever, headache, depression, and chills), gastrointestinal tract effects (nausea, vomiting, and diarrhea), and rash. Oral effects include taste changes, reactivation of herpes labialis, and excessive salivation.

DENTAL HYGIENE CONSIDERATIONS

1. Counsel the patient as to the proper application of the antiviral or antifungal drug.
2. Make sure that the patient knows how to take or apply the drug and understands the importance of completing drug therapy.
3. Counsel the patient on the correct use of oral dose forms of antifungal drugs. Encourage the patient to brush his or her teeth, rinse, and swallow after using an antifungal drug such as nystatin and clotrimazole. Both products contain sugar.
4. Counsel the patient on the appropriate application of topical antiviral drugs.
5. Be aware of drug interactions and the clinical implications of patients taking drugs to treat hepatitis or HIV.

CLINICAL SKILLS ASSESSMENT

1. Name the least toxic antifungal agent useful in the treatment of oral candidiasis. State three dose forms useful in dentistry and describe their pros and cons.
2. State two agents (other than those from question 1) used to treat oral candidiasis. State one problem with each agent. Explain when administration of each is appropriate.
3. Describe the reason for the difficulty associated with the treatment of herpes simplex labialis with antiviral agents. Describe any useful clinically proved effect of either topical or systemic use in dentistry.
4. Explain the significance of a patient taking AZT, ddI, ddC, d4T, NVP, and ritonavir.
5. Describe the serious adverse reactions associated with AZT.
6. Describe how drug combinations are used to manage HIV.
7. List the therapeutic use of two different interferons.
8. Describe the mechanism of action of the different groups of antiviral drugs.

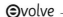

Please visit http://evolve.elsevier.com/Haveles/pharmacology for review questions and additional practice and reference materials.

9 Local Anesthetics

LEARNING OBJECTIVES

1. Discuss the history and reasons for the use of local anesthetics in dentistry.
2. Explain the mechanism of action, pharmacokinetics, pharmacologic effects, and adverse reactions of local anesthetics.
3. Describe the types and workings of each of the drugs used in local anesthetic solutions and summarize the factors involved in the choice of a local anesthetic.
4. Briefly discuss the use of and types of topical anesthetics used in dentistry.

Local anesthetics: most often used drugs in dentistry.

No drugs are used more often in the dental office than the local anesthetic agents. Because their use can become routine, it is easy to forget that these agents have a potential for systemic effects in addition to the desired local effects. Dentists and, in some states, dental hygienists are responsible for the administration of local anesthetic agents in certain situations. With this duty comes the need for an in-depth knowledge of the local anesthetic agents.

HISTORY

First local anesthetic: cocaine

"Painless" dentistry, through the use of a local anesthetic, is a relatively recent development. It began with the observation that the indigenous people of the South American Andes chewed certain leaves that made them feel better. The active ingredient of the leaves was cocaine, isolated by Niemann in 1860. He noted that tasting this substance produced not only the loss of taste but also of the sensation of pain (Figures 9-1 and 9-2). In 1884, Koller noted that cocaine instilled in the eye produced complete anesthesia. Its use in eye surgery was immediately adopted. During this time, Sigmund Freud was also experimenting with cocaine and its effects on the central nervous system (CNS). CNS stimulation, toxicity, and the potential for abuse were quickly recognized as major problems with the widespread use of cocaine as a local anesthetic.

The search for a more acceptable local anesthetic for dentistry continued. Einhorn synthesized procaine in 1905, but it was not until many years later that its use in dentistry became common. In 1952, the amide lidocaine (Xylocaine) was released, and mepivacaine (Carbocaine) was released in 1960. More recently, bupivacaine (Marcaine) has been made available for dental use. The search for the perfect local anesthetic agent continues.

IDEAL LOCAL ANESTHETIC

Although local anesthesia can be produced by several different agents, many are not clinically acceptable. The ideal local anesthetic should possess certain properties (Box 9-1). No local anesthetic agent in use today meets all of these requirements, although many acceptable agents are available.

OW!!!

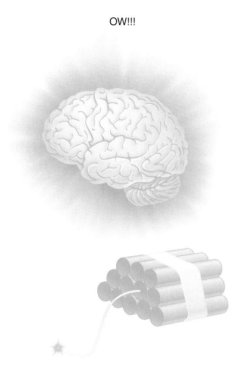

FIGURE 9-1

The conduction of nerve impulses that lead a patient to experience pain can be compared to a fuse. The fuse is the "nerve," and the dynamite is the "brain." If the fuse is lit and the flame reaches the dynamite, an explosion occurs and the patient experiences pain. (From Malamed SF: *Handbook of local anesthesia,* ed 5, St Louis, 2004, Mosby.)

CHEMISTRY

Local anesthetic agents are divided chemically into two major groups: the esters and the amides (Table 9-1). A few agents fall outside these two groups and are called other. The clinical importance of this division is associated with potential allergic reactions. A patient who has an allergy to one group is more likely to exhibit a hypersensitivity reaction to other agents within the same group. Cross-hypersensitivity between the amides and the esters is unlikely. The structure of local anesthetics is composed of the following three parts:

1. Aromatic nucleus (R)

2. Linkage (either an ester or an amide, followed by an aliphatic chain, R)

N

3. Amino group

The aromatic nucleus *(R)* is lipophilic (lipid soluble), and the amino group is hydrophilic (water soluble). The esters are largely metabolized in the plasma and the amides in the liver.

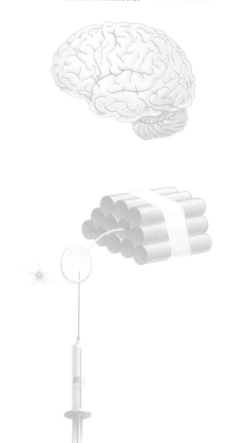

FIGURE 9-2

Using the same example as in Figure 9-1, local anesthetic is placed at some point between the pain stimulus and the brain ("dynamite"). The nerve impulse travels up to the point of the local anesthetic application and then "dies," never reaching the brain. Thus the patient does not experience pain. (From Malamed SF: *Handbook of local anesthesia,* ed 5, St Louis, 2004, Mosby.)

BOX 9-1   PROPERTIES OF THE IDEAL LOCAL ANESTHETIC
• Potent local anesthesia
• Reversible local anesthesia
• Absence of local reactions
• Absence of systemic reactions
• Absence of allergic reactions
• Rapid onset
• Satisfactory duration
• Adequate tissue penetration
• Low cost
• Stability in solution (long shelf life)
• Sterilization by autoclave
• Ease of metabolism and excretion

MECHANISM OF ACTION

Action on Nerve Fibers

Interfere with function of the neurons

A resting nerve fiber has a large number of positive ions (cations) on the outside (electropositive) and a large number of negative ions (anions) on the inside (electronegative). The nerve action potential results in the opening of the sodium channels

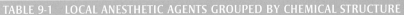

TABLE 9-1   LOCAL ANESTHETIC AGENTS GROUPED BY CHEMICAL STRUCTURE

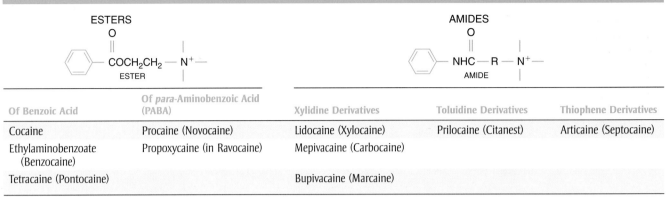

Of Benzoic Acid	Of *para*-Aminobenzoic Acid (PABA)	Xylidine Derivatives	Toluidine Derivatives	Thiophene Derivatives
Cocaine	Procaine (Novocaine)	Lidocaine (Xylocaine)	Prilocaine (Citanest)	Articaine (Septocaine)
Ethylaminobenzoate (Benzocaine)	Propoxycaine (in Ravocaine)	Mepivacaine (Carbocaine)		
Tetracaine (Pontocaine)		Bupivacaine (Marcaine)		

FIGURE 9-3
An action potential involves opening both Na^+ and K^+ channels.

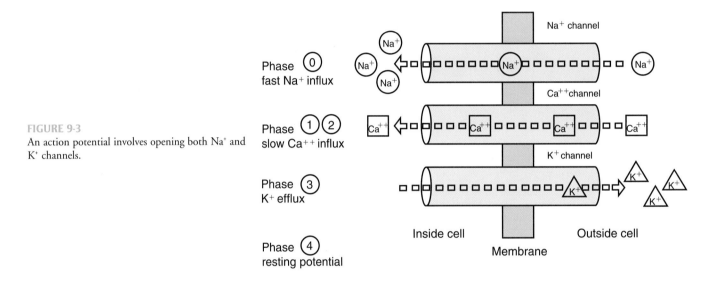

Phase ⓪
fast Na^+ influx

Phase ① ②
slow Ca^{++} influx

Phase ③
K^+ efflux

Phase ④
resting potential

Na^+ channel

Ca^{++} channel

K^+ channel

Inside cell   Outside cell

Membrane

BOX 9-2   MECHANISM OF ACTION = BLOCKADE OF VOLTAGE-GATED SODIUM CHANNELS

1. Membrane potential = −90 to −60 mV
2. Excitatory impulse
3. Na^+ channels open
4. Na^+ flows in (depolarizes membrane [+40 mV])
5. Na^+ channels close
6. K^+ channels open
7. K^+ flows out
8. K^+ channels close
9. Na^+/K^+ exchange
10. Repolarizes membrane (−95 mV)

---

and an inward flux of sodium, resulting in a change from the −90-mV potential to a +40-mV potential (Figure 9-3 and Box 9-2). The outward flow of potassium ions repolarizes the membrane and closes the sodium channels. Local anesthetics attach themselves to specific receptors in the nerve membrane. After combining with the receptor, the local anesthetics block conduction of nerve impulses (thus the term nerve block) by decreasing the permeability of the nerve cell membrane to sodium ions. This then decreases the rate of depolarization of the nerve membrane,

increases the threshold for excitability, and prevents the propagation of the action potential. Local anesthetics may reduce permeability by competing with calcium for the membrane binding sites and by preventing the onset of nerve conduction.

Ionization Factors

Ionization equilibrium depends on pH and pK_a.

The local anesthetic agents are weak bases occurring equilibrated between their two forms, which are the fat-soluble (lipophilic) free base and the water-soluble (hydrophilic) hydrochloride salt (Figure 9-4). The proportion of drug in each form is determined by the pK_a^* of the local anesthetic and the pH of the environment. In the acidic pH of the dental cartridge (4.5), the proportion of the drug in the ionized form increases, thereby increasing solubility. Once injected into the tissues (pH 7.4), the amount of local anesthetic in the free-base form increases. This provides for greater tissue (lipid) penetration. In the presence of an acidic environment, such as infection or inflammation (pH lower), the amount of free base is reduced (more in ionized form), which is one reason dental anesthesia with a local anesthetic is more difficult when

---
*pH at which half is in each form (salt and base equal).

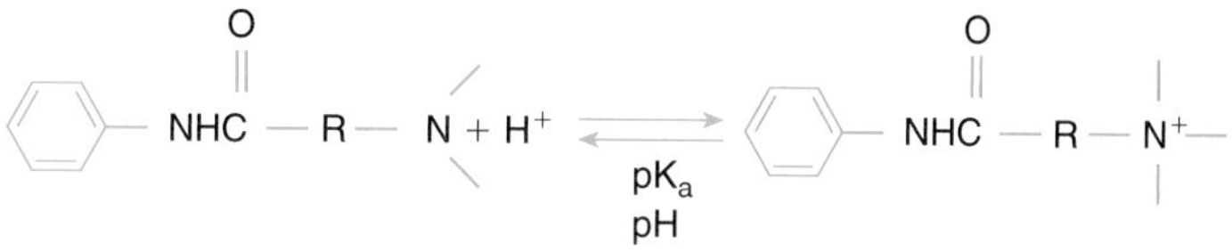

$$\text{benzene-NHC(O)}-R-N+H^+ \underset{\underset{pH}{pK_a}}{\rightleftharpoons} \text{benzene-NHC(O)}-R-N^+-$$

or written simply as

$$RN + H^+ \rightleftharpoons RNH^+$$

Free base	**Salt**
• Viscid liquids or amorphous solids	• Crystalline solids
• Fat soluble (lipophilic)	• Water soluble (hydrophilic)
• Unstable	• Stable
• Alkaline	• Acidic
• Uncharged, nonionized	• Charged, cation (ionized)
• Penetrates nerve tissue	• Active form at site of action
• Form present in tissue (pH 7.4)	• Form present in dental cartridge (pH 4.5–6.0)

FIGURE 9-4

Properties of base and salt forms of local anesthetics.

infection is present. Other reasons include dilution by fluid, inflammation, and vasodilation in the area. Although the free-base form is needed to penetrate the nerve membrane, it is the cationic form that exerts blocking action by binding to the specific receptor site.

PHARMACOKINETICS

Absorption

> Systemic absorption greater, especially with inflammation

The absorption of a local anesthetic depends on its route. When it is injected into the tissues, the rate of absorption depends on the vascularity of the tissues. This is a function of the degree of inflammation present, the vasodilating properties of the local anesthetic agent, the presence of heat, or the use of massage. It is important to reduce the systemic absorption of a local anesthetic when it is used in dentistry. With reduced systemic absorption, the chance of systemic toxicity is reduced. To reduce absorption, a vaso-constrictor is added to the local anesthetic. The vasoconstrictor reduces the blood supply to the area, limits systemic absorption, and reduces systemic toxicity.

With topical application, especially on the mucous membranes or if the surface is denuded, absorption can approximate that produced by intravenous (IV) injection. Absorption is also determined by the proportion of the agent present in the free-base form (nonionized).

Distribution

After absorption, local anesthetics are distributed throughout the body. Highly vascular organs have higher concentrations of anesthetics. Local anesthetics cross the placenta and blood-brain barrier. The lipid solubility of a particular anesthetic affects the potency of the agent. For example, bupivacaine, used as a 0.5% solution, is about 10 times more lipid soluble than lidocaine used as a 2% solution.

Metabolism

> Metabolism
> Esters: plasma
> Amides: liver

The local anesthetic agents are metabolized differently, depending on whether they are amides or esters. Esters are hydrolyzed by plasma pseudocholinesterases and liver esterases. Procaine is hydrolyzed to *para*-aminobenzoic acid (PABA), a metabolite that may be responsible for its allergic reactions. Some patients who have an atypical form of pseudocholinesterase that does not allow them to hydrolyze these esters may exhibit an increase in systemic toxicity if an ester is administered.

Amide local anesthetics are metabolized primarily by the liver. In severe liver disease or with alcoholism, amides may accumulate and produce systemic toxicity. A small amount of prilocaine is metabolized to orthotoluidine, which can produce methemoglobinemia if given in very large doses. By reducing hepatic blood flow, cimetidine can interfere with the metabolism of the amides. (This is usually unimportant in dentistry because only one dose is given. No accumulation can result if repeated doses are not administered.)

Excretion

The metabolites and some unchanged drug of both esters and amides are excreted by the kidneys. With end-stage renal disease, both parent drug and metabolites can accumulate.

PHARMACOLOGIC EFFECTS

Peripheral Nerve Conduction (Blocker)

The main clinical effect of the local anesthetics is reversible blockage of peripheral nerve conduction. These agents inhibit the movement of the nerve impulse along the fibers, at sensory endings, at myoneural junctions, and at synapses. Therefore they may have wide-reaching effects on many kinds of nerves. Because they do not penetrate the myelin sheath, they affect the myelinated fibers only at the nodes of Ranvier. The local anesthetics affect the small, unmyelinated fibers first and the large, heavily myelinated fibers last. This is probably related to the ability of these agents to penetrate to their site of action.

The losses of nerve function are listed in Box 9-3. This listing is in the order in which the senses are typically lost, but some individual variation occurs among patients. In some patients, the pain sensation is lost before the cold sensation. The functions of the individual nerves return in reverse order.

Antiarrhythmic

Local anesthetics have a direct effect on the cardiac muscle by blocking cardiac sodium channels and depressing abnormal cardiac pacemaker activity, excitability, and conduction. They also depress the strength of cardiac contraction and produce arteriolar dilation, leading to hypotension. These properties make them useful intravenously in the treatment of arrhythmias.

ADVERSE REACTIONS

The adverse reactions and toxicity of the local anesthetics are directly related to the plasma level of drug.

Considering the widespread use of these agents, their potential for danger must be minimal. Deaths from local anesthetics are difficult to document, but dental-related mortality is even rarer. Table 9-2 lists the maximal safe doses for common local anesthetics. Factors that influence toxicity include the following:

BOX 9-3   COMMON ORDER OF NERVE FUNCTION LOSS
1. Autonomic
2. Cold
3. Warmth
4. Pain
5. Touch
6. Pressure
7. Vibration
8. Proprioception
9. Motor

- *Drug:* Both the inherent toxicity of the particular local anesthetic and the amount of vasodilation it produces can contribute to toxicity.
- *Concentration:* The higher the concentration injected, the more drug that enters the systemic circulation.
- *Route of administration:* Inadvertent IV injection can produce extremely high blood levels. Even topical administration can produce high blood levels and lead to toxicity.
- *Rate of injection:* The faster the injection is made, the lower the chance that the local area can accept the volume injected. The operator, who has control over this variable, may find that counting the seconds is helpful.
- *Vascularity:* The presence of inflammation, infection, or vasodilation produced by the agent will increase the vascularity and therefore the systemic toxicity.
- *Patient's weight:* The same dose administered to a child and an adult will produce different blood levels because of their differences in weight.
- *Rate of metabolism and excretion:* Amides may accumulate with liver disease; both amides and their metabolites and ester metabolites may accumulate in renal disease.

Children, elderly individuals, and debilitated persons are more susceptible to the adverse reactions of the local anesthetic agents. The symptoms of an overdose of the local anesthetic agents are directly proportional to the blood level attained.

Toxicity

The two main systems affected by local anesthetic toxicity are the CNS and the cardiovascular system.

◆ CENTRAL NERVOUS SYSTEM EFFECTS

CNS stimulation may occur before CNS depression. CNS stimulation caused by depression of the inhibitory fibers results in restlessness, tremors, and convulsions. CNS depression caused by depression of both the inhibitory and facilitative fibers results in respiratory and cardiovascular depression, and coma follows.

◆ CARDIOVASCULAR EFFECTS

The local anesthetic agents can produce myocardial depression and cardiac arrest with peripheral vasodilation. The usual concentrations that are achieved with administration of dental anesthesia would not be expected to result in any of these adverse

TABLE 9-2 MAXIMUM SAFE DOSE* (MSD) OF LOCAL ANESTHETICS				
Local Anesthetic (Concentration)	Epinephrine	Dose (mg/lb)	ABSOLUTE MAXIMUM	
			mg	No. of Cartridges
Lidocaine 2%	1:50,000	2 (3.5)*	200 (500)*	5.5
	1:100,000	2 (3)*	300 (500)*	8.5
	1:200,000	2 (3)	300 (500)*	8.5
Mepivacaine 3%	None (plain)	2 (3)*	300 (400)*	5.5
Mepivacaine 2%	1:20,000†	2 (3)*	300 (400)*	11
Prilocaine 4%	None (plain) and 1:200,000	2.7	400	5.5
Bupivacaine 0.5%	1:200,000	0.6	90	10
Articaine 4%	1:200,000	3.2	500	7

*Manufacturer's recommendations.
†Vasoconstrictor—levonordefrin.

reactions, although deaths have been reported with the use of lower doses of anesthetic. It is postulated that the effect of these agents on heart conduction may produce a fatal arrhythmia.

Local Effects

Local effects can occur with the administration of local anesthetic agents. This is most commonly the result of physical injury caused by the injection technique or the administration of an excessive volume too quickly to be accepted by the tissues. Occasionally, a hematoma may be produced.

Malignant Hyperthermia

| Malignant hyperthermia not related to amides |

Malignant hyperthermia is an inherited disease that is transmitted as an autosomal dominant gene with reduced penetration and variable expression. Its symptoms include an acute rise in calcium, which produces muscular rigidity, metabolic acidosis, and extremely high fever. Its mortality rate is about 50%. Treatment of malignant hyperthermia includes supportive measures and the administration of dantrolene (Dantrium). In the past, it was thought that the amide local anesthetics might precipitate malignant hyperthermia, but currently they are no longer implicated. Patients with a family history of malignant hyperthermia can be given amide local anesthetic agents. Halothane, the inhalation anesthetic, and succinylcholine, the neuromuscular blocking agent, are the most common agents precipitating malignant hyperthermia.

Pregnancy and Nursing Considerations

Elective dental treatment should be rendered before a patient becomes pregnant. If dental treatment is needed, however, most sources suggest that lidocaine may be administered to a pregnant woman. Fetal bradycardia has been reported when larger doses are administered to the mother near term. Both lidocaine and prilocaine are in Food and Drug Administration (FDA) pregnancy category B, whereas mepivacaine, articaine, and bupivacaine are category C drugs.

If a local anesthetic is needed, lidocaine in the smallest effective dose should be used. Usual doses of local anesthetics given to nursing mothers will not affect the health of the normal nursing infant.

Allergy

| Probably no allergies to amides |

Allergic reactions that result from local anesthetics have been reported, and they range from rash to anaphylactic shock. An allergy history should be elicited from each patient before a local anesthetic agent is chosen. Esters have a much greater allergic potential; in fact, there is some question about whether amides can produce allergic reactions at all. Cross-allergenicity exists between the esters but does not seem to occur between the amides in the xylidine and toluidine groups.

Patients giving a history of allergies to all local anesthetic agents may be "tested" by giving them an amide by injection. Of course, before contemplating administering this test, trained emergency personnel, equipment, and drugs should be assembled. Use of skin testing to determine local anesthetic allergies is unreliable because it can give both false-positive and false-negative results.

Another approach to treating a patient with a history of allergies to all the local anesthetic agents is to use the antihistamine diphenhydramine (Benadryl) as a local anesthetic. Antihistamines, because of their similarity in structure to local anesthetics, have some local anesthetic action. Diphenhydramine (Benadryl) in a concentration of 1% plus 1:100,000 epinephrine is recommended to be given by injection to produce a block. There is no prepared product available, so this combination must be prepared from its constituents. Histories of allergic reactions to local anesthetics may have been the result of the preservative methylparaben. It is no longer present in any local anesthetic dental cartridges.

Local anesthetics with vasoconstrictors also contain a sulfite that serves as an antioxidant. In sulfite-sensitive patients, the sulfites may produce a hypersensitivity reaction that exhibits itself as an acute asthmatic attack. This reaction is the same as the "salad bar" syndrome, a hypersensitivity reaction to sulfites. In the past, certain restaurant foods offered at salad bars, such as lettuce, contained sulfites to prevent browning. Sulfites were used to help the lettuce and other greens retain their green color. Some restaurant menus still describe salad bars as "sulfite free." Deaths of hypersensitive asthmatics who ate in restaurants have been reported. The nature of the reaction involves bronchoconstriction and anaphylactic reactions. A patient with an allergy to "sulfa" drugs does not exhibit cross-hypersensitivity with sulfites. Appendix D discusses the implications of a sulfite hypersensitivity in more detail.

COMPOSITION OF LOCAL ANESTHETIC SOLUTIONS

In addition to the local anesthetic agent, local anesthetic solutions usually contain several other ingredients such as the following:

- *Vasoconstrictor:* A vasoconstrictor, such as epinephrine, is added to local anesthetic solutions to retard absorption, reduce systemic toxicity, and prolong its duration of action.

| Sulfites: asthmatic hypersensitivity reaction |

- *Antioxidant:* An antioxidant (sodium metabisulfite, sodium bisulfite, or acetone sodium bisulfite) is included in local anesthetic solutions to retard oxidation of the epinephrine. The antioxidants, such as sodium bisulfite or metabisulfite, prolong shelf life. Asthmatic dental patients who are given local anesthetic agents with a vasoconstrictor, which also contains a sulfite agent, should be watched for symptoms of wheezing or chest tightness.

- *Sodium hydroxide:* Sodium hydroxide alkalinizes, or adjusts, the pH of the solution to between 6 and 7.

- *Sodium chloride:* Sodium chloride makes the injectable solution isotonic.

- *Methylparaben and propylparaben:* Methylparaben and propylparaben are preservatives added to multidose parenteral solutions to prevent bacterial growth. Unlike multidose vials, dental cartridges are single-use containers and do not contain methylparaben. In the past, this preservative was added to dental cartridges. (A question one might ask is, "Why was methylparaben added to a dental cartridge?" Perhaps the manufacturer had a big vat of solution prepared for the multidose vials, which need a preservative, and used the same solution to fill the dental cartridges.) The parabens may be responsible for some allergic reactions attributable to local anesthetic agents reported in the past. No dental cartridge currently contains methylparaben.

LOCAL ANESTHETIC AGENTS

Many local anesthetic agents are available with similar pharmacologic and clinical effects and systemic toxicity. Commonly used local anesthetics are discussed next, and dental issues associated with local anesthetics are listed in Box 9-4. Table 9-3 lists the local anesthetics available in dental cartridges. For clinical applications, lidocaine with epinephrine 1:100,000 is the usual choice. The question to be answered is, "Under what conditions would a local anesthetic other than lidocaine with epinephrine 1:100,000 be indicated?"

Amides

The amide local anesthetic agents are the only class of anesthetics used parenterally. Esters are occasionally used topically. The relative lack of allergenicity of the amides is probably responsible for this use.

◆ LIDOCAINE

> Lidocaine with epinephrine is good for almost all dentistry.

An amide derivative of xylidine introduced in 1948, lidocaine (LYE-doe-kane) (Xylocaine, Octocaine) quickly became an anesthetic standard to which other local anesthetics were compared. It has a rapid onset, which is related to its tendency to spread well through the tissues. Lidocaine 2% with vasoconstrictor provides profound anesthesia of medium duration. It is the local anesthetic solution most commonly used in dental offices.

No cross-allergenicity between the amide lidocaine, other available amides, or esters has been documented. Some patients appear to experience some sedation with lidocaine, and in toxic reactions one is likely to observe CNS depression initially rather than the CNS stimulation characteristic of other local anesthetics (Figure 9-5).

Adverse reactions include hypotension, positional headache, and shivering. Lidocaine is used for topical, infiltration, block, spinal, epidural, and caudal anesthesia. It is also used intravenously to treat cardiac arrhythmias during surgery.

BOX 9-4 INSTRUCTIONS FOR PATIENTS RECEIVING LOCAL ANESTHETICS

- Patients should be advised to tell the dental practitioner if they are feeling anxious, nervous, or if they are having heart palpitations.
- Most of these symptoms can be avoided by lowering the dose or switching to another local anesthetic.
- Some local anesthetics may cause drowsiness.
- Patients should use caution if an opioid analgesic or antianxiety drug is also prescribed.
- Avoid driving or doing anything that requires thought or concentration
- Have the patient avoid eating or drinking very hot or cold foods or drinks. The local anesthetic may make it difficult for the patient to detect temperature changes.

TABLE 9-3   LOCAL ANESTHETIC COMBINATIONS AVAILABLE IN DENTAL CARTRIDGES

Local Anesthetic	%	Vasoconstrictor	Concentration
Lidocaine (Xylocaine, Octocaine)	2	Epinephrine	1:50,000
			1:200,000
	2	Epinephrine	1:100,000
Mepivacaine (Carbocaine, Isocaine)	3	Plain	—
	2	Levonordefrin	1:20,000
Prilocaine (Citanest)	4	Plain	—
Prilocaine (Citanest Forte)	4	Epinephrine	1:200,000
Bupivacaine (Marcaine)	0.5	Epinephrine	1:200,000
Articaine (Septocaine)	4	Epinephrine	1:100,000
			1:200,000

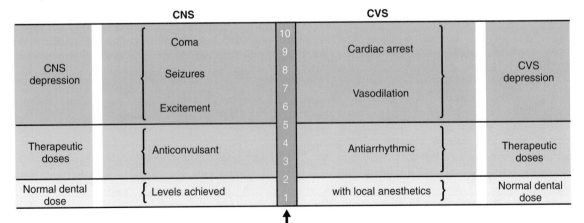

FIGURE 9-5

Relationship between levels of local anesthesia in serum and the pharmacologic and adverse effects. *CNS*, Central nervous system; *CVS*, cardiovascular system.

In dentistry, lidocaine 2% with 1:100,000 epinephrine is used for infiltration and block anesthesia. Lidocaine is used for topical anesthesia as a 5% ointment, a 10% spray, and a 2% viscous solution. When used topically, its onset is rapid (2 to 3 minutes). Lidocaine with epinephrine 1:100,000 provides a 1- to 1.5-hour duration of pulpal anesthesia. Soft tissue anesthesia is maintained for 3 to 4 hours. Lidocaine with epinephrine 1:50,000 is used for hemostasis during surgical procedures. Rebound vasodilation (β effect) can be expected after the α effect (vasoconstriction) has occurred. A new dose form of lidocaine is a patch that is applied to the mucosal membranes for local anesthesia. It provides good anesthesia, but its maximal effect occurs after about 10 minutes, which is probably too long to wait.

◆ MEPIVACAINE

> To avoid vasoconstrictor, one should use mepivacaine plain.

Another amide derivative of xylidine is mepivacaine (me-PIV-a-kane) (Carbocaine, Polocaine, or Isocaine). Introduced in 1960, its rate of onset, duration, potency, and toxicity are similar to those of lidocaine. No cross-allergenicity between the amide mepivacaine, other currently available amides, or the esters has been documented.

Mepivacaine is not effective topically; however, it is used for infiltration, block, spinal, epidural, and caudal anesthesia. The usual dose form in dentistry is a 2% solution with the addition of 1:20,000 levonordefrin (Neo-Cobefrin) as the vasoconstrictor. Because mepivacaine produces less vasodilation than lidocaine, it can be used as a 3% solution without a vasoconstrictor (called *plain*). It can be used for short procedures when a vasoconstrictor is contraindicated (not often). Caution should be exercised when using the increased concentrations of the local anesthetic without a vasoconstrictor because systemic toxicity is more likely. Except in unusual cases, the benefit of a shorter duration does not warrant eliminating the vasoconstrictor, especially when the concentration of the drug is increased.

◆ PRILOCAINE

> *Ortho*-toluidine can induce methemoglobinemia.

Prilocaine (PRILL-loh-kane) (Citanest, Citanest Forte) is related chemically and pharmacologically to both lidocaine and mepivacaine. Chemically, lidocaine and mepivacaine are xylidine derivatives, whereas prilocaine is a toluidine derivative. Prilocaine appears to be less potent and less toxic than lidocaine and has a slightly longer duration of action. It has been shown to produce satisfactory local anesthesia with low concentrations of epinephrine and without epinephrine.

Although toxicity of prilocaine is 60% of that occurring with lidocaine, several cases of methemoglobinemia have been reported after its use. Prilocaine is metabolized to *ortho*-toluidine and in large doses, can induce some methemoglobinemia. A very large dose (greater than the maximal safe dose) would be required to produce clinical symptoms: cyanosis of the lips and mucous membranes and occasionally respiratory or circulatory distress. Although the small doses required in dental practice are not likely to present a problem in healthy, nonpregnant adults, prilocaine should not be administered to patients with any condition in which problems of oxygenation may be especially critical. Drugs that affect the hemoglobin, such as acetamino-

phen, may exacerbate the adverse reaction. Methemoglobinemia can be reversed by IV methylene blue.

Prilocaine is used for infiltration, block, epidural, and caudal anesthesia. It is available in dental cartridges as a 4% concentration both with and without 1:200,000 epinephrine.

Prilocaine's niche in dentistry involves situations in which the desired duration of action is somewhat longer than that obtained with mepivacaine (without and with). Prilocaine plain has a duration of action slightly longer than mepivacaine plain, and prilocaine with epinephrine has a duration of action slightly longer than lidocaine with epinephrine. The other potential advantage of prilocaine is that the concentration of epinephrine (1:200,000) is lower than in other local anesthetic amide combinations. Therefore, if prilocaine with epinephrine were to be used, the patient would be exposed to half of the amount of epinephrine as with lidocaine with epinephrine 1:100,000.

◆ BUPIVACAINE

> Bupivacaine: prolonged duration

Bupivacaine (byoo-PIV-a-kane) (Marcaine) is an amide type of local anesthetic related to lidocaine and mepivacaine. It is more potent but less toxic than the other amides. The major advantage of bupivacaine is its greatly prolonged duration of action. It is indicated in lengthy dental procedures when pulpal anesthesia of greater than 1.5 hours is needed or when postoperative pain is expected (e.g., endodontics, periodontics, or oral surgery). After sensation begins to return, a period of reduced or altered sensation (analgesia) may last several hours. Compared with lidocaine with epinephrine, the onset of bupivacaine with epinephrine is slightly longer, but its duration is at least twice that of lidocaine. It is available in dental cartridges as a 0.5% solution with 1:200,000 epinephrine. It should not be used in patients prone to self-mutilation (mental patients or children younger than 12 years). During its early use in anesthesiology and obstetrics, fatal unresuscitable cardiac arrests occurred. The doses used for obstetrics were much higher than those used in dentistry. After the maximal doses for obstetrics were lowered, these cardiac arrests essentially disappeared. Because much lower maximal doses are recommended for dental procedures, these adverse reactions are very unlikely to occur in dental practice. Bupivacaine has been used for infiltration, block, and peridural anesthesia.

◆ ARTICAINE

Articaine (Septocaine) was approved for use in the United States in 2000 and has been used in Europe since the mid-1970s. Its delay in the United States was a result of the addition of methylparaben to both multidose vials and single-dose cartridges. In the late 1990s, Septodont, a Canadian pharmaceutical company, submitted a methylparaben-free formulation for approval in the United States in 1995 and it was finally approved in 2000.

Articaine differs from other amide local anesthetics because it is derived from thiophene. This allows for greater lipid solubility and ability to cross lipid barriers such as nerve membranes. It has been suggested that this mechanism may account for its enhanced action compared with other local anesthetics. Articaine also differs from other amide local anesthetics because it has an extra ester linkage. This extra linkage causes articaine to be hydrolyzed by plasma esterase. Only 5% to 10% of articaine is metabolized by the liver, the other 90% to 95% is metabolized in the blood. Its major metabolite is articainic acid and it is unclear how active this metabolite is.

Articaine is excreted by the kidneys, 40% to 70% as articainic acid, 2% to 5% unchanged, and 4% to 15% as articainic acid glucuronide, which also appears to be inactive. The half-life of articaine is approximately 20 minutes compared with lidocaine, which is approximately 90 minutes. Articaine's shorter half-life is the result of its metabolism by plasma esterases. Other amides are metabolized by the liver and have much longer half-lives. Because of its rapid metabolism, articaine may be a safer drug to reinject later on during a dental visit. This would be especially true if all of articaine's metabolites were inactive.

Despite its short half-life and apparent safety, articaine is a 4% solution with a toxic dose of 7 mg/kg for the average healthy adult. Because lidocaine is only a 2% solution with the same maximal dose, the average patient can tolerate twice as much lidocaine as compared with articaine before the maximal dose is reached. In addition, articaine, like prilocaine, in very high doses may cause methemoglobinemia. It should be noted that no reported cases of methemoglobinemia have been reported with articaine in doses recommended for dental local anesthesia. Lastly, articaine rarely causes paresthesia after a mandibular block when the 4% solution is used.

Articaine is used for local, infiltrative, and conductive anesthesia. It is available as a 4% concentration with 1 : 100,000 epinephrine in a 1.7 ml dental cartridge unlike the more common 1.8 ml dental cartridge. It has become the most widely used local anesthetic in just about every country in which it has been introduced. Its relative lack of significant active metabolites makes it more desirable in patients that may need to be reinjected. This lowers the risk for toxicity. Although clinical trials have not shown that articaine is better than available local anesthetics, many of these clinical trials show that articaine slightly outperformed the local anesthetics with which it was compared.

Esters

There are currently no esters available in a dental cartridge. Esters, such as benzocaine, are commonly used topically.

◆ PROCAINE

Procaine (PROE-kane) (Novocain) is a PABA ester. Procaine is used as an antiarrhythmic agent (procainamide) and is combined with penicillin to form procaine penicillin G. Procaine is not used in dentistry today because of the high rate of allergic reaction. The allergic reaction is usually a result of PABA and not procaine.

◆ PROPOXYCAINE

Propoxycaine (proe-POX-i-kane) (Ravocaine), another ester of PABA, is not available in a dental cartridge.

◆ TETRACAINE

Tetracaine (TET-ra-kane) (Pontocaine), an ester of PABA, has a slow onset and long duration and is generally estimated to have at least 10 times the potency and toxicity of procaine. In view of this drug's high toxicity and the rapidity with which it is absorbed from mucosal surfaces, great care must be exercised if it is used for topical anesthesia. Dermatologic reactions include contact dermatitis, burning, stinging, and angioedema. A maximal dose of 20 mg is recommended for topical administration. Tetracaine is available in various sprays, solutions, and

ointments for topical application. The concentration of tetracaine in most topical preparations is 2%.

Other Local Anesthetics

◆ DYCLONINE

Dyclonine (DYE-kloe-neen) (Dyclone) is a topical local anesthetic that is neither an ester nor an amide. Its side effects involving the cardiovascular system and CNS are similar to those of the other local anesthetics. Dyclonine may produce slight irritation and stinging when applied. Patients can exhibit allergic reactions to dyclonine, but cross-allergenicity with other local anesthetics would not be expected because of its unique structure. The onset of local anesthesia is 2 to 10 minutes, and its duration is 30 to 60 minutes. The solution and topical product are available as 0.5% and 1% concentrations.

◆ BENZONATATE

Benzonatate (ben-ZOE-na-tate) (Tessalon Perles) is a tetracaine congener (a near relative) indicated in the management of nonproductive cough. It is a topical anesthetic that acts on the respiratory stretch receptors, which produces its antitussive properties. Because the drug's local anesthetic activity can reduce the patient's gag reflex, care should be taken when working within the mouth to prevent foreign particles from entering the throat. Side effects include sedation, headache, dizziness, rash, gastrointestinal upset, and nasal congestion. It is used to treat cough.

VASOCONSTRICTORS

Overview

| Vasoconstriction keeps anesthetic in area injected. |

The vasoconstricting agents are included in local anesthetic solutions for many reasons (Box 9-5).

The vasoconstrictors are members of the autonomic nervous system drugs called the *adrenergic agonists* or *sympathomimetics* (see Chapter 4).

When a local anesthetic solution does not contain a vasoconstrictor, the anesthetic drug is more quickly removed from the injection site and distributed into systemic circulation than if the solution contained a vasoconstrictor. Plain (without vasoconstrictor) anesthetics will exhibit a shorter duration of action and result in a more rapid buildup of a systemic blood level. Therefore any anesthetic given without a vasoconstrictor is more likely to be toxic than those given with a vasoconstrictor. Any advantage gained by eliminating the vasoconstrictor (shorter duration and increased possible systemic effect of the vasocon-

---

BOX 9-5   REASONS FOR USE OF VASOCONSTRICTING AGENTS IN LOCAL ANESTHETICS

Vasoconstricting agents in local anesthetics are used because they do the following:
1. Prolong the duration of action.
2. Increase the depth of anesthesia.
3. Delay systemic absorption.
4. Reduce the toxic effect in the systemic circulation.
5. Reduce the bleeding in the area of injection and improve visibility at surgical site.

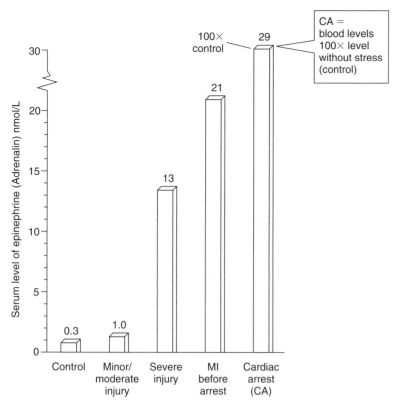

FIGURE 9-6

Blood levels of endogenous epinephrine during rest; with minor, moderate, or severe injury; myocardial infarction (*MI;* before arrest); and cardiac arrest *(CA)*.

strictor) must be weighed against the potential for adverse effects from the epinephrine.

The decision about whether epinephrine should be used in a patient is made by weighing the risks and the benefits. Figure 9-6 shows the amount of epinephrine at rest and during mild-to-severe stress, and Figure 9-7 compares the dose for anaphylaxis and dental use.

A sufficient concentration must be used to keep the local anesthetic localized at its site of action and provide adequate depth, duration, and low systemic toxicity of the anesthetic. It has been shown that 1:100,000 and 1:200,000 produce about the same amount of vasoconstriction and the same distribution of the local anesthetics. No justification exists for the use of epinephrine in a concentration greater than 1:200,000, except in cases in which local hemostasis is needed (1:50,000 is used). Lidocaine is available with 1:100,000 epinephrine, although the weaker concentration has been shown to produce similar results.

In the 1940s, the literature stated that dental local anesthetics containing vasoconstrictors should not be used in patients with cardiovascular disease. This recommendation stemmed from the fear that the vasoconstrictor would elevate the blood pressure too much. It is now known that a patient can produce endogenous epinephrine far in excess of that administered in dentistry in the presence of inadequate anesthesia, which sometimes occurs when vasoconstrictors are avoided. Medical consults often recommend that epinephrine be avoided because physicians are more familiar with the doses used in medicine (0.5 to 1.0 mg) rather than the dental dose (0.018 mg/cartridge [1.8 ml] of 1:100,000) of epinephrine (see Figure 9-7).

Patients with uncontrolled high blood pressure, hyperthyroidism, angina pectoris, and cardiac arrhythmias and those who

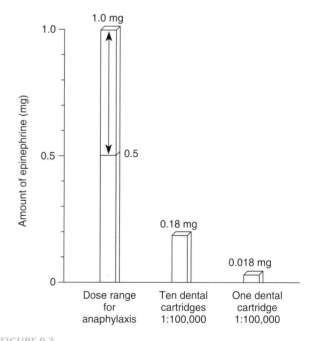

FIGURE 9-7

Histogram showing the dose range of epinephrine for anaphylaxis and the doses provided in dental cartridges.

have had a myocardial infarction or cerebrovascular accident in the past 6 months should make an appointment for elective dental treatment after their medical condition is under control. For patients who have had a myocardial infarction or cerebrovascular accident, that would be 6 months after the cardiovas-

TABLE 9-4   VASOCONSTRICTORS: MAXIMUM SAFE DOSE (MSD) IN NORMAL AND CARDIAC PATIENTS

| | | | MAXIMUM SAFE DOSE | | | | |
| | | | Normal Adult | | Cardiac Patient | | |
Drug	Concentration	Relative Pressor Potency	mg	No. of Cartridges	mg	No. of Cartridges	Approximate % of (α/β) Activity
Epinephrine (Adrenalin)	1:50,000	1	0.2	5	0.04	1	50/50
	1:100,000	1	0.2	11	0.04	2	50/50
	1:200,000	1	0.2	22	0.04	4	50/50
Levonordefrin (Neo-Cobefrin)	1:20,000	1/5	1.0	11	0.2 or 1.0*	2 or 11*	75/25

*Data from Malamed SF: *Handbook of local anesthesia*, ed 5, St Louis, 2004, Mosby.

cular or cerebrovascular event.. Those undergoing general anesthesia with a halogenated hydrocarbon inhalation anesthetic should be monitored for arrhythmias if epinephrine (including epinephrine-soaked retraction cords) is used for its hemostatic effect (used commonly with halothane). If arrhythmias occur, antiarrhythmic agents are administered.

> Epinephrine cardiac dose: 0.04 mg

Patients with cardiovascular disease who are able to withstand elective dental treatment can receive epinephrine-containing local anesthetic agents. The anesthetic should be administered in the lowest possible dose by means of the best technique, including aspiration and a very slow injection rate to minimize systemic absorption. Maximal cardiac doses should not be exceeded in patients with severe cardiovascular disease. Table 9-4 lists the maximal safe dose of epinephrine for the healthy patient (0.2 mg) and the cardiac patient (0.04 mg); the number of cartridges each of these doses represents is included. For example, the cardiac patient could be given two cartridges of 1:100,000 epinephrine without exceeding the cardiac dose.

Drug Interactions

> Significant drug interactions with epinephrine: tricyclic antidepressants and nonselective β-blockers

Selected drug interactions of epinephrine are listed in Table 9-5. Of the most important drug interactions with epinephrine, two are clinically significant and two are not. The two epinephrine drug interactions that are most likely to be clinically significant are those with tricyclic antidepressants and nonselective β-blockers. With tricyclic antidepressants, administration of epinephrine may produce an exaggerated increase in pressor response (increased blood pressure). With the nonselective β-blockers, hypertension and reflex bradycardia may be exhibited. These are not absolute contraindications to the use of epinephrine, but patients taking these agents should be monitored for symptoms of alterations in their blood pressure. The two drug interactions that are commonly mentioned but are not usually clinically significant are with monoamine oxidase inhibitors (MAOIs) and phenothiazines. Epinephrine can be given to patients taking MAOIs because epinephrine is eliminated primarily by reuptake and secondarily by catechol *O*-methyltransferase (COMT) rather than by monoamine oxidase (MAO). If any small interaction exists, it would be the result of "denervation hypersensitivity." In contrast to epinephrine, the indirect-acting sympathomimetic agents (e.g., pseudoephedrine) should be avoided in patients taking MAOIs because they are inactivated in significant amounts by MAO. The drug interaction between epinephrine and phenothiazines occurs

TABLE 9-5   DRUG INTERACTIONS OF EPINEPHRINE

Medical Drug Group	Examples	Potential Outcomes
Tricyclic antidepressants	Amitriptyline (Elavil) Imipramine (Tofranil)	Pressor response to IV EPI markedly enhanced
β-Blockers, nonselective	Pindolol (Visken) Propranolol (Inderal) Timolol (Blocadren)	Hypertension and reflex bradycardia
Antidiabetics	Tolbutamide (Orinase) Chlorpropamide (Diabinese)	Blood glucose increased
Interactions *not* Significant in Dentistry		
Phenothiazines	Chlorpromazine (Thorazine)	Reverse pressor response of EPI; avoid using EPI to raise BP
MAOI	Phenelzine (Nardil) Tranylcypromine (Parnate)	EPI not inactivated by MAO

BP, Blood pressure; *EPI*, epinephrine; *IV*, intravenous; *MAO*, monoamine oxidase; *MAOI*, monoamine oxidase inhibitor.

because the phenothiazines are α-blockers, and when an α and β agonist (epinephrine) is given, the β effects (vasodilation) predominate. Therefore, if epinephrine is used for its vasopressor effect (to raise the blood pressure), the blood pressure is likely to decrease. When epinephrine is used in a local anesthetic solution, it is not being given for its vasopressor effect, so this interaction is not clinically significant.

CHOICE OF LOCAL ANESTHETIC

> One should choose two local anesthetic solutions.

Practitioners should choose a few local anesthetic solutions to use, depending on the duration of local anesthesia desired and the side effects that must be avoided. Box 9-6 lists the local anesthetics by their durations of action, including both pulpal and soft tissue anesthesia. Figures 9-8 and 9-9 illustrate the durations of action of local anesthetic agents for soft tissue and pulpal anesthetics, respectively. Several properties of local anesthetic agents determine their differences in pharmacokinetics. Table 9-6 lists these physical properties for some local anesthetics. For example, the pK$_a$

is related to the onset of action. With a lower pK_a, the local anesthetic is distributed more in the base form and so is better absorbed. The duration of action of the local anesthetic is primarily related to its protein-binding capacity. Its lipid solubility may also play some part. The duration is unrelated to the local anesthetic's half-life because its action is terminated when the drug is removed from the receptor. The lipid solubility deter-

mines the potency of a local anesthetic agent. The vasodilating property of a local anesthetic can affect both the potency and duration of action. One should note that the vasodilating effect of lidocaine (1) is more than that of mepivacaine (0.8) and prilocaine (0.5). Because mepivacaine and prilocaine have less vasodilating effect, they can be used without vasoconstrictor. In contrast, lidocaine (1) and bupivacaine (2.5) produce too much vasodilation to be used without a vasoconstrictor. The dental practitioner should become familiar with a short-, an intermediate-, and a long-acting agent. The duration of the procedure and any patient-specific information will determine the anesthetic of choice. Table 9-7 lists some common contraindications to the use of local anesthetic agents.

TOPICAL ANESTHETICS

Benzocaine, an ester, is the most commonly used topical anesthetic; lidocaine, an amide, is the second most commonly used. Some topical anesthetics are listed in Table 9-8. Comparison among the agents should take into account their onset, duration of action, and allergenic potential. The patient should be instructed to avoid eating for 1 hour after application to oral mucosa so that the gag reflex can become fully functional.

Amides

◆ LIDOCAINE

Lidocaine (Xylocaine) is available as the base or hydrochloride salt. The base is preferred when large areas of the mucosal surfaces are ulcerated, abraded, denuded, or erythematous. The hydrochloride salt is water soluble and penetrates the tissue better. Therefore its propensity for systemic absorption is greater than with the base. Lidocaine base is available as a jelly and an oral topical solution, and hydrochloride is available as an ointment, an oral topical, and an oral aerosol. Concentration

---

BOX 9-6 CATEGORIES OF DURATION OF ACTION OF LOCAL ANESTHETIC AGENTS (PLAIN AND WITH A VASOCONSTRICTOR)

General Categories

Short Duration (Pulpal = 30 min)	*Intermediate Duration (Pulpal 30-60 min)*	*Long Duration (Pulpal >90 min)*
Lidocaine plain (without)	Mepivacaine with	Bupivacaine with
Mepivacaine plain (without)	Prilocaine plain (block) (without)	
Prilocaine plain (infiltration)	Prilocaine with (60-90 min)	
	Articaine with (60-90 min)	

Pulpal and Soft Tissue

Local Anesthetics	*Pulpal (min)*	*Soft Tissue (hr)*
Lidocaine with	60	3-5
Mepivacaine without (plain)	40 (20)*	2-3
Mepivacaine with	60-90	3-5
Prilocaine without (plain)	60 (10)*	2-4 (1.5-2)*
Prilocaine with	60-90 (45-60)*	3-8 (2-4)†
Bupivacaine with	90-180	4-9 (12)
Articaine with	60-90	3-4

*With infiltration.
†With 1:200,000 epinephrine.

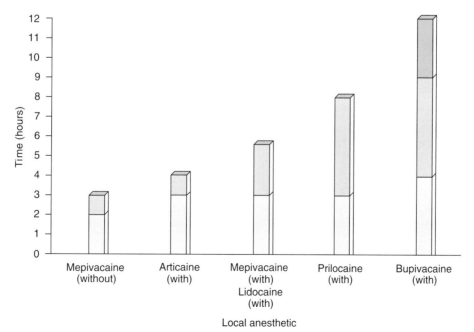

FIGURE 9-8
Duration of anesthesia in soft tissue after a nerve block.

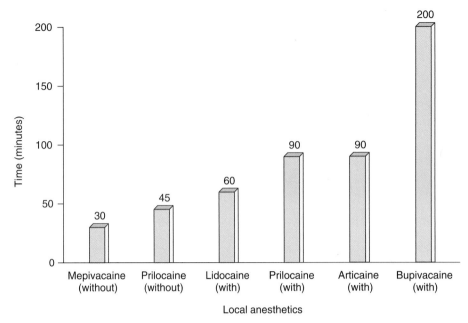

FIGURE 9-9
Duration of pulpal anesthesia after a nerve block.

TABLE 9-6	PHYSICAL PROPERTIES OF LOCAL ANESTHETICS				
Local Anesthetic	pK$_a$*	Vasodilating†	T ½‡	Lipid Solubility§	Protein Binding‖(%)
Lidocaine	7.9	1	90	2.9	65
Mepivacaine	7.6	0.8	90¶	0.8	75
Prilocaine	7.9	0.5	80	0.9	55
Bupivacaine	8.1	2.5	76	27.5	95
Articaine	7.8	Uncertain	20	1.5	54

*pK$_a$, Dissociation constant; rate of onset.
†Vasodilating lidocaine given value of 1.
‡Half-life (min).
§Lipid solubility oil/water solubility; intrinsic potency, increased penetrability.
‖Protein binding duration of action.
¶Estimated.

of the creams ranges from 2% to 5%. Viscous lidocaine (2%) is available for oral rinse to manage aphthous lesions or reduce gagging.

♦ LIDOCAINE AND PRILOCAINE (INJECTION-FREE LOCAL ANESTHESIA)

More often than not, the fear of injection prevents many people from seeking necessary dental treatment. Either the thought of the injection or the injection itself can be painful and upsetting. The combination of lidocaine and prilocaine gel (Oraqix) applied into the periodontal pocket offers pain relief during scaling and root planing procedures. The combination of lidocaine and prilocaine, in the gel form, provides a duration of action of approximately 20 minutes. Its onset of action is approximately 30 seconds after application. Lidocaine provides rapid anesthesia, and prilocaine has a slower onset of action. The combination appears to be well tolerated. The more common side effects include pain, soreness, irritation, edema or redness at the area of application, and taste changes.

Esters

♦ BENZOCAINE

Benzocaine (BEN-zoe-kane) (Hurricaine, Anbesol, Benzodent, or Orabase-B), an ester of PABA, cannot be converted to a water-soluble form for injection. Because it is poorly soluble, it is poorly absorbed and lacks significant systemic toxicity. Local reactions reported include burning and stinging. Dermatologic reactions have included angioedema and contact dermatitis, which can occur if the operator does not wear gloves (an unacceptable practice today). Benzocaine is available in dental products and in many over-the-counter (OTC) products for teething, sunburn, hemorrhoids, or insect bites (up to 20% for many but not all). Benzocaine is used in many dental offices, although a hypersensitivity reaction is possible.

♦ COCAINE

Cocaine (koe-KANE) is a naturally occurring ester of benzoic acid that is potent and extremely toxic. Its onset of action is less

TABLE 9-7   CONTRAINDICATIONS TO THE USE OF LOCAL ANESTHETIC COMBINATIONS

Categories	Situation	Preferred Anesthetic
History of allergy	To amides (very unlikely)	Amides, with informed consent
	To esters	Amide
	Sulfa	Any
	Sulfite hypersensitivity (asthma)	Any without vasoconstrictor
Choice of local anesthetic agent	Pregnancy	Lidocaine
	Congenital cholinesterase deficiency	Amides
	Malignant hyperthermia	Any amide
	Methemoglobinemia	Any but prilocaine
	Severe renal disease	Any, but limit dose
	Severe liver disease	Any, but limit dose
Vasoconstrictor limits	Very severe cardiovascular disease	Limit to cardiac dose
	Untreated (or drug treated) hyperthyroidism	Limit to cardiac dose
	Tricyclic antidepressants	Limit to cardiac dose
	β-Blockers, nonselective	Limit to cardiac dose

BOX 9-7   HOW TO PREVENT TOXIC REACTIONS FROM SURFACE ANESTHESIA

1. Know the relative toxicity of the drug being used.
2. Know the concentration of the drug being used.
3. Use the smallest volume.
4. Use the lowest concentration.
5. Use the least toxic drug to satisfy clinical requirements.
6. Limit the area of application (avoid sprays).

BOX 9-8   SAMPLE CALCULATION TO DETERMINE AMOUNT OF ANESTHETIC IN 2% SOLUTION

Amount of local anesthetic in a 2% solution:

$$2\% = \frac{2\text{ gm}}{100\text{ ml}} \times \frac{2000\text{ mg}}{\text{gm}} = \frac{2000\text{ mg}}{100\text{ ml}} = \frac{20\text{ mg}}{1\text{ ml}} = 20\text{ mg/ml}$$

Amount in one cartridge:

$$1\text{ cartridge} = \frac{20\text{ mg}}{\text{ml}} \times \frac{1.8\text{ ml}}{\text{cartridge}} = \frac{36\text{ mg}}{\text{cartridge}}$$

TABLE 9-8   SELECTED TOPICAL LOCAL ANESTHETICS

	Local Anesthetic Agent	Dosage Forms	Concentration (%)	Maximum Dose (mg)	Peak (min)	Duration (min)	Chemical Group
Lidocaine	Xylocaine	Spray, ointment, solution, viscous, jelly	2-10	750	2-5	15-45	Amide
Benzocaine	Hurricaine Orajel Mouth-Aid Maximum Strength Anbesol Americaine Anesthetic lubricant	Liquid, gel, cream, spray, ointment	7.5-20	5000	1	15-45	Esters
Tetracaine (Pontocaine, in Cetacaine)		Solution	0.5-2	50	3-8	30-60	
Cocaine		Has no dental use, highly abused					
Dyclonine (Dyclone)		Solution	0.5-1	100	<10	<60	Other

than 1 minute, and its peak is within 5 minutes. Its duration of action is about 30 minutes. Although cocaine has ideal pharmacokinetics, the systemic absorption and subsequent CNS stimulation and its great potential for abuse make the use of cocaine as a local anesthetic untenable. Its CNS effects are discussed in Chapter 25. It has no dental application.

Precautions in Topical Anesthesia

Some local anesthetics are absorbed rapidly when applied topically to mucous membranes. To avoid toxic reactions from surface anesthesia, the dental health care provider should consider many factors (Box 9-7).

DOSES OF LOCAL ANESTHETIC AND VASOCONSTRICTOR

The amounts of local anesthetic and vasoconstrictor contained in a certain volume of solution can be calculated from the concentration of that solution. The local anesthetic percent, for example, 2%, may be expressed as seen in Box 9-8. Box 9-9 shows how to calculate the amount of epinephrine.

The dental health care provider should be able to determine the number of milligrams of both local anesthetic and vasoconstrictor given in any clinical situation. The maximal safe dose for each component should not be exceeded.

Each dose should be recorded in the patient's chart as soon as possible after the injection. The information placed in the

BOX 9-9   SAMPLE CALCULATION FOR AMOUNT OF EPINEPHRINE PER CARTRIDGE

Amount of epinephrine in a milliliter of a 1:100,000 anesthetic:

$$1:100,000 = \frac{1 \text{ gm}}{100,000 \text{ ml}} \times \frac{1000 \text{ mg}}{1 \text{ gm}} = \frac{1000 \text{ mg}}{100,000 \text{ ml}}$$

$$= \frac{1 \text{ mg}}{100 \text{ ml}} \times \frac{1000 \text{ µg}}{1 \text{ mg}} = \frac{1000 \text{ µg}}{100 \text{ ml}} = \frac{10 \text{ µg}}{\text{ml}}$$

Amount of epinephrine in one cartridge:

$$\frac{10 \text{ µg}}{\text{ml}} \times \frac{1.8 \text{ ml}}{\text{cartridge}} = \frac{18 \text{ µg}}{\text{cartridge}} \times \frac{0.001 \text{ mg}}{\text{µg}} = \frac{0.018 \text{ mg}}{\text{cartridge}}$$

chart should include the strength of both ingredients and the volume of solution used or the number of milligrams of each given. For example, if a patient were given one cartridge of lidocaine 2% with 1:100,000 epinephrine, the chart would read: lidocaine 2% with epinephrine 1:100,000 1.8 ml, or lidocaine 36 mg with epinephrine 0.018 mg.

One reason for including this information in the chart is to minimize questions that might arise later if the patient or a future practitioner has concerns about the treatment. Because of the increasing incidence of lawsuits against dentists and hygienists, maintaining a complete chart to prevent any ambiguity is extremely important.

CLINICAL SKILLS ASSESSMENT

1. Name the properties of the ideal local anesthetic.
2. Differentiate between the two major chemical groups of local anesthetic agents.
3. Contrast the allergenicity and metabolism of the ester and amide local anesthetics.
4. List the systemic adverse reactions to the local anesthetics.
5. List five injectable local anesthetic agents and give their composition.
6. Explain the presence in a dental cartridge of agents other than the local anesthetic.
7. State the rationale for the inclusion of vasoconstricting agents in local anesthetic solution.
8. State the maximal safe dose of the two vasoconstrictors used in dentistry for both the normal patient and the cardiac patient.
9. Explain the rationale for use of Oraqix in a dental practice.

⊖volve ─────────────────────────────

10 General Anesthetics

LEARNING OBJECTIVES

1. Summarize the history of general anesthesia in dentistry.
2. Describe how general anesthesia works and the stages and planes involved.
3. Compare and contrast the classifications of general anesthesia.
4. Discuss the use of nitrous oxide in dentistry, including how it works, the pharmacologic effects, adverse reactions, and contraindications.
5. Name and describe several types of halogenated hydrocarbons.
6. Identify and describe several other types of general anesthesia.

> Reversible loss of consciousness and insensibility to painful stimuli

The state of general anesthesia is produced by a heterogeneous group of potent central nervous system (CNS) depressants. They produce a reversible loss of consciousness and insensibility to painful stimuli. Contemporary general anesthetic techniques use balanced anesthesia that uses a combination of drugs to minimize adverse reactions, taking into account the patient's physical status and preanesthetic and postanesthetic needs. Respiratory depression and loss of protective reflexes are associated with general anesthesia; thus the patient must be constantly monitored and evaluated. Because of the variety of anesthetic agents and techniques used, special training and a complete working knowledge of the pharmacology of each anesthetic is essential.

> Hospital: General anesthesia
> Dental office: Conscious sedation

The hospital operating room provides the optimal setting for procedures requiring general anesthesia because of the ready availability of monitors for vital signs, resuscitative equipment, and trained anesthesia personnel. However, oral and maxillofacial surgeons have used general anesthetic drugs in their offices for many years with an excellent safety record. Nitrous oxide, because it is not a complete anesthetic, is not useful alone as a general anesthetic. In the dental office, it is commonly employed to allay patient anxiety. Other general anesthetic drugs, in less than anesthetic doses, are now used to provide conscious sedation in the dental office. In today's practice, the dental health team should have an understanding of the principles of general anesthesia because it is an indispensable tool for the needs of special patients and for extensive oral and maxillofacial surgery.

HISTORY

The original methods to produce general anesthesia involved either strangulation or cerebral concussion. Later, opium, belladonna, hemp, and alcohol were used to render patients unconscious. During this time, the surgeries were "quick and dirty." Nitrous oxide was discovered in 1776, and 20 years later Sir Humphrey Davy suggested that the administration of nitrous oxide might be useful in surgery.

Gardner Quincy Colton, a traveling showman, began giving public demonstrations of "laughing gas" (nitrous oxide) for 25 cents admission (similar to the "hits" of nitrous oxide placed in balloons that are sold in New Orleans). Horace Wells, a dentist, attended one of Colton's lectures, at which a drug clerk volunteered to receive the gas. A fight commenced, and the clerk gashed his leg; under Wells' questioning, the clerk said that he felt no pain. The next day Wells extracted one of his own teeth after having administered nitrous oxide and felt no pain.

| Dentists Wells and Morton recognized nitrous oxide and ether's uses. |

Wells began using nitrous oxide in his own dental practice. Finally, he persuaded William T. G. Morton, a former dental partner who was studying medicine, to arrange a demonstration of nitrous oxide before the Harvard University medical faculty. During the demonstration, the patient awoke too soon and began screaming. Nitrous oxide's low potency accounted for its failure (it is an incomplete anesthetic without anoxia).

Soon after, ether was manufactured and ether "jags" (sort of like parties) were held. Morton practiced administering these drugs to himself and the family dogs and cats. His demonstration of the use of ether began with the surgeon turning to Morton and stating, "Well, sir, your patient is ready." After using ether successfully to anesthetize the patient, Morton said to the surgeon, "Here's your patient!" The surgeon replied, "Gentlemen, this is no humbug."

In the following months, Morton attempted to patent ether and spent the remainder of his life futilely trying to collect claims for compensation from the U.S. government. Both Wells and Morton committed suicide because they did not get credit for their "finds." Although the accomplishments of these dentists were not recognized during their lifetimes, the medical and dental professions today applaud their contribution to methods of alleviating pain.

About the middle of the 1800s, true general anesthetics were discovered in the United States.

MECHANISM OF ACTION

Overview

Many theories have been proposed to explain the mechanism of action of the various general anesthetic agents, but unfortunately none of them does so completely. It may seem relatively simple to say that these drugs are CNS depressants. However, the way in which they depress the normal functions of the CNS is complicated by the lack of knowledge of the physiologic and biochemical events of arousal and unconsciousness. Proposed mechanisms for the action of different general anesthetics involve an increase in the threshold for firing, facilitation of inhibitory γ-aminobutyric acid (GABA), and a decrease in duration of opening of nicotinic receptor-activated cation channels. The increase in the threshold or hyperpolarization is a result of the activation of the potassium channels.

Stages and Planes of Anesthesia

| Guedel described four stages and planes of anesthesia. |

The degree of CNS depression produced by general anesthetics must be carefully titrated to avoid excessive cardiorespiratory depression. In 1920, Guedel described a system of stages and planes to describe the effects of anesthetics (Table 10-1). Although Guedel's classification applied to the effects produced by ether when using the open drop method of administration, modern anesthetic techniques seldom show these exact stages. However, the four stages are briefly described because Guedel's terminology is still used to describe the depth of anesthesia.

TABLE 10-1 STAGES AND PLANES OF ANESTHESIA

Stage and Plane	Patient Response
Stage I: Analgesia	1. Patient is unresponsive 2. Reduced sensation to pain 3. Can still respond to commands 4. Reflexes are present 5. Regular respiration 6. Some amnesia 7. Loss of consciousness (end of stage)
Stage II: Delirium or excitement	1. Unconsciousness 2. Amnesia 3. Involuntary movement and excitement 4. Irregular respiration 5. Increased muscle tone 6. Sympathetic stimulation: tachycardia, mydriasis, hypertension
Stage III: Surgical anesthesia	1. Return to regular respiration, muscle relaxation, and normal heart and pulse rates 2. Divided into four planes
Stage IV: Respiratory or medullary paralysis	1. Cessation of respiration 2. Subsequent circulatory failure 3. Respiration must be artificially maintained

Copyright 1996 Elena Bablenis Haveles.

Induction is the term used to refer to the quick change in the patient's state of consciousness from stage I to stage III, as follows:

1. *Stage I analgesia* is characterized by the development of analgesia or reduced sensation to pain. The patient is conscious and can still respond to command. Reflexes are present, and respiration remains regular. Some amnesia may also be evident. Nitrous oxide, as used in the dental office, maintains the patient in stage I. The end of this stage is marked by the loss of consciousness.

2. *Stage II delirium or excitement* begins with unconsciousness and is associated with involuntary movement and excitement. Respiration becomes irregular, and muscle tone increases. Sympathetic stimulation produces tachycardia, mydriasis, and hypertension. This can be an uncomfortable time for the patient because emesis and incontinence can occur. As the depth of anesthesia increases, the patient begins to relax and proceeds to stage III. To ensure the patient's comfort and safety, it is important to have a smooth and rapid induction. The ultrashort-acting barbiturates accomplish this readily. When balanced anesthesia is used, the patient does not pass through each stage as listed. Adjunct drugs reduce the side effects of each of the drugs used during surgery.

3. *Stage III surgical anesthesia* is the stage in which most major surgery is performed. This stage is further divided into four planes that are differentiated based on eye movements, depth of respiration, and muscle relaxation. The onset of stage III (planes I and II) is typically characterized by the return of regular respiratory movements, muscle relaxation, and normal heart and pulse rates. Reflexes associated with the eye disappear during planes I and II. Vomiting reflex stops during stage II, but swallowing reflex is maintained until stage III, plane I. Plane III is associated with decreased skel-

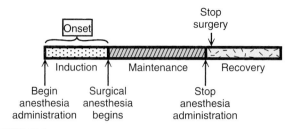

FIGURE 10-1
Levels of anesthesia: induction, maintenance, and recovery.

etal muscle tone, dilated pupils, tachycardia, and hypotension. Beginning in plane III and progressing to plane IV, stage III is characterized by intercostal muscle paralysis (diaphragmatic breathing remains), absence of all reflexes, and extreme muscle flaccidity. If the depth of anesthesia is allowed to increase, the patient will rapidly progress to the last stage with cessation of all respiration.

4. *Stage IV respiratory or medullary paralysis* is characterized by complete cessation of all respiration (diaphragmatic respiration is the last to go) and subsequent circulatory failure. At this point, pupils are maximally dilated and blood pressure falls rapidly. If this stage is not reversed immediately, the patient will die. Respiration must be artificially maintained.

Modern anesthetic techniques now use more rapidly-acting agents than those associated with the four stages of Guedel. Flagg's approach, used to describe the levels of anesthesia (Figure 10-1), includes the following categories:

1. *Induction:* The induction phase encompasses all the preparation and medication necessary for a patient up to the time the operation begins, including preoperative medications, adjunctive drugs to anesthesia, and anesthetics required for induction.

2. *Maintenance:* The maintenance phase begins with the patient at a depth of anesthesia sufficient to allow surgical manipulation and continues until completion of the procedure.

3. *Recovery:* The recovery phase begins with the termination of the surgical procedure and continues through the postoperative period until the patient is fully responsive to the environment.

ADVERSE REACTIONS

Risk of general anesthesia must always be compared with the benefit of surgery.

The goals of surgical anesthesia are good patient control, adequate muscle relaxation, and pain relief. To produce anesthesia, potent CNS depressants are given in relatively high doses, and many combinations of drugs are used in balanced anesthesia. The hazards encountered with the administration of general anesthetics are summarized in Table 10-2.

GENERAL ANESTHETICS
Classification of Anesthetic Agents

The general anesthetic agents can be classified according to their chemical structure or route of administration. Table 10-3 categorizes the agents according to their routes of administration.

TABLE 10-2 ADVERSE REACTIONS TO GENERAL ANESTHETICS

System	Effect/Comment
Cardiovascular system	Cardiovascular collapse Cardiac arrest
Arrhythmias	Ventricular fibrillation with halogenated hydrocarbons
Blood pressure	Hypertension (stage II) Hypotension
Respiration	Depressed respiration (stage III) Respiratory arrest (stage IV) Laryngospasm with ultrashort-acting barbiturates "Boardlike" chest with neuroleptanalgesia
Explosions/flammability	Cyclopropane Ether
Teratogenicity (either male or female exposure)	Chronic exposure fetal abnormalities Spontaneous abortions
Hepatotoxicity (repeated exposure)	Operating room personnel Halogenated hydrocarbons
Other	Headache, fatigue, irritability, addicting

◆ INHALATION ANESTHETICS

Inhalation agents can be divided into gases and volatile liquids. The liquids are vaporized and carried to the patient in the form of gas. The inhalation agents are often used in combination, using oxygen as a carrier gas.

Volatile anesthetics: liquids that easily evaporate

The volatile general anesthetics are liquids that evaporate easily at room temperature because of their low boiling points. They are classified chemically as halogenated hydrocarbons because they contain fluorine, chlorine, or bromine in their structure. These are potent agents with limited solubility in body tissues, and they have successfully replaced the use of ether in anesthesia. Both methoxyflurane and halothane are used infrequently; enflurane and isoflurane are the more popular volatile liquids in current use.

◆ PHYSICAL FACTORS

The concentration of anesthetic in the inspired mixture is proportional to its partial pressure or tension. The depth of anesthesia produced is a function of the tension (partial pressure) of the anesthetic agent in the brain. The most important physical factors that influence brain anesthetic tension are the tension of the anesthetics in the inspired gases, the rate and volume of delivery of anesthetics to the lungs, and the anesthetic's solubility in body tissues. Induction can be hastened with high initial anesthetic concentrations and hyperventilation. As anesthesia depth develops, both the concentration and rate of delivery are reduced to maintenance levels.

Table 10-4 gives the physical properties of some of the anesthetics. The solubility in blood is expressed by the blood/gas partition coefficient. The less soluble the anesthetic is in body tissues, the more rapid the onset and recovery. The low solubil-

TABLE 10-3	CLASSIFICATION OF GENERAL ANESTHETICS BY ROUTE OF ADMINISTRATION		
	INHALATION AGENTS		
Gases	Volatile Liquids		**INTRAVENOUS AGENTS**
Nitrous oxide	**Halogenated hydrocarbons** • Chloroform* • Trichloroethylene* • Halothane (Fluothane)		**Barbiturates** • Methohexital (Brevital) • Thiamylal (Surital) • Thiopental (Pentothal)
Cyclopropane*	**Halogenated ethers** • Methoxyflurane (Penthrane) • Enflurane (Ethrane) • Isoflurane (Forane) **Ethers** • Diethyl ether (ether)*		**Dissociative** • Ketamine (Ketalar) **Opioids** • Morphine • Fentanyl (Sublimaze) • Sufentanil (Sufenta) • Alfentanil (Alfenta) **Neuroleptanalgesia** • Fentanyl with droperidol (Innovar) **Benzodiazepines** • Diazepam (Valium) • Midazolam (Versed) **Others** • Etomidate (Amidate) • Propofol (Diprivan)

*Of historic interest only.

TABLE 10-4	PHYSICAL PROPERTIES OF SELECTED INHALATION GENERAL ANESTHETICS		
	Blood:Gas Partition Coefficient*	MAC† (%)	Comments
Nitrous oxide	(0.47); very low solubility in blood; quick onset	Need >100%	Incomplete anesthetic, rapid onset and recovery
Halothane	(2.3); longer induction and recovery	0.75	Intermediate onset and recovery
Methoxyflurane	(12); high solubility in blood; slow onset	0.16; small % anesthetized	Slow onset and recovery

*Partition coefficient (relative distribution by area; blood, brain, gas).
†MAC, Minimal alveolar concentration (amount that anesthetizes 50% of people).

ity of nitrous oxide (0.47) correlates well with its rapid onset and recovery. This physical factor allows the anesthesiologist to adjust quickly the desired level of anesthesia. In contrast, halothane, with its higher solubility (2.30), has a longer induction and recovery and changes in level of anesthesia occur more slowly.

The term *minimum alveolar concentration* (MAC) is used to compare the potency of general anesthetic inhalation agents. MAC is defined as the minimal alveolar concentration of an anesthetic at 1 atmosphere required to prevent 50% of patients from responding to a supramaximal surgical stimulus. The MAC of nitrous oxide is greater than 100, whereas halothane has a MAC of 0.75, isoflurane of 1.15, and enflurane of 1.68. The lower MAC values indicate the more potent anesthetics. The volatile anesthetics are given in combination with nitrous oxide to reduce the concentration of each while improving MAC values.

♦ INTRAVENOUS ANESTHETICS

The intravenously administered general anesthetics are a diverse group of CNS depressants that include the opioids, the ultra-short-acting barbiturates, and the benzodiazepines. Although most injectable general anesthetics are administered intravenously, one agent, ketamine, can also be given intramuscularly. These drugs find their greatest utility in induction of general anesthesia but may occasionally be used as single agents for short procedures. Although they offer the advantage of convenience, the depth and duration of anesthesia are less easily controlled compared with the inhalation agents. Certain drugs of this group are used in less than anesthetic doses to produce conscious sedation (reflexes retained).

Nitrous Oxide

Nitrous (NYE-trus) oxide (N_2O) is a colorless gas with little or no odor and is the least soluble in blood of all the inhalation anesthetics. Because of its low potency (MAC >100), nitrous oxide used alone is unsatisfactory as a general anesthetic agent. However, if anesthesia is first induced with a rapidly acting intravenous (IV) agent and nitrous oxide-oxygen (O_2) combination (N_2O-O_2) is administered in combination with a volatile anesthetic, excellent balanced anesthesia is produced. This synergistic combination permits the use of reduced doses of the more potent inhalation anesthetics. N_2O-O_2 is given throughout most surgical procedures that necessitate the use of general anesthesia because it reduces the concentration of other agents needed to obtain the desired depth of anesthesia.

Provides anxiety relief

Administration of N_2O-O_2 has become a primary part of dental office anxiety reduction procedures. This use should not be confused with general anesthesia because the intent is to provide for a lightly sedated and relaxed patient. When nitrous oxide is properly administered, the patient remains conscious with the protective reflexes intact. Nitrous oxide provides anxiety relief coupled with analgesia. Thus the N_2O-O_2 sedation technique may be adopted to offer increased patient cooperation and comfort in a wide range of dental office procedures. The dental practitioner should be thoroughly familiar with this use of nitrous oxide. The dentist (and in some states the hygienist) may legally administer nitrous oxide.

Onset rapid: a few minutes

N_2O-O_2 sedation technique involves increasing the concentration of nitrous oxide to titrate the patient to a desired level of sedation. The gas mixture is delivered to the patient by flowmeters that control both the volume flow and the ratio of nitrous oxide to oxygen. Starting with 100% oxygen for 2 to 3 minutes, nitrous oxide is gradually added in 5% to 10% increments until the patient response indicates that the desired level of sedation has been achieved. Once the nitrous oxide is added, onset occurs rapidly within 3 to 5 minutes. Table 10-5 shows the typical responses observed with increasing concentrations of nitrous oxide. The percent of nitrous oxide required for patient comfort is variable and may range from 10% to 50% (average 35%).

At the termination of a N_2O-O_2 sedation procedure, the patient should be placed on 100% oxygen for at least 5 minutes. Recovery occurs rapidly as nitrous oxide is quickly removed from the tissues. If the mask is removed without the oxygen recovery period and the patient allowed to breathe room air, a phenomenon known as *diffusion hypoxia* may result. This occurs because of the rapid outward flow of nitrous oxide accompanied by oxygen and carbon dioxide. The loss of carbon dioxide, a stimulant to respiratory drive, could decrease ventilation with resultant hypoxia. Patients may complain of headache or other side effects if this occurs. Recovery with 100% oxygen avoids this problem.

As has been implied, the N_2O-O_2 technique has sufficient advantages to recommend its consideration in many dental procedures. Among its advantages are the following:
- *Rapid onset:* Because of the poor solubility of nitrous oxide in blood, it has a rapid onset of action (<5 minutes).
- *Easy administration:* No injection is required to obtain an effect. The patient merely breathes through his or her nose.
- *Close control:* The proper depth of sedation can be maintained by adjusting the percentage of nitrous oxide administered.
- *Rapid recovery:* Recovery is obtained rapidly with a full return to presedative psychomotor capacity. Thus the need for the

TABLE 10-5 SIGNS AND SYMPTOMS IN RESPONSE TO NITROUS OXIDE AND OXYGEN CONSCIOUS SEDATION

Concentration of N_2O (%)	Response
10-20	Body warmth Tingling of hands and feet
20-30	Circumoral numbness Numbness of thighs
20-40	Numbness of tongue Numbness of hands and feet Droning sounds present Hearing distinct but distant Dissociation begins and reaches peak Mild sleepiness Analgesia (maximum concentration of 30%) Euphoria Feeling of heaviness or lightness of body
30-50	Sweating Nausea Amnesia Increased sleepiness
40-60	Dreaming, laughing, giddiness Further increased sleepiness, tending toward unconsciousness Increased nausea and vomiting
50 and over	Unconsciousness and light general anesthesia

From Clark M, Brunick A: *Handbook of nitrous oxide and oxygen sedation,* ed 3, St. Louis, 2008, Mosby.
N_2O, Nitrous oxide.

patient to be accompanied to the dental appointment can often be eliminated.
- *Acceptability for children:* Nitrous oxide is a valuable adjunct in managing some apprehensive children. However, it cannot be used when a child's behavior is openly defiant or hysterical, and it is not a substitute for good behavioral management techniques. The analogy of "going into space" can be effective.
- *Relaxed dental team:* The N_2O-O_2 technique not only will offer comfort to the patient and increase the acceptance of dental procedures but also will afford more relaxed treatment, that is, the dental team should be less tense and fatigued at the end of the office day.

◆ PHARMACOLOGIC EFFECTS

Central Nervous System Sedation. Sedation is the main pharmacologic effect of nitrous oxide on the CNS, resulting in analgesia and amnesia. Although there is sensory depression, auditory perception is not affected to the same degree. Therefore a tranquil, quiet environment is required for N_2O-O_2 analgesic procedures. The use of personal audio input may be useful.

Cardiovascular Effects. Peripheral vasodilation is produced by nitrous oxide administration. This property may facilitate venipuncture should an IV route be desired after starting the N_2O-O_2.

Gastrointestinal Effects. Nausea and vomiting with N_2O-O_2 analgesia are uncommon but can occur. The patient should eat a light meal before the appointment but should be warned to avoid a large meal within 3 hours of the appointment.

Changing the concentration of nitrous oxide slowly and monitoring the patient closely can minimize this response. When nitrous oxide is administered slowly, its effects may be evaluated according to Table 10-5 and are summarized as follows:

- The best indicator of the degree of sedation is the patient's response to questions. The patient may exhibit slurred speech or a slow response. One should not evaluate only as anesthesia is adjusted. The dental practitioner should perform repeated evaluations throughout the dental procedure. Examples of evaluations are asking the patient to "open your mouth" or "move one finger" and noting the patient's response (can be slow, but the patient should respond).
- The patient is relaxed and cooperative and reports a feeling of euphoria. Local anesthetic injections elicit little if any response at this time. Analgesia produced by nitrous oxide is variable but can be equivalent to morphine injection in patients.
- The patient is easily able to maintain an open-mouth position in the desired plane.
- The patient's eyes may be closed but can be opened easily.
- The respiration, pulse rate, and blood pressure are within normal limits.

In addition to the features already mentioned, the patient often indicates that the time frame the procedure occupied in his or her consciousness has been dramatically decreased. The operating time may appear to the patient to be one-third or one-half as long as it is in reality. This can be especially beneficial in long procedures, particularly in dental schools. Interesting audio input acts as a distractor for both hearing and feeling sensations.

♦ ADVERSE REACTIONS

Be smart; think; monitor patient.

Invariably, complications that have occurred with the use of N_2O-O_2 techniques have been the result of misuse or faulty installation of equipment. Obviously, an installation that crossed oxygen and nitrous oxide lines could be disastrous if nitrous oxide were given under the assumption that it was oxygen. (This has occurred, and taking off the mask would have saved the patient's life.) Cases of dentists abusing N_2O, including use of solely N_2O, and taping the mask to the face have resulted in reported deaths.

O_2: Green tank N_2O: Blue tank

All cylinders are now colored in a standardized manner. Nitrous oxide cylinders are blue, and oxygen cylinders are green. The cylinders are also "pin coded" to prevent inadvertent mixing of cylinders and lines.

Equipment with built-in safety features is now available. Modern equipment has built-in features that allow no more than 70% of N_2O to be dispensed. Oxygen, in the gaseous mixture, must be dispensed at concentrations of 30% or higher during the sedation period. The inhalation administration equipment in every dentist's office should automatically limit the percentage of nitrous oxide that can be administered and have a fail-safe system that shuts down the nitrous oxide if the oxygen runs out.

The combination of nitrous oxide with other sedative regimens can increase the potential danger of causing a general anesthetic state. The limits of this sedation technique must be understood by every member of the dental health team. If inhalation sedation is combined with other modes of sedation, the entire dental staff must be trained and prepared for the possibility that general anesthesia might be produced.

♦ CONTRAINDICATIONS AND DENTAL ISSUES

Respiratory Obstruction. Because the nasal passages are used for gaseous exchange, upper respiratory obstruction or a stuffy nose is an absolute contraindication to this technique. Other respiratory diseases must also be carefully evaluated.

Chronic Obstructive Pulmonary Disease. In the normal person, the drive for ventilation (breathing) is stimulated by an elevation in the partial pressure of carbon dioxide (Pa_{CO_2}). The partial pressure of oxygen (Pa_{O_2}) can vary widely without stimulating ventilation in the normal patient. Patients with chronic obstructive pulmonary disease (COPD) have compromised ventilation; thus they experience a gradual rise in Pa_{CO_2} over time. Because this mechanism becomes resistant to this stimulus, a new stimulant emerges—the partial pressure of Pa_{CO_2}. The patient's ventilation is then driven by a decrease in Pa_{O_2}. If a patient with COPD is given oxygen and the Pa_{O_2} rises, the stimulant to breathing is removed and there is the possibility of inducing apnea. For patients with COPD American Society of Anesthesiologists Levels III and IV, it is suggested that oxygen be limited to less than 3 L/min. Another recommendation is that patients with severe COPD should be given oxygen by nasal cannula during a dental appointment, especially if pain or stress is expected (increased oxygen demand).

Emotional Instability. Because patients may experience euphoria or an altered sensorium with nitrous oxide analgesia, a patient's emotional instability is a relative contraindication to its use. Patients taking psychotherapeutic medication must be carefully evaluated before nitrous oxide is used. These medications include phenothiazines, tricyclic antidepressants, and lithium. Fanciful dreams occurring during a procedure may be interpreted on recovery as having actually occurred; therefore a female staff member must be in attendance when a female patient is being treated by a male dentist or dental hygienist and nitrous oxide is used. Aberrant sensations may lead to unfounded accusations unless this requirement is strictly enforced. This is required to minimize legal liability (record in chart).

Pregnancy Considerations. Safety of the use of nitrous oxide

Pregnant dental practitioners should determine levels in dental operatory before exposure.

in pregnant patients or administration by pregnant operators is in question. Although no direct correlation has yet been found, several epidemiologic studies cast doubt on the safety of exposure to nitrous oxide during pregnancy. The incidence of spontaneous abortion or miscarriages is higher in female operating personnel chronically exposed to anesthetic agents or in wives of male operators. Women exposed to high levels of nitrous oxide (>5 hours/week) were significantly less fertile than unexposed women. This is especially important to female dentists and dental hygienists because dental operatories have been found to have higher concentrations of gases than even hospital operating rooms (poorer ventilation).

Dental health care workers should be aware of the concentration of nitrous oxide that is present in the dental operatories in which they practice. Machines are available that monitor the concentration of nitrous oxide. Scavenger systems that can retrieve much of the expired gas can be installed, and turnover of the room air can be increased. Checking of the nitrous oxide concentration in the dental operatory should be repeated, especially if the use changes or personnel are pregnant.

Abuse. The dental team should be knowledgeable about the potential hazards associated with the abuse of nitrous oxide. Case histories describing the chronic abuse of nitrous oxide (self-administration) have reported examples of nitrous-induced neuropathy. Symptoms include numbness and paresthesia of the hands or legs that progresses to more severe neurologic symptoms with continued abuse. Nitrous oxide has been shown to reduce the activity of methionine synthetase, the enzyme involved with the function of vitamin B_{12}. Thus it appears that the chronic abuse of nitrous oxide and attendant neurologic symptoms may be related to its effect on the utilization of vitamin B_{12}. Liver and kidney problems have also been mentioned in association with nitrous oxide abuse. The profile of the average dentist who abuses nitrous oxide is male, white, and in his 40s. He has abused many drugs in the past (polydrug abuser) and has previously self-administered nitrous oxide "therapeutically." As his abuse progresses, he spends more time at the office alone. The number of missed appointments with patients increases, and his attention is focused on issues other than his patients (using the drug again).

Situations that determine that abuse has begun include self-using nitrous oxide, using nitrous oxide for anything other than dental anxiety, using nitrous oxide during lunch or after work, sneaking nitrous oxide use, missing appointments, not keeping promises, and having problems with family or money.

Halogenated Hydrocarbons

◆ HALOTHANE

Halothane (HA-loe-thane) (Fluothane) has a fruity, pleasant odor and is nonflammable and nonexplosive. Both induction and recovery are relatively rapid. The MAC for halothane is 0.77 but is improved to 0.29 when combined with 70% nitrous oxide. Because halothane is nonirritating to bronchial mucous membranes, it is considered safe for use on asthmatics. As with the other volatile agents, the halothane dose must be carefully regulated to prevent overt respiratory depression. Muscle relaxation is incomplete, and peripheral neuromuscular blocking drugs, such as *d*-tubocurarine, are required. Halothane also depresses renal function and can cause uterine muscle relaxation.

Halothane's effects on the cardiovascular system are manifested by increased vagal activity producing bradycardia and peripheral vasodilation that lowers the blood pressure. It sensitizes the myocardium to the cardiac stimulatory effects of injected epinephrine and norepinephrine, leading to serious cardiac arrhythmias such as ventricular fibrillation (Figure 10-2).

During surgery, epinephrine is used with halothane and cardiac rhythm is monitored. If arrhythmias occur, antiarrhythmics are administered.

Evidence indicates a causal relationship between halothane use and postanesthetic hepatitis. Approximately 15% of halothane is metabolized in the liver, and these metabolites have been suggested as a cause of liver damage. Although halothane has proved to be a reliable and effective general anesthetic for many years, the occurrence of this adverse effect has diminished its popularity. For this reason, halothane is contraindicated in patients in whom a previous exposure to halothane or other halogenated hydrocarbons has been followed by postanesthetic liver toxicity. Patients with impaired liver function should be treated only with care.

◆ ENFLURANE

Enflurane (EN-floo-rane) (Ethrane) is a halogenated ether anesthetic with a pleasant smell. Induction and recovery are rapid because of its low tissue solubility. The MAC is 0.57 when combined with nitrous oxide. Enflurane depresses respiration, but this effect is controlled with assisted ventilation. It provides good analgesia and muscle relaxation, but supplemental muscle relaxants are still required. The heart is depressed, and blood pressure is reduced. Myocardial sensitization to injected epinephrine is less than that associated with halothane.

Adverse effects associated with enflurane use include alteration in electroencephalographic activity; thus excessive motor activity may occur during anesthesia. Careful regulation of anesthetic depth prevents such muscular activity. Enflurane is metabolized less than other volatile agents, which may account for the absence of hepatotoxicity. Enflurane also produces a transient depression of renal function.

◆ ISOFLURANE

A drug chemically related to enflurane is isoflurane (eye-soe-FLURE-ane) (Forane). Its low tissue solubility allows for rapid induction and recovery. Isoflurane has a slightly pungent smell, limiting the induction concentration, which otherwise could provoke coughing. When isoflurane is combined with 70% nitrous oxide, the MAC is 0.5. The pharmacologic effects of isoflurane are similar to those of the other halogenated ethers and include respiratory depression, reduced blood pressure, and muscle relaxation. Only a small amount of isoflurane undergoes metabolism, and liver toxicity does not seem to be a problem. Limited if any myocardial sensitization to injected epinephrine occurs. Nausea, vomiting, and shivering on recovery are comparable to responses to other anesthetic agents. The most undesirable side effect is respiratory acidosis associated with deeper levels of anesthesia. Isoflurane has proved to be a useful and popular drug for general anesthesia.

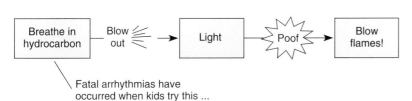

FIGURE 10-2
Hydrocarbon inhalation can produce fatal arrhythmias.

◆ DESFLURANE AND SEVOFLURANE

> Desflurane requires special vaporizer.

The newest halogenated hydrocarbons include desflurane and sevoflurane. They have the advantage of having low blood/gas partition coefficient so that they have a more rapid onset and a shorter duration of action than the other halogenated hydrocarbon anesthetics. Unfortunately, they have other difficulties. Desflurane's low volatility requires a special vaporizer. Because it induces cough and laryngospasm, it cannot be used for induction. Its recovery, despite its physical properties, does not appear to be faster than that of older agents. Sevoflurane is chemically unstable when exposed to carbon dioxide absorbents, producing a potentially nephrotoxic compound. Because it releases fluoride (F⁻) when metabolized, renal damage may occur.

Other General Anesthetics

◆ ULTRASHORT-ACTING BARBITURATES

The ultrashort-acting barbiturates used include methohexital (meth-oh-HEX-i-tal) sodium (Brevital), thiopental (thye-oh-PEN-tal) sodium (Pentothal), and thiamylal (thye-AM-i-lal) sodium (Surital). Although the basic pharmacology of the barbiturates is discussed in Chapter 11, certain facts about these drugs are discussed here.

These ultrashort-acting agents have a rapid onset of action (about 30 to 40 seconds) when given intravenously. Figure 10-3 demonstrates the percentage of the dose in each tissue over time. One should note that the dose begins in the blood, rapidly goes to the brain (lipid soluble), redistributes to lean tissues (muscles with high vascularity), and finally moves to the fat (lipid soluble, but low perfusion). If repeated doses are given, as is often the case during anesthesia, the drug accumulates in body tissues, resulting in prolonged recovery.

If these drugs are used as the sole anesthetic for short procedures, the patient will respond to painful stimuli. Because no analgesia is observed with doses that allow the patient to breathe spontaneously, the intravenously administered barbiturates function more effectively when used with a local anesthetic agent as part of a balanced anesthetic technique.

A serious complication with the use of IV barbiturates occurs when the solution is accidentally injected extravascularly or intraarterially. Symptoms with extravascular infiltration can range from tissue tenderness to necrosis and sloughing. Intraar-

terial injection is extremely dangerous and can lead to arteriospasm associated with ischemia of the arm and fingers and severe pain.

Other complications with ultrashort-acting barbiturates include laryngospasm and bronchospasm. In some patients, hiccoughs, increased muscle activity, and delirium occur on recovery. Premedication with atropine or opioids has proved reasonably effective in reducing these recovery problems.

The absolute contraindications to the use of ultrashort-acting barbiturates include an absence of suitable veins for administration, status asthmaticus, porphyria, or known hypersensitivity. The dose should be adjusted, and caution should be taken in patients with asthma or hepatic, renal, or cardiovascular impairment. These drugs can be used alone by trained and qualified practitioners for very short dental procedures or as part of a balanced anesthesia to induce surgical anesthesia (going from stage I to stage III). Because these drugs are potent anesthetics, they should be administered only by qualified individuals, with resuscitation equipment readily available.

◆ PROPOFOL

> Patient feels good; used for day surgery

One of the general anesthetics unrelated to any other general anesthetic is propofol (PROE-po-fole) (Diprivan). It is an IV anesthetic that produces an onset of anesthesia in 30 seconds (similar to the barbiturates) and a duration of action of about 5 minutes. Patients "feel better" and begin ambulation sooner than with other agents. It produces little vomiting and may have antiemetic effects. Propofol can be used for induction and for maintenance of balanced anesthesia. It is popular for outpatient surgery. Propofol is metabolized in the liver by conjugation to glucuronide and sulfate and excreted in the kidneys with a half-life of 30 to 60 minutes.

Propofol can produce a marked decrease in blood pressure during induction because it produces vasodilation. Apnea occurs in 50% to 80% of patients given propofol. Bradycardia and pain at the injection site can occur. Gastrointestinal adverse reactions have been reported. Hypersensitivity reactions involving hypotension, flushing, and bronchospasm occurred when propofol was dissolved in the original vehicle (polyoxyethylated castor oil) (Cremophor), but this reaction does not occur when it is dissolved in a fat emulsion (Intralipid) or soybean oil. Propofol is a relatively costly anesthetic.

◆ KETAMINE

> Chemically related to phencyclidine (PCP); produces dissociative anesthesia

The anesthetic ketamine (KEET-a-meen) (Ketalar) is related chemically to phencyclidine (PCP), a hallucinogen. The anesthetic state ketamine produces has been given the name *dissociative anesthesia* because ketamine appears to disrupt association pathways in the brain. Under ketamine, the patient appears to be catatonic and has amnesia; ketamine produces analgesia without actual loss of consciousness.

Ketamine may be given intravenously or intramuscularly, with a rapid (1 to 2 minutes) onset of action occurring with either route. It is distributed first to lipid tissues then to more vascular areas. Pharyngeal and laryngeal reflexes remain active, and there is little respiratory change. Ketamine increases cerebral blood flow and stimulates the heart to increase cardiac output. Because excessive salivation is a common finding with ketamine,

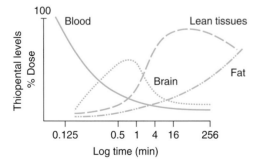

FIGURE 10-3

Thiopental concentrations in various tissues: fat, muscle (lean tissues), blood, and brain.

atropine is a necessary premedication. Muscle tone may increase during its use.

The principal drawback to the use of ketamine is the occurrence of "emergence phenomena," including delirium and hallucinations during recovery. This happens most often in adults, older children, and drug abusers. Reactions of this type can be minimized if visual and auditory stimuli are reduced during recovery. Small doses of an ultrashort-acting intravenously administered barbiturate or benzodiazepine have been used to control the recovery problem. Specific contraindications include a history of cerebrovascular disease, hypertension, and hypersensitivity to the drug. Psychiatric problems present a relative contraindication. Because protective reflexes of the pharynx and larynx are active, care should be taken not to stimulate the pharynx. This increase in reflexes in the throat may discourage use in dentistry.

◆ OPIOIDS

The opioids (OH-pee-oyds) have long been used as adjunctive drugs to general anesthesia in preanesthetic medication and to provide analgesia during and after a surgical procedure. Now opioids are used as anesthetic agents as well. The opioids used include morphine, fentanyl (Sublimaze), sufentanil (Sufenta), and alfentanil (Alfenta). These drugs do not significantly alter cardiovascular function or peripheral resistance. Prolonged respiratory depression is the major disadvantage and requires careful attention to ventilatory function throughout the anesthetic period. Reversal of this depression can be produced by the opioid antagonist naloxone.

◆ DROPERIDOL PLUS FENTANYL

The term *neuroleptanalgesia* refers to the so-called wakeful anesthetic state produced by the combination of a neuroleptic drug, droperidol (Inapsine), and a potent opioid analgesic, fentanyl (Sublimaze). Droperidol produces marked sedation and a catatonic state. It is a close relative of haloperidol, an antipsychotic agent. The combination of drugs is marketed as Innovar and is usually given intravenously for a rapid onset. Adding nitrous oxide results in *neuroleptanesthesia*. Return to consciousness appears to be rapid, but the effects of droperidol are long lasting and recovery is slow.

The adverse effects can be serious and include those that would normally be associated with the opioids and major tranquilizers. Respiratory depression and extrapyramidal tremors have occurred. This combination of drugs should be used with great care, especially in patients with pulmonary insufficiency and parkinsonism. A boardlike chest, associated with intercostal muscle paralysis and requiring ventilatory support, has occurred in some patients using IV opioids. Fentanyl is sometimes used as a sole agent for sedation.

◆ BENZODIAZEPINES

The anxiolytic benzodiazepines have been an integral part of conscious sedation and preanesthetic medication for years. Diazepam (Valium) has been used intravenously for many years. Midazolam (Versed), which is water soluble, does not need a solvent for solution, so one of diazepam's major side effects, thrombophlebitis, can be avoided. Other advantages include that it has a shorter duration of action and produces more amnesia than diazepam. Parenteral lorazepam is also available for similar uses. The benzodiazepines find their greatest applica-

tion as adjunctive drugs in the balanced anesthesia technique or for conscious sedation. They are discussed in detail in Chapter 11.

BALANCED GENERAL ANESTHESIA

The goals of surgical anesthesia are good patient control, adequate muscle relaxation, and pain relief. There are many agents that can produce general anesthesia. Each drug has its own adverse reaction profile. The many specific steps in Guedel's classification were developed for describing the effects obtained when ether was used alone. When balanced anesthesia is used, the patient readily passes from stage I to stage III (surgical anesthesia), skipping over the signs of stage II. The ultrashort-acting IV barbiturates accomplish this readily. These barbiturates are combined with the N_2O-O_2 in combination, which are then administered along with a volatile inhalation anesthetic (e.g., halogenated hydrocarbons). If local anesthetic blocks are administered before oral surgery procedures, the depth of general anesthesia can be lighter.

DENTAL HYGIENE CONSIDERATIONS

1. Review the patient's medication/health history for evidence of contraindications with nitrous oxide to include medical conditions and medications.
2. Check equipment before use to ensure that it works properly.
3. Several states now allow dental hygienists to administer nitrous oxide. Table 10-5 reviews patient response at different concentrations of nitrous oxide.
4. Patient response is the best indicator for degree of sedation.
5. Make sure that the patient's blood pressure and pulse are always within normal limits.
6. Encourage the patient to refrain from making any major decisions while still feeling sedated from any of the anesthetics.

CLINICAL SKILLS ASSESSMENT

1. Name and describe the four stages of anesthesia.
2. State the pharmacologic effects of the general anesthetics.
3. Describe the effects observed with varying concentrations of nitrous oxide.
4. What are the adverse reactions associated with nitrous oxide?
5. List the contraindications to the use of nitrous oxide.
6. State the potential hazards associated with the general anesthetic agents.
7. Describe which general anesthetics would be useful in the following situations:
   a. A patient with anxiety.
   b. A patient requiring oral surgery.
8. Explain the rationale for the use of several agents during general anesthesia.

◉**volve** ─────────────────────────

Please visit http://evolve.elsevier.com/Haveles/pharmacology for review questions and additional practice and reference materials.

11 Antianxiety Agents

LEARNING OBJECTIVES

1. Discuss the value of patient relaxation in dentistry.
2. Describe the mechanism of action, interactions, and dental relevance of the benzodiazepines and barbiturates.
3. Name and briefly describe the mechanism of action of the nonbenzodiazepine-nonbarbiturate sedative-hypnotics and the nonbenzodiazepine-nonbarbiturate receptor agonists.
4. Name a melatonin receptor agonist and summarize its actions.
5. Explain the workings of the centrally acting muscle relaxants and how they are used.
6. Discuss some general precautions about which the dental practitioner should be aware with the use of antianxiety agents.

> Dental professionals often do not recognize or relate to a patient's stress level while treatment is being provided.

Both the dentist and the dental hygienist recognize the value of a relaxed patient. Often, patient anxiety is sufficiently reduced by a calm, patient, confident, and understanding attitude on the part of the dental health care workers. However, individual responses to dental treatment vary widely, ranging from total relaxation and even sleeping to severe apprehension and the inability to approach the dental office, much less the dental chair. Each dental patient should be provided with the most pleasant experience possible within the limits of safety. When the patient is relaxed, appointments can be more productive, and the dentist, hygienist, and patient all benefit.

Dental professionals, because of their familiarity with all of dentistry's components and ramifications, often do not understand the basis of anxiety in the dental patient. Often, dental health care workers lack empathy and even commonly blame or fault the patient for his or her discomfort. Members of the dental team often become defensive because they do not feel comfortable and do not know how to manage these intense feelings. By acting perturbed, the dental team reinforces the patient's negative feelings about the dental appointment. A dental practitioner who decides that anxiety control is only necessary for the first third of a dental appointment does not understand patient anxiety and its treatment.

Many patients who require dental care never go to the dental office because of fear and apprehension. A common misconception is that dental patients who express anxiety are just "looking for drugs." The average dental patient who is being treated for dental anxiety during the appointment does not get the opportunity to abuse antianxiety agents. The appropriate use of antianxiety agents might encourage more patients to seek needed dental treatment. If, to treat many nervous dental patients, an occasional patient who was "seeking" antianxiety agents obtains them, that is an appropriate balance in the use of antianxiety agents. It would be unlikely for a person in search of drugs to sit for an hour in the dental chair, have dental treatment performed, and then pay for the treatment just to obtain one tablet of an antianxiety drug that was taken in the dental office. However, prescribing 20 tablets of an antianxiety drug for a patient nervous about getting dentures would be inappropriate.

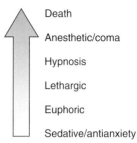

FIGURE 11-2
Sedative-hypnotics. Range of effects with increasing doses.

The normal sedative dose (calms normal patient without dental appointment) is not expected to produce calmness in a dental patient, but the hypnotic dose (that which induces sleep in the normal patient) can often produce the desired degree of sedation before dental treatment.

This chapter discusses some of the agents that can be used to allay anxiety—primarily, the benzodiazepines. Nitrous oxide, which is used in dentistry as an antianxiety agent, is discussed in Chapter 10 because it is classified as a general anesthetic. It is very useful in decreasing apprehension during the dental appointment and is underused in many dental practices. Some drugs with properties of both the antihistamines and phenothiazines, such as hydroxyzine and promethazine, have weak antianxiety properties and are discussed in Chapter 18.

DEFINITIONS

The sedative-hypnotic agents can produce varying degrees of central nervous system (CNS) depression, depending on the dose administered. A small dose will produce mild CNS depression described as sedation (reduction of activity and simple anxiety). This level of CNS depression has some anxiolytic effects. A larger dose of the same drug, the hypnotic dose (inducing sleep), will produce greater CNS depression. Thus the same drug may be either a sedative or a hypnotic, depending on the dose administered. In even larger doses, sedative-hypnotics may produce anesthesia and eventually death (Figure 11-2).

This chapter discusses the benzodiazepines, barbiturates, and the nonbenzodiazepine-nonbarbiturate sedative-hypnotics. The benzodiazepines are discussed first because they are used most often.

BENZODIAZEPINES

The benzodiazepines (ben-zoe-dye-AZ-e-peens) are the most commonly prescribed antianxiety drugs. The members of this group differ mainly in their onset and duration of action, dose, and dose forms available.

Chemistry

These drugs are named benzodiazepines because of their structure: a 1,4-benzodiazepine nucleus. Chlordiazepoxide (klor-dye-az-e-POX-ide) (Librium), the first derivative, was synthesized in 1955. After its success, thousands of other benzodiazepine derivatives were screened for psychopharmacologic activity. As a

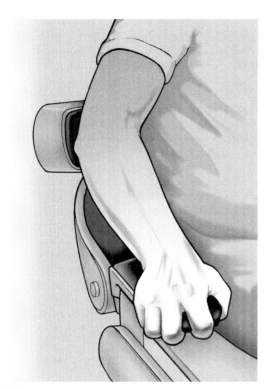

FIGURE 11-1
White-knuckle syndrome indicates that a patient is not in a relaxed state. (From Clark MS, Brunick A: *Handbook of nitrous oxide and oxygen sedation,* ed 3, St Louis, 2008, Mosby.)

It is necessary to objectively assess the patient's anxiety on both the first and subsequent visits. A patient who is clutching the dental chair arms and has white knuckles is not in a relaxed state (Figure 11-1). By questioning and observing the patient, a determination can be made about the need for antianxiety agents. Thus the patient can feel comfortable and relaxed during subsequent dental appointments. The dental health professional should remember that whatever procedure is performed, he or she has performed it many times. However, for many patients, this may be their first experience with the procedure, and their reactions may be altered by their interpretation of what is happening (e.g., "that sharp, pointy thing is going to hurt!" or "what are those gunlike weapons?").

Of the agents discussed in this chapter, the dental team will most commonly use orally administered drugs to provide relaxation for the anxious patient. Intravenous (IV) administration is used infrequently because it requires more training and experience than most general dentists possess. Most states require a separate certificate to administer IV agents or to provide conscious sedation, and the malpractice insurance is much more expensive. Although orally administered sedatives provide inconsistent or poorly predictable results, practitioners should become familiar with one or two drugs and use them repeatedly. In the long run, this practice will produce greater benefits than changing from drug to drug.

The dose of a particular antianxiety agent effective for a particular patient is vastly variable, involving both intrapatient and interpatient variation. Predicting the correct dose is a guess at best. The amount needed is poorly related to the degree of the patient's anxiety or the dental procedure to be performed.

TABLE 11-1   BENZODIAZEPINES AND MISCELLANEOUS SEDATIVE-HYPNOTIC AGENTS

Drug Name Generic (Trade)	INDICATION DOSE (mg/d)		ONSET OF ACTION		Peak (hr)	Half-Life (hr)	FDA Pregnancy Category
	Sleep	Anxiety	Category	(min)			
Benzodiazepines							
Alprazolam		1-4	I	45-60	1-2	6-27	D
Chlordiazepoxide (Librium)		15-100	I	15-45	0.5-4	5-30	D
Clonazepam (Klonopin)*	0.5		I	20-60	1-2	18-50	C
Clorazepate (Tranxene)		15-60	F	30-60	1-2	40-50	C
Diazepam (Valium)†	5-10	4-40	VF	15-45	0.5-2	20-80	D
Estazolam (ProSom)	1-2				0.5-2	10-19	X
Flurazepam (Dalmane)	30		I	15-45	0.5-1	2.3	D
Halazepam (Paxipam)		60-160	S		1-3	14	D
Lorazepam (Ativan)‡	1-4	1-10	I	15-45	1-6	10-20	D
Midazolam (Versed)‡§		Titrate	F	PO 30	PO 0.5-1	2-7	D
			F	IV 1-5	IV 3-5 min	2-6	
Oxazepam (Serax)	15-30	30-120	S	45-90	2-4 (1-2)	5-20	C
Quazepam (Doral)	15				1-2	39	X
Temazepam (Restoril)	15-30		S	25-60	2-3	4-18	X
Triazolam (Halcion)	0.125-0.5		F	15-30	2, 0.5-2	1.5-5	X
Nonbenzodiazepine-Benzodiazepine Receptor Agonists							
Zolpidem (Ambien)	10				0.5-2	1.5-4.5	B
Zolpidem (Ambien CR)	12.5			30	1.5	1.5-4.5	B
Zaleplon (Sonata)	10-20			15-30	1	1	C
Eszopiclone (Lunesta)	2-3			15-30	1	6	C
Nonbenzodiazepine-Nonbarbiturate Sedative-Hypnotics							
Chloral hydrate (Noctec)	500-1000			30			C
Melatonin Receptor Agonist							
Ramelteon (Rozerem)	8			15-30	0.5-1.5	1-2.6	C

I, Intermediate; *F*, fast; *VF*, very fast; *S*, slow.
*Used as an adjunct to treat certain kinds of seizures.
†Injectable form contains propylene glycol—can produce thrombophlebitis.
‡Available parenterally.
§Midazolam administered intravenously in United States; intravenous form can be given orally.

result of this search, diazepam (Valium) was synthesized in 1959 and marketed in 1963. Many benzodiazepines are now available (Table 11-1).

Pharmacokinetics

The benzodiazepines are well absorbed when administered by the oral route. The rapid onset of action of the benzodiazepines is related to their lipid solubility. Diazepam, which is highly lipid soluble, has a quick onset and is concentrated in the adipose tissue. Storage in adipose tissue prolongs the action of lipid-soluble benzodiazepines. The benzodiazepines are available in the following dose forms: tablets, capsules, oral solution, rectal gel, and injectable forms. The intramuscular (IM) route, for benzodiazepines other than midazolam, gives slow, erratic, and unpredictable results. In contrast, the IV route, for those available in parenteral form, produces a rapid, predictable response that makes them ideal for conscious sedation. Once a benzodi-

azepine is absorbed, the rate at which it crosses into the cerebrospinal fluid (CSF) through the blood-brain barrier depends on protein binding, lipid solubility, and the ionization constant of the compound. Most benzodiazepines are highly protein bound and are present in the un-ionized, lipid-soluble form. They easily cross the blood-brain and placental barriers to produce an effect in the CNS and on the fetus (Food and Drug Administration [FDA] categories D or X), where they can accumulate with repeated doses.

After absorption, the benzodiazepines are metabolized in the liver by either phase II metabolism or phase I followed by phase II metabolism. Phase I metabolism is decreased in the elderly, in patients taking certain drugs that inhibit hepatic metabolism, and in the presence of hepatic disease. Phase I metabolism results in active metabolites that, with repeated administration, can accumulate. The half-lives of these drugs range from 2 to 200 hours (see Table 11-1).

Benzodiazepines that undergo only phase II metabolism are much less affected by drugs or hepatic disease. Age does not seem to affect phase II metabolism. However, caution should still be used when prescribing these drugs for elderly persons.

Mechanism of Action

| Benzodiazepines facilitate GABA-mediated transmission. |

Benzodiazepines enhance or facilitate the action of the neurotransmitter γ-aminobutyric acid (GABA), a major inhibitory transmitter in the CNS. It acts in the limbic, thalamic, cortical, and hypothalamic levels of the CNS. Benzodiazepines act as agonists at the benzodiazepine receptor site, thereby reducing the symptoms of anxiety.

Pharmacologic Effects

The pharmacologic effects of the benzodiazepines have qualitatively similar actions but vary in potency.

◆ BEHAVIORAL EFFECTS

The clinical effects of these agents in humans are anxiety and panic reduction at lower doses and production of drowsiness and sleep at higher doses. Repeated doses of benzodiazepines reduce rapid eye movement (REM) sleep. Usual doses produce a marked reduction in stages 3 and 4 sleep (deep sleep), which, after long-term use, can interfere with restorative sleep.

◆ ANTISEIZURE EFFECTS

The benzodiazepines, such as diazepam, have antiseizure activity (i.e., they increase the seizure threshold). Diazepam, used parenterally, has been shown to be an effective antiseizure drug for the prevention of seizures associated with local anesthetic toxicity and for the treatment of status epilepticus. Clonazepam, an oral benzodiazepine, is used in combination with other antiseizure drugs to manage partial seizures. The benzodiazepines prevent the spread of seizures in tissues surrounding the anatomic seizure focus (when such a focus exists) but have little effect on the discharges at the focus itself.

◆ MUSCLE RELAXATION

Like all CNS depressants, benzodiazepines can produce relaxation of skeletal muscles. Some studies show benzodiazepines to be superior to other skeletal muscle relaxants for relief of musculoskeletal pain; other studies show the pain relief effect to be no better than aspirin or placebo. Benzodiazepines are effective for muscle spasticity secondary to pathologic states such as cerebral palsy or paraplegia.

Adverse Reactions

In general, benzodiazepines used alone have a wide margin of safety. They all have similar adverse effects but differ in their frequency. Agents with long-elimination half-lives tend to accumulate and produce more side effects.

◆ CENTRAL NERVOUS SYSTEM EFFECTS

The most common side effect attributed to benzodiazepines is CNS depression manifested as fatigue, drowsiness, muscle weakness, and ataxia. These side effects are more likely to occur in elderly persons. The patient may also experience lightheadedness and dizziness. Tolerance to this effect occurs over time. Paradoxical CNS stimulation that produces talkativeness, anxiety, nightmares, tremulousness, hyperactivity, and increased muscle

spasticity can occur. This reaction is more common in psychiatric patients, and benzodiazepines should be discontinued if this reaction occurs.

When benzodiazepines are used in dentistry to produce conscious sedation, this side effect of CNS depression is used as the primary effect. The amount of the benzodiazepine used to provide conscious sedation is titrated to the patient's response. The appearance of ptosis is used as an initial endpoint for the dose administered. These agents have a rapid onset of action and an initial effect of 45 minutes to 1 hour.

Diazepam was the most common benzodiazepine used parenterally until newer benzodiazepines were developed. Diazepam's long half-life and its metabolism to an active metabolite prolonged its duration of action. Its effect lasted past the dental appointment time and even into the next day.

Midazolam, a water-soluble benzodiazepine, is metabolized primarily to inactive metabolites. This produces an advantage for its IV use over diazepam in conscious sedation. Because these benzodiazepines are inactivated either by metabolism or by metabolism of their active metabolites, the duration and depth of sedation can be magnified by administration of drugs that inhibit the hepatic microsomal enzymes. Agents that inhibit these enzymes include cimetidine and erythromycin.

| "Roofies" are used before date rape; amnesia makes prosecution difficult. |

A potent benzodiazepine named flunitrazepam (flew-nye-TRAY-ze-pam) (Rohypnol) is a benzodiazepine available in Europe but not the United States. Acquired illegally from Europe or Mexico, this benzodiazepine, nicknamed "roofies," is being used inappropriately in the United States and has been secretly administered to women who were then "date raped." The muscle flaccidity and amnesia produced by this agent make it difficult for the victim to resist or to testify later. Increasing the penalty for possession of this agent is being considered.

◆ ANTEROGRADE AMNESIA

It can be easily demonstrated that parenteral benzodiazepines, such as diazepam and midazolam, produce amnesia beginning when the drug is taken. This effect is used to therapeutic advantage in patients scheduled for an unpleasant dental procedure. Clinical use has produced episodes of amnesia that can sometimes last several hours and can occur with several benzodiazepines. Oral triazolam seems to have a greater likelihood to produce amnesia than other oral benzodiazepines. Patients should be warned not to sign important papers or make important decisions after benzodiazepines are administered. The mechanism of amnesia results from an impairment of consolidation processes that store the information in the brain.

◆ RESPIRATORY EFFECTS

Usual doses of benzodiazepines have no adverse effect on respiration. However, doses of diazepam administered for outpatient dental procedures have been occasionally reported to produce respiratory depression. An isolated case of apnea after IV diazepam has also been observed. These respiratory effects are more common in elderly patients. The minimal respiratory depression can be exacerbated by opioids or alcohol.

◆ CARDIOVASCULAR EFFECTS

Therapeutic doses of benzodiazepines have no adverse effect on circulation. The relief of anxiety may result in a fall in blood pressure and pulse rate. The pulse rate has also been reported to rise (tachycardia) and then return to normal after a few minutes.

♦ VISUAL EFFECTS

Benzodiazepines are contraindicated in angle-closure (narrow angle) glaucoma and can produce other visual changes such as diplopia, **nystagmus**, and blurred vision. They may be used in treatment of wide-angle glaucoma, which is the most common kind of glaucoma.

♦ DENTAL EFFECTS

The benzodiazepines have been reported to produce xerostomia, increased salivation (note that these are opposite effects), swollen tongue, and a bitter or metallic taste.

♦ THROMBOPHLEBITIS

Parenteral diazepam can produce thrombophlebitis. Because diazepam is poorly soluble in water, the vehicle propylene glycol is used to solubilize it. The vehicle is responsible for the thrombophlebitis. The incidence is lower when the IV **infusion** is given in the antecubital space rather than the dorsum of the hand (more blood and faster blood flow). Because midazolam is soluble in water and propylene glycol is not used to solubilize it, it is much less likely to produce this effect. With parenteral use, apnea, hypotension, bradycardia, and cardiac arrest have been reported. These are more frequent with rapid administration. Equipment for respiratory and cardiovascular assistance must be available if these agents are to be used parenterally (e.g., conscious sedation in the dental office). Special training of the dental team administering benzodiazepines is required.

♦ OTHER EFFECTS

Benzodiazepines can affect the gastrointestinal tract, producing cramps or pain, and the genitourinary tract, producing difficulty in urination. They can also produce allergic reactions, including skin rash or itching.

♦ PREGNANCY AND LACTATION CONSIDERATIONS

An increased risk of congenital malformation in infants of mothers taking benzodiazepines in the first trimester has been reported. **Cleft lip and palate**, microencephaly, and gastrointestinal and cardiovascular abnormalities were greater in the group taking benzodiazepines. Most of these agents are classified as FDA pregnancy category D drugs; triazolam and temazepam are in FDA pregnancy category X (see Chapter 24).

Near-term administration of benzodiazepines to the mother has resulted in floppy infant syndrome. This syndrome includes hypoactivity, hypotonia, hypothermia, apnea, and feeding problems. Because these agents are seldom absolutely needed (except for epilepsy), they should be avoided in women who are or may become pregnant and in nursing mothers. Before administering a benzodiazepine, the pregnancy status of the female patient should be determined. The first trimester, often before the patient knows that she is pregnant, is the time benzodiazepines are more likely to be teratogenic or cause problems in the fetus.

Abuse and Tolerance

♦ OVERVIEW

Benzodiazepines can be abused, and physical dependence and tolerance have been documented. Physiologic addiction can occur if large doses are taken over an extended period. However, their abuse and addiction potential is less than that of the other sedative-hypnotic agents such as the barbiturates.

Prolonged intake of large doses of benzodiazepines can result in a degree of CNS tolerance. Cross-tolerance also exists between the benzodiazepines and other CNS depressants. This may explain why benzodiazepines can be substituted for ethyl alcohol to relieve the symptoms of delirium tremens precipitated by acute alcohol withdrawal.

| Very wide therapeutic index |

One advantage of benzodiazepines over barbiturates is their wider therapeutic index, or range of safe dose. Overdose poisoning with these drugs has been rare and appears to be difficult to achieve when used alone, although apnea has rarely been reported. In most instances, excessively large doses must be ingested to produce respiratory or central vasomotor depression. Combining benzodiazepines with other CNS depressants can reduce the safety so that the combination can be lethal. The addition of alcohol can result in coma, respiratory depression, hypotension, or hypothermia.

♦ TREATMENT OF OVERDOSE

| Chronic use in insomnia is not recommended. |

Rarely does the ingestion of a benzodiazepine alone result in severe symptoms. Supportive therapy should be undertaken if symptoms result. With recent ingestion, emesis may be induced. Activated charcoal and a saline cathartic may be administered. The patient's respiration and blood pressure should be monitored.

To reverse some of the effects of a benzodiazepine, flumazenil (floo-MA-zee-nill) (Romazicon), a benzodiazepine antagonist available for IV administration, may be used. It has been shown to reverse the sedating and psychomotor effects, but reversing the respiratory depression produced by the benzodiazepines is incomplete. The amnesia is not consistently reversed. It has an initial half-life of about 10 minutes and a terminal half-life of about 60 minutes. Side effects include pain at the injection site, agitation, and anxiety. An increase in inadequate analgesia does not occur. Some patients became resedated before the end of 3 hours when high doses of long-acting benzodiazepines were ingested (the antagonist wore off before the agonist had been metabolized and excreted). Administering flumazenil to benzodiazepine-dependent individuals could precipitate withdrawal symptoms (similar to naloxone to opioids).

Drug Interactions

Like other antianxiety agents, benzodiazepines interact in an additive fashion with other CNS depressants, notably alcohol, barbiturates, anticonvulsants, and phenothiazines. Because diazepam and desmethyldiazepam are cytochrome P-450 2C enzyme substrates, enzyme inducers may increase their metabolism and enzyme stimulators may decrease their metabolism.

Smoking reduces the effectiveness of the benzodiazepines. The tars produced by smoking cigarettes stimulate the hepatic microsomal enzymes in the liver. The increased number of liver enzymes increases the rate of metabolism of the benzodiazepines, so a higher dose of a benzodiazepine is required to produce the same effect.

Drugs, such as cimetidine, disulfiram, isoniazid, and omeprazole, may increase the effects of benzodiazepines. Valproic acid may displace diazepam from binding sites, which may result in an increase in sedative effects. Selective serotonin reuptake inhibitors (e.g., fluoxetine, sertraline, or paroxetine) have greatly increased diazepam levels by altering its clearance. Benzodiazepines may reduce the effectiveness of levodopa, and parkinsonism has been exacerbated in these patients. Benzodiazepines may increase the effect of digoxin, phenytoin, and probenecid.

Medical Uses

Benzodiazepines are useful in short-term treatment of anxiety, panic attacks, insomnia, and alcohol withdrawal. They are used for the acute treatment of seizures. Some neuromuscular diseases can be treated with the benzodiazepines. They are used in conscious sedation, general anesthesia, or during surgery.

ANXIETY CONTROL

Generalized anxiety disorder and panic disorder are common indications for use of benzodiazepines in general medicine. Anxiety produces a physiologic response resembling fear, with manifestations including restlessness, tension, tachycardia, and dyspnea. Most well-controlled clinical trials have shown that the antianxiety effect of benzodiazepines is better than those of placebo, barbiturates, and meprobamate. Benzodiazepines also produce less sedation than the classic sedative-hypnotic agents.

◆ INSOMNIA MANAGEMENT

| For dental anxiety | If insomnia is a manifestation of
anxiety, sleep will usually improve when a benzodiazepine is administered at bedtime as an antianxiety drug. The benzodiazepines are preferable to the barbiturates as hypnotics because the risk of physical addiction or serious poisoning is much less. The efficacy of the benzodiazepines in the treatment of chronic insomnia has not been demonstrated past 1 month.

The occasional use of the benzodiazepines within controlled limits can be useful. For example, limiting the number of tablets to 10 per month for insomnia will limit tolerance, dependence, and withdrawal. Underlying causes of insomnia, such as depression or alcoholism, should be identified and treated. Nonaddicting agents, such as trazodone, may be useful in the treatment of insomnia, and unlike the benzodiazepines, no tolerance or dependence is produced even with chronic use. Nonpharmacologic management of sleep disorders (Box 11-1) should be instituted before any benzodiazepine is prescribed. Several patients with new prescriptions for "sleeping pills" have discussed the pot of coffee they drink after dinner. (What is wrong with this picture?)

◆ TREATMENT OF EPILEPSY (SEIZURES)

Diazepam or lorazepam is the drug of choice for treatment of repetitive, intractable seizures (status epilepticus) that require IV therapy. They are also used for treatment of seizures caused by local anesthetic toxicity. Orally administered diazepam is of little value, even as a maintenance anticonvulsant. Oral clonazepam is used as an adjunct to other anticonvulsants for some difficult-to-control types of seizures. It is also used in the management of mood disorders.

◆ TREATMENT OF ALCOHOLISM

The benzodiazepines are used in the treatment of the alcohol withdrawal syndrome. Administration of an adequate amount of a benzodiazepine can prevent the emergence of the signs and

---

BOX 11-1   NONPHARMACOLOGIC MANAGEMENT OF SLEEP DISORDERS

Before patients are given agents to treat insomnia, they should be questioned about their sleep hygiene habits. Insomnia can be a result of many organic, psychological, or situational causes. The following is a list of several habits that should be developed to minimize insomnia:

- Regular bedtime regardless of whether sleepy
- Remain in bed no more than 20 minutes without sleeping
- Get up if not sleeping and perform a quiet activity
- Regular awakening at 6 am even if sleep only began at 5 am
- Limit sleeping to fewer hours, go to bed later, get up earlier
- Exercise during the day (not within 3 hours of bedtime)
- Light snack (warm milk) at bedtime
- No naps during the day regardless of sleep problems
- Avoid caffeine within 8 hours of bedtime (cola, sodas [check label for caffeine], coffee, and tea)
- No smoking within 8 hours of bedtime
- Get ready for bed by engaging in quiet activities such as reading or listening to music. Use "noise" to disguise noise by listening to white noise.

Repeated use of a sedative-hypnotic leads to tolerance and a need for an increased dose to produce the same effect. Most agents become increasingly less effective with regular use. These agents can also alter sleep architecture (rapid eye movement [REM] sleep).

The normal sleep cycle involves several stages. Latency is the time it takes to get to sleep. Sleeping is distributed between REM sleep (30%) and non-REM (NREM) sleep. NREM sleep has four stages.

Benzodiazepines reduce the latency, REM sleep, and NREM sleep stages 3 and 4, while increasing stage 2. When benzodiazepines have been used chronically and are discontinued, rebound REM sleep often occurs, resulting in an increase in vivid dreams. Some patients continue to take benzodiazepines because they do not want to experience these scary dreams.

---

symptoms of acute alcohol withdrawal, such as agitation and tremor. It has not been shown that they prevent hallucinations or delirium tremens.

◆ CONTROL OF MUSCLE SPASMS

Benzodiazepines are used to control the muscle spasticity that accompanies various diseases such as multiple sclerosis and cerebral palsy. They are used for the relief of pain and spasm of back strain. Studies have suggested that the benzodiazepines are more effective than other muscle relaxants such as methocarbamol, carisoprodol, and chlorzoxazone.

Management of the Dental Patient Taking Benzodiazepines

The dental implications of the benzodiazepines are described in Box 11-2.

◆ DENTAL PROCEDURES

| Ensure that the patient has a responsible driver before releasing. | Orally administered diazepam has been shown to be more effective than placebo in allaying apprehension in patients undergoing restorative procedures. It is used in combination with other agents such as opioids and anticholinergic agents. If diazepam is used for the initial treatment of patients with dental anxiety, it is hoped that future appointments may be completed successfully without benzodiazepine increases. For preoperative dental anxiety, a ben-

---

BOX 11-2   MANAGEMENT OF THE DENTAL PATIENT TAKING BENZODIAZEPINES

- Additive CNS depression with other CNS depressants (including alcohol).
- Avoid in addicts or women who could be pregnant (women 11-63 years of age).
- Keep track of exact number prescribed and usage rate in patient's chart.
- Use glucuronidated type in elderly patients and in patients on cimetidine.
- Warn patient about sedation and amnesia.
- Match onset and duration with dental procedure requirements.
- Make sure patient has arranged for transportation to and from dental appointment.

CNS, Central nervous system.

zodiazepine should be chosen that has a fast onset of action and a relatively short half-life. This reduces the patient's waiting time and allows resumption of normal functions as soon as possible. The dose used should be in the range of the usual hypnotic dose (see Table 11-1). Examples of agents used for dental anxiety might include triazolam (trye-AY-zoe-lam) (fast onset and short half-life) and diazepam (very fast onset but long half-life). Lorazepam (lor-A-ze-pam) or alprazolam (al-PRAY-zoe-lam) (intermediate onset but relatively short half-lives) could also be used, especially in the elderly. Midazolam (MID-ay-zoe-lam) is available for parenteral (Versed injection) and oral (Versed syrup) use in the United States and is used to sedate children. The parenteral midazolam product can be administered orally to sedate children. Patients given either oral or parenteral benzodiazepines should not be allowed to operate a motor vehicle, and the dental staff should ensure that a driver is present before dismissing the patient.

◆ PREMEDICATION

The benzodiazepines have been used before surgical procedures to allay anxiety. They may be used orally or parenterally. The amnesia that occurs with parenteral administration is especially useful during stressful dental procedures. Diazepam is used as a premedication before general anesthesia, endoscopy, cardioversion, gastroscopy, sigmoidoscopy, and cystoscopy.

◆ CONSCIOUS SEDATION

Conscious sedation using the benzodiazepines is usually accomplished by IV administration. Diazepam, lorazepam, or midazolam, given intravenously, provides muscle relaxation and anterograde amnesia (amnesia occurs to events after the injection) during dental procedures. Although amnesia quickly follows the IV injection of diazepam and midazolam, it depends on several variables. Amnesia may be expected to persist for up to 45 minutes; therefore postoperative instructions should be provided in writing. Benzodiazepines available for parenteral administration (diazepam, midazolam, and lorazepam) are used for conscious sedation. The patient maintains reflexes, but time perception is lost and amnesia reduces the patient's memory. Because parenteral benzodiazepines have been associated with respiratory depression and arrest when used for conscious sedation, they require continuous monitoring of respiratory and cardiac function. Emergency drugs, equipment, and personnel must be available. Because some states and insurance companies are placing controls on the use of IV sedation in dentistry, those dentists without additional training cannot use conscious sedation. Additional training is now a requirement before dentists can administer parenteral benzodiazepines.

BARBITURATES

Barbiturates (bar-BI-tyoo-rates), the original sedative-hypnotic agents, are chemically related to each other and have similar pharmacologic effects. The barbiturates differ from each other mainly in their onset and duration of action (Table 11-2). Because these agents have been used for years, the problems with their use have been well documented. Barbiturates have long been associated with a high rate of abuse and complete cardiovascular and respiratory depression with overdose. Because the benzodiazepines have a much more acceptable safety profile, they have almost completely replaced barbiturates in clinical use for treating anxiety and insomnia. Barbiturates are still used as anticonvulsants and to induce general anesthesia.

Chemistry

The clinically useful barbiturates are formed by substitution of R groups (organic groups) on the barbiturate nucleus sites A and B. Another modification of the barbiturate nucleus involves replacing the oxygen atom with a sulfur atom site C. Compounds with the S-substitution are effective as IV agents such as thiopental.

Pharmacokinetics

Barbiturates are well absorbed orally and rectally. Because the injectable solutions are highly irritating, the IM route is avoided and the drugs are used intravenously. The IV agents are inactivated mainly by redistribution from their site of action in the CNS to the muscles and finally to adipose tissue. The short- and intermediate-acting barbiturates are rapidly and almost completely metabolized by the liver. Long-acting barbiturates are largely excreted through the kidneys as the free drug. Patients with liver damage may have an exaggerated response to short- and intermediate-acting agents, and patients with renal impairment may have an accumulation of the long-acting agents.

Mechanism of Action

Barbiturates produce their effect by enhancing GABA-receptor binding. They prolong the opening of the chloride channels. In higher doses, they may also act directly on the chloride channels without GABA presence. This mechanism is less specific than that of the benzodiazepines, which may account for their ability to induce surgical anesthesia and produce pronounced generalized CNS depressant effects.

Pharmacologic Effects

◆ CENTRAL NERVOUS SYSTEM DEPRESSION

The principal effects of the barbiturates are on the CNS. When normal doses of these agents are administered, relaxation occurs and the electroencephalogram (EEG) speeds up. With larger doses, the inhibitory fibers of the CNS are depressed, resulting in disinhibition and euphoria. If excitation occurs at this point, it is a result of depression of the inhibitory pathways. Anxiety

TABLE 11-2	BARBITURATES		
Barbiturate Group	Route of Administration	Onset*	Duration† of Action (hr)
Ultrashort Acting			
Methohexital (Brevital)	IV	Immediate	Minutes
Thiopental sodium (Pentothal)	IV	Immediate	Minutes
Short Acting			
Pentobarbital (Nembutal)	PO, IM, IV, rectal	10-15 min	3-4
Secobarbital (Seconal)	PO, IM, IV, rectal	10-15 min	3-4
Immediate Acting			
Amobarbital (Amytal)	PO, IM, IV, rectal	40-60 min	6-8
Butabarbital (Butisol)	PO	40-60 min	6-8
Long Acting			
Phenobarbital (Luminal)	PO, IM, IV	30-60 min	10-16
Mephobarbital (Mebaral)	PO	30-60 min	10-16

IM, Intramuscular; *IV,* intravenous; *PO,* orally.
*Onset = time until the drug's action begins.
†Duration = length of drug's action.

relief cannot be separated from the sedative effects. When higher doses are administered, hypnosis can be produced. The administration of even higher doses can result in anesthesia, with respiratory and cardiovascular depression and finally arrest. This progressive CNS depression parallels that caused by most CNS depressants, including general anesthetics (see Chapter 10).

The CNS depression produced by the barbiturates is additive with other agents that produce this effect. For example, a patient who drinks an alcoholic beverage or is given an opioid analgesic will show additive CNS depression.

◆ ANALGESIA

Barbiturates have no significant analgesic effects. Even doses that produce general anesthesia do not block the reflex response to pain. Patients in pain may become agitated and even delirious if barbiturates are administered without analgesic agents.

◆ ANTICONVULSANT EFFECT

The barbiturates possess anticonvulsant action. The long-acting agents such as phenobarbital are used in the treatment of epilepsy (see Chapter 16).

Adverse Reactions

◆ SEDATIVE OR HYPNOTIC DOSES

In the usual therapeutic doses, barbiturates are relatively safe. However, one should be aware that CNS depression may be exaggerated in elderly and debilitated patients or in those with liver or kidney impairment. In some patients, especially the elderly, barbiturates can have an idiosyncratic effect, causing stimulation instead of sedation. Barbiturates can cause fetal harm if administered to a pregnant woman.

◆ ANESTHETIC DOSES

With higher doses, barbiturate concentrations attained in the blood can be lethal. High concentrations are used for intubation or very short procedures. Coughing and laryngospasm have

been reported with IV use of barbiturates. High doses may reversibly depress liver and kidney function, reduce gastrointestinal motility, and lower body temperature.

◆ ACUTE POISONING

When barbiturates are prescribed, the possibility that acute poisoning can occur must be considered. Although a lethal dose can only be approximated, severe poisoning will follow the ingestion of 10 times the hypnotic dose, and life is seriously threatened when more than 15 times the hypnotic dose is consumed. The cause of death when an overdose occurs is respiratory failure. The treatment includes conservative management and treatment of specific symptoms.

Chronic Long-Term Use

Chronic use of barbiturates can lead to physical and psychological dependence. Long-term use produces a state similar to alcohol intoxication. The barbiturate addict becomes progressively depressed and is unable to function. Tolerance develops to most effects of barbiturates but not to the lethal dose. Therefore a larger and larger dose must be used to produce an effect, and this dose can approximate the lethal dose. Cross-tolerance occurs among barbiturates and between the barbiturates and nonbarbiturate sedative-hypnotic agents. Chapter 25 discusses the abuse of the barbiturates.

Contraindications

The use of barbiturates is absolutely contraindicated in patients with intermittent porphyria or a positive family history of porphyria. This is because barbiturates can stimulate and increase the synthesis of porphyrins, which are already at an excessive level in this metabolic disease. In fact, the barbiturates have been reported to precipitate an acute attack of porphyria.

Drug Interactions

Because barbiturates are potent stimulators of liver microsomal enzyme production, they are involved in many drug interac-

BOX 11-3 BARBITURATE DRUG INTERACTIONS
Barbiturates Reduce These Drugs' Effects
Acetaminophen
β-Blocker
Birth control pills
Chlorpromazine
Doxycycline
Estrogens
Griseofulvin
Phenytoin
Quinidine
Steroids
Tricyclic antidepressants
Warfarin
Barbiturate's Effect Enhanced by These Drugs
Disulfiram
Propoxyphene
Phenytoin
Enhanced or Additive CNS Depressant Effect
Alcohol
CNS depressants
Opioid analgesics
MAOIs

CNS, Central nervous system; *MAOIs,* monoamine oxidase inhibitors.

tions. These enzymes are responsible for the metabolism of many drugs, so an increase in these enzymes could increase the rate of drug destruction and decrease the duration of action. For example, if an epileptic patient who is currently receiving phenytoin (Dilantin) is subsequently given phenobarbital, the phenobarbital stimulates the liver microsomal enzymes that destroy the phenytoin and the phenobarbital more rapidly, which could cause convulsions. This drug interaction requires repeated doses and is not significant with a single dose. Some barbiturate drug interactions are listed in Box 11-3.

Uses

The therapeutic uses of barbiturates are determined by their duration of action (see Table 11-2). The ultrashort-acting agents, such as thiopental (thye-oh-PEN-tal), are used intravenously for the induction of general anesthesia. For very brief procedures, they may be used alone. For more extensive procedures, they are used to induce stage III surgical anesthesia (see Chapter 10).

The short- and intermediate-acting agents have little medical use. Benzodiazepines have replaced them for insomnia and anxiety relief. The short-acting agents were popular agents of abuse because of their fast onset of action.

The long-acting barbiturates, such as phenobarbital (fee-noe-BAR-bi-tal), are used for the treatment of epilepsy.

NONBENZODIAZEPINE-NONBARBITURATE SEDATIVE-HYPNOTICS

Chloral Hydrate

Chloral hydrate (KLOR-al HYE-drate) (Noctec) is an inexpensive, orally effective sedative-hypnotic drug with a rapid onset (20 to 30 minutes) and fairly short duration of action (about 4

hours). Therapeutic doses do not produce pronounced respiratory or cardiovascular depression. An exaggerated effect occurs in patients with advanced liver or kidney disease. Large doses or long-term use may produce peripheral vasodilation and hypotension with some degree of myocardial depression. Gastric irritation can be minimized by taking chloral hydrate in diluted solutions with milk or food. The highly irritating effect of chloral hydrate on the mucosa can produce aspiration, especially in struggling children. Its disagreeable odor and taste can be partially masked in a flavored syrup. As with all sedative-hypnotic agents, psychologic or physical dependence may follow prolonged use of this drug.

Chloral hydrate has been used in dentistry for the preoperative sedation of children. The child's hypnotic dose of chloral hydrate, when used alone, is 50 mg/kg, up to a maximum of 1 gm. Benzodiazepines are a safer choice for sedation of children. Because of its high incidence of gastrointestinal adverse effects and its ability to cause vasodilation and hypotension, this drug is rarely used in children.

Buspirone

Buspirone (byoo-SPYE-rone) (BuSpar) is unique in structure and action. It is the only member of this anxiolytic group. Its onset of action is about 1 week. It is discussed separately because of its unique structure and pharmacology. Its mechanism of action is unknown, but it is believed to be related to interactions with neurotransmitters in the CNS, including serotonin (5-HT$_{1A}$), dopamine, and cholinergic and α-adrenergic receptors. Buspirone undergoes first-pass metabolism and has a half-life of 2 to 4 hours.

The pharmacologic effect of buspirone is called *anxioselective* because of its selective anxiolytic action without hypnotic, anticonvulsant, or muscle-relaxant properties. It produces much less CNS depression than other sedative-hypnotic agents and does not affect driving skills. Some patients experience nervousness or insomnia. Buspirone does not produce tolerance or dependence. It does not appear to be addicting and there is no withdrawal syndrome. Because of the mechanism by which buspirone produces its anxiolytic effect, most patients prefer the benzodiazepines.

NONBENZODIAZEPINE-BENZODIAZEPINE RECEPTOR AGONISTS

Zolpidem (Ambien), zaleplon (Sonata), and eszopiclone (Lunesta) are a new class of drugs that are not benzodiazepines but appear to bind to benzodiazepine receptors and decrease sleep latency with little effect on sleep stages. All of these drugs are thought to have agonist effects on GABA. These drugs are used to treat insomnia only. They are controlled substances and have the potential to cause both physical and psychologic dependence.

Zolpidem

Zolpidem (zole-PI-dem) is a hypnotic agent that was recently developed and is indicated for the short-term management of insomnia. Its structure is unlike the benzodiazepines. In contrast to some sedative-hypnotic agents that act at all benzodiazepine (BZ) receptors, zolpidem interacts with the GABA$_A$ receptor at the BZ$_1$ receptor. Although zolpidem retains its hypnotic and anxiolytic effects, its receptor specificity gives zolpidem

TABLE 11-3 CENTRALLY ACTING SKELETAL MUSCLE RELAXANTS

Drug	Comments	Dose (mg)
Carisoprodol (Soma)	Tachycardia, flushing	350 tid-qid
Chlorzoxazone (Parafon Forte DSC)	GI distress, hypersensitivity, CNS depression	250-750 tid-qid
Methocarbamol (Robaxin)	CNS depression, GI distress, rash	1000-1500 qid
Orphenadrine (Norflex)	Xerostomia, GIT, vision changes	100 bid
Cyclobenzaprine (Flexeril)	Sedation (40%), xerostomia (30%)	10 tid
Diazepam (Valium)	Benzodiazepine	5-10 bid-tid

bid, Twice per day; *CNS,* central nervous system; *GI,* gastrointestinal; *GIT,* gastrointestinal tract; *qid,* 4 times per day; *tid,* 3 times per day.

fewer muscle relaxant and anticonvulsant effects. It may be less likely to produce depression of sleep stages 3 and 4. Side effects include headache, drowsiness, dizziness, and diarrhea. Myalgia, arthralgia, sinusitis, and pharyngitis have been reported. Amnesia may also occur. Withdrawal can occur if abruptly stopped after 1 to 2 weeks of use. Rebound insomnia may be experienced. Its quicker onset of action makes it useful to initiate sleep. Because of its fast onset of action, it should be taken immediately before bedtime. Patients should not drive while taking this drug until they see what kind of effect it has on them.

Zolpidem may be used in dentistry if the patient is having difficulty falling asleep the night before a dental appointment. This drug is usually used for persons with chronic insomnia.

Zolpidem is also available as Ambien CR, a controlled-release dose form. There have been reports of behavioral and emotional changes in patients taking Ambien CR. Patients have reported a decrease in inhibition similar to that seen with alcohol and other CNS depressant drugs. Amnesia, anxiety, and a worsening of depression have been reported in patients taking Ambien CR.

Zaleplon

Zaleplon is a rapid-acting hypnotic that is less potent and has a shorter duration of action than zolpidem. It does not appear to decrease premature awakenings or increase total sleep time, but it appears to have a lower risk of next-day residual effects, even with middle of the night use. It does not appear to affect driving the morning after nighttime administration. Zaleplon can cause anterograde amnesia.

Eszopiclone

Eszopiclone is the newest agent of this class available in the United States. It has the longest half-life of the three, but comparative clinical data are lacking. A 6-month trial with eszopiclone found no development of tolerance. Anterograde amnesia has been reported with this drug. Some patients have reported an unpleasant taste while taking this drug. Because of its long half-life, eszopiclone could impair driving the morning after nighttime administration.

MELATONIN RECEPTOR AGONIST

Ramelteon (Rozerem) has been approved by the FDA for the treatment of insomnia characterized by difficulty falling asleep. This drug is an indenofuran derivative that is highly selective for melatonin type 1 (MT_1) and melatonin type 2

(MT_2) receptors. Studies in animals indicate that the MT_1 receptor regulates sleep and the MT_2 receptor may mediate the phase-shifting effects of melatonin on a 24-hour biologic clock. In clinical trials, ramelteon produced small, statistically significant improvements on sleep latency but had little effect on sleep maintenance.

The most common adverse effects reported during clinical trials included somnolence, dizziness, fatigue, headache, and insomnia. It is not a controlled substance like the benzodiazepines and the nonbenzodiazepine-benzodiazepine receptor agonists (NBRAs), and there have been no reports of tolerance, rebound insomnia, or withdrawal effects. The long-term safety of ramelteon is unknown.

CENTRALLY ACTING MUSCLE RELAXANTS

Drugs classified as centrally acting muscle relaxants (Table 11-3) exert their effects on the CNS to produce skeletal muscle relaxation.

Pharmacologic Effects

Some degree of sedative effect is exhibited by all the CNS muscle relaxants because their action is on the CNS. Xerostomia is common with these agents.

Clinical tests have shown that the sedative effects dominate over the "selective" muscle relaxant activity. When administered intravenously in humans, these agents have been shown to be useful in treating muscle spasm and producing muscle relaxation for certain orthopedic procedures. When these agents are given orally, they do not produce the flaccidity obtainable with IV administration. Thus, until better studies are produced, the beneficial effects of these drugs can be logically ascribed to their sedative action. They are used for back and neck pain and in patients with muscle spasms related to a car accident.

Individual Centrally Acting Muscle Relaxants

◆ OVERVIEW

Centrally acting skeletal muscle relaxants exert their muscle-relaxing properties indirectly by producing CNS depression. They act in the CNS and have no direct effect on striated muscle, the motor endplate, or nerve fibers. They do not directly relax tense skeletal muscles.

They share many common side effects, including gastrointestinal upset, sedation, and dizziness (results of CNS depression). All of the muscle relaxants have the potential to produce allergic reactions. Most of these agents can produce xerostomia, and the dental health care worker should question the patient about self-treatment for this adverse effect.

Structurally related to the tricyclic antidepressants, cyclobenzaprine (sye-kloe-BEN-za-preen) (Flexeril) is considered to be the strongest muscle relaxant. Because sedation occurs in about 40% of the patients taking cyclobenzaprine, it is the most sedating muscle relaxant. It also is most likely to produce xerostomia with an incidence of 30%. (This demonstrates typical effects and adverse reactions of drugs: the more pharmacologic effect [wanted], the more adverse reactions [unwanted].)

A relative of meprobamate is carisoprodol (kar-eye-soe-PROE-dole) (Soma). Chlorzoxazone (klor-ZOX-a-zone) (Paraflex) may discolor the urine purple-red. The patient should be warned about this harmless property. Other muscle relaxants include methocarbamol (meth-oh-KAR-ba-mole) (Robaxin) and orphenadrine (or-FEN-a-dreen) (Norflex). Diazepam (Valium), a benzodiazepine, also possesses muscle-relaxant properties and is used for spastic muscles such as occurs in multiple sclerosis. Table 11-3 lists the muscle relaxants that function via the brain and their selected side effects and usual doses.

◆ USE

The muscle relaxants are all indicated as an adjunct to rest and physical therapy for relief of muscle spasm associated with acute painful musculoskeletal conditions. Questions about their efficacy still linger in the literature. They are also used in the treatment of temporomandibular disorder (TMD) because relaxation of the muscles is helpful to the symptoms. The success of muscle relaxants in the management of TMD has not been documented.

MISCELLANEOUS AGENTS

Baclofen

Baclofen (BAK-loe-fen) (Lioresal) inhibits both monosynaptic and polysynaptic reflexes at the spinal level. It also inhibits GABA, but whether this is related to its action is unknown. It is indicated for spasticity from multiple sclerosis or spinal cord injuries or diseases. Baclofen has been used to treat trigeminal neuralgia, although it is not FDA approved for this purpose. Drowsiness, weakness, headache, and insomnia have been reported. Nausea, dry mouth, taste disorder, and urinary frequency have been seen. Lowering of the seizure threshold and an increase in ovarian cysts in rats have also occurred.

Tizanidine

Tizanidine (tye-ZAN-i-deen) (Zanaflex) is a short-acting muscle relaxant. It is a centrally acting α-adrenergic receptor agonist (like clonidine) that increases presynaptic inhibition of motor neurons. Like clonidine, it can produce sedation, drowsiness, hypotension, and xerostomia.

Dantrolene

Dantrolene (DAN-troe-leen) (Dantrium) affects the contractile response of the skeletal muscle by acting directly on the muscle itself. It dissociates the excitation-contraction coupling, probably by interfering with the release of calcium from the sarcoplasmic reticulum. It is indicated in the treatment of spasticity from upper motor neuron disorders such as spinal cord injury, cerebral palsy, or multiple sclerosis. It is also used orally to prevent and intravenously to treat malignant hyperthermia brought on by succinylcholine or inhalation of general anesthetics. The hepatotoxicity it produces is more common with higher doses and in older female patients taking concomitant medications. This agent may cause drowsiness or photosensitivity.

GENERAL COMMENTS ABOUT ANTIANXIETY AGENTS

Analgesic-Sedative Combinations

The use of an analgesic and a sedative-hypnotic agent to provide concomitant sedation and analgesia is rational for several reasons (Box 11-4).

Both sedation and analgesia can be obtained from the opioid analgesics alone. However, it is not desirable to prescribe an opioid to add sedation to analgesia unless the analgesic potency is required. In cases in which anxiety is an important component in pain relief, either a nonopioid or opioid can be used concomitantly with a sedative. This combination may be prescribed separately, although a few fixed-dose products are available. A combination of a sedative with an analgesic is available in butalbital compound (Fiorinal) or butalbital/acetaminophen (Fioricet). If the patient's pain is more severe, then an opioid and a sedative-hypnotic agent can be prescribed. The previously mentioned agents are available mixed with codeine (#3 contains 30 mg codeine) to make Fiorinal #3. In a dental patient in whom anxiety is magnifying the pain reaction, the prescribing of a combination agent might be useful.

Special Considerations

> Psychological management must accompany use of antianxiety agents.

Certain generalizations should be kept in mind when discussing the use of the antianxiety agents. The dental practitioner plays an important role in helping the patient understand the possible effects of the drugs used to allay anxiety. The patient may raise questions about these agents, and their effects should be explained. Dental patients who are to use antianxiety agents should be driven to and from the dental appointment.

Drugs are not to be used as a substitute for patient management. The practitioner should not rely exclusively on drugs to provide a calm and cooperative patient. The dental team should exhibit a confident and relaxed manner. A pleasant, soothing office atmosphere is of great importance in relaxing an anxious patient. Appropriate use of music of the patient's choice can reduce anxiety. Drugs should not be substituted for patient education or for the proper psychological approach to patient care.

When an agent for anxiety relief is required, the selection of the specific drug should be based on knowledge of the advan-

---

BOX 11-4	RATIONALE FOR USE OF ANALGESIC-SEDATIVE COMBINATIONS

- Relief of both anxiety and pain is often required in one patient.
- Sedatives potentiate analgesic agents.
- Sedatives may induce excitation when given without an analgesic to patients with uncontrolled pain.
- Anxiety can lower the pain threshold.

tages and disadvantages of the agents available and an understanding of the needs and contraindications related to the case at hand.

Precautions

Regardless of the antianxiety agent selected, the following precautions pertain:

- Patients with impaired elimination may experience exaggerated effects of these medications. These persons include the young, the elderly, the debilitated, and those with liver or kidney disease.
- Depression caused by all sedative-hypnotics will add to depression caused by other CNS depressants that the patient may be taking. The patient should be made aware of this, particularly in regard to alcohol; over-the-counter (OTC) sleep aids may also be a potential source of hazard.
- The patient should understand that the drug prescribed will make it unsafe to perform acts requiring full alertness and muscle coordination such as driving a car. The patient should be accompanied by a responsible adult who can drive the patient home. The patient should be warned against signing any important papers or documents. These cautions are particularly important if the patient has not taken the drug previously and consequently his or her response is less predictable.
- Psychic and physical dependence has been observed with almost all drugs used to allay anxiety. The dentist should realize that these drugs have abuse potential and should limit their use accordingly. This is particularly important in regard to the treatment of chronic conditions or persons with a history of addiction or alcoholism.
- Suicide may be attempted by taking sedative-hypnotic drugs. Consequently, the amount of drug prescribed should be limited to the minimum required to accomplish the therapeutic objective. With benzodiazepines, the therapeutic index is wide unless mixed with alcohol.
- These drugs should never be administered to pregnant women or those who may be pregnant unless the potential benefit to the mother outweighs the risk to the fetus.
- Sedatives do not provide analgesia. In fact, the use of a sedative without adequate pain control may cause the patient to become highly excited and act irrationally. However, sedatives may potentiate the effect of an analgesic taken concomitantly.

DENTAL HYGIENE CONSIDERATIONS

1. Review the patient's medication/health history for any contraindications.
2. These medications are sedating, so it is best to try to avoid other sedating medications. If this is not possible, counsel the patient about the increased risk for sedation.
3. Encourage the patient to have someone drive him or her to and from the appointment.
4. Encourage the patient to refrain from any activity that requires thought or concentration.
5. Encourage the patient to go home, if possible, and rest until the remaining sedation clears up.
6. Review Boxes 11-1, 11-2, and 11-4.

CLINICAL SKILLS ASSESSMENT

1. What are some of the nonpharmacologic methods of helping a patient deal with her anxiety?
2. The dentist decides to prescribe diazepam, which is to be taken the night before her appointment and approximately 1 hour before her appointment. What is the rationale for using benzodiazepines to treat anxiety?
3. What are the adverse reactions associated with benzodiazepines?
4. Is memory loss a problem with benzodiazepines? What should a patient be told?
5. Should a patient be concerned about becoming addicted to benzodiazepines? Why or why not?
6. What should a patient be told about the medication that the dentist has chosen?
7. Name two major pharmacologic effects of barbiturates.
8. Describe the major adverse reactions of barbiturates.
9. Name the one absolute contraindication to the use of barbiturates.
10. Describe the mechanism of the most important drug interaction of barbiturates.
11. State the potential advantages of the NBRAs.
12. Explain why chloral hydrate is still used by some dentists as premedication for children.
13. What is the rationale for combining a sedative-hypnotic drug with an analgesic?

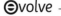 volve

Please visit http://evolve.elsevier.com/Haveles/pharmacology for review questions and additional practice and reference materials.

12 Vitamins and Minerals

LEARNING OBJECTIVES

1. Explain the body's need for vitamins and minerals.
2. Summarize and explain how vitamins are classified.
3. Name and describe the water- and fat-soluble vitamins—sources, recommended amounts, roles, deficiencies, adverse reactions, and clinical considerations.
4. Describe the sources, recommended amounts, roles, deficiencies, and toxicity of the minerals iron, zinc, and calcium.
5. Discuss the clinical considerations of vitamins and minerals and provide several examples of their relevance to dental treatment.

> Vitamins are essential in small quantities for the maintenance of cell structure and metabolism.

The vitamins (VYE-ta-mins), which are essential in small quantities for the maintenance of cell structure and metabolism, are a group of low-molecular-weight compounds. In normal quantities, a vitamin is used to replace that vitamin which is deficient. Vitamins are also used to treat problems not associated with vitamin deficiency. When used as such, they are regarded as drugs. However, few situations exist for which there is proof that vitamins are useful for the treatment of any condition except vitamin deficiency.

Vitamins are classified into two large groups: water soluble and fat soluble. The water-soluble vitamins include the B vitamins and vitamin C. The fat-soluble vitamins are vitamins A, D, E, and K. Vitamins act in three different ways: as coenzymes, antioxidants, or hormones. The water-soluble vitamins act as coenzymes, acting with a specific enzyme that catalyzes a specific reaction. Vitamins C and E act as antioxidants, and vitamin A and D act as hormones. Table 12-1 lists the common names of the vitamins and their deficiencies.

MEASUREMENTS OF VITAMIN NEEDS

Since the early 1940s, the Food and Nutrition Board of the National Academy of Sciences has been reviewing research to determine dietary recommendations. The original recommended daily allowance (RDA) was designed with the goal of preventing the diseases produced by the deficiency of a certain nutrient. These values were meant to be used to make recommendations for populations (e.g., school lunches or nursing homes) rather than specific people. These RDAs are not synonymous with an individual's requirement. Individual requirements are influenced by many factors, including but not limited to physical characteristics, dietary habits, sex, pregnancy, lactation, and age. However, the RDAs are set high enough to allow for many variations in patient needs. During the subsequent years, because no other values were available, the RDAs began to be used (inappropriately) to address specific patient needs.

Since the discovery of vitamins, dietitians have been searching the literature for evidence for the vitamin needs of individuals and populations. After the release of the last published RDAs in 1989, a discussion of inappropriate use of the former RDAs was begun. Agreement was reached that the use of this one number did not cover all the needs for nutrition information. In 1993 the Food and Nutrition

TABLE 12-1   VITAMINS AND THEIR DEFICIENCIES

Vitamin	Name	Deficiency	Therapeutic Use
Water Soluble			
B_1	Thiamine	Beriberi, Wernicke's encephalopathy with alcoholism	Converted to thiamine pyrophosphate in the liver
B_2	Riboflavin	Glossitis, cheilitis	Converted into FMN and FAD
B_3	Niacin (nicotinic acid)	Pellagra	Antihyperlipidemic; flushing
B_6	Pyridoxine		
B_{12}	Cyanocobalamin	Pernicious anemia	Watch with gout, needs intrinsic factor to be orally absorbed
B_9	Folacin (folic acid)	Megaloblastic anemia	Treat deficiency
C	Ascorbic acid	Scurvy	Antioxidant
Fat Soluble			
A	Retinoic acid, retinal, retinol (from plant carotene)	Night blindness	Topical/systemic for acne—analogs
D	Cholecalciferol,* calcitriol (Rocaltrol), ergocalciferol† (Calciferol), dihydrotachysterol (Hytakerol)	Rickets, osteomalacia	Renal disease—preformed 1,25(OH)$_2$ cholecalciferol; osteoporosis in combination with calcium
E	Tocopherol (α, β, γ)		Antioxidant (combined with selenium), for cardiovascular disease
K	Phytonadione, menadione	Bleeding	Hepatic cirrhosis

FAD, Flavin adenine dinucleotide; *FMN,* flavin mononucleotide; *NAD,* nicotinamide adenine dinucleotide; *NADP,* NAD phosphate.
*Called vitamin D$_3$.
†Form found in vitamin pills, vitamin D$_2$, product of sun on skin.

Board initiated a review process, beginning with a symposium. This process of reviewing the literature to determine the appropriate recommendations reflecting the current research began and continues today. The new RDAs are designed not only to prevent deficiency diseases but also to minimize chronic diseases such as heart disease.

The original term, *RDAs* (old), that was used as reference for years has been divided into different, more specific recommendations. The definitions of the five newer terms appear in Box 12-1. Dietary reference intakes (DRIs) are used to develop diets for healthy people. The DRIs for individual vitamins and minerals began to be compiled and released. In 1997, the DRIs for vitamin D, magnesium, and fluoride were completed, and in 1998, the B vitamins were addressed and recommendations released. Currently, the recommendations available are divided between the RDAs, and if that is unknown, the adequate intake

(AI). In general, the AI for a specific agent is less than the RDA because the RDA allows for some variation.

WATER-SOLUBLE VITAMINS

Ascorbic Acid (Vitamin C)

Ascorbic (a-SKOR-bik) **acid,** or vitamin C, chemically is a sugar acid that readily undergoes oxidation to form dehydroascorbic acid. Because of this ability, ascorbic acid is an effective reducing agent. The active isomer is *l*-ascorbic acid.

◆ SOURCE

Good natural sources of ascorbic acid include citrus fruits, green peppers, tomatoes, strawberries, broccoli, raw cabbage, baked potatoes, and papaya (Figure 12-1). Some food products are fortified with vitamin C. Ascorbic acid is absorbed in the ileum by a Na$^+$-dependent carrier-mediated mechanism.

Because of its ability to be easily oxidized, ascorbic acid is readily destroyed through cooking, and as much as 50% of the ascorbic acid content of foods can be lost in this manner.

◆ RECOMMENDED DIETARY ALLOWANCE

The RDA of ascorbic acid for a healthy female adult is 75 mg and 90 mg for a healthy male adult. During pregnancy and lactation, stress, or tobacco smoking, the need for this vitamin increases.

◆ ROLE

The metabolic role of ascorbic acid is probably related to the fact that ascorbic acid and dehydroascorbic acid form a readily reversible oxidation-reduction system. It is thought that this

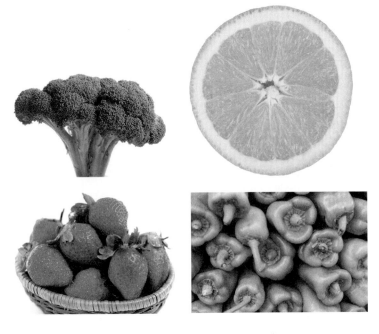

FIGURE 12-1
Good source of vitamin C includes citrus fruits such as oranges, green peppers, broccoli, and strawberries. (Copyright 2009 Jupiterimages Corporation.)

vitamin plays a role in biologic oxidations and reductions in cellular respirations. Ascorbic acid also plays a definite role in connective tissue metabolism because it is required for the formation of collagen. The function of ascorbic acid can be dramatically demonstrated in the wound-healing process. Scorbutic wounds have a decrease in mature collagen fibrils associated with an accumulation of mucopolysaccharides or ground substance around a matrix of precollagenous fibers. The absence of mature collagen results in abnormal healing that reduces the tensile strength of the wound.

◆ DEFICIENCY

Scurvy

The deficiency of ascorbic acid produces a condition termed *scurvy*. The manifestations of scurvy occur because of the inability of the connective tissue to produce and maintain intercellular substances such as collagen, bone matrix, dentin, cartilage, and vascular endothelium.

The functions of vitamin C include the following:
- Collagen formation
- Synthesis of epinephrine and norepinephrine
- Synthesis of carnitine, a protein that facilitates transport of fatty acids into mitochondria for β oxidation

The following are manifestations of defective connective tissue formation in vitamin C deficiency:
- Impaired wound healing resulting from a lack of collagen
- Inadequate response to infections
- Alterations in the integrity of capillary walls, manifested as hemorrhages in skin, mucous membranes, muscles, lungs, joints, and gingivae (spongy, edematous, inflamed)
- Lack of formation of bone matrix, resulting in disorganization of epiphyseal line, weakening of bones, pathologic fractures, and resorption of alveolar bone with loosening and loss of teeth

Because humans and other primates cannot synthesize vitamin C, they must obtain it daily from their diet.

Diets completely deficient in vitamin C are unusual, and there are few cases of serious vitamin C deficiency (scurvy). After a prolonged period (4 to 5 months) without vitamin C, humans have symptoms of weakness, anorexia, suppressed growth, anemia, lower resistance to infection and fever, swollen and inflamed gums, loosened teeth, swollen wrists and ankle joints, petechial hemorrhages, fracture of ribs at costochondral junctions, and hemorrhaging resulting from capillary fragility in joints, muscle, and intestines.

◆ ADVERSE REACTIONS

Untoward effects have been reported with the use of megadoses of vitamin C. A daily intake of 1 gm of vitamin C may cause precipitation of oxalate stones in the urinary tract. For this reason, unwarranted use of large quantities of vitamin C is discouraged. A rebound scurvy has been reported in adults and infants who received megadoses that were then stopped abruptly.

◆ CLINICAL CONSIDERATIONS

As long ago as 1942, the suggestion was made that vitamin C could be therapeutically beneficial in preventing the common cold. Linus Pauling reviewed the available data and indicated that vitamin C has a substantial beneficial effect in preventing and treating the common cold. Other investigators reviewed the data and concluded that little if any evidence existed to suggest the effectiveness of vitamin C in either preventing or treating the common cold. Based on current evidence, unrestricted use of ascorbic acid for these purposes cannot be advocated.

Another Pauling hypothesis suggested that large quantities of vitamin C may suppress neoplastic cellular proliferation. He indicated that vitamin C should be used in the management of all types of cancer. Other investigators have been unable to verify his claim.

Because vitamin C enhances the absorption of iron, iron is either combined with vitamin C or taken with orange juice to treat iron deficiency anemia.

B-Complex Vitamins

The water-soluble vitamins, except for vitamin C, are known as the B-complex vitamins. On a functional basis, these vitamins may be subdivided into the following three classes:

1. Those that primarily release energy from carbohydrates and fats (thiamine, pyridoxine, niacin, riboflavin, pantothenic acid, and biotin)
2. Those that among other functions catalyze the formation of red cells (folic acid, vitamin B_{12})
3. Those that have not been shown to be required in human nutrition (choline and inositol)

A close interrelationship among the B-complex vitamins exists. If a deficiency of one of them occurs, it will impair the utilization of others. Also, the signs and symptoms of a deficiency of individual B vitamins are similar. This is probably because a deficiency of a single member of the B complex seldom occurs. A diet deficient in one B vitamin is usually lacking in other B vitamins. Figure 12-2 shows some examples of good sources of B-complex vitamins.

◆ THIAMINE (VITAMIN B₁)

Thiamine (THYE-a-min) (vitamin B_1) is an essential water-soluble vitamin in humans. It is converted in the liver to its active coenzyme form, thiamine pyrophosphate (TPP).

Source. Thiamine is present in foods of both animal and vegetable origin. The best sources are pork, whole grain and enriched breads, cereals and pastas, seeds of legumes such as peas, dried brewer's yeast, and wheat germ (see Figure 12-2). The vitamin tends to be destroyed if heated to about 100° C; therefore significant amounts of this vitamin may be lost if foods are cooked too long above this temperature.

Recommended Dietary Allowance. The RDA for thiamine is 1.2 mg for adult men (ages 14 to >70 years) and 1.1 mg for adult women (ages 19 to >70 years). Table 12-2 lists RDAs for other groups. Thiamine requirements parallel the caloric or carbohydrate content of the diet.

Role. TPP plays a principal role in intermediary metabolism. It is a coenzyme required for the oxidative decarboxylation of α-ketoacids. In this role, TPP is sometimes referred to as cocarboxylase.

Deficiency. The severe deficiency of thiamine leads to a condition known as *beriberi*. Characteristics of beriberi are peripheral neuritis, muscle weakness, paralysis of the limbs, enlargement of the heart, tachycardia, and edema (typical of wet beriberi). Gastrointestinal tract effects include loss of appetite and intestinal **atony**, and constipation may also be present. The symptoms of mild thiamine deficiency are less characteristic. They include fatigue and apathy, loss of appetite, moodiness and irritability, pain and paresthesias in the extremities, slight edema, decreased blood pressure, and lowered body temperature.

Possible oral manifestations of thiamine deficiency are burning tongue, ageusia (loss of taste functions of the tongue), and hyperesthesia of the oral mucosa.

The most common cause of thiamine deficiency in the United States is alcoholism. Both poor appetite and the effect of alcohol on the nerves may exacerbate this problem. Both Wernicke's encephalopathy and Korsakoff's psychosis can result if a severe deficiency exists.

Adverse Reactions. Thiamine is usually nontoxic, even in large parenteral doses. However, in patients who are hypersensitive to thiamine, pruritus, sweating, nausea, respiratory distress with hypotension, vascular collapse, and death have occurred.

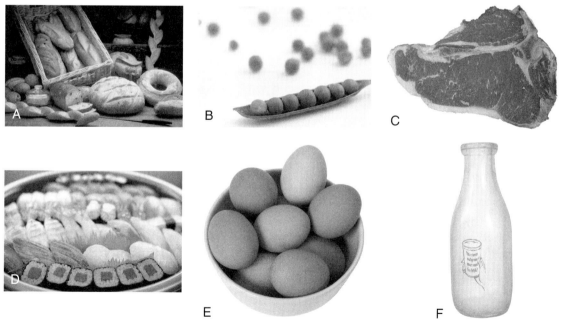

FIGURE 12-2

Examples of foods containing various B-complex vitamins. **A,** Whole-grain and enriched breads provide vitamins B_1, B_3, and B_6, folic acid, pantothenic acid, and biotin. **B,** Peas and other legumes are good sources of thiamine (vitamin B_1), niacin (vitamin B_3), and pyridoxine (vitamin B_6). Riboflavin (vitamin B_2) is present in leafy green vegetables. **C,** Meat is a rich source of several vitamins, including riboflavin, niacin, pyridoxine, folic acid, cyanocobalamin, pantothenic acid, and biotin, whereas fish provides niacin (**D**). **E,** Eggs contain riboflavin, pyridoxine, cyanocobalamin, pantothenic acid, and biotin. **F,** Riboflavin, cyanocobalamin, and biotin are found in dairy products such as milk and cheese. (Copyright 2009 Jupiterimages Corporation.)

TABLE 12-2 DIETARY REFERENCE INTAKES: RECOMMENDED DIETARY ALLOWANCES AND ADEQUATE INTAKES OF SELECTED VITAMINS AND ELEMENTS

Life Stage	Vitamin A (µg/d)*	Vitamin C (mg/d)	Vitamin D (µg/d)†	Vitamin E (mg/d)‡	Vitamin K (µg/d)	Thiamine (mg/d)	Riboflavin (mg/d)	Niacin (mg/d)§	Vitamin B6 (mg/d)	Folate (µg/d)	Vitamin B12 (µg/d)	Calcium (mg/d)	Iodine (µg/d)	Iron (mg/d)	Magnesium (mg/d)	Phosphorous (mg/d)	Selenium (µg/d)	Zinc (mg/d)
Infants																		
0-6 mo	400	40	5	4	2	0.2	0.3	2	0.1	65	0.4	210	110	0.27	30	100	15	2
7-12 mo	500	50	5	5	2.5	0.3	0.4	4	0.3	80	0.5	270	130	**11**	75	275	20	3
Children																		
1-3 yr	**300**	**15**	5	**6**	30	**0.5**	**0.5**	**6**	**0.5**	**150**	**0.9**	500	**90**	**7**	**80**	460	**20**	**3**
4-8 yr	**400**	**25**	5	**7**	55	**0.6**	**0.6**	**8**	**0.6**	**200**	**1.2**	800	**90**	**10**	**130**	500	**30**	**5**
Males																		
9-13 yr	**600**	**45**	5	**11**	60	**0.9**	**0.9**	**12**	**1.0**	**300**	**1.8**	1300	**120**	**8**	**240**	1250	**40**	**8**
14-18 yr	**900**	**75**	5	**15**	75	**1.2**	**1.3**	**16**	**1.3**	**400**	**2.4**	1300	**150**	**11**	**410**	1250	**55**	**11**
19-30 yr	**900**	**90**	5	**15**	120	**1.2**	**1.3**	**16**	**1.3**	**400**	**2.4**	1000	**150**	**8**	**400**	700	**55**	**11**
31-50 yr	**900**	**90**	5	**15**	120	**1.2**	**1.3**	**16**	**1.3**	**400**	**2.4**	1000	**150**	**8**	**420**	700	**55**	**11**
51-70 yr	**900**	**90**	10	**15**	120	**1.2**	**1.3**	**16**	**1.7**	**400**	**2.4**	1200	**150**	**8**	**420**	700	**55**	**11**
>70 yr	**900**	**90**	15	**15**	120	**1.2**	**1.3**	**16**	**1.7**	**400**	**2.4**	1200	**150**	**8**	**420**	700	**55**	**11**
Females																		
9-13 yr	**600**	**45**	5	**11**	60	**0.9**	**0.9**	**12**	**1.0**	**300**	**1.8**	1300	**120**	**8**	**240**	1250	**40**	**8**
14-18 yr	**700**	**65**	5	**15**	75	**1.0**	**1.0**	**14**	**1.2**	**400**	**2.4**	1300	**150**	**15**	**360**	1250	**55**	**9**
19-30 yr	**700**	**75**	5	**15**	90	**1.1**	**1.1**	**14**	**1.3**	**400**	**2.4**	1000	**150**	**18**	**310**	700	**55**	**8**
31-50 yr	**700**	**75**	5	**15**	90	**1.1**	**1.1**	**14**	**1.3**	**400**	**2.4**	1000	**150**	**18**	**320**	700	**55**	**8**
51-70 yr	**700**	**75**	10	**15**	90	**1.1**	**1.1**	**14**	**1.5**	**400**	**2.4**	1200	**150**	**8**	**320**	700	**55**	**8**
>70 yr	**700**	**75**	15	**15**	90	**1.1**	**1.1**	**14**	**1.5**	**400**	**2.4**	1200	**150**	**8**	**320**	700	**55**	**8**
Pregnancy																		
14-18 yr	**750**	**80**	5	**15**	75	**1.4**	**1.4**	**18**	**1.9**	**600**	**2.6**	1300	**220**	**27**	**400**	1250	**60**	**12**
19-30 yr	**770**	**85**	5	**15**	90	**1.4**	**1.4**	**18**	**1.9**	**600**	**2.6**	1000	**220**	**27**	**350**	700	**60**	**11**
31-50 yr	**770**	**85**	5	**15**	90	**1.4**	**1.4**	**18**	**1.9**	**600**	**2.6**	1000	**220**	**27**	**360**	700	**60**	**11**
Lactation																		
14-18 yr	**1200**	**115**	5	**19**	75	**1.4**	**1.6**	**17**	**2.0**	**500**	**2.8**	1300	**290**	**10**	**360**	1250	**70**	**13**
19-30 yr	**1300**	**120**	5	**19**	90	**1.4**	**1.6**	**17**	**2.0**	**500**	**2.8**	1000	**290**	**9**	**310**	700	**70**	**12**
31-50 yr	**1300**	**120**	5	**19**	90	**1.4**	**1.6**	**17**	**2.0**	**500**	**2.8**	1000	**290**	**9**	**320**	700	**70**	**12**

From Otten JJ, Hellwig JP, Meyers LD, eds: *Dietary reference intakes: the essential guide to nutrient requirements*, Washington, DC, 2006, National Academics Press.
This table presents Recommended Dietary Allowances (RDAs) in **bold** type and Adequate Intakes (AIs) in ordinary type.
*Retinal activity equivalents (RAEs): 1 RAE = 1 µg retinol, 12 µg β-carotene, 24 µg α-carotene, or 24 µg β-cryptoxanthin.
†As cholecalciferol. 1 µg cholecalciferol = 40 IU vitamin D.
‡α-Tocopherol equivalents (TEs): 1 mg/day α-tocopherol = 1-α-TE.
§Niacin equivalents: 1 mg of niacin = 60 mg tryptophan; 0-6 months = preformed niacin (not niacin equivalents).

Clinical Considerations. For treatment of a variety of manifestations of thiamine deficiencies, including beriberi and peripheral neuritis, which is also associated with pellagra, thiamine is used. In acute Wernicke's encephalopathy, which occurs in some chronic alcoholics, thiamine is administered intravenously. It can temporarily correct certain rare genetic metabolic disorders (maple syrup urine disease and subacute necrotizing encephalomyelopathy). It has also been used as an insect repellent, but there is no evidence of its effectiveness.

◆ RIBOFLAVIN (VITAMIN B₂)

Riboflavin (RYE-boe-flay-vin) (vitamin B₂) is a water-soluble vitamin composed of flavin and D-ribitol.

Source. Riboflavin is abundant in both plants and animals. However, dairy products and meat (especially organ meats such as liver) are the best sources of this vitamin. It is also present in green leafy vegetables and yeast. Riboflavin is relatively stable to heat, and cooking will not cause an appreciable loss. It is destroyed by ultraviolet radiation.

Recommended Dietary Allowance. The RDA for riboflavin ranges from 1.1 (adult women) to 1.2 mg (adult men). Table 12-2 lists the requirements for other groups. Requirements for riboflavin usually parallel caloric intake or metabolic body size.

Role. Riboflavin functions in the body as a component of two flavoprotein coenzymes, riboflavin phosphate (flavin mononucleotide [FMN]) and flavin adenine dinucleotide (FAD). Flavoprotein coenzymes in turn are proteins that act as electron acceptors and are involved in a variety of oxidation-reduction reactions. Riboflavin is also indirectly involved in maintaining the integrity of the erythrocytes.

Deficiency. Symptoms of riboflavin deficiency usually involve the lips, tongue, and skin. Sore throat and angular stomatitis (cheilosis) appearing as an ulceration with painful fissuring at the corners of the mouth are early and frequent findings. The lips may be either unusually red or whitish because of desquamation. Later, glossitis can occur, with the dorsum of the tongue becoming pebbly or granular. Contact with food or drink may produce pain or a burning sensation on the tongue. In some instances, the tongue may become magenta or purplish-red. Excessive salivation and enlargement of the salivary glands may occur. Skin manifestations include a greasy, scaling inflammation around the nose, cheeks, and chin. Involvement of the scrotum and the vulva is frequent. Other manifestations of a severe riboflavin deficiency are normocytic, normochromic anemia and neuropathy.

Adverse Reactions. Riboflavin has not been associated with any toxicity.

Clinical Considerations. Riboflavin deficiency is most likely to be seen in alcoholics, economically deprived individuals, or patients with severe gastrointestinal disease that causes loss of appetite, vomiting, and malabsorption syndromes. Oral contraceptives and probenecid may be associated with an increased need for riboflavin. The manifestations of riboflavin deficiency are difficult to distinguish from those of other B-vitamin deficiencies because of the similarities in syndromes. The discovery of a deficiency of riboflavin warrants the use of a multivitamin because deficiency of several vitamins often coexists. The ease of measuring riboflavin in the urine has prompted its use as a marker in drug studies to measure compliance.

◆ NIACIN OR NICOTINIC ACID (VITAMIN B₃)

Niacin (NYE-a-sin), or nicotinic acid, is converted in the body to niacinamide or nicotinamide, its active form, to serve as a vitamin. These water-soluble organic compounds have the ability to alleviate a deficiency syndrome known as *pellagra.*

Source. Good sources of niacin are lean meats, fish, liver, poultry, legumes, and whole grains. Pellagra was at one time a common disease of the southeastern United States among persons subsisting on a diet exclusively of corn products because corn is extremely low in tryptophan, a precursor of this vitamin. Beans are often used in combination with corn to rectify this deficiency.

Recommended Dietary Allowance. Niacin requirement in the diet is somewhat dependent on both caloric and protein intake. Because tryptophan, an amino acid found in dietary protein, is metabolized to niacin in the body, intake of protein would reduce the amount of vitamin needed in the diet. The recommended dietary allowance for niacin is 16 mg niacin equivalents (NE) for men (1 NE is equal to 1 mg of niacin or 60 mg of tryptophan) and 14 mg NE for women. Oral doses of 15 to

20 mg of niacin daily are sufficient as a dietary supplement if patients have normal gastrointestinal absorption.

Role. Nicotinic acid, like riboflavin, plays a key role in metabolism by participating in a variety of oxidation-reduction reactions (transfer of electrons). In the body, it is converted into two active forms, the coenzymes nicotinamide adenine dinucleotide (NAD) and nicotinamide adenine dinucleotide phosphate (NADP). This vitamin serves as an essential coenzyme for dehydrogenases involved in the Krebs cycle. The Krebs cycle is responsible for anaerobic carbohydrate metabolism and lipid and protein metabolism.

> 3 Ds:
> 1. Dermatitis
> 2. Diarrhea
> 3. Dementia

Deficiency. The clinical syndrome produced by niacin deficiency is pellagra, so named because the skin becomes rough (Latin: *pelle,* skin; *agra,* rough). Early symptoms are an erythematous cutaneous eruption on the back of the hands, glossitis, and stomatitis. In advanced stages, pellagra can be diagnosed by the classic "three Ds": dermatitis, diarrhea, and dementia. The dermatitis consists of redness, thickening, and roughening of the skin, followed by scaling desquamation and depigmentation. Diarrhea is caused by atrophy of the gastrointestinal tract mucosal epithelium, followed by inflammation of the mucosal lining of the esophagus, stomach, and colon. The dementia results from regressive changes in the ganglion cells of the brain and tracts of the spinal cord. Death may also result.

During the course of pellagra, symptoms are evident in the oral cavity. A burning sensation occurs throughout the oral mucosa. The lip and lateral margins of the tongue are initially reddened and swollen. In the later stages, the entire dorsal surface of the tongue becomes red and swollen. In acute stages, vascular hyperemia, proliferation, hypertrophy, and atrophy occur successively in the papillae. Papillary loss may ultimately become complete, with the tongue surface becoming beefy red. Deep penetrating ulcers may appear on the tongue surface. In the gingiva, desquamative epithelial degeneration may occur, exposing the tissue to infection, inflammation, and fibrinous exudation. Gingivitis caused by pellagra is characterized by ulcers in the interdental papillae and marginal gingiva. Excessive salivary secretion with enlargement of the salivary glands also occurs.

Niacin deficiency occurs most often in poverty-stricken areas of the world because of inadequate intake. Deficiency may also arise from chronic alcoholism, gastrointestinal disturbances, pregnancy, hyperthyroidism, and infections.

> Aspirin prevents flushing and pruritus.

Adverse Reactions. Side effects that occur from ingestion of large doses of niacin include cutaneous flushing, pruritus, and gastrointestinal distress. These side effects can be reduced by administering an aspirin one-half hour before the niacin is ingested. Other adverse reactions include increased sebaceous gland action and increased gastrointestinal motility. With chronic use, dry skin, xerostomia, hyperuricemia, peptic ulcer, blurred vision, nervousness, panic, and hyperglycemia can occur. Abnormal liver function tests, prothrombin time, and hypoalbuminemia have been reported.

Clinical Considerations. Niacin or nicotinic acid and niacinamide are used as a vitamin in the treatment of pellagra. Only high-dose niacin is useful in the treatment of hyperlipidemias. It reduces plasma cholesterol, triglycerides, very-low-density lipoproteins (VLDL), low-density lipoproteins (LDL), and chylomicrons. These effects are dose-dependent. Niacin can also be used in combination with other lipid-lowering agents, so that a lower dose of each may be used.

◆ PYRIDOXINE (VITAMIN B₆)

Pyridoxine (peer-i-DOX-een) is one of three different pyridoxine derivatives known as vitamin B₆. The other two derivatives, pyridoxal and pyridoxamine, are chemically similar.

Source. Vitamin B₆ is present in most foods of both plant and animal origin. Good sources of this vitamin include whole grain cereals, meat, legumes, eggs, and some vegetables. These similar foods are the sources of many of the B vitamins.

Recommended Dietary Allowance. The RDA for vitamin B₆ varies from 1.0 to 1.7 mg daily for men and women ages 9 to older than 70 years (see Table 12-2).

Role. To exert physiologic activity, all three forms of vitamin B₆ are converted to pyridoxal phosphate in the body. Pyridoxal phosphate is the active coenzyme form of vitamin B₆ and participates in all metabolic reactions that require the vitamin. Pyridoxal phosphate acts as a coenzyme in a variety of metabolic transformations of amino acids, including transamination and decarboxylation.

B₆: cheilosis, stomatitis, glossitis

Deficiency. Vitamin B₆ deficiency is rare because of the widespread distribution of this vitamin in food. The characteristics of vitamin B₆ deficiency resemble those of riboflavin, niacin, and thiamine deficiencies. These include angular cheilosis, stomatitis, dermatitis, and erythema of the nasolabial folds. The dorsal mucosa of the tongue seems to be unusually sensitive to a single deficiency or mixed deficiencies of the B vitamins. Specifically, glossitis resulting from pyridoxine deficiency has been described in which the tongue's surface is smooth, slightly edematous, painful, and purplish.

Adverse Reactions. Pyridoxine is usually nontoxic. When it is given parenterally in large doses, peripheral neuritis may be produced.

Clinical Considerations. Vitamin B₆ can interact with other therapeutically useful drugs. For example, isoniazid (INH), a drug used to treat tuberculosis, inhibits the action of vitamin B₆ by blocking both the formation and the reaction involving pyridoxal phosphate, the active coenzyme. INH-induced vitamin B₆ deficiency can be prevented or treated by the administration of pyridoxine. For this reason, patients taking INH usually also take vitamin B₆. Long-term administration or high doses of steroids can require administration of folic acid. Because the anticonvulsants, such as carbamazepine and phenytoin, interfere with the absorption and storage of folic acid, patients taking these medications are given pyridoxine (see Table 12-4).

Vitamin B₆ administration can cancel the therapeutic and side effects of levodopa, a drug used to treat Parkinson's disease. If carbidopa, a peripheral decarboxylase inhibitor, is administered simultaneously with levodopa (the combination is Sinemet), pyridoxine may be administered concomitantly. In practice, Sinemet is currently used almost exclusively rather than levodopa alone.

Certain other drugs, such as cycloserine, hydralazine, and pyrazinamide, may produce a pyridoxine deficiency. Estrogenic steroids can produce vitamin B₆ deficiency in women. About 20% of women taking oral contraceptive agents can be shown to have a biochemical pyridoxine (B₆) deficiency. Usual RDAs seem to be enough to prevent this situation, and women taking birth control pills should routinely be encouraged to take supplemental pyridoxine.

The use of pyridoxine for many conditions has not been shown to be effective in well-controlled trials (premenstrual syndrome, acne, vertigo, tardive dyskinesia, asthma, or alcohol intoxication).

◆ FOLIC ACID

Folic acid (FOE-lik) (pteroylglutamic acid, folacin, folate) is a form of the water-soluble vitamin B₉.

Source. Significant sources of folic acid include glandular meats such as liver, some fruits and vegetables, wheat germ, and yeasts. Because availability of folic acid from foods is highly variable, a wide margin of safety is allowed in the RDA.

Recommended Dietary Allowance. The RDA for folic acid is 400 μg daily for healthy, nonpregnant, or nonlactating adults.

Role. The biologically active form of folic acid is the reduced derivative tetrahydrofolic acid, which is formed enzymatically in the body. Tetrahydrofolic acid functions primarily in the transfer and utilization of one-carbon groups.

Certain microorganisms synthesize their own folic acid from *para*-aminobenzoic acid (PABA). The sulfonamides exert their bacteriostatic effect by antagonizing PABA and thereby interfering with the biosynthesis of folic acid in these organisms. This antagonism has no effect on humans because they require preformed folic acid and do not synthesize their own.

Megaloblastic anemia

Deficiency. Folic acid deficiency, the most common deficiency in the United States, produces megaloblastic anemia, which is indistinguishable from that caused by vitamin B₁₂ deficiency. Other symptoms include weakness, weight loss, loss of skin pigmentation, and mental irritability. As with riboflavin deficiency, oral manifestations of folic acid deficiency include glossitis, angular cheilosis, and gingivitis. The glossitis begins with swelling and pallor of the tongue followed by desquamation of the papillae and accompanied by minute ulcers with fiery red borders.

Some causes of folic acid deficiency are inadequate diet, pregnancy, malabsorption syndrome, and chronic alcoholism. Pregnant women need supplemental synthetic folacin and should not rely solely on dietary sources. The absorption of folate decreases during pregnancy and in patients taking oral contraceptives.

Several drugs have been reported to produce folic acid deficiencies, including the anticonvulsants, oral contraceptives, and nitrofurantoin. Some drugs act as folic acid antagonists (e.g., pyrimethamine, trimethoprim) (see Table 12-4). The anticonvulsants produce a deficiency by interfering with the conversion of folate to a form of the vitamin that can penetrate the brain. Some cancer chemotherapy agents prevent the formation of tetrahydrofolic acid and interfere with DNA synthesis. Folic acid is not an antidote to an overdose from a folic acid antagonist (e.g., methotrexate); leucovorin calcium is used.

Adverse Reactions. Folic acid is relatively nontoxic. Allergic reactions have been reported rarely and include rash, itching, and respiratory difficulty.

Clinical Considerations. Although the administration of folic acid will cause remission of the hematologic effects of pernicious anemia, it will not prevent the neurologic effects caused by a deficiency of vitamin B₁₂. Therefore folic acid can mask a vitamin B₁₂ deficiency. For this reason the Food and Drug

Administration (FDA) has limited the dose of folic acid per tablet that can be purchased without a prescription to 0.4 mg in normal vitamin supplements and 0.8 mg for pregnant or lactating women (over-the-counter [OTC] prenatal vitamins). The use of folic acid several months before conception and early in pregnancy can help prevent neural tube defects.

♦ CYANOCOBALAMIN (VITAMIN B₁₂)

Vitamin B₁₂: cyanocobalamin

Cyanocobalamin (sye-an-oh-koe-BAL-a-min) (vitamin B₁₂) is a chemically complex substance that contains four extensively substituted pyrrole rings surrounding an atom of cobalt. A cyanide molecule is attached to the cobalt, thus the name *cyanocobalamin.* Vitamin B₁₂ is heat stable at a neutral pH but is readily destroyed by heat at an alkaline pH.

Source. The only sources of vitamin B₁₂ in nature are certain microorganisms that synthesize the vitamin. When vegetable produce is contaminated with these microorganisms, the produce possesses the vitamin. Animals depend on synthesis within their own intestinal tracts. Human vitamin B₁₂, synthesized within the gastrointestinal tract, is not available for absorption.

Good sources of vitamin B₁₂ include foods of animal origin such as liver, meat, milk, cheese, and eggs. Vegans (strict vegetarians who do not eat animal or dairy products) can become deficient because they do not eat these foods. In recent years, some vegetable products, such as soy milk, have been fortified with vitamin B₁₂.

Vitamin B₁₂ is absorbed from the distal ileum by a receptor-mediated process. Without the presence of intrinsic factor, a protein-binding factor that aids in the absorption of vitamin B₁₂, it cannot be well absorbed. This system is saturated by about 3 mg of vitamin B₁₂. With very large doses of oral vitamin B₁₂ (1 mg) daily, the vitamin may be absorbed independent of intrinsic factor. Absorption of vitamin B₁₂ is decreased by damage to the stomach or ileum.

Recommended Dietary Allowance. The RDA of vitamin B₁₂ is 2.4 μg, with an additional 2.6 μg and 2.8 μg during pregnancy and lactation, respectively. Oral doses between 1 and 25 μg are adequate if the gastrointestinal absorption is normal. In pernicious anemia, a maintenance injection of vitamin B₁₂ is recommended once a month for life.

Role. Vitamin B₁₂ serves as a coenzyme for the hydrogen transfer and isomerization process required in the conversion of methylmalonyl-CoA to succinyl-CoA. Thus vitamin B₁₂ is important in the metabolism of fats and carbohydrates.

Megaloblastic anemia

Deficiency. The symptoms of vitamin B₁₂ deficiency include inadequate hematopoiesis, gastrointestinal tract disturbances, inadequate myelin synthesis, and generalized debility. The lack of this vitamin affects the cells that are most actively dividing such as those in the bone marrow and gastrointestinal tract. The erythroblasts do not undergo proper division, resulting in megaloblastic anemia. Atrophic changes occur in the alimentary canal. The synthesis of abnormal fatty acids, which are then incorporated into cell membranes, may produce the neurologic manifestations of deficiency, including peripheral neuropathies and spinal cord and organic brain syndromes. The patient suffers from weakness, numbness, and difficulty in walking, which are symptoms that fluctuate with remission and relapses. The skin may have a distinctive lemon-yellow hue.

The most common cause of vitamin B₁₂ deficiency is pernicious anemia, an autoimmune disease that prevents the production of intrinsic factor. The secretory cells in the gastric mucosa do not produce intrinsic factor, and thus vitamin B₁₂ is very poorly absorbed. With a gastrectomy, usually for the treatment of peptic ulcer in the "old days," intrinsic factor secretion ceases. It then takes 3 to 6 years for a vitamin B₁₂ deficiency to develop. Other causes of vitamin B₁₂ deficiency include inadequate dietary intake, malabsorption syndromes, and gastric bypass surgery.

Sore and red tongue, atrophy of papillae

Pernicious anemia results in several oral manifestations (see Color Plate 3). Recurrent attacks of soreness and burning of the tongue occur followed by glossitis, at the peak of which the tongue is extremely painful and red. Atrophy of the filiform and fungiform papillae is a common occurrence. Involvement of the circumvallate papillae may cause diminution of taste. Painful, bright red lesions may occur in the buccal and pharyngeal mucosa and undersurface of the tongue.

Adverse Reactions. Even large doses of vitamin B₁₂ are usually nontoxic. Diarrhea, itching, urticaria, and swelling have occasionally been reported. If intrinsic factor is given with the vitamin B₁₂, an allergy to hog protein (a source of exogenous intrinsic factor) may be exhibited.

Clinical Considerations. As mentioned previously, patients who are strict vegetarians (rarely) or who have had a gastrectomy can exhibit the symptoms of vitamin B₁₂ deficiency. Ingestion of other agents can alter the absorption of vitamin B₁₂. For example, vitamin C may destroy the vitamin B₁₂ levels in food. Pregnancy and use of the sweetener sorbitol increase vitamin B₁₂ absorption. Absorption of vitamin B₁₂ is decreased in persons with pyridoxine deficiency, iron deficiency, or hypothyroidism. Sustained-release potassium and anticonvulsants may decrease the absorption of vitamin B₁₂. Vitamin B₁₂ has also been used, without any proof of efficacy, to treat trigeminal neuralgia, psychiatric disorders, and fatigue. Because intrinsic factor is not required for absorption from an intramuscular (IM) site, vitamin B₁₂ can be administered intramuscularly (100 μg/month) in the absence of intrinsic factor. An oral dose of 1 mg daily is equivalent to the 100 μg/month intramuscularly. Because oral administration of vitamin B₁₂ is unreliable, the IM route is preferred.

♦ PANTOTHENIC ACID

Pantothenic acid is another compound required to form acetyl-CoA. The active form of pantothenic acid is a component of the more complex compound, coenzyme A.

Source. Pantothenic acid is a part of all living material. Egg yolk, bran, yeast, and beef liver are excellent sources.

Recommended Dietary Allowance. It is suggested that a daily dietary intake of 5 to 7 mg is adequate for adults with normal gastrointestinal absorption. Table 12-3 lists the estimated safe and adequate daily dietary intake (ESADDI) for pantothenic acid.

Role. The physiologically active form of pantothenic acid is incorporated into coenzyme A, which serves as a coenzyme in various metabolic reactions; some of these reactions involve the transfer of acetyl (two-carbon) groups. Pantothenic acid is required for gluconeogenesis and synthesis of fatty acids and sterols and steroid hormones. Both pantothenic acid and thiamine are required for the oxidative decarboxylation of pyruvate

TABLE 12-3   DIETARY REFERENCE INTAKES: TOLERABLE UPPER INTAKE LEVELS FOR SELECTED VITAMINS AND ELEMENTS*

Age Group (yr)	VITAMINS		TRACE ELEMENTS					
	Biotin (µg)	Pantothenic Acid (mg)	Copper (µg)	Manganese (mg)	Fluoride (mg)	Magnesium (µg)	Chromium (µg)	Molybdenum (µg)
Infants								
0-6 mo	ND	ND	ND	ND	0.7	ND	ND	ND
7-12 mo	ND	ND	ND	ND	0.9	ND	ND	ND
Children								
1-3 yr	ND	ND	1000	2	1.3	65	ND	300
4-8 yr	ND	ND	3000	3	2.2	110	ND	600
Males, Females								
9-13 yr	ND	ND	5000	6	10	350	ND	1100
14-18 yr	ND	ND	8000	9	10	350	ND	1700
19-70 yr	ND	ND	10,000	11	10	350	ND	2000
>70 yr	ND	ND	10,000	11	10	420	ND	2000
Pregnancy								
14-18 yr	ND	ND	8000	9	10	350	ND	1700
19-50 yr	ND	ND	10,000	11	10	350	ND	2000
Lactation								
14-18 yr	ND	ND	8000	9	10	350	ND	1700
19-50 yr	ND	ND	10,000	11	10	350	ND	2000

From Otten JJ, Hellwig JP, Meyers LD, eds: *Dietary reference intakes: the essential guide to nutrient requirements*, Washington, DC, 2006, National Academics Press.
*A tolerable upper intake level is the highest level of daily nutrient intake that is likely to pose no risk of adverse health effects to almost all individuals in the general population.
ND, Not determinable because of a lack of data on adverse effects in this age group and concern with regard to lack of ability to handle excess amounts. To prevent high levels of intake, the source of intake should be food only.

to produce acetyl-CoA. Pantothenic acid also functions as part of a glucose-carrier system to facilitate absorption through the intestinal mucosa. It is essential for normal epithelial function.

Deficiency. Because clinical deficiencies of pantothenic acid are extremely rare in humans, they are produced experimentally in humans only by using a pantothenic acid antagonist. Deficiency may develop in patients with liver disease or who drink excessive alcohol. The symptoms of pantothenic acid deficiency include fatigue, headache, malaise, nausea, abdominal pain, burning feeling of hands and feet, and cramping of leg muscles.

Clinical Considerations. Pantothenic acid has been used to treat gastrointestinal tract paralysis after surgery because it apparently promotes gastrointestinal motility. Although a deficiency of pantothenic acid produces gray hair in black rats, there is absolutely no evidence that taking pantothenic acid reverses gray hair in humans.

◆ BIOTIN

Biotin was initially demonstrated to be an essential growth factor for yeast, and it was later isolated from both yeast and egg yolk.

Source. Although biotin is present in almost all foods, good sources include liver, cow's milk, egg yolk, and yeast. It is also synthesized by the microflora in the intestinal tract, so the amount of biotin excreted in the feces can actually exceed the intake.

Recommended Dietary Allowance. Although no minimum daily requirement of biotin has been established, the suggested adequate daily dietary intake for adults is 25 to 35 mg. Table 12-3 lists the RDA for biotin.

Role. Biotin is a coenzyme required in metabolism in carbon dioxide fixation reactions, β-carboxylation, and deamination.

Deficiency. Biotin deficiency is extremely rare but can occur with long-term parenteral nutrition. A biotin deficiency can be induced by eating large quantities of raw egg white. Avidin, a component of egg white, combines with biotin in the gastrointestinal tract and prevents its absorption. If the egg white is cooked, the avidin is denatured and has no activity. When biotin deficiency is experimentally induced by concurrent administration of large amounts of raw egg white containing avidin, symptoms include loss of appetite, mental depression, hyperesthesia of the skin, nausea, malaise, and dry dermatitis.

Clinical Considerations. Because the amount of biotin synthesized in the intestines is related to the number of microorganisms present, antiinfective agents, such as the sulfonamides or tetracyclines, can produce a biotin deficiency. Two types of infant dermatitis respond to biotin therapy.

Other B Vitamins

Vitamin B_{15} and vitamin B_{17}, also known as pangamic acid and amygdalin (Laetrile), respectively, have been shown to be neither vitamins nor important in human nutrition.

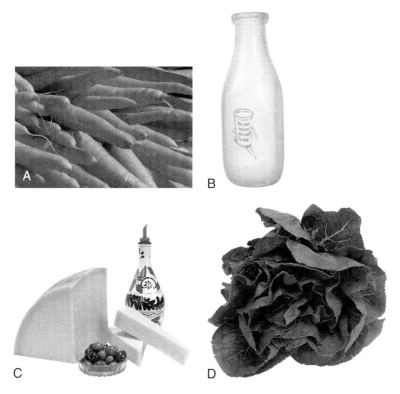

FIGURE 12-3
Examples of foods containing fat-soluble vitamins. **A,** Carrots are a rich source of carotenes, which provide the body with vitamin A, also found in milk (**B**) and some cheeses (**C**). Dairy products also contribute to the body's absorption of vitamin D. **C,** Vegetable oils are the best sources of vitamin E, whereas spinach (**D**) is rich in vitamins A, E, and K. (Copyright 2009 Jupiterimages Corporation.)

Neither choline (KOE-leen) nor inositol (EYE-nos-e-tal) has been demonstrated to be required in the human diet. They serve as lipotropic agents and prevent fatty infiltration of the liver. Choline serves as a precursor to acetylcholine. In humans, no deficiency for either choline or inositol has been demonstrated. Deficiencies of choline (in rats) and inositol (in mice) have been produced.

FAT-SOLUBLE VITAMINS

Fat-soluble vitamins include vitamins A, D, E, and K. Figure 12-3 provides some examples of good sources of fat-soluble vitamins.

Vitamin A

| Vitamin A₁ and A₂: retinoids |

Vitamin A, which is an essential fat-soluble compound, is necessary for normal growth and for maintaining the health and integrity of certain epithelial tissues. The term *vitamin A* represents a group of retinoids (e.g., vitamin A₁ [retinol], vitamin A₂ [3-dehydroretinol]) and carotenoids. The retinoids include both naturally occurring and synthetic analogs of vitamin A. By cleavage of the carotene molecule, two molecules of vitamin A aldehyde (retinal) are formed.

◆ SOURCE

| Retinoids are found in orange-colored fruits and vegetables (e.g., carrots). |

Vitamin A₁ occurs naturally in saltwater fish and animal tissues. Vitamin A₂ is found in freshwater fish. Preformed vitamin A is found in milk, liver, and some cheeses. Margarine can be fortified with vitamin A. However, carotenes provide the greatest source of vitamin A in most diets. Carotenes are found in various pigmented fruits, such as apricots, peaches, tomatoes, and watermelon, and in vegetables such as carrots, pumpkins, broccoli, spinach, and sweet potatoes. A dark green, yellow, or orange color indicates that a vegetable or fruit has carotene.

◆ RECOMMENDED DIETARY ALLOWANCE

The adult RDA for vitamin A is 700 to 1300 retinol equivalents (RE). One RE is equal to 1 μg of retinol or 6 μg of β-carotene.

◆ ROLE

Vitamin A is essential for the maintenance of the photoreceptor mechanism of the retina; the integrity of the epithelia, such as the mucous membranes of the eye, and the mucosa of the respiratory, gastrointestinal, and genitourinary tracts; and lysosome stability. Vitamin A plays a significant role in maintaining the integrity and controlling differentiation and possibly the normal permeability of the cell membrane and the membrane subcellular particles. Vitamin A deficiency decreases the activity of osteoblasts and odontoblasts, thereby reducing the growth of bones and teeth. In contrast, excessive doses of vitamin A accelerate bone and cartilage resorption and new bone formation.

◆ DEFICIENCY

| Night blindness |

The human liver may store enough vitamin A to meet physiologic demands for as long as a year, and therefore a deficiency of this vitamin is rare. Deficiencies, if they do occur, generally result from inadequate intake of the vitamin; a malabsorption syndrome, especially biliary tract disease; or severe liver disease. Deficiency of the vitamin leads to impaired vision in dim light, called *night blindness* (nyctalopia). It also results in keratinization of mucosa and cornea. Corneal keratinization leads to impairment of vision, called *xerophthalmia*. Irritation and inflammation may occur on the cornea, a condition called *keratomalacia*. Keratinization may also occur in the oral cavity and mucosa. The normal defense mechanisms of ciliary movement and mucous production are impaired, producing irritation and inflammation of these surfaces. Loss of the senses of taste and smell also occurs in vitamin A deficiency. Deficiency of vitamin A during pregnancy and infancy contributes to the development of enamel hypoplasia and caries in primary teeth.

♦ TOXICITY

Excessive intake of vitamin A results in a toxic condition called *hypervitaminosis A*. The characteristics of this toxic reaction include itching skin, desquamation, coarse or absent hair, painful subcutaneous swellings, gingivitis, hyperirritability, and limitation of motion. Hyperostosis in the bone is easily demonstrated on radiography. In infants, headache from increased intracranial pressure, gastrointestinal distress, jaundice, and hepatomegaly may occur. Because the margin of safety of vitamin A intake is large, a toxic reaction can occur only after long-term daily ingestion of more than 50,000 RE.

Acute poisoning has been reported in both infants and adults. After ingestion of lesser amounts by infants, increased intracranial pressure with bulging fontanel and vomiting was reported. When the Vikings landed in Iceland, they ingested polar bear liver, a rich source of vitamin A, and died from acute poisoning.

♦ PREGNANCY CONSIDERATIONS

The use of or exposure to excess retinoids (vitamin A or its analogs) during pregnancy can have serious teratogenic effects. Excessive doses of both vitamin A and the analogs etretinate and isotretinoin are classified as FDA pregnancy category X drugs (see discussion of FDA category drugs in Chapter 24). Other retinoids, such as adapalene (Differin) and tretinoin (Retin-A), are FDA category C drugs because the equivalent amount of vitamin A absorbed is substantially below the RDA.

♦ VITAMIN A ANALOGS

Tretinoin (TRET-i-noyn) (Retin-A), the acid form of vitamin A, is a topical product that causes skin peeling and is used to treat acne. Another indication is the treatment of wrinkles. Erythema, desquamation, and unusual sun sensitivity can occur.

Isotretinoin (eye-soe-TRET-i-noyn) (13-cis-retinoic acid, Accutane) is used orally for treatment of severe cystic acne. Side effects include corneal opacities; abnormal liver function tests; elevated plasma triglycerides; and rarely, pseudotumor cerebri. It is highly teratogenic (FDA category X) and should not be used without adequate birth control measures. Remission of acne can remain after the drug has been withdrawn.

Like all vitamin A analogs, these agents are contraindicated in anyone who might become pregnant within the next few years, and they are FDA pregnancy category X drugs. Side effects are similar to those of hypervitaminosis A and relate to the mucocutaneous, musculoskeletal, hepatic, and central nervous systems. Oral manifestations include gingival bleeding, inflammation, and xerostomia with its concomitant implications. A drug interaction with alcohol exists because they can both produce hypertriglyceridemia. Tetracyclines may increase the potential for a rare side effect, pseudotumor cerebri.

Vitamin D

♦ SOURCE

Vitamin D is a collective term used to refer to both vitamin D_2 and vitamin D_3, two closely related sterols. Vitamin D_3 (cholecalciferol [koh-lee-kal-SIF-e-role]) is produced in the skin of mammals by the action of sunlight (ultraviolet rays) on its precursor, 7-dehydrocholesterol. Cholecalciferol (vitamin D_3) is also present in some foods and is added as a supplement to dairy products. Ergocalciferol (er-goe-kal-SIF-e-role) (vitamin D_2), the vitamin D found in plants, is the form of vitamin D used in vitamin supplements. Vitamin D_2 is produced by the commercial irradiation (by ultraviolet light) of ergosterol.

♦ RECOMMENDED DIETARY ALLOWANCE

The adequate daily dietary intake of vitamin D is 5 μg/day for children and 5 to 15 μg/day for adults.

♦ ROLE

Vitamin D promotes normal mineralization of bone by stimulating intestinal absorption of calcium and decreasing the excretion from the kidney.

♦ DEFICIENCY

Rickets

The deficiency of vitamin D produces inadequate absorption of calcium and phosphate with a decrease in plasma calcium. Parathyroid hormone secretion is stimulated, which removes calcium from the bone to restore plasma levels. In children, this deficiency results in rickets, a disease involving a decreased mineralization of newly formed bone and cartilage tissue. Children with rickets have bones that are unusually soft and easily bent, compressed, or fractured. Under the stress and strain of weight-bearing, the gross deformities of rickets, including spine curvature and bowing of the legs, become evident. Because of the excess formation of osteoids, a squared appearance of the head occurs. Collapse of the ribs and protrusion of the sternum (pigeon breast syndrome) are also seen. Bone pain and muscle weakness may be present.

Vitamin D deficiency during pregnancy or in young children may result in enamel hypoplasia, but the teeth may remain caries free. In adults, vitamin D deficiency produces a disease state called osteomalacia. In general, there is decreased bone density because of inadequate mineralization, which results in an excess of osteoid matrix. Because of the weakness of the bones, pathologic fractures and deformities of weight-bearing bones occur. This happens most often during times of increased calcium use such as pregnancy or lactation. Persons with malabsorption syndromes, alcoholics, those adhering to a low-fat diet, strict vegetarians, and those undergoing anticonvulsant therapy or using sedatives or tranquilizers are more prone to vitamin D deficiency.

♦ TOXICITY

The symptoms of hypervitaminosis D, which may result from either long-term or short-term ingestion of excessive quantities of vitamin D, are caused by abnormal calcium metabolism. The signs and symptoms of vitamin D toxicity include weakness, fatigue, headache, nausea, vomiting, and diarrhea. With prolonged hypercalcemia, calcification of the blood vessels, heart, lung, and kidney can occur. Continued ingestion of large doses in a normal adult is likely to produce hypervitaminosis D.

◆ CLINICAL CONSIDERATIONS

Vitamin D is used to prevent and treat rickets. It is also used to treat chronic hypocalcemia, hypophosphatemia, osteodystrophy, and osteomalacia. Dihydroxycholecalciferol (calcitriol, 1,25 $[OH]_2D_3$) and dihydroxyergocalciferol ($[OH]_2D_2$) do not require activation by the kidneys and are used for hypocalcemia in patients with chronic renal failure undergoing dialysis. Because of the need for a functioning kidney to activate vitamin D, the patient is given the preformed active vitamin D. Exogenous dihydrotachysterol (DHT), a close isomer of vitamin D, is hydroxylated in the liver to 25-hydroxy-DHT.

◆ OSTEOPOROSIS

> Highest risk: Female, thin, white, smoker

Normal bone is continuously being made and broken down in response to various stimuli. Osteoporosis occurs when the equilibrium between the resorption and formation of bone becomes negative. The loss of bone mass predisposes the patient to fractures. Patients who develop osteoporosis are much more likely to sustain fractures of their bones, including vertebra or hip, which often reduces their quality of life. The thin, white or Asian woman who smokes is most likely to develop osteoporosis. Patients taking chronic corticosteroids develop osteoporosis earlier. The most common occurrence of osteoporosis is in postmenopausal women because of inadequate sex hormones. Calcium intake of the equivalent of 1200 to 1500 mg of elemental calcium is recommended for postmenopausal women. Weight-bearing exercise may modulate osteoporosis. Estrogen replacement therapy (ERT) reduces the risk of osteoporosis, and recent evidence has determined that the minimum dose of estrogen for this effect is 0.3 mg (0.625 mg was previously recommended). Some women fear the side effects of estrogens, including an increased risk of breast cancer (small increase in risk) and increased risk of uterine cancer (nullified by using progestin with the estrogen). Therefore they do not take supplemental estrogens and osteoporosis is not prevented.

Calcium supplementation is encouraged to prevent osteoporosis in postmenopausal women. Osteoporosis is more effectively prevented when adequate intake of calcium begins in their 20s and 30s.

Three new drugs are indicated for the management of osteoporosis and have been recently released. The bisphosphonates include alendronate and etidronate.

Alendronate (Fosamax), a third-generation bisphosphonate, has been shown to inhibit osteoclastic activity and reduce bone turnover. Under the influence of alendronate, bone formation is greater than bone resorption. It can produce an increase in bone density and reduces fractures for a 5-year period. It is taken on an empty stomach with plain water with instructions to refrain from lying down for 30 minutes thereafter. With higher doses, there is a potential for gastrointestinal adverse reactions. Salicylates can increase the gastrointestinal side effects.

Etidronate (Didronel) has been shown to increase bone mass and reduce the incidence of fractures for at least 2 years. It has been shown to increase the bone mass slightly.

Calcitonin (Miacalcin) is administered by intranasal inhalation. It has been shown to increase spinal bone mass in postmenopausal women with osteoporosis. Further study is needed to define the appropriate therapeutic use of these agents.

Although it is known that fluoride can stimulate bone formation, the use of sodium fluoride in the treatment of osteoporosis is controversial.

Vitamin E

There are eight naturally occurring tocopherols possessing vitamin E activity. α-Tocopherol is the most active tocopherol. α-Tocopherol is found in wheat, sunflower, cottonseed, and olive oils. Although the metabolic role of vitamin E is not understood, it is known that this vitamin functions as an antioxidant.

◆ SOURCE

The best sources of vitamin E are vegetable oils such as soybean, corn, and cottonseed oils. Other sources include fresh greens and vegetables.

◆ RECOMMENDED DIETARY ALLOWANCE

It has been estimated that a daily intake of 10 to 20 mg of vitamin E will keep the vitamin E serum level within a normal range. The Food and Nutrition Board of the National Academy of Sciences recommends between 8 and 10 α-tocopherol equivalents (TE) for adults per day (see Table 12-2).

◆ ROLE

The action of vitamin E is probably exerted via its antioxidant effect. It prevents the oxidation of vitamins A and C, protects polyunsaturated fatty acids in membranes from attack by free radicals, and protects red blood cells against hemolysis. Vitamin E increases the absorption and utilization of vitamin A and protects against hypervitaminosis A.

Vitamin E is being intensely studied for its effect on clotting and on prevention of thromboses. It can be shown to interfere with clotting, but the exact mechanism is unknown (may be related to inhibition of prostaglandins). The evidence of vitamin E's role in cardiovascular disease is strengthened because studies have shown a decrease in both myocardial infarction and stroke.

◆ DEFICIENCY

Deficiency of vitamin E, produced in laboratory animals, can affect the reproductive, muscular, cardiovascular, and hematopoietic systems. Vitamin E deficiency in male rats has resulted in reproductive failure and sterility; in the pregnant female rat, it has led to fetal death and resorption.

In humans, vitamin E has been used for the treatment of sterility and habitual abortion, but there is no conclusive evidence that this vitamin provides any beneficial effect in these conditions. Although vitamin E has been used to treat several cardiovascular diseases, there is no scientific rationale for this use.

A deficiency of vitamin E can occur in malabsorption syndromes and in premature infants with impaired absorption ability. A deficiency of vitamin E has also been reported to cause anemia resulting from a decreased erythrocyte life span and abnormal hematopoiesis. Oxidizing agents can more easily hemolyze the erythrocytes from vitamin E–deficient animals.

◆ TOXICITY

Vitamin E is generally thought to have low toxicity. Levels of vitamin E greatly in excess of the normal dietary requirements have been administered to human subjects with no apparent adverse effect. Nausea, diarrhea, fatigue, weakness, and rash have occurred rarely. Recently, there have been concerns raised about the safety of vitamin E, particularly in doses greater than 400 IU/day. Evidence suggests that regular use of high-dose vitamin E supplements may increase the risk of death.*

♦ CLINICAL CONSIDERATIONS

Vitamin E therapy has been recommended for treatment of a wide variety of human diseases that are similar to conditions of vitamin E deficiency. Vitamin E has been used for many indications in which documentation is poor such as intermittent claudication and protection against certain air pollutants. Other researchers have found that vitamin E supplementation had no effect on work performance, sexuality, or general well-being. At present, no therapeutic use of vitamin E has been proved by controlled scientific studies, with the exception of hemolytic anemia of the newborn.

Pharmacologic doses of vitamin E (used as a drug) have been used as an antioxidant in premature infants exposed to high concentrations of oxygen to reduce the incidence and severity of retinopathy and bronchopulmonary dysplasia. Vitamin E has been used to treat both β-thalassemia and sickle cell anemia with questionable success. The usual dose of vitamin E for its protective cardiovascular effect is 400 IU.

Vitamin K

Vitamin K was originally found to be a fat-soluble substance present in hog liver fat and alfalfa. Large quantities of the vitamin are also found in the feces of most species of animals. At least two distinct natural substances possess vitamin K activity: vitamin K_1 and vitamin K_2. Vitamin K_2 consists of several substances, with menaquinone-4 being the most active form. Vitamin K_1 (phytonadione [fye-toe-na-DYE-one], phytyl-menaquinone, phylloquinone) is found in plants. Vitamin K_2 (menaquinone, multi-prenyl-menaquinone) is synthesized by gram-positive bacteria present in the gastrointestinal tract. Both Vitamins K_1 and K_2 require bile salts for absorption from the intestines.

♦ SOURCE

Vitamin K occurs in green vegetables, such as alfalfa, cabbage, and spinach, and in egg yolk, soybean oil, and liver. Vitamin K is synthesized by gram-positive bacteria, and the microorganisms in the intestinal flora can provide humans with some vitamin K. Synthetic vitamin K is a form of vitamin K that has activity similar to that of naturally occurring vitamin K.

♦ RECOMMENDED DIETARY ALLOWANCE

The adequate daily dietary intake for vitamin K is 60 to 120 μg for males and 60 to 90 μg for females. Generally, the normal diet and intestinal bacteria provide all the necessary vitamin K.

♦ ROLE

Vitamin K is essential for the hepatic synthesis of four of the clotting factors: II (prothrombin), VII, IX, and X. Without adequate clotting factors, normal blood clotting does not occur.

---

*Data from Miller ER III, Pastor-Barriuso R, Dalal D, et al: Meta-analysis: high-dosage vitamin E supplementation may increase all-cause mortality, *Ann Intern Med* 142(1):37, 2004.

♦ DEFICIENCY

A vitamin K deficiency can produce hypoprothrombinemia. In the absence of this vitamin, bleeding will result. With a severe deficiency of vitamin K, the smallest trauma may produce hemorrhage. The most common sites of hemorrhage are operative wounds, skin (petechial bleeding), mucous membranes in the intestinal tract, and serosal surfaces. Ecchymoses, epistaxis, and hematuria are also common.

| Antibiotics can reduce vitamin K production. |

A vitamin K deficiency is usually caused by an inadequate intake or absorption (lack of bile salts) of the vitamin or by decreased normal bacterial flora resulting from prolonged antibiotic use. The newborn can have vitamin K deficiency because the intestinal organisms have not yet been established.

♦ TOXICITY

The naturally occurring vitamins K_1 and K_2 are essentially nontoxic in massive doses, and vitamin K (menadione) must be administered in large doses before toxicity can be demonstrated. It has been implicated in producing hemolytic anemia in newborns and hemolysis in persons suffering from glucose-6-phosphate dehydrogenase (G6PD) deficiency. Hypersensitivity reactions can occur.

♦ CLINICAL CONSIDERATIONS

Anticoagulant drugs such as warfarin competitively antagonize vitamin K and interfere with the production of prothrombin (II) and factors VII, IX, and X. Vitamin K, in the form of phytonadione, is used to treat excessive hypoprothrombinemia caused by warfarin toxicity. It is ineffective in reversing the hypoprothrombinemia caused by severe liver disease.

In patients with severe hepatic disease, a deficiency of clotting factors can result in a prolonged prothrombin time without therapy. Vitamin K is administered to these patients, and their prothrombin time is measured before surgery. Other measures to help clotting include fresh frozen plasma or platelets.

SELECTED MINERALS

Table 12-3 lists the ESADDIs of selected minerals. Less information is available on minerals than on vitamins; selected minerals are discussed: iron, zinc, and calcium. Figure 12-4 provides examples of good sources of these minerals.

Iron

| Fe = iron |

Although iron (Fe) is widely distributed throughout the human body, it is principally found as hemoglobin. Approximately 80% of the iron in the body is functional or "essential" iron (e.g., in hemoglobin [70%] and myoglobin [10%]), whereas 10% to 20% remains as storage or "nonessential" iron (in ferritin and hemosiderin).

♦ SOURCE

Good sources of iron include organ meats such as liver and heart, wheat germ, brewer's yeast, egg yolks, oysters, red meats, and dried beans. Breads, flours, and cereals are commonly enriched with iron. Cooking utensils made of iron can raise the iron

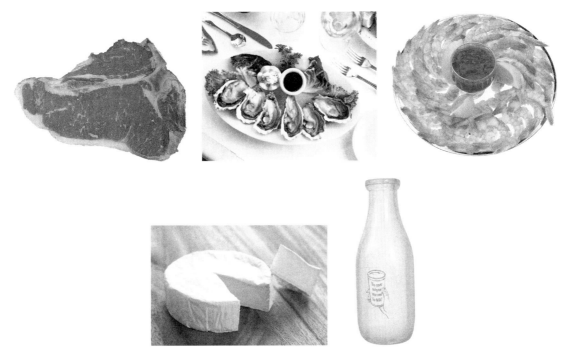

FIGURE 12-4
Examples of foods containing the minerals iron, zinc, and calcium. Iron is found in oysters, red meats, and egg yolks. Meat and seafood are the best sources of zinc, whereas dairy products, such as milk and cheese, and shrimp are rich in calcium. (Copyright 2009 Jupiterimages Corporation.)

content of foods if the foods prepared in them are acidic. The percentage of iron absorbed from foods varies considerably, with absorption from meats being better. Numerous factors affect absorption, such as other foods eaten concomitantly, the bulk in the diet, the size of the dose of iron, the body's need, and the presence of achlorhydria. The H_2-receptor antagonists (H$_2$-RA) and proton pump inhibitors (PPIs) can reduce the absorption of iron. If iron supplements are taken, they should be ingested at different times than the intake of these agents that increase pH.

◆ RECOMMENDED DIETARY ALLOWANCE

The body carefully conserves its iron, and there is no mechanism for its excretion. Excess ingestion of iron over a long period may produce iron toxicity. The iron level is regulated by limiting its absorption from the intestinal tract. However, because iron is contained in each cell, when body cells are lost, iron is also lost. Women must replace the extra iron lost during menstruation. The RDA for iron is about 8 mg of iron per day for males and about 8 to 27 mg of iron daily for females to replace loss. Replacement of a donated pint of blood requires an additional 0.7 mg of absorbed iron daily for 1 year. Two percent to 10% of ingested iron is absorbed, and therefore men need about 1 mg of absorbed iron and women about 2 mg of absorbed iron each day. A pregnant woman's need for iron cannot be met by the usual American diet or the 18-mg supplement recommended for women. For this reason, 27 mg of iron is recommended for pregnant women. Of course, if they have iron deficiency anemia, the requirement is higher.

◆ ROLE

The basic function of iron is to allow the movement of oxygen and carbon dioxide from one tissue to another. Iron accom-
plishes this task by being a part of both hemoglobin and myoglobin. Iron is also a component of enzymes involved in the uptake and release of oxygen and carbon dioxide, and therefore it is essential for protein metabolism.

◆ DEFICIENCY

Because the body is so efficient in conserving iron, a deficiency can occur only with growth, blood loss, or inadequate intake during pregnancy or lactation. The requirements of younger women cannot easily be reached without a supplement. Preschool children, adolescents, and elderly persons are also often found to be deficient in iron, probably because of inadequate intake.

Iron deficiency produces microcytic and hypochromic anemia. The symptoms are nonspecific but include pallor, irritability, fatigue, decreased resistance to infection, and sore mouth. Anemia, a decrease in the quality or quantity of red blood cells, can be measured by laboratory tests.

Before treatment, patients with iron deficiency anemia should be checked for any sources of bleeding to rule out chronic problems such as colon cancer. After ruling out problems, iron deficiency is treated by the concurrent administration of adequate iron salt, usually in tablet form. Ascorbic acid, which increases the absorption of iron may be used concomitantly (e.g., take iron tablets with orange juice). When the hemoglobin becomes normal, which may require months, there is no reason to continue therapy if the diet has improved or the cause of the deficiency has been removed (e.g., by control of excessive bleeding).

Although iron has many salt forms, no product has been shown to be superior to another, but the dose of elemental iron must be calculated based on the specific salt. Because ferrous sulfate (FER-us SUL-fate) contains about 30% iron, 200-mg tablets contain about 60 mg of iron. If side effects occur, ferrous gluconate (FER-us GLOO-koe-nate) may be substituted, but the 300-mg (12% iron) tablets contain about 36 mg of iron. (Of course these will have fewer side effects because they have less iron.) Other preparations, including sustained-release products, have no advantage and in some cases may actually be less effective than ferrous sulfate. The actual amount of iron needed can be calculated based on the results of a laboratory test.

♦ TOXICITY

Complaints of gastrointestinal distress are common, even with therapeutic doses of iron. However, with an acute overdose, bleeding into the intestine can occur, resulting in shock or even death. Poisoning of children with iron has occurred and iron products, like all medications, should be placed out of the reach of children. Treatment of an acute overdose of iron involves removing the iron by gastric lavage and introducing phosphate into the stomach to decrease the iron's solubility. Chelating agents, such as deferoxamine, which form a complex with iron, can be used if warranted.

With prolonged administration of iron, the intestinal mucosa, which normally regulates iron absorption, can be overcome. When an excess of iron accumulates, it produces hemochromatosis, a deposition of hemosiderin, in the organs. An iron overload can also occur with frequent blood transfusions. (Hemoglobin in blood is released, and the iron is conserved within the body.) As with the treatment of acute overdose, chelating agents can be used to treat chronic toxic effects from iron. Removing a pint of blood from the patient weekly can also be used to remove iron from the body.

Zinc

Zinc has only recently been recognized as a mineral the body requires.

♦ SOURCE

The best sources of zinc are seafood and meat. Cereals and legumes also contain zinc, but it is more poorly absorbed from these foods because of the presence of phytic acid, which interferes with intestinal absorption.

♦ RECOMMENDED DIETARY ALLOWANCE

The RDA of zinc for adults is 11 mg for men and 8 mg for women.

♦ ROLE

Zinc is required to transport carbon dioxide in the blood and eliminate it in the lungs. It is essential in the utilization of alcohol, and it rids the body of lactic acid formed during exercise. It is also a component of insulin.

At least 59 enzymes involved in digestion or metabolism contain zinc or need it to function. Zinc plays an integral part in some enzymatic reactions and is a catalyst for others.

♦ DEFICIENCY

Only in 1961 was zinc deficiency recognized in humans. A delay in sexual maturity, slow healing of wounds, and slowed growth are associated with this deficiency. In zinc-deficient rats, fetuses were either resorbed or born with congenital malformations. In humans, zinc-deficient mothers gave birth to low-birth-weight infants or infants with suggested malformations of the central nervous system. Both sexes have shown retarded gonadal development, and with severe deficiency, reproduction is impossible. In view of the drop in serum zinc produced by the oral contraceptives, speculation concerning subsequent pregnancies would be natural. A deficiency of zinc also stunts growth.

Change in taste and smell

Hypogeusia, anorexia, and hyposmia have been reported in conjunction with zinc deficiency. Zinc seems to be essential to the growth and differentiation of the taste buds. It may also be a part of a "growth factor" for taste buds, appropriately named *gustin*. It may soon become routine to measure the zinc in saliva to correlate it with body zinc levels.

♦ TOXICITY

Long-term studies must be conducted to determine the effect of chronic zinc toxicity. Excessive intake of zinc has impaired the lymphocyte and polymorphonuclear leukocyte functions in healthy persons. Nausea, vomiting, fever, and diarrhea have been reported to follow acute ingestion.

♦ CLINICAL CONSIDERATIONS

Although it has long been known that zinc participates in wound healing, there is no known advantage to the administration of zinc in patients who have no zinc deficiency. The use of zinc supplements to promote wound healing is currently being studied for periodontal surgery. Zinc has also been used, without documented evidence, to treat acne, arthritis, and Wilson's disease. Zinc gluconate lozenges have been shown to reduce the duration of the common cold. Zinc lozenges are available OTC.

Calcium

Calcium, the fifth most prevalent element in the body, is present in bones, teeth, and extracellular fluids. The level of calcium in the serum must be maintained within a narrow concentration to prevent serious problems.

♦ SOURCE

Dairy products are the best source of calcium in the diet. These include milk, cheese, yogurt, and cottage cheese. Other good sources of calcium are sardines with bones, tofu, and shrimp.

♦ RECOMMENDED DIETARY ALLOWANCE

The adequate daily dietary intake of calcium is from 1000 to 1300 mg for the adult. Pregnant and nursing women require 1000 to 1300 mg daily, depending on age. The recommended intake of calcium in postmenopausal women is 1200 mg per day. Postmenopausal women who add estrogen replacement therapy reduce their chance of exhibiting osteoporosis. Weight-bearing exercise also helps to prevent osteoporosis. Adequate vitamin D intake should be evaluated. Before a patient ingests exogenous calcium, the patient's diet should be evaluated to determine the baseline intake of calcium from food. Supplemental calcium should be taken to adjust the intake of calcium to 1500 mg. For example, if a diet analysis finds that the patient is taking 600 mg of calcium (two glasses of skim milk), then the calcium supplementation should be 900 mg for the postmenopausal woman.

♦ **ROLE**

Calcium is essential for the function of the nervous, muscular, and skeletal systems and for cell membrane and capillary permeability. It is needed for skeletal muscle contraction, cardiac function, renal function, membrane integrity, and blood coagulation. The skeleton is a reservoir of calcium for the body. Parathyroid hormone, calcitonin, and vitamin D regulate calcium concentrations in the body.

♦ **DEFICIENCY**

A deficiency of calcium can occur when both calcium and vitamin D are withheld. Mobilization from the bone keeps tissue levels nearly normal. If levels in the blood fall, tetany, paresthesias, muscle cramps, and convulsions can result.

♦ **ADVERSE REACTIONS**

Oral calcium may be irritating to the gastrointestinal tract. It may cause constipation. Hypercalcemia may result if large doses of calcium are given to patients with chronic renal failure. Calcium can complex with tetracycline and the quinolones and inactivate them. Their oral administration should be separated by at least 2 hours.

♦ **CLINICAL CONSIDERATIONS**

Calcium is used to treat a deficiency of calcium and secondary to low calcium levels. When calculating the RDA of calcium, the amount of elemental calcium, not the total weight of the calcium salt, must be used. For example, 1250 mg of calcium carbonate provides 500 mg of elemental calcium (40% Ca), whereas 500 mg of calcium gluconate provides 45 mg of elemental calcium (9%). So calcium gluconate has 90 mg of elemental calcium per gram, and calcium carbonate has 400 mg of elemental calcium per gram. Before choosing a calcium supplement, the labels of each product must be carefully compared. It is interesting that on the label of one bottle of calcium the weight of salt (1250 mg Ca [CO_3]$_2$) is printed in BIG letters and the weight of the elemental calcium (Ca) is in small letters.

Calcium may be used parenterally to elevate the serum calcium in an emergency. It is also used during cardiopulmonary resuscitation, in the treatment of hyperkalemia with secondary cardiac toxicity, and to treat hypermagnesemia.

DRUG-INDUCED VITAMIN DEFICIENCIES

Drugs from a large variety of drug groups have the ability to produce vitamin deficiency. Some actually produce a deficiency, whereas others tend to lower the levels of some vitamins. Table 12-4 lists drugs and the vitamin deficiencies they produce.

INH, a drug used for management of tuberculosis, can produce a neuropathy resulting from vitamin B_6 deficiency, so patients taking INH are given concomitant vitamin B_6. Patients taking the anticonvulsant phenytoin (Dilantin) may exhibit vitamin D deficiency because phenytoin stimulates the liver microsomal enzymes, resulting in an increase in vitamin D metabolism and a decrease in its blood levels. It may be necessary to give vitamin D to patients taking phenytoin. Folic acid levels may fall in patients taking phenytoin, but folic acid supplemen-

TABLE 12-4   DRUG-INDUCED VITAMIN DEFICIENCIES

Drug(s)	Potential Deficiency
Methotrexate (MTX)	Folic acid
Isoniazid (INH)	Pyridoxine (B_6)
Sulfasalazine	Folic acid
Trimethoprim	Folic acid
Anticonvulsants	Vitamin D
Phenytoin	Folic acid
Birth control pills (oral contraceptives)	Vitamin A; B vitamins: thiamine (B_1), riboflavin (B_2), pyridoxine (B_6), folic acid, and vitamin B_{12}; vitamins C and E
Levodopa	Pyridoxine (vitamin B_6)
Smoking	Vitamin C
Colchicine	Vitamin B_{12}
Alcohol	Vitamin B_{12}

tation may lower the blood level of the anticonvulsant, requiring an increase in its dose.

Certain drugs, such as oral contraceptives, tend to induce a deficiency of vitamins B_1 and B_2 and folic acid. The exact mechanism by which these vitamin deficiencies occur is not known, but an interference with absorption of the vitamin is a postulate. Drugs that produce a folic acid deficiency include methotrexate, sulfonamides, and triamterene. The anticonvulsants phenytoin, valproic acid, and phenobarbital are associated with folic acid deficiency.

DENTAL HYGIENE CONSIDERATIONS

1. Help evaluate the patient for vitamin deficiencies.
2. Be aware that water-soluble vitamin and mineral deficiencies have many oral manifestations.
3. Talk with the patient about the patient's dietary intake or any health problems.
4. Encourage the patient to see his or her health care provider for appropriate therapy.

CLINICAL SKILLS ASSESSMENT

1. What are some sources of vitamin C?
2. Are there any toxicities to vitamin C and if so, what are they?
3. What are the clinical uses of vitamin C?
4. How does vitamin C work?
5. How could vitamin C deficiency be treated?
6. Can any drugs cause a vitamin C deficiency? If so, what are they?
7. Why were the recommended dietary allowances developed?
8. Compare and contrast fat-soluble and water-soluble vitamins.
9. What are the toxicities and deficiencies of vitamin A?

10. Who is at risk for vitamin D deficiency and what are its signs and symptoms?

11. What are the sources of vitamin K and what are its signs and symptoms of deficiency?

12. What are the B vitamins and who is at risk for vitamin B deficiency?

13. What are the oral manifestations of vitamin B deficiency?

14. What are choline and inositol and what is their function?

15. What are sources of calcium and who is at risk for deficiency? Include signs and symptoms of deficiency.

16. What is zinc and what is its relevance to maintaining a healthy diet and body?

⊖volve _____

Please visit http://evolve.elsevier.com/Haveles/pharmacology for review questions and additional practice and reference materials.

Oral Conditions and Their Treatment

LEARNING OBJECTIVES

1. Name several common infectious lesions of the oral cavity and summarize the treatments for each.
2. Describe immune reactions resulting in canker sores and lichen planus and discuss the treatments for each.
3. Name several oral conditions that result from inflammation and the measures used to treat them.
4. Discuss treatment options for xerostomia and name several other possible drug-induced oral side effects.
5. Discuss the pharmacologic agents most commonly used to treat oral lesions.

The dental health care worker is the first professional that patients visit when they notice a lesion in the oral cavity. Patients often ask the dental care provider, "What is this? How do I get rid of it? How long will it take to go away? Why do I have it? Is it cancer?" Patients who have even visited several physicians may appear at the office with commonly seen oral lesions. The first step is the diagnosis. Obtaining an in-depth history of the problem (by listening and asking open-ended questions) and examining the lesion can often result in a diagnosis or potential diagnoses. Depending on the diagnosis, the lesion may require only reassurance, palliative treatment, specific treatment, or even surgical intervention.

This chapter discusses a few of the more common oral lesions and medications used for the treatment of these conditions. Before discussing individual oral lesions, commonly used treatments for several types of lesions are discussed.

INFECTIOUS LESIONS

Acute Necrotizing Ulcerative Gingivitis

ANUG: Vincent's infection

Acute necrotizing ulcerative gingivitis (ANUG), which is also called *Vincent's infection* and *trench mouth*, has both bacteriologic (spirochetes) and environmental (stress, debilitation) factors (see Color Plate 4). ANUG is a spreading ulcer associated with a distinctive odor; the ulcerated area begins at the interdental papillae.

Good oral hygiene is the cornerstone of treatment, but other modalities have been recommended. Mouthwashes, such as hydrogen peroxide, or saline rinses assist by their flushing action. If pain or an elevated temperature accompanies ANUG, then aspirin or acetaminophen can be recommended. If eating is difficult, food supplements (Meritene, Sustacal, or Sustagen) may be used instead of meals. Vitamin supplementation is useful only if the patient has a vitamin deficiency. The food supplements mentioned contain the required vitamins and minerals. Antibiotics should be considered only if the patient is immunosuppressed or there is evidence of systemic involvement (see Table 7-1). Antibiotics useful for the immunosuppressed patient with ANUG include penicillin VK and metronidazole. Topical chlorhexidine gluconate, active against gram-positive and gram-negative organisms and *Candida* organisms, is used as a rinse for ANUG. The majority of

ANUG cases respond dramatically to local treatment (oral prophylaxis with scaling).

Herpes Infections

◆ OVERVIEW

Herpes simplex, herpes labialis: fever blister, cold sore

Primary herpetic gingivostomatitis (see Color Plates 5, 6, and 7), or primary herpes, is the manifestation of the initial herpes infection. Occurring principally in infants and children, it is caused by the **herpes simplex** virus (HSV). Because it is often associated with or follows other infections, it is also known as a *fever blister* or *cold sore*. The painful lesions may appear throughout the oral mucosa. Beginning as an erythematous area, numerous ulcers with a circumscribed area of erythema appear. The ulcers can coalesce to form larger irregular ulcers with gray centers. Other signs of herpes include the formation of vesicles that become scabbed. Systemic symptoms that are more severe in infants can develop and in some cases, can be life threatening.

Without treatment, herpes is self-limiting in the patient with normal immunity. Approximately 80% to 90% of the adult population has been exposed to HSV. HSV-1 is involved in most oral lesions, and transmission is usually not sexual. HSV-2 is usually responsible for genital herpes and is transmitted sexually. Both HSV-1 and HSV-2 can spread to other parts of the body, for example, the eyes, genitals, and fingers (herpetic whitlow). When the lesions are in the vesicle stage, they are contagious and the virus can survive for several hours on surfaces (one should think about possibilities in the dental office).

After the primary episode, the patient may experience recurrent outbreaks (cold sores or fever blisters) that occur at irregular and variable intervals. Events that may precipitate a herpetic outbreak include sunlight (ultraviolet light), hormonal changes such as menstruation, lip pulling, a rubber dam, biting an anesthetized lip, emotional stress, or other infections (e.g., a viral respiratory infection). One should repeatedly apply petroleum jelly to the lips and be careful when manipulating the lips to minimize the trauma from a dental appointment. The effectiveness of the antiviral drugs varies depending on whether the outbreak is a primary episode or recurrence and whether the patient is immunocompromised or nonimmunocompromised.

◆ TREATMENT

The treatment of herpes may include an antiviral agent, depending on the patient and the episode. Many instances of herpes simplex are not affected by antiviral therapy. Adequate clinical trials determine whether an antiviral agent should be prescribed.

Symptomatic treatment of lesions includes swishing the mouth with topical diphenhydramine (DPH) (Benadryl) elixir or viscous lidocaine and spitting it out. Antiviral agents, such as acyclovir, valacyclovir, and penciclovir, are useful in certain herpes simplex infections (Table 13-1).

Acyclovir. Acyclovir is available as tablets, capsules, oral suspension, ointment, cream, and parenteral forms. This discussion is limited to the oral and topical products; parenteral products are not discussed in-depth.

The approved indications for oral acyclovir include the treatment of primary and recurrent HSV in the immunocompromised patient. In the nonimmunocompromised patient, oral acyclovir is indicated for both treatment of the primary (first episode) outbreak and prophylaxis. Used prophylactically, it reduces the number and severity of recurrent outbreaks. Acyclovir should not be used prophylactically to prevent minor outbreaks because excessive use may lead to resistant strains of herpes.

Oral acyclovir proved effective when taken prophylactically.

Administration of oral acyclovir can be used before situations known to precipitate herpes lesions, such as a ski trip or wedding (stress), or a dental appointment that will produce trauma. The usual prophylactic dose of acyclovir is 400 mg twice a day (bid). It has yet to be shown that oral acyclovir produces a significant clinical effect in the treatment of recurrent lesions in the immunocompetent patient. It may shorten the time to healing or the pain by a small amount.

Topical acyclovir ointment does not affect the course of recurrent herpes in the immunocompetent patient. This may be a result of poor penetration or delay in applying the ointment. Cell damage may be irreversible by the time symptoms are noticed. Topical acyclovir cream was recently approved to treat herpes labialis in immunocompetent patients.

The incidence of resistance of the herpes organisms to acyclovir is increasing. If herpes lesions fail to respond to therapy,

---

TABLE 13-1   DOSING OF FDA-APPROVED ANTIVIRAL AGENTS IN THE MANAGEMENT OF HERPES LABIALIS

Drug	Indication	Dosing
Acyclovir topical cream (Zovirax)	Treatment of recurrent herpes labialis in adults and adolescents 12 years and older	Apply 5 times a day for 4 days
Acyclovir systemic ointment (Zovirax)	Treatment of herpes labialis in immunocompromised patients	Apply q3h 6 times a day for 7 days
Valacyclovir systemic (Valtrex)	Treatment of herpes labialis	2 g orally every 12 hours for 1 day
Famciclovir (Famvir)	Treatment of herpes labialis in adults	1500 mg PO single dose
Penciclovir topical (Denavir)	Recurrent herpes labialis in immunocompetent patients	Apply q2h while awake for 4 days
Docosanol 10% topical cream (Abreva)	Nonprescription treatment for herpes labialis	Apply 5 times daily

FDA, Food and Drug Administration; *PO*, Orally.

the virus should be tested for susceptibility to acyclovir. Resistant strains have been identified, especially in human immunodeficiency virus (HIV)-positive patients taking chronic acyclovir. This is the same principle that produces antibiotic resistance in the general population.

> Penciclovir: reduces lesion duration and viral shedding by 0.7 days

Penciclovir. Penciclovir (Denavir), which is available only topically, has been shown to reduce by one-half day the duration and pain of lesions on the lips and face associated with both primary and recurrent herpes simplex. The advantages of penciclovir over acyclovir are that penciclovir can achieve a higher concentration within the cell and it remains in the cells longer. Table 13-1 summarizes the indications for the antiviral agents.

Famciclovir and Valacyclovir. Both famciclovir and valacyclovir are prodrugs that are converted to active antiviral agents. They are indicated in the treatment of acute localized varicella-zoster infections and recurrent genital herpes in immunocompetent adults. Valacyclovir is also indicated for the treatment of herpes labialis. Ganciclovir is indicated for serious cytomegalovirus retinitis in immunocompromised patients. It may be effective in some acyclovir-resistant organisms.

> Diphenhydramine or lidocaine topically

Treatment of Symptoms. Palliative treatment involves treating the patient's symptoms. In a primary episode of herpes, fever may be managed by the administration of acetaminophen or by sponging the affected area with tepid water. The discomfort associated with herpes may be relieved by swishing diphenhydramine. This product is available under many trade names, for example, Diphen Cough, Diphenhist, Genahist, and Siladryl. All of these products are alcohol-free liquids. Perhaps the most commonly available product is Benadryl. The strength of all the products is 12.5 mg of the active ingredient per 5 ml (1 teaspoonful). Other agents, such as viscous lidocaine (Xylocaine) or combinations of diphenhydramine with kaolin (Kaopectate), calcium carbonate (Maalox Quick Dissolve), or simethicone (Mylanta Gas), are recommended for use in the oral cavity. Because antihistamines, such as diphenhydramine, have a structure similar to local anesthetics, they have some local anesthetic action and can therefore reduce the pain.

Sodium carboxymethylcellulose paste (Orabase plain or with benzocaine) may reduce discomfort. Food supplements may be used if intake of food is impossible (because of oral discomfort). These remedies are the same as those used for patients receiving cancer chemotherapy agents. Corticosteroids are contraindicated because they suppress the cellular immunity that inhibits viral infections.

Candidiasis (Moniliasis)

Candidiasis, a fungal infection caused by *Candida albicans,* often affects the oral and vaginal mucosa. Candidiasis occurs when the organisms multiply and predominate. Because *Candida* is part of the normal oral flora, it is always present in small numbers. When other flora are suppressed, *Candida* can predominate.

> Candidiasis often secondary to broad-spectrum antibiotics

When a patient presents with oral candidiasis, it is important that the dental health care worker search exhaustively for potential predisposing factors. Systemic antibiotic treatment, especially with broad-spectrum antibiotics such as tetracycline, can predispose a patient to candidiasis. A dental health care worker may be the first professional to diagnose HIV-positive patients or those with acquired immunodeficiency syndrome (AIDS) (see Color Plate 8).

Although candidiasis can appear in several different forms, the lesions are typical and can usually be diagnosed by clinical appearance. They may be confirmed by culture. Topical products available to treat oral candidiasis include nystatin products (aqueous suspension, vaginal tablets [used as lozenges], and lozenges [pastilles]) or clotrimazole troches (see Chapter 8).

With chronic candidiasis (see Color Plate 9), ketoconazole tablets taken orally once daily can be used. Systemic alternatives include either fluconazole or itraconazole. All are effective, but they should be continued for at least 2 weeks and/or at least 2 to 3 days past the time when the symptoms have disappeared.

Angular Cheilitis/Cheilosis

> Angular cheilitis: cracks in corners of mouth

Angular cheilitis appears as simple redness, fissures, erosion, ulcers, and crusting located at the angles of the mouth, which may or may not be painful (see Color Plate 10). Most cases of cheilitis are associated with a mixed infection. Often, *C. albicans* infection is present, and not uncommonly both *Candida* and gram-positive bacteria, such as streptococci and/or staphylococci, also invade the lesion.

Predisposing factors may include moisture from drooling (moist areas are more likely to be infected with fungus). In the past, a decrease in vertical dimension was thought to contribute to angular cheilitis, but recent evidence has not shown this to be true.

Depending on the presentation of the patient's lesion, therapy is addressed toward treating the secondary infection(s). If *Candida* organisms are present, treatment with an antifungal agent (see Chapter 8) is indicated. Examples of topical antifungal agents include nystatin, clotrimazole, or miconazole. If inflammation is present, some practitioners prescribe a combination of an antifungal agent mixed with a topical steroid (e.g., Mycolog [nystatin (Mycostatin) plus triamcinolone acetonide (Kenalog)]). One concern, which may or may not be clinically significant, about using steroids with a fungal infection is that steroids inhibit the inflammatory reaction associated with cellular immunity (this is the reaction that normally fights fungal infections).

If a bacterial overgrowth is suspected, the organisms responsible are usually similar to staphylococci and streptococci. To treat this bacterial infection, systemic penicillinase-resistant penicillins, such as dicloxacillin, are indicated (see Chapter 7). A relatively new agent, mupirocin (Bactroban), is a topical antibacterial useful in the treatment of staphylococcal and streptococcal infections. Using mupirocin (see Chapter 7) decreases the likelihood of adverse reactions, and mupirocin is as effective as systemic penicillinase-resistant penicillins. A topical antifungal agent and mupirocin can be used concomitantly if both are indicated.

Although rarely produced by a deficiency of vitamin B_6 (pyridoxine) or B_2 (riboflavin), cheilosis can result from deficiencies of these vitamins. Vitamin B supplements would be useful, but only if a vitamin deficiency exists.

Alveolar Osteitis

Dry socket increases with birth control pills, smoking, and diabetes.

Alveolar osteitis, or "dry socket," occurs in 2% to 3% of all tooth extractions, most commonly in the lower molar region, where the incidence is considerably higher than in other areas. Alveolar osteitis is thought to be caused by loss or necrosis of the blood clot that has formed in the extraction site, exposing the underlying bone. The exposed bone produces severe pain. Predisposing factors include oral contraceptive use and menstrual cycle phase. Smoking, especially after extraction, can increase the likelihood of dry socket. Inhaling on a cigarette produces a negative pressure in the oral cavity that may dislodge the clot.

Infection, swelling, elevated temperature, lymphadenopathy, and a foul odor may be present. Treatment consists of rinsing with saline water and debridement, placement of a pack, analgesics, and supportive therapy. Although there is some indication that local placement of antibiotics may reduce the incidence of dry socket, aseptic techniques, proper suturing techniques, and minimal trauma should be used as prophylactic measures. Most literature does not recommend the use of prophylactic antibiotics. If infection is present, antibiotics are indicated (treatment not prophylaxis). Antibiotics may be indicated in patients at high risk for infection.

IMMUNE REACTIONS

Recurrent Aphthous Stomatitis

RAS: canker sore

Recurrent aphthous stomatitis (RAS), which is sometimes referred to as a canker sore, is a common oral lesion occurring in about 20% of the population. It is seen after 20 years of age and has an unknown etiology, although an involvement of the immune system is suspected.

RAS presents clinically as a few small to many large ulcers. These ulcers can even coalesce into giant ulcers. Although three distinct types have been clinically identified—minor, major, and herpetiforme—the most common form of aphthous ulcers is the minor type (see Color Plates 11 and 12).

The etiology of aphthous stomatitis involves an immunologic component and may be associated with a focal immune dysfunction in which T lymphocytes play a significant role. There is a decreased ratio of T-helper (CD4+) cells to T-suppressor/cytotoxic (CD8+) cells. An increase in the CD8 cells is seen. The oral mucosa is destroyed by lymphocytes.

Many hypotheses have been considered concerning the etiology of RAS, including the following: an allergenic/hypersensitivity reaction (endogenous [autoimmune], exogenous [hyperimmune]), genetic, hematologic, hormones, infection, nutrition, and nonspecific events such as trauma and stress. Another hypothesis is that it is a hypersensitivity reaction to the sodium lauryl sulfate present in many over-the-counter (OTC) products, including most toothpastes (Table 13-2).

◆ CORTICOSTEROIDS

Steroids have been the mainstay of therapy for RAS for many years. Topical steroids, such as fluocinonide or betamethasone, are used to reduce the inflammation associated with the lesions. Topical corticosteroids are available in different strengths and

TABLE 13-2   TOOTHPASTES (DENTIFRICES) THAT DO NOT CONTAIN SODIUM LAURYL SULFATE*

Dentifrice	American Dental Association Approved
Arm & Hammer Dental Care Baking Soda Tooth Powder	No
Platinum Whitening Toothpaste with Fluoride	No
Pycopay Tooth Powder	No
Sensodyne Gel, Cool Mint	No
Sensodyne-SC Toothpaste	Yes

*Many products with almost identical names made by the same company do contain sodium lauryl sulfate. Mr. Toms contains sodium lauryl sulfate. The ingredients are listed on toothpaste tubes.

potencies (see Chapter 19). The amount of antiinflammatory action present depends on the strength of the steroid; however, the possibility for adverse reactions associated with the corticosteroids increases with increased strength of the steroid. Creams or gels are more easily applied than ointments (greasy base), but gels, because they contain alcohol, can cause burning. Examples of topical steroids are triamcinolone acetonide, clobetasol, and fluocinonide.

Another base, carboxymethylcellulose paste (Orabase), is a plasticized base that hardens into a plastic-like plaster. Steroids are incorporated into this paste, which is applied after drying the area. Patient opinions differ with respect to this base. Some like its plastic consistency and covering of the lesion, but others dislike the soft, shell-like inflexible lump of base. Orabase is available plain or mixed with either hydrocortisone or triamcinolone acetonide.

In severe cases of RAS, a short course of systemic steroids (40 mg/day) may be indicated.

◆ APHTHASOL

Aphthasol reduces duration of aphthous ulcers by 0.7 days.

Aphthasol (Aphthasol) is a new drug used topically in treatment of aphthous ulcers. It is applied four times daily and can produce a decrease in the duration of both healing and pain by 0.7 days.

◆ DIPHENHYDRAMINE

DPH alone is now preferred because of its local anesthetic action. Tetracycline suspension mixed with nystatin and DPH has been advocated.

◆ IMMUNOSUPPRESSIVES

Immunosuppressives: last resort

As a last resort, immunosuppressive agents, such as azathioprine (Imuran), methotrexate (Rheumatrex), and cyclosporine (Sandimmune), have been used to treat severe aphthous ulcers. Other immunomodulating agents, such as thalidomide and interferon, also have been used. Whether thalidomide is effective in the treatment of aphthous ulcers and suppression of recurrences is controversial. Some studies found a positive effect, whereas others found none. Thalidomide was previously approved for use in Europe for insomnia in pregnant women. It was later found that as little as one tablet, taken on a certain day of gestation, could produce phocomelia (missing arm and/ or leg bones). It is currently used in certain South American countries to treat leprosy in men. Not unexpectedly, some thalidomide has been inappropriately transferred to women and teratogenic effects have been produced. The risk of teratogenic effects must be weighed against thalidomide's potential beneficial effects. The United States has approved thalidomide for use only with very limited distribution.

Tetracycline has been used in the past, but current thinking is that adding tetracycline suspension to mixtures does not add to the therapeutic effect. Chlorhexidine (Peridex) has been used to manage this condition.

Lichen Planus

Lichen planus is a skin condition (see Color Plate 13) that often involves lesions on the oral mucous membranes. The oral lesions are present without the skin lesions in 65% of the cases. Lichen planus can present in three forms: striated, plaquelike, and erosive (contains the atrophic and bullous subtypes). The most characteristic type is hypertrophic lichen planus; this lesion has a white lacelike pattern that intersects to form a reticular pattern.

Symptoms of pain vary between no pain and extreme pain, depending on the presence of ulceration. The etiology of lichen planus is unknown, but current hypotheses include a viral infection, an autoimmune disease, and a hypersensitivity reaction to an unknown agent. The treatment for lichen planus depends on symptoms and includes oral and topical steroids, oral retinoids, and immunosuppressants.

MISCELLANEOUS ORAL CONDITIONS
Geographic Tongue

With geographic tongue, the tongue may have lesions that typically appear to be a map of the world with the lesions appearing to be the continents. Usually, the lesions are ringed with erythema and their centers are white. There are changes in the patterns over time, and they may even disappear. The etiology of geographic tongue is unknown, but the condition may be related to hormonal changes, stress, infection, psoriasis, or autoimmune diseases. Often, the burning becomes severe when eating spicy foods or drinking alcohol. Treatment includes reassurance and avoidance of irritating food and alcohol.

Burning Mouth or Tongue Syndrome

Burning mouth or tongue syndrome has been called glossodynia and glossopyrosis (*pyro,* burn). With this syndrome, the oral cavity commonly appears normal, but the patient gives a history of experiencing a discomfort described as pain or a burning sensation that increases in severity through the day.

Glossodynia is a painful tongue and is divided into two types: with and without observable alterations on the tongue. It can be caused by many conditions, both local and systemic. Because the tongue is sensitive, small inflammation of fungiform papillae or small trauma from a tooth can be extremely painful. Other visible changes in the tongue are atrophy of the filiform papillae and generalized redness. Burning, stinging, or itching may occur.

The nature of the psychological component in this disease is unclear, but it is known that the presence of chronic disease can lead to depression and anxiety. Patients often are concerned that the cause of their problem may be related to malignancy. Scientific study must be done to determine its cause.

The etiology of burning tongue has not been elucidated, but numerous hypotheses have been proposed, including xerostomia, candidiasis, acid reflux, nutritional deficiency (B_{12}, folate, or iron), immunologic reaction, hormonal changes, allergic reaction, inflammatory process, psychogenic reaction, or an idiopathic reaction. (The variety of hypotheses indicates that the cause of burning tongue has not yet been determined.)

The treatment of burning tongue syndrome depends on the particular etiology the practitioner believes in. Some clinicians treat the patient as they would if the patient had candidiasis. Others test for vitamin deficiencies. Palliative therapy involves using topical DPH to relieve the symptoms. Tricyclic antidepressants, such as amitriptyline, can be used on a trial basis, beginning with a dose of 10 mg at bedtime and slowly increasing the amount until an effective dose is achieved. Amitriptyline is used for two effects. It is thought that depression may play a role in this syndrome, and the amitriptyline may treat the depression. However, this is unlikely because the dose used is not an antidepressant dose and the onset of action is much quicker than the antidepressant effect of amitriptyline. The second mechanism of amitriptyline's proposed effect is that amitriptyline is acting as an adjunct in the management of chronic pain. Amitriptyline has been shown to be effective in chronic pain. Additional studies are needed to determine whether any psychotropic agents might be effective in treating burning tongue.

INFLAMMATION
Pericoronitis

Pericoronitis is inflammation of the tissue around the crown of the tooth. This term, most commonly applied to partially erupted third molars, refers to an inflammatory response that is produced when food and bacteria become trapped between the operculum and the tooth. Periodontal pockets can become painful and swell. If the condition is observed early in its course, debridement with saline irrigation and the use of warm saline rinses will rectify the situation. With severe pericoronitis, debridement is still the primary treatment. If the affected tooth is to be extracted, extraction can prevent further episodes of pericoronitis. With erupting third molars, repeated episodes may occur. Analgesics can be used for the discomfort. Infection, usually managed by local treatment, may rapidly spread in debilitated patients and should be aggressively treated with antibiotics.

Postirradiation Caries

Changes in saliva after irradiation therapy and lack of proper plaque control can rapidly accelerate the rate of dental caries. Generalized cervical decay within the first year after radiation therapy can result. Meticulous oral hygiene, reinforced by the hygienist, short duration between subsequent recall appointments, artificial salivas, and self-application of sodium fluoride gel four times daily in a bite guard are recommended.

Root Sensitivity

Sensitivity of exposed root surfaces may be precipitated by heat, cold, and sweet or sour foods. Occlusal trauma may produce irritation to the exposed dentinal tubules; occlusal adjustment is the treatment. Roots exposed by periodontal surgery, extensive root planing, or accumulation of plaque and its byproducts are more difficult to manage. Applications of glycerin with burnishing, sodium fluoride, stannous fluoride, fluoride varnish, and adrenal steroids have been used in the dental office in an attempt to reduce root sensitivity.

Adequate clinical trials for these products are lacking. The patient may use home brushing with concentrated sodium chloride and 0.4% stannous fluoride. Sodium fluoride gel may also be self-applied in a bite guard. Desensitizing toothpastes have helped some patients, but controlled clinical trials with sufficient patient populations are lacking. Current research indicates that root sensitivity due to recession, bleaching, or abrasion may be successfully treated with amorphous calcium phosphate.

Actinic Lip Changes

Long-term exposure of the lip to the sun can cause irreversible tissue changes known as actinic cheilitis. These sun-related changes occur near the vermilion border of the lips and can progress to malignancy. Sunscreen preparations with higher (greater than 15) sun protective factors should be applied before sun exposure and reapplied as needed. If keratotic changes have occurred, treatment is topical 5-fluorouracil (5-FU), an antineoplastic agent that promotes sloughing of the skin (bad layers of cells are sloughed off). A topical steroid (see Chapter 19) may be used to relieve the irritation produced by 5-FU.

Stomatitis

Stomatitis is an inflammation of the mucus lining the cheeks, gums, tongue, lips, throat, and roof or floor of the mouth. Stomatitis is caused by poor oral hygiene, by poorly fitted dentures, from mouth burns from hot food or drinks, or by conditions that affect the entire body such as medications, allergic reactions, radiation therapy, or infections. Treatment is based on its cause and usually includes good oral hygiene. If stomatitis is a result of mouth burns, then it should resolve on its own.

DRUG-INDUCED ORAL SIDE EFFECTS

Drug-induced oral side effects can be produced by a wide variety of drugs. Different kinds of lesions can be produced with the same drug, and the same kind of lesion can be produced by different agents. Some drugs that can cause changes in the oral cavity are listed in Box 13-1. Common oral side effects include xerostomia, drug-induced lichenoid-like reaction, and hypersensitivity reactions.

The most commonly listed oral side effect of drugs is xerostomia. Many drugs have been stated to produce xerostomia, but the effect is variable, depending on the patient and the dose of the drug. An extensive list of xerostomia-producing drugs is available in Appendix E.

Xerostomia

Xerostomia, or dryness of the mouth, may result from a drug (e.g., atropine), a disease (e.g., Sjögren's syndrome [see

Color Plate 14]), age, or radiation. Radiation therapy to the head and neck affects the salivary glands so that the consistency of saliva is altered and its volume is reduced substantially.

Many different groups of drugs produce xerostomia (Appendix E). For example, the anticholinergics and other drugs with anticholinergic side effects are likely to produce xerostomia. With xerostomia, the patient has a dry mouth. Saliva washes the teeth; xerostomia produces an increase in the incidence of caries, especially Class V lesions.

Treatment of xerostomia consists of the following:

- *Caries prevention:* The use of fluoride trays and gels and other topical agents to counteract the formation of caries should be recommended and demonstrated.
- *Artificial saliva:* Artificial saliva may be suggested for use in these patients. Table 13-3 lists selected drug groups and examples most likely to produce dry mouth.
- *Home care:* The use of fluoride rinses or trays containing fluoride to deliver fluoride should be recommended before extensive caries occur. Drinking water or chewing sugarless gum should be encouraged in place of gum and candies containing sugar.
- *Change in medication or reduction in dose:* With some drug groups, such as antidepressants, there are drugs that produce significant xerostomia and others that produce much less xerostomia. For example, the antidepressant amitriptyline produces a significant amount of xerostomia, whereas a different antidepressant, sertraline, produces much less. Any medication change must be coordinated with the patient's physician and would depend on many factors.
- *Pilocarpine:* Cholinergic agents (P+), such as pilocarpine, can stimulate an increase in saliva in patients with functioning parotid glands. Chapter 4 discusses its dose and adverse effects.
- *Cevimeline hydrochloride (Evoxac):* Cholinergic agonist that binds to muscarinic receptors and increases the secretion of salivary glands. This drug is approved by the FDA for the treatment of dry mouth in persons with Sjögren's syndrome. Adverse effects include excessive salivation, lacrimation, urination, and defecation.

Sialorrhea

Certain drugs may produce an increase in saliva termed *sialosis, sialism,* or *sialorrhea.* One example is the cholinergic agent pilocarpine.

Hypersensitivity-Type Reactions

Hypersensitivity reactions may be hyperimmune responses triggered by an antigenic component of the drug or its metabolite. Contact stomatitis is more localized when gum and candy are responsible and is more diffuse with toothpaste use. The buccal mucosa and the lateral borders of the tongue are often involved. Even cinnamon-flavored products have been implicated in hypersensitivity reactions. The potential for a hypersensitivity reaction is determined by the particular drug, the frequency of administration, the route of administration (antibiotics administered topically are more likely to produce hypersensitivity reactions than those given parenterally), and the patient's immune system (immunoglobulin E [IgE]).

BOX 13-1   ORAL SIDE EFFECTS OF DRUGS

Discoloration
Intrinsic
Tetracycline/doxycycline
Minocycline
Excessive fluoride (fluorosis)

Extrinsic
Stannous fluoride (extrinsic)
Chlorhexidine (extrinsic)
Liquid iron (extrinsic)

Sialorrhea (Ptyalism)
Cholinergics
    Pilocarpine
Cholinesterase inhibitors
    Neostigmine
Ethionamide
Iodides
Ketamine
Lithium
Aldosterone
Apomorphine
Mercurials
Niridazole
Nitrazepam

Sialosis
Propylthiouracil (PTU)
Methimazole
Iodides
Isoprenaline
Methyldopa
Oxyphenbutazone
Sulfonamides

Gingival Bleeding
Warfarin (Coumadin)
Ticlopidine (Ticlid)
Quinidine
Aspirin

Xerostomia*
Antihypertensives
    Clonidine—centrally acting
    Diuretics
Psychotropic
    Antipsychotics
    Antidepressants
Antihistamines
Anticholinergics
Anticonvulsants
Laxatives
Muscle relaxants
    Cyclobenzaprine

Taste Changes*
Metronidazole
Angiotensin-converting enzyme (ACE)
    inhibitors
Penicillamine
Griseofulvin
Gold salts

Gingival Enlargement
Anticonvulsants
    Phenytoin
    Sodium valproate
    Phenobarbital
Cyclosporine
Calcium channel blockers
    Nifedipine
    Diltiazem
Verapamil

Systemic Lupus Erythematosus
Antiarrhythmics
    Procainamide
    Quinidine
Hydralazine
Isoniazid
Anticonvulsants
    Hydantoins
    Ethosuximide
Lithium
Thiouracil

Parotitis
Cardiovascular drugs
    Methyldopa
    Guanethidine
    Clonidine
    Bretylium
    Carisoprodol
    Methocarbamol
    Orphenadrine
Opioids
Sedative-hypnotics

Erythema Multiforme
Antiinfectives
    Penicillins
    Tetracyclines
    Sulfonamides
    Clindamycin
Anticonvulsants

Stomatitis
Antineoplastic agents
    Nitrogen mustard
    Methotrexate
    5-Fluorouracil
    6-Mercaptopurine
    Chlorambucil
    Doxorubicin
    Daunorubicin
    Bleomycin
Antiarthritic
    Penicillamine
    Gold salts
Local application
    Aspirin
    Valproic acid (inside capsule)
Gentian violet

Pigmentation
Amalgam (e.g., tattoo)
Antineoplastics
    Cisplatin
    Doxorubicin
Oral contraceptives
Minocycline
Antimalarials

Candidiasis
Broad-spectrum antibiotics
Corticosteroids

Sialoadenitis
Phenylbutazone
Oxyphenbutazone
Nitrofurantoin
Isoproterenol
Iodine (iodides)
α-Methyldopa

Caries
Xerostomia-producing agents
Sugar-containing medications

Muscle-Related Effects
Dystonic reactions
Antipsychotic agents
Metoclopramide
Cisapride
Bruxism
    Amphetamines

*Additional information can be located in Appendix E.

Oral Lesions That Resemble Autoimmune-Type Reactions

♦ LICHENOID-LIKE ERUPTIONS

Many drugs are associated with eruptions that resemble lichen planus. Box 13-2 lists some drugs that have been associated with this type of reaction. The most common drug implicated is hydrochlorothiazide (HCTZ). Others include β-blockers and antimalarials.

♦ LUPUS-LIKE REACTIONS

Oral manifestations can occur with systemic lupus erythematosus. These lesions may also be produced by a variety of drugs, including antiarrhythmic agents and anticonvulsants.

TABLE 13-3 AGENTS THAT PRODUCE XEROSTOMIA (DRY MOUTH)

Drug Group	Examples
Anticholinergics*	dicyclomine, hyoscyamine sulfate, trihexyphenidyl
Antihypertensives*	methyldopa, clonidine, prazosin
Antipsychotics*	haloperidol, thiothixene, phenothiazines, thioridazine
Tricyclic antidepressants*	amitriptyline, desipramine
Antihistamines	diphenhydramine, chlorpheniramine maleate, hydroxyzine
Adrenergic agents	phenylpropanolamine, pseudoephedrine
Diuretics	Dyazide, hydrochlorothiazide
Benzodiazepines	alprazolam, diazepam, triazolam

*Most likely to produce xerostomia.

◆ ERYTHEMA MULTIFORME–LIKE LESIONS

Some drugs (e.g., anticonvulsants) can produce lesions that resemble those of erythema multiforme.

Stains

Staining of teeth may occur either as the teeth are formed or in a few cases in adult teeth. The tetracyclines are incorporated into forming teeth and thereby stain the teeth (see Color Plate 15). Today, this adverse reaction is well known and pregnant women or very small children are not given tetracycline. With adults, both intrinsic and extrinsic stains may occur. Minocycline is thought to produce a blue-gray coloration to the bone in adult teeth. Chlorhexidine rinse and liquid iron preparations can also cause extrinsic staining.

Gingival Enlargement

Gingival hyperplasia, now known as *gingival enlargement* (see Color Plates 16 and 17), has been renamed because hyperplasia is not the sole process that occurs in the gums. Gingival enlargement can occur in relation to several drug groups; the most common three are the following:

- *Phenytoin (Dilantin):* Chapter 16 discusses phenytoin and gingival enlargement. The rate of occurrence varies with the patient population, but almost half of the patients exhibit this reaction. Occurrence of gingival enlargement in patients taking phenytoin may be dose related. Oral hygiene practices affect its incidence and severity.
- *Cyclosporine:* Cyclosporine is the antirejection drug used for every patient who has had a kidney transplant and for patients receiving many other transplants. Cyclosporine is associated with gingival enlargement.
- *Calcium channel blockers (CCB):* CCBs are used for hypertension and congestive heart failure and have been associated with gingival enlargement.
- *Others:* Other implicated drugs include some anticonvulsants such as carbamazepine (Tegretol) and valproic acid (Depakene).

BOX 13-2 DRUGS ASSOCIATED WITH LICHENOID ERUPTIONS

Heavy Metals
Arsenic
Bismuth
Gold salts
Mercury (in amalgam)
Palladium

Antihypertensives
Methyldopa

β-Blockers
Labetalol
Oxprenolol
Practolol
Propranolol

Diuretics
Thiazides
Furosemide
Spironolactone

Antiarrhythmics
Quinidine
Procainamide

Angiotensin-Converting Enzyme (ACE) Inhibitors
Captopril
Enalapril

Calcium Channel Blockers
Nifedipine

Ulcerative Colitis Agents
Sulfasalazine
Mesalazine

Antimalarials
Chloroquine
Hydroxychloroquine
Quinacrine (Atabrine)
Quinine
Levamisole

Antitubercular Agents
Streptomycin
Pyrimethamine
p-Aminosalicylic acid (PAS)
Ethambutol
Isoniazid

Antiinfectives
Tetracycline
Demeclocycline
Ketoconazole

Antineoplastic Agents
Hydroxyurea
5-Fluorouracil

Sulfonylureas
Chlorpropamide
Tolbutamide
Tolazamide

Psychotropics
Phenothiazines
Chlorpromazine
Lithium

Others
Nonsteroidal antiinflammatory agents (NSAIDs)
Carbamazepine
Allopurinol
Triprolidine
Penicillamine
Dapsone

COMMON AGENTS USED TO TREAT ORAL LESIONS

Corticosteroids

For many oral lesions, especially those with a component of inflammation or immune response, corticosteroids are used. Depending on the severity of the lesions, the topical corticosteroids would be selected based on their potency. Weak, intermediate, and potent corticosteroids are used in turn until an agent is effective. The proper strength of steroid is the least potent that will ameliorate the lesion (see the steroid topical chart in Chapter 19). Hydrocortisone cream 1% is a low-potency topical steroid available OTC. The 2.5% hydrocortisone cream is available by prescription. Triamcinolone acetonide (TAC) is more potent than hydrocortisone and is in the middle range of potency of the steroids. It is available as 0.025%, 0.1%, and 0.5 %; the first two strengths are classified as moderate, and 0.5% is stronger. Fluocinonide (Lidex) is more potent than TAC and is available as a 0.05% cream or solution. Clobetasol (Temovate), 0.05% cream or solution, is in the most potent group. The latter would be used only if the other agents were ineffective.

If topical corticosteroid therapy is ineffective or if the condition is severe, then systemic corticosteroids may be indicated. When systemic steroids are used, prednisone is the most commonly used. There is little reason to use other agents because all corticosteroids have virtually the same effect. When dosing systemic steroids, the dose begins high (usually between 40 and 60 mg of prednisone per day) and is then tapered, depending on the progress of the lesions. In some cases, chronic systemic corticosteroids are required to control the oral lesion. When systemic steroids are used chronically, their adverse reactions must be managed (i.e., osteoporosis, fluid retention, diabetes, hypertension, and the manifestations of moon face, buffalo hump, and abdominal striae).

Palliative Treatment

Palliative treatment is treatment designed to make the patient more comfortable. Agents that reduce the pain of the oral cavity can be topical and systemic. Topical agents are applied by swishing the liquid around in the mouth. These agents include a local anesthetic agent (viscous lidocaine) (see Chapter 9) and an antihistamine with local anesthetic properties (DPH elixir) (see Chapter 18).

Many combination products have been prescribed, but their benefit over plain DPH elixir is controversial. Mixtures of diphenhydramine, lidocaine, and magnesium-aluminum hydroxide have been advocated. Systemic analgesics can often provide relief from a painful oral lesion. Topical and systemic agents may be used together for an additive effect. One concern with the use of topical local anesthetics is that reduction in the sensations from the throat could lead to choking. This can be minimized by avoiding eating directly after application. If isolated lesions are present, the anesthetic can be painted on the lesion using a cotton-tipped swab.

DENTAL HYGIENE CONSIDERATIONS

1. Recognize the clinical manifestations of the various oral conditions.
2. Conduct a thorough medication/health history because many drugs and physical disorders can cause or aggravate oral conditions.
3. Be familiar with the therapies for the various oral conditions.
4. Educate the patient about the appropriate therapy once the dentist has made the diagnosis and prescribed the appropriate therapy.
5. Educate the patient about appropriate ways to avoid offending causes of some of the oral conditions.

CLINICAL SKILLS ASSESSMENT

1. Name two ways to reduce alveolar osteitis.
2. Describe three causes of xerostomia and name several drugs that can produce this effect.
3. Explain the management of xerostomia, including preventive measures.
4. State the best way to prevent actinic lip changes.
5. Describe the treatment of a patient with ANUG.
6. Describe two appropriate treatments for RAS.

⊖volve ─────────────────────────────

Please visit http://evolve.elsevier.com/Haveles/pharmacology for review questions and additional practice and reference materials.

14 Hygiene-Related Oral Disorders

LEARNING OBJECTIVES

1. Discuss the nonpharmacologic therapies that are effective in preventing caries.
2. Discuss the proper methods that patients should use when brushing and flossing.
3. Discuss the role of fluoride in preventing caries.
4. Differentiate between acute and chronic fluoride toxicity and know how to treat both.
5. Compare and contrast both professionally applied and at-home fluoride preparations.
6. Discuss the proper methods that patients should use regarding at-home fluoride preparations.
7. Discuss the proper method for administering professionally applied fluoride preparations.
8. Discuss the pathophysiology and incidence of gingivitis.
9. Compare and contrast the available treatments for gingivitis.
10. Discuss the pathophysiology of tooth hypersensitivity.
11. Compare and contrast the at-home and in-office therapies for the treatment of tooth hypersensitivity.
12. Discuss the dental hygiene considerations associated with caries, gingivitis, and tooth hypersensitivity.

Oral disorders or diseases are among the most prevalent diseases in American society. Each year, dental disorders result in 7 million days of lost work. Among Americans, 50% require oral health care or treatment and almost 80% have some form of periodontal disease. Furthermore, 68% of children aged 12 to 17 have experienced tooth decay and the average adult has 21.5 decayed or filled tooth surfaces. Less than 60% of adults over the age of 65 years visit an oral health care provider during a given year. Also, almost 44% of Americans 75 years and older have lost all of their permanent teeth; however, this percentage is decreasing. The increasing number of older persons with their own, natural teeth has many dental implications.[1]

Poor or improper oral hygiene is a direct cause of dental caries, gingivitis, and halitosis. Nonprescription products for preventing and treating hygiene-related oral disorders are available in pharmacies, food stores, and other retail outlets. Dental hygienists are in the forefront on educating the public about the proper use of these products and their role in preventing hygiene-related oral disorders.

DENTAL CARIES

> Highest caries risk: persons with poor oral hygiene

Approximately 20% of the general population has experienced dental caries. The incidence of dental caries in children has decreased over the past decades.[2] This decrease has been attributed to fluoridation of public water supplies, dentifrices, and mouth rinses, not improved oral hygiene. Despite

BOX 14-1   RISK CATEGORIES FOR DENTAL CARIES
Low Risk: All Age Groups • No risk factors for caries* • No incipient or cavitated primary or secondary carious lesions during the past 3 years **Moderate Risk: <6 Years of Age** • No incipient or cavitated primary or secondary carious lesions during the past 3 years; however, the patient has at least one risk factor for caries* • One or two incipient or cavitated primary or secondary carious lesions during the past 3 years **High Risk: <6 Years of Age** • Any incipient or cavitated primary or secondary carious lesions during the past 3 years, **or** the patient has multiple risk factors for caries* • Low socioeconomic background, suboptimal fluoride exposure, xerostomia **High Risk: >6 Years of Age** • Three or more incipient or cavitated primary or secondary carious lesions during the past 3 years • Presence of multiple risk factors for caries* • Suboptimal fluoride exposure, xerostomia

*High titers of cariogenic bacteria, poor oral hygiene, prolonged nursing (bottle or breast), developmental or acquired enamel defects, genetic abnormality of the teeth, multisurface restorations, chemotherapy, radiation therapy, eating disorders, alcohol or drug abuse, irregular dental care, orthodontic appliances, or cariogenic diet all increase the risk for developing caries.

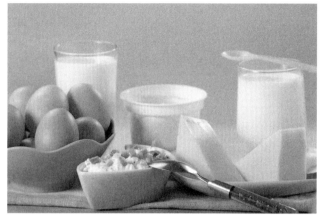

FIGURE 14-1
Dairy products can have a cariostatic effect. Proteins in these foods raise pH levels and can inhibit bacterial growth. (Image from www.BigStock-Photo.com. Copyright 2009 Teresa Kasprzycka.)

improvements in these areas, dental caries are a public health concern and prevention programs should not be ignored but encouraged. Patients at highest risk for caries are those with poor oral hygiene. Patients at increased risk include those with orthodontic appliances, xerostomia, gum recession, and tobacco use. Box 14-1 gives a more detailed overview of the risk criteria for caries.

Dental caries is considered to be an infectious disease that affects the calcified tissue of the teeth. Certain plaque bacteria generate acid from dietary carbohydrates, causing acid demineralization of tooth enamel, which then leads to the formation of carious lesions. Plaque buildup is directly related to the incidence of oral disease. If left untreated, these lesions can destroy the tooth.

Carious lesions start slowly on the enamel surface and initially produce no clinical symptoms. Once demineralization of the tooth progresses through the enamel to the soft dentin, the destruction process proceeds at a much faster pace. At this point, the patient becomes aware of the problem either by directly noticing the carious lesion or by experiencing sensitivity to hot and cold stimuli. If left untreated, the lesion can damage the dental pulp and lead to necrosis of vital pulp tissue.

Prevention

The key to preventing dental caries is good dental plaque control. Reducing the amount and frequency of refined carbohydrates, plaque removal, and fluoride use can reduce the incidence of dental caries. Antiplaque products aid in the mechanical removal of plaque and slow or inhibit its buildup on teeth. Two methods are available to remove plaque from the teeth: mechanical and chemical management. Mechanical methods include brushing and flossing, and chemical methods include specific drug products to prevent or remove plaque buildup. The dental hygienist should teach the patient that the best way to ensure healthy teeth and gingival tissues is to mechanically remove plaque by brushing at least twice daily and by flossing at least once a day.

◆ NONPHARMACOLOGIC THERAPIES

Dietary Measures. One of the easiest ways, although in some ways the most difficult, to prevent caries is to avoid highly cariogenic foods. Foods with higher water content, those that stimulate saliva flow, and foods high in protein are less cariogenic. Proteins in dairy products raise pH levels and can inhibit bacterial growth (Figure 14-1). Noncariogenic sugar substitutes, such as sorbitol, xylitol, and aspartame, can help reduce the risk for developing caries.

Mechanical Measures. Toothbrushes, floss, oral irrigating devices, and specialty aids are the primary types of plaque removal devices.

Toothbrushes. Both manual and electric toothbrushes are available for plaque removal. The proper frequency and method of brushing often vary from patient to patient. Although there are no definite guidelines as to how often patients should replace a toothbrush, it is recommended that the average life of a toothbrush is 3 months. Wear and tear and bacterial accumulation lead to increased plaque buildup instead of plaque removal. Box 14-2 describes the proper method of brushing.

Dental Floss. Interdental plaque removal can help decrease the incidence of proximal caries, gingival inflammation, and periodontal pocketing. Proper flossing techniques require some finger dexterity and practice. Box 14-3 describes the proper method of flossing.

◆ PHARMACOLOGIC THERAPIES

Pharmacologic management of plaque and calculus enhances the mechanical removal by either acting directly on plaque bacteria or by disrupting plaque so that it can be removed mechanically.

- Brush at least twice daily.
- Place a small amount of toothpaste to the toothbrush.
- If using powder, apply the powder to a wet toothbrush making sure to cover all bristles.
- Powder must be applied twice.
- Use a gentle scrubbing motion and angle the toothbrush at a 45-degree angle against the gumline to make sure that the tips of the bristles do the work.
- Do not use excessive force.
- Excessive force can lead to gingival recession and tooth hypersensitivity.
- Brush for at least 1 minute.
- Gently brush the tongue to reduce debris, plaque, and bacteria that can cause oral hygiene problems.
- Do not swallow paste or powder.
- Rinse the mouth and expectorate the water.

BOX 14-3   GUIDELINES FOR PROPER USE OF DENTAL FLOSS

- Have the patient pull out approximately 18 inches of floss from its container and wrap most of it around the middle finger.
- Wrap the remaining floss around the middle finger of the opposite hand until approximately 1 inch of floss remains visible.
- Use a gentle gliding motion and place the floss between two teeth until it reaches the gumline.
- When at the gumline, curve the floss into a C-shaped curve against one tooth and gently slide the floss into the space between the gum and tooth until the patient feels resistance.
- Hold the floss tightly against one tooth and gently scrape the side of the tooth while moving the floss away from the gumline.
- Repeat this process until all teeth have been flossed.

Fluoride. Fluoride is the most commonly used agent used to reduce demineralization and remineralize decalcified areas. The type and amount of fluoride that a person receives depends on his or her risk for developing caries (see Box 14-1). Those with a low risk for caries only require fluoridated dentifrices. Additional, professionally applied fluoride is not recommended in this group because of insufficient evidence regarding any beneficial gains. Patients considered to have a moderate-to-high risk for caries benefit from professionally applied fluoride products. According to the American Dental Association (ADA), only adults with active caries in the last 3 years with risk factors for caries should receive professionally applied fluoride products.

Mechanism of Action. Fluoride is thought to work by two different means. Fluoride ions interact with mineralized tissue, including bones and teeth. Once incorporated into developing teeth, fluoride systemically reduces the solubility of dental enamel by enhancing the development of fluoridated hydroxyapatite, thereby forming the stable compound, calcium fluoride, at the enamel surface. This chemical structure facilitates the remineralization of early carious lesions during repeated cycles of demineralization and remineralization. This same action is thought to occur when topical fluoride is administered. The second action of the fluoride ion is thought to occur on the individual microorganisms in biofilm. Topically applied stannous fluoride (SnF) inhibits bacterial enzyme systems and alters the acid production that would result in demineralization of tooth structure.

| TABLE 14-1 | DOSING SCHEDULE FOR FLUORIDE SUPPLEMENT DEPENDENT ON WATER FLUORIDE ION CONCENTRATIONS IN DRINKING WATER |

	Fluoridation Concentrations in Drinking Water (ppm)		
	<0.3	0.3-0.6	>0.6
Child's Age (yr)	Dosing Schedule for Fluoride Supplements (mg/day)*		
6 months to 3	0.25	0	0
3 to 6	0.5	0.25	0
6 to 16	1	0.5	0

Data from Council on Scientific Affairs, American Dental Association: Intervention: fluoride supplementation. In ADA Council on Access, Prevention and Interprofessional Relations: Caries diagnosis and risk assessment, *J Am Dent Assoc* 126 (6 Suppl):19-S, 1995.
*2.2 mg of NaF = 1 mg fluoride ion.

Toxicity. As with any drug, side effects can occur with fluoride. Nausea and vomiting have been reported in children who have swallowed some of their fluoride treatment. Both acute and chronic toxicity can occur with fluoride use. Acute toxicity is a result of fluoride overdose and is a medical emergency. Chronic fluoride toxicity occurs over time and is treated with medical management.

> Acute toxicity: medical emergency

Acute Toxicity. Acute toxicity of fluoride occurs with a single overdose of fluoride. Signs and symptoms of acute toxicity include nausea, vomiting, diarrhea, intestinal cramping, profuse salivation, black stools, progressive hypotension, and cardiac abnormalities. Death can occur as the result of cardiovascular and respiratory collapse.

Immediate treatment is necessary and includes inducing vomiting and binding fluoride in the gastrointestinal tract to prevent systemic absorption. A designated member of the oral health care team should call 911 for emergency medical treatment. Other team members should induce emesis to get the fluoride out of the stomach. Milk will bind to fluoride and prevent systemic absorption. Monitor patient vital signs and prepare for cardiopulmonary resuscitation (CPR) until emergency help arrives.

> Chronic toxicity is treated esthetically.

Chronic Toxicity. Drinking water with more than 2 ppm of fluoride can lead to fluorosis of tooth enamel during the age of tooth mineralization. Dental fluorosis or mottled tooth enamel is the most common sign of chronic fluoride toxicity during tooth development. The resultant color changes in tooth enamel are a result of hypomineralization of the outer one-third of the tooth enamel. Children that drink water with at least 1 ppm of fluoride and ingest fluoride supplements are at risk for developing chronic toxicity. Table 14-1 reviews the current recommendations of the American Academy of Pediatrics, American Academy of Pediatric Dentistry, and the ADA Council on Access, Prevention, and Interpersonal Relations regarding fluoride supplementation and drinking water fluoridation. The treatment of chronic toxicity is one of esthetics and includes bleaching the anterior teeth and covering the anterior teeth with porcelain restorations.

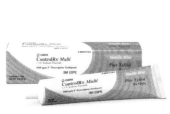

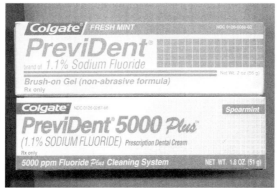

FIGURE 14-2

Sample prescription fluoride products. (Courtesy Dr. Mark Dillenges. From Darby ML, Walsh MM: *Dental hygiene: theory and practice,* ed 3, St Louis, 2010, Saunders.)

TABLE 14-2	FLUORIDE CONCENTRATIONS OF PROFESSIONALLY APPLIED PREPARATIONS
Preparation	Fluoride Concentration (ppm)
Solution, Foam, Gels, and Varnish: In-Office Applications	
Sodium 2%	9050
Sodium varnish 5%	22,600
APF 1.23%	12,300
Prescription Gels: Daily Home Use	
Sodium 1.1%	5000
0.4% SnF and 1.1% NaF in APF	5000

SnF, stannous fluoride; *NaF,* sodium fluoride; *APF,* acidulated phosphate fluoride.

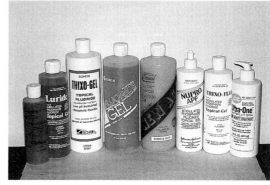

FIGURE 14-3

Examples of topical fluoride gels for professional application. (From Darby ML, Walsh MM: *Dental hygiene: theory and practice,* ed 3, St Louis, 2010, Saunders.)

Fluoride Preparations. Fluoride preparations can be organized into two groups: those applied by the dental hygienist and those applied by the patient.

Professionally Applied Fluoride Topical Agents. Currently accepted agents for professional application are sodium fluoride (NaF) and acidulated phosphate fluoride (APF). Both types of fluoride are equally efficacious in preventing caries. NaF is recommended when restorations are present because of the damage caused by acids. Topically administered fluoride products must remain in contact with the tooth surface for a specified amount of time to allow the chemical change to develop. It is recommended that fluoride applications remain in place for 4 minutes. The ionic exchange lasts for about 30 minutes, which is why the patient is instructed to refrain from eating or drinking for at least 30 minutes after fluoride applications. Topical fluoride applications only last for approximately 5 to 8 weeks because fluoride leaches from the enamel and returns to preapplication levels. Daily applications of low concentration–fluoride dentifrices help maintain fluoride levels in tooth structure.

Annual 4-minute in-office topical fluoride applications reduce tooth decay in permanent teeth of children living in nonfluoridated areas by 26%. Some topical fluoride products are marketed as 1-minute in-office applications. However, clinical trials have not proved that they are as effective as the 4-minute applications. The ADA has given its Seal of Acceptance only to the 4-minute application products.

The concentration of fluoride products varies, and selected products are listed in Table 14-2 and shown in Figures 14-2 and

BOX 14-4	IN-OFFICE ADMINISTRATION OF TOPICAL FLUORIDE PRODUCTS

- Keep the patient in an upright, seated position.
- Place a properly functioning saliva ejector in the floor of the mouth.
- Use the right size tray for the patient.
- Provide the patient with a napkin to catch oral fluids during fluoride application.
- Use a ribbon of gel or foam to cover no more than half the tray's depth.
- Advise the patient to not swallow the fluoride.
- Have the patient lean his or her head forward so fluids will flow to the front of the mouth.
- After the manufacturer's recommended time period of application, remove the tray and suction oral fluids and excess fluoride; wipe the teeth, tongue, and mucosa thoroughly with gauze; and have the patient expectorate for 1 minute.
- Advise the patient to refrain from eating or drinking for at least 30 minutes after the applications.

14-3. Box 14-4 reviews the administration of professionally applied fluoride products. The higher the fluoride concentration, the better the anticariogenic effect. Products with higher fluoride concentrations are recommended for those patients with widespread decay or at increased risk for caries. Patients undergoing head and neck radiation therapy often require higher concentrations of fluoride.

The following are summaries of various professionally applied topical agents:

- *Topical NaF* is available as a viscous gel or foam and is stable in a 2% solution. It comes in several different flavors, is nonirritating to surrounding tissue, and does not stain teeth or restorations. All NaF agents have a neutral pH of 7.0 and are ideal for porcelain or composite restorations or sealants. NaF is applied twice yearly for 4 minutes. A concentrated 2% NaF rinse is available for in-office use. Patients swish the product for 30 seconds and then expectorate. This treatment is applied four times a year.
- *APF 1.23%:* The pH of this product is 3.5, which makes it acidic. Increasing the acidity of the fluoride increases the uptake of fluoride by the tooth enamel. APF products are applied every 6 to 12 months following oral prophylaxis. APF is stable, nonirritating to surrounding tissue, does not discolor teeth or restorations, and causes a slight astringent taste in the mouth. This product is indicated for those patients taking medications on a chronic basis that contain sugar. APF is contraindicated in patients with porcelain, composite, glass ionomer restorations, or sealants.
- *SnF* is only available in a two-part rinse that contains SnF 1.64% and APF 0.3%. The manufacturer recommends a 60-second pretreatment rinse with APF to enhance stannous uptake, followed by a 60-second rinse with SnF. It should be noted that this product is not endorsed by the ADA.
- *NaF varnish* with a 5% sodium fluoride concentration is currently available for use in the United States as a dentin-desensitizing agent and as a cavity liner. The U.S. Food and Drug Administration (FDA) has not approved the varnish for its anticaries effect. However, the use of fluoride varnish for caries prevention has been endorsed by the ADA.

NaF varnish has several advantages over the 4-minute in-office application. The varnish can be applied without prior oral prophylaxis, stays on the enamel longer than topical fluorides, and can be applied if saliva is present. It dries quickly (within 10 seconds) and is slowly released into saliva so there is less systemic absorption, which reduces the risk of toxicity. Finally, application time is short, well tolerated, and safe. NaF varnish is applied to the occlusals or the smooth surface of teeth and leaves a yellow color on the occlusal surface. Varnishes are available as a one-time application formulation and must be mixed in the dispensing cup. It is applied with a small brush and dries quickly so the patient does not gag. The patient should not eat for 2 hours after the application and should not brush his or her teeth for 1 day after the varnish has been applied. Toothbrushing can remove the newly applied varnish. Varnishes are applied two to four times a year. High-risk individuals should have the varnish applied every 3 to 6 months. NaF is a relatively safe product. The product dries quickly, and over time, small amounts are released into the systemic circulation. Preschool and school-aged children treated with NaF varnish suffered no adverse effects on renal function or increased plasma fluoride levels.

Patient-Applied Topical Fluoride Preparations. Patient-applied topical fluoride preparations help to maintain the fluoride applied during oral prophylaxis and help to prevent, stop, and reverse the caries process. Home fluoride products should be used daily at low concentrations. With the exception of dentifrices, rinses and gels come with the warning to expectorate after using and should not be used in children younger than 6 years of age.

Following are summaries of the general types of patient-applied fluoride preparations.

- *Dentifrices:* Almost 98% of all dentifrices or toothpastes available in the United States contain some form of fluoride. Table 14-3 reviews several of the products available in the United States (Figure 14-4). The vast majority of fluoridated dentifrices with ADA acceptance for their anticaries effect contain 0.243% of NaF, which provides 1100 ppm fluoride. Products that also contain triclosan 0.3% carry ADA approval for its effects against gingivitis. Patients should brush at least twice daily. Studies have shown that children between the ages of 10 to 15 years that brush three times daily with a fluoride dentifrice have a 46% reduction in the decayed-missing-filled rate compared to those that only brush once a day (21%). Children should use a pea-sized amount of toothpaste to minimize fluoride ingestion.
- *Gels:* Fluoride gels are prescription gels that the patient self-applies at home (see Table 14-2). The gels are applied for 1 to 2 minutes with a toothbrush or they can be placed in a custom-fitted tray. The gels are intended for adults at high risk for caries, although they can be used in school-aged children. They are often recommended for people undergoing head and neck radiation.
- *Rinses:* Mouth rinses with plaque- or calculus-control ingredients are indicated as adjunct to proper flossing and brushing with a fluoride dentifrice (Table 14-4 and Figure 14-5). Mouth rinses may be cosmetic or therapeutic and both contain surfactants, humectants, flavor, coloring, water, and therapeutic ingredients. Alcohol is added to mouth rinses to provide bite and freshness and to enhance flavor, solubilize other ingredients, and contribute to the mouth rinse's cleansing action and antibacterial activity. Flavors add taste and breath freshening. Surfactants are foaming agents that help remove debris. Cosmetic mouth rinses freshen the breath and remove debris. The primary purpose of cosmetic mouth rinses is to eliminate or suppress mouth odor of local origin in healthy individuals. Cosmetic mouth rinses are minty or spicy, medicinal or alcoholic, and contain any of the following ingredients: glycerin (tastes sweet and is soothing to the oral mucosa), benzoic acid (antimicrobial agent), and zinc chloride/citrate (astringent that neutralizes bad breath).

> Dental hygienists should be aware that mouth rinses may mask pathologic conditions.

A concern with cosmetic mouth rinses is that they may mask pathologic conditions. Patients may confuse oral malodor associated with periodontal disease, oral infections, or respiratory infections with bad breath. If bad breath persists after proper toothbrushing and rinsing, patients should be instructed to contact their oral health care provider.

Since the 1990s, the number of mouth rinses promoted for their antiplaque activity has increased dramatically. Ingredients for plaque control include aromatic oils, such as thymol, eucalyptol, menthol, and methyl salicylates, and agents with antimicrobial activity, such as quaternary ammonium compounds. Phenols control plaque by destroying bacterial cell walls, inhibiting bacterial enzymes, and extracting bacterial lipopolysaccharides. Cetylpyridinium chloride is a cationic surfactant capable of bactericidal activity, although it does not penetrate plaque well. Domiphen bromide is similar to cetylpyridinium.

Mouth rinses are generally safe when used as directed. A burning sensation and oral irritation have been reported. Unsu-

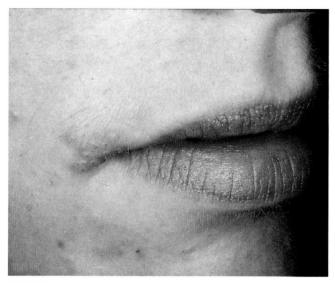

PLATE 1
Herpes labialis 12 hours after onset.

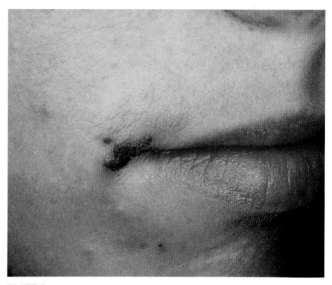

PLATE 2
Herpes labialis 48 hours after onset.

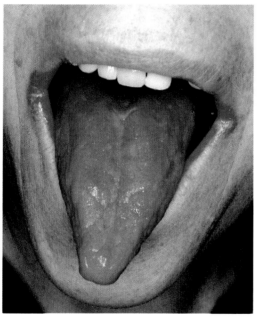

PLATE 3
Pernicious anemia. Note the angular cheilitis and depapillation of the tongue in a patient with pernicious anemia.

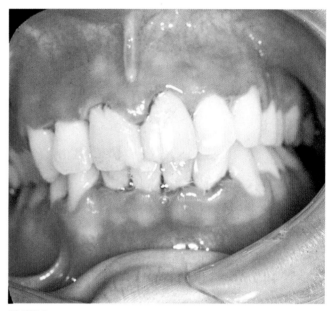

PLATE 4
Necrotizing ulcerative gingivitis.

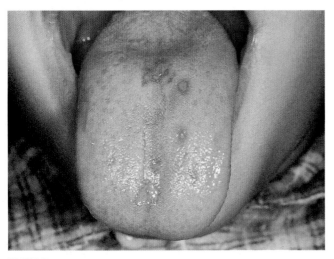

PLATE 5
Primary herpetic gingivostomatitis in a child.

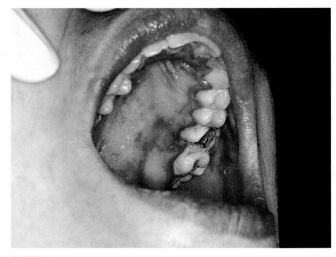

PLATE 6
Primary herpetic gingivostomatitis in an adolescent. Note the painful, swollen gingiva.

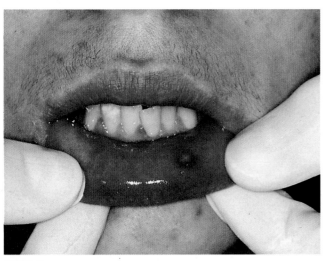

PLATE 7
Primary herpetic gingivostomatitis in an adolescent.

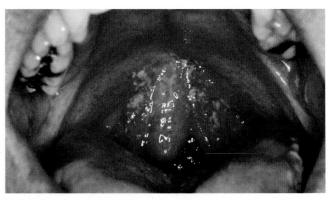

PLATE 8
Candidiasis in a patient with human immunodeficiency virus (HIV) infection. Removable white plaques are present on the mucosa of the soft palate.

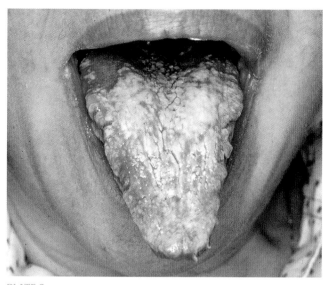

PLATE 9

Chronic hyperplastic candidiasis. The white appearance of the tongue did not wipe off, and it disappeared with antifungal treatment.

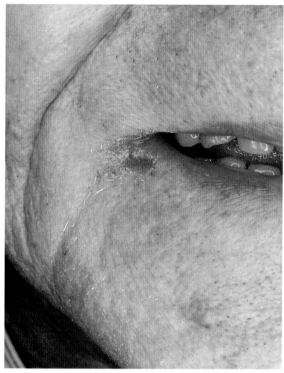

PLATE 10   Angular cheilitis.

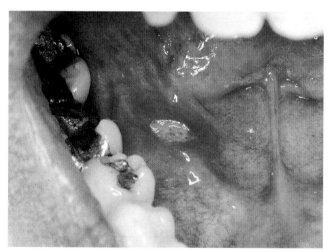

PLATE 11

Example of a minor aphthous ulcer.

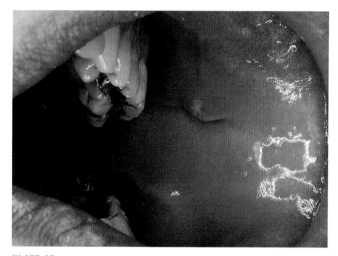

PLATE 12

Minor aphthous ulcer on the buccal mucosa on the papilla of Stensen's duct.

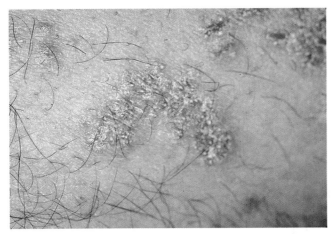

PLATE 13
Skin lesions of lichen planus.

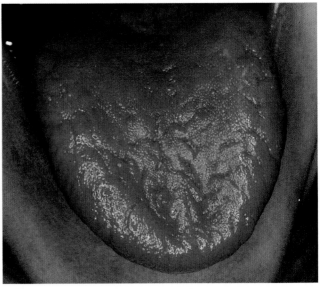

PLATE 14
Sjögren's syndrome. The patient had severe xerostomia. The filiform papillae are lacking.

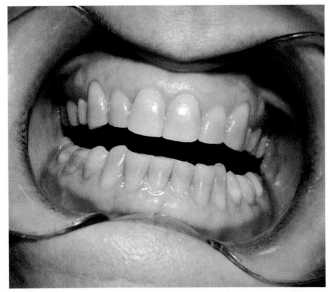

PLATE 15
Discoloration of teeth caused by tetracycline ingestion.

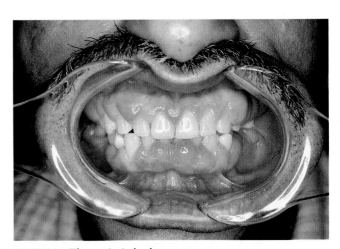

PLATE 16   Fibrous gingival enlargement.

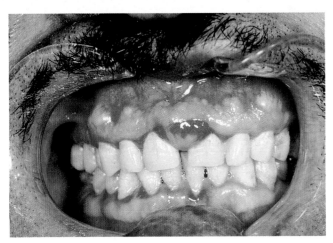

PLATE 17
Inflamed gingival enlargement.

TABLE 14-3   SELECTED DENTIFRICES

Trade Name	Primary Ingredients	Fluoride Concentration (ppm)
Fluoride Toothpastes		
Aquafresh Extra Fresh Toothpaste	Calcium carbonate, hydrated silica, sodium monofluorophosphate (fluoride 0.15%)	850-1150
Colgate Toothpaste	Dicalcium phosphate dehydrate, sodium monofluorophosphate (fluoride 0.15%)	850-1150
Crest Cavity Protection Gel	Hydrated silica, sodium fluoride (0.15%)	850-1150
Tartar-Control Toothpastes		
Colgate Baking Soda and Peroxide Tartar Control Toothpaste	Hydrated silica, sodium monofluorophosphate (fluoride 0.15%), pentasodium triphosphate, tetrasodium pyrophosphate	850-1150
Crest Tartar Protection Gel/Toothpaste	Silica, sodium fluoride (fluoride 0.15%), tetrapotassium pyrophosphate, disodium pyrophosphate, tetrasodium pyrophosphate	850-1150
Antiplaque/Antigingivitis Toothpastes		
Colgate Total Toothpaste	Hydrated silica, sodium bicarbonate, sodium fluoride (fluoride 0.14%), triclosan 0.3%	850-1150
Crest Multicare Toothpaste	Hydrated silica, sodium fluoride (fluoride 0.15%), sodium bicarbonate, tetrasodium pyrophosphate	
Sodium Laurel Sulfate–Free Toothpastes		
Biotène Dry Mouth Toothpaste	Lactoperoxidase, glucose oxidase, lysozyme, sodium monofluorophosphate 0.15%	850-1150
Sensodyne Original Flavor Toothpaste	Potassium nitrate 5%, sodium fluoride (fluoride 0.13%)	850-1150
Botanical-Based Toothpastes		
Dr. Burt's	Peppermint, coconut oil, lavender oil, rosemary, eucalyptus, comfrey	
Tom's of Maine	Peppermint, spearmint, orange, mango, fennel, carrageenan, propolis, cassia, myrrh, cinnamon	
Viadent Original	Zinc citrate trihydrate (2%), sodium monofluorophosphate (0.13% w/v fluoride ion)	

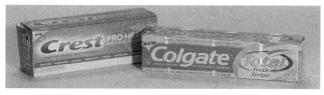

FIGURE 14-4
Sample sodium fluoride dentifrices that have the American Dental Association (ADA) Seal of Acceptance for dental caries prevention. (Courtesy Dr. Mark Dillenges. From Darby ML, Walsh MM: *Dental hygiene: theory and practice,* ed 3, St Louis, 2010, Saunders.)

pervised use is contraindicated in persons with mouth irritations or ulcers. These products should be kept out of the reach of children. The alcohol content in mouth rinses ranges from 0% to 27% with most products containing 14% to 27% alcohol. Ingestion of alcohol-containing mouth rinses poses a great danger for children. In case of accidental ingestion, the caregiver should seek professional assistance or contact a poison control center. Children's products also contain fluoride. Box 14-5 reviews the proper guidelines for using home topical fluoride treatments.

Xylitol. Xylitol is a natural product found in plants that looks and tastes like sucrose but is not fermented by cariogenic bacteria. Xylitol has been found to reduce the levels of *Streptococcus*

mutans in plaque and saliva, inhibit the attachment of biofilm to teeth, and prevent the transmission of oral bacteria from mother to child. Xylitol is a five-carbon sugar alcohol and cannot be digested by bacteria. Xylitol interferes with the metabolism of *S. mutans* as it is transported into the cell. Once in the cell, it may stay bound to the transport protein. The degree of antibacterial effect depends on the amount of xylitol ingested and frequency of use. More often than not, chewing gum is the delivery vehicle. Several clinical trials have demonstrated the beneficial effects of chewing xylitol-based gum. Box 14-6 lists available products that contain xylitol.

Chlorhexidine. Chlorhexidine gluconate 0.2% is a bis-biguanide local antiinfective that is used to kill *S. mutans* bacteria and reduce the harmful effects of biofilm. Chlorhexidine mouth rinse, 10 ml/day for 2 weeks every 2 to 3 months, is effective in reducing the incidence of caries (Figure 14-6).

GINGIVITIS

Gingivitis is the result of the accumulation of supragingival bacterial plaque. If this plaque buildup is not controlled, the plaque grows and invades subgingival spaces. If left untreated, chronic gingivitis can lead to severe periodontal disease or

TABLE 14-4   SELECTED MOUTH RINSES

Trade Name	Primary Ingredients
Cosmetic Mouth Rinses	
Biotène	Lysozyme, lactoferrin, glucose oxidase, lactoperoxidase
Lavoris	Zantate, clove oil, zinc chloride
Targon	Polyethylene glycol 40, hydrogenated castor oil
Therapeutic Mouth Rinses	
Crest Pro-Health Rinse	Cetylpyridinium chloride 0.07%
Listerine Tartar Control Antiseptic	Sodium lauryl sulfate, tetrasodium pyrophosphate
Scope	Cetylpyridinium chloride, domiphen
Fluoridated Mouth Rinses	
ACT for Kids	Sodium fluoride 0.05%, cetylpyridinium chloride
Oral-B Anti-Cavity Rinse	Sodium fluoride 0.05%
Botanical-Based Mouthwashes	
Glyoxide	Carbamide peroxide
Listerine	Thymol, eucalyptol, methyl salicylates, menthol
Tom's of Maine	Peppermint, spearmint, cinnamon, fennel, aloe vera, witch hazel

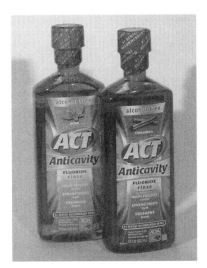

FIGURE 14-5
Sample over-the-counter 0.05% sodium fluoride rinses with the ADA Seal of Acceptance. (Courtesy Dr. Mark Dillenges. From Darby ML, Walsh MM: *Dental hygiene: theory and practice,* ed 3, St Louis, 2010, Saunders.)

periodontitis. Gingivitis is the mildest form of periodontal disease and the most common.

Prevention

Preventive measures for gingivitis are similar to those for caries.

The prevention of gingivitis depends on calculus prevention and plaque control. Therefore many of the same products used to prevent caries are also used to

BOX 14-5   GUIDELINES FOR USING AT-HOME TOPICAL FLUORIDE PREPARATIONS

- Topical fluoride rinses should be used no more than once per day.
- Brush teeth with a fluoride dentifrice before rinsing.
- Pour 10 ml of a fluoride rinse into a calibrated measuring cup and then place in the mouth.
- Rinse vigorously for approximately 60 seconds.
- Spit out the fluoride rinse. Do not swallow the rinse.
- If brushing with a fluoride gel, brush the teeth and allow the gel to remain on the teeth for 60 seconds then expectorate.
- Do not eat or drink for 30 minutes after the treatment.
- Supervise children as necessary to make sure that they do not swallow the fluoride preparation.
- Instruct children younger than 12 years of age on the importance of good rinsing techniques.

Data from Fairbrother KJ, Heasman PA: Anticalculus agents, *J Clin Periodontol* 27:285-301, 2000; and Whitaker AL: Prevention of hygiene-related oral disorders. In Berardi RR et al, eds: *Handbook of nonprescription drugs,* ed 16, Washington, DC, 2009, American Pharmacists Association.

BOX 14-6   SELECTED XYLITOL-CONTAINING PRODUCTS

- Ice Breakers Ice Cubes
- Starbucks Peppermint flavor
- Epic Mints
- ElimiTaste
- Zapp!
- Trident with Xylitol
- Eco-DenT Between

prevent gingivitis. Active antigingivitis ingredients in dentifrices, mouth rinses, and other plaque removal products include SnF, triclosan, cetylpyridinium chloride, and stabilized SnF.

Brushing and flossing are the first line of defense in treating and preventing gingivitis. Brushing, flossing, and rinsing twice a day dramatically reduce plaque buildup. Gum massage is also recommended.

◆ CHLORHEXIDINE

Chlorhexidine: adjunct therapy used for a limited time

Chlorhexidine is active against both gram-positive and -negative bacteria and has some antifungal activity. It is a safe product that does not appear to succumb to bacterial resistance. Chlorhexidine binds to the bacterial cell membrane and increases its permeability, which results in cell death. Chlorhexidine rinse is used in persons with periodontal disease. It is not used prophylactically but as an adjunct therapy for up to 6 months. It is discontinued when the periodontal disease is under control. Chlorhexidine rinse 0.2% is used twice daily. Patients rinse for 30 seconds with 15 ml of chlorhexidine twice a day. The most common adverse effects include tooth and mucosal staining, bitter taste, taste alteration, increased calculus formation, and mucosal irritation. It is best for the patient to rinse after eating in the morning and before bedtime because of the taste changes. Sodium laurel sulfate reduces the antimicrobial effect of chlorhexidine, and they should be administered at least 30 minutes apart.

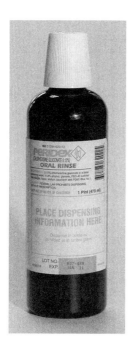

FIGURE 14-6

FIGURE 14-6
Example of a 0.12% chlorhexidine gluconate mouth rinse. (From Darby ML, Walsh MM: *Dental hygiene: theory and practice,* ed 3, St Louis, 2010, Saunders.)

♦ ESSENTIAL OILS

The antigingivitis mouth rinse that contains thymol, menthol, and eucalyptol has been shown to reduce gingivitis and plaque. In a recent clinical trial, an essential oil mouth rinse plus brushing and flossing was found to be effective in reducing interproximal bleeding. When compared to chlorhexidine, the essential oil mouth rinse produced similar results to chlorhexidine at the end of 6 months of therapy, whereas chlorhexidine showed improvements at the end of the first 3 months.

♦ TRICLOSAN

Triclosan is a natural substance that has antibacterial efficacy that reduces plaque and gingivitis. Research has shown that triclosan is more effective than fluoridated products in reducing gingivitis. Triclosan carries the ADA Seal of Acceptance as an antigingivitis agent. The only dentifrice product in the United States containing 0.3% triclosan, copolymer, and 0.243% NaF is Colgate Total. It has no side effects and is safe to use.

TOOTH HYPERSENSITIVITY

Oral pain and discomfort are among the most common oral health disorders that affect people in the United States. Tooth hypersensitivity, or dentinal hyperalgesia (DH), is characterized by a short, sharp pain that comes from exposed dentin in response to thermal, chemical, or physical stimuli that cannot be attributed to any other type of dental defect or disease. Severe attrition and gingival recession as a result of abrasions, erosions, abfraction, and abnormal tooth development can lead to tooth hypersensitivity. Tooth hypersensitivity can occur after teeth whitening treatments when the root surfaces are exposed. Bleaching can increase the risk for sensitivity.

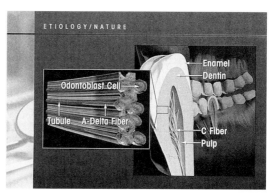

FIGURE 14-7
Structure of a dentinal tubule. (Courtesy Osprey Communications, Inc., Stamford, Conn.)

Pathophysiology

Two processes are necessary for the development of DH: the dentin must become exposed through the loss of gingival recession or enamel and the dentin tubules must be open to the oral cavity and the pulp (Figure 14-7). This occurs when the smear layer of the dentin tubular plugs is removed and the outer orifice of the tubule is opened and exposed to stimuli. When heat, cold, pressure, or acid touch exposed dentin or reach an open tubule, fluid flow in the dentinal tubule increases, causing increased stimulation of the nerves and resulting in pain.

> Both internal (reflux) and external (drugs, foods, or drinks) acids lead to dental erosion.

Dental erosion, which affects tooth enamel, is a result of both intrinsic and extrinsic acid. Extrinsic sources of acid include medication, foods, and drink. Citrus juices, carbonated drinks, wines, and ciders put the patient at risk for tooth hypersensitivity. The most common cause of intrinsic acid production is gastric reflux.

Treatment

The goals of treating tooth hypersensitivity are to alter the damage of the tooth surface using the appropriate dentifrice and to stop abrasive toothbrushing practices. The choice of therapeutic agent should be based on effectiveness, caries risk, amount of tooth structure present, patient acceptance, cost, and esthetics. Treatment for acute DH includes placing a barrier between the exposed nerve at the area where the pulp interfaces with the dentin tubule and the opening of the exposed dentin tubules that opens to the oral cavity. Desensitizing agents seal the dentin tubules and prevent irritants from stimulating the nerves when topically applied to the dentin.

♦ AT-HOME THERAPIES

The most common therapy for at-home use is desensitizing toothpaste (Table 14-5 and Figure 14-8). The vast majority of desensitizing toothpastes contain 5% potassium nitrate. Potassium ions are thought to diffuse along dentin tubules and decrease the excitability of intradental nerves by altering their membrane potential and decreasing repolarization.

♦ IN-OFFICE THERAPIES

Professionally applied products include fluorides (NaF, SnF), potassium oxalate, and adhesives and resins (Figure 14-9). Their effects are temporary because they do not adhere to the dentin surface.

TABLE 14-5   SELECTED DESENSITIZING TOOTHPASTES*

Trade Name	Active Ingredients
Crest Pro-Health	Stannous fluoride 0.454%, sodium hexametaphosphate
Orajel Sensitive Pain-Relieving Toothpaste for Adults	Potassium nitrate 5%, sodium monofluorophosphate 0.20%
Crest Sensitivity Protection	Potassium nitrate 5%, sodium fluoride 0.243%

*These toothpastes have earned the American Dental Association (ADA) Seal of Acceptance for Desensitization.

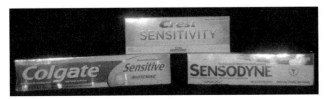

FIGURE 14-8
Examples of desensitizing dentifrices. (From Darby ML, Walsh MM: *Dental hygiene: theory and practice,* ed 3, St Louis, 2010, Saunders.)

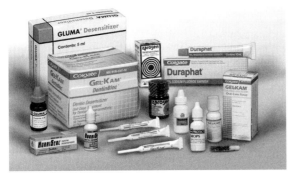

FIGURE 14-9
Examples of professionally applied desensitizing agents. (From Darby ML, Walsh MM: *Dental hygiene: theory and practice,* ed 3, St Louis, 2010, Saunders.)

Fluorides. NaF is thought to work by the formation of insoluble calcium fluoride within the dentin tubules. ADA-accepted products for desensitization include 33.3% SnF applied as a paste or solution and burnished over the sensitive dental area. NaF therapy is not permanent and must be repeated for an extended effect.

Oxalates. Oxalate products reduce dentin permeability and occlude the tubules. Several clinical trials have demonstrated its efficacy, but other trials have found that it is no better than placebo.

Adhesives and Resins. Adhesive products differ from other in-office therapies in that they provide longer-lasting desensitization. They include cavity varnishes, bonding agents, and restorative resin materials. Cavity varnishes provide a protective barrier between the dentin tubules and the oral environment. However, acids will dissolve them and they will need to be reapplied. Restorations seal the tubule, which provides an opportunity for permanent protection.

DENTAL HYGIENE CONSIDERATIONS

The primary objective of patient-centered oral health care is the removal of plaque to prevent caries and gingivitis. Most patients need only follow product instructions and self-care measures provided by the dental hygienist.

Patient Education for Caries and Gingivitis
Nondrug Therapies
- Avoid cariogenic foods that contain more than 15% sugar.
- Eat low-cariogenic foods such as foods with high water contents (fresh fruit), foods that stimulate saliva flow, and foods high in protein.
- Alcohol and tobacco use can cause caries and gingivitis.
- Hormonal changes during pregnancy can cause gingivitis.
- Consider incorporating gum massage as an antigingivitis measure.

Plaque Removal
Brushing Teeth
- Mechanically remove plaque buildup by brushing teeth at least twice daily (see Box 14-2).
- Use a toothbrush with nylon bristles.
- Replace the toothbrush when the bristles show signs of wear and tear.
- For children younger than 2 years of age, clean teeth with a soft cloth and massage the gums.
- Use only regular strength fluoride toothpastes in children ages 2 to 6 years.
- For preschool children, place a pea-size amount of toothpaste on the toothbrush and brush the child's teeth until they can do it themselves.
- Teach children how to rinse the mouth and spit out toothpaste or mouth rinse and to avoid swallowing fluoride.
Flossing Teeth
- Floss teeth at least once a day (see Box 14-3).

Mouth Rinse and Gels
- Teach children how to rinse with mouth rinses and to avoid swallowing fluoride (see Boxes 14-4 and 14-5).
- Teach adults and children not to swallow mouth rinses.

Patient Education for Tooth Hypersensitivity
The objectives for the patient regarding self-care of tooth hypersensitivity are to repair the damaged tooth surface using the appropriate home or in-office therapy and to stop abrasive brushing. Again, most patients will obtain positive results by following product instructions and the dental hygienist's recommendations.

Patient Self-Care
- Use soft-bristled toothbrushes and brush by applying light pressure to the teeth and gums.
- Use a toothpaste for sensitive teeth and brush at or near the receding gumline.
- Note that relief may not be observed for several days to weeks.
- The better the plaque removal the quicker the sensitivity will resolve.
- Use prescription and nonprescription products as directed by the oral health care provider.

REFERENCES

1. Harris NO, Garcia-Godoy F: *Primary preventive dentistry*, ed 6, Stamford, Conn, 2004, Appleton & Lange.
2. ten Cate JM: Fluorides in caries prevention and control: empiricism or science, *Caries Res* 38:254-257, 2004.

BIBLIOGRAPHY

Weck Marciniak M: Oral and pain discomfort. In Beredi RR, Ferreri SP, Hume AL, et al: *Handbook of nonprescription drugs*, ed 16, Washington, DC, 2009, pp 602-623.

Whitaker AL: Prevention of hygiene-related disorders. In Beredi RR, Ferreri SP, Hume AL, et al: *Handbook of nonprescription drugs*, ed 16, Washington, DC, 2009, pp 581-600.

CLINICAL SKILLS ASSESSMENT

1. Describe the two ways to minimize the risk for dental caries.
2. Describe the mechanism of action of fluoride in preventing caries.
3. Describe the signs of acute fluoride toxicity and chronic fluoride toxicity.
4. How is acute fluoride toxicity managed?
5. What directions should be given to the patient for topical home-use fluoride products?
6. What directions should be given to the patient following fluoride varnish applications?
7. How is xylitol used to prevent dental caries?
8. How should 0.2% chlorhexidine be used?
9. What are the adverse effects of chlorhexidine rinse?
10. What are the contributing factors to dentin hypersensitivity?
11. Compare and contrast in-office and home-use desensitization products.

volve

Please visit http://evolve.elsevier.com/Haveles/pharmacology for review questions and additional practice and reference materials.

DRUGS THAT MAY ALTER DENTAL TREATMENT

15 Cardiovascular Drugs

LEARNING OBJECTIVES

1. Identify several dental issues in the treatment of patients with cardiovascular disease.
2. Describe heart failure and identify drugs commonly used to treat it, including the mechanisms of action, pharmacologic effects, adverse reactions, and uses of each.
3. Define *arrhythmia* and *dysrhythmia* and describe how the heart maintains its normal rhythm.
4. Describe the mechanisms of action, pharmacologic effects, adverse reactions, and uses of antiarrhythmic agents and identify the issues to consider in dental treatment.
5. Define angina pectoris and describe the types of drugs used to treat it; identify the dental implications of these drugs.
6. Describe the various types of antihypertensive agents, including the mechanisms of action, pharmacologic effects, adverse reactions, and uses of each. Also identify potential drug interactions and the dental implications of these drugs.
7. Define *hyperlipidemia* and *hyperlipoproteinemia* and summarize the types of drugs used to restore cholesterol homeostasis in the body.
8. Describe the role of warfarin in blood coagulation and the potential adverse reactions and interactions associated with its use.
9. Identify several other drugs that affect blood coagulation.

Cardiovascular disease affects many dental patients.

The term *cardiovascular disease* refers to a variety of diseases of the heart and blood vessels. Examples of these diseases include hypertension, angina pectoris, coronary artery disease, cerebrovascular accident (CVA), and heart failure (HF). Although cardiovascular disease is the leading cause of death in the United States, patients with cardiovascular disease are now living longer, more productive lives because of cardiac care units, comprehensive drug therapy, and intensive screening procedures. This explains why cardiovascular disease affects such a large proportion of the dental patient population.

The dental health care worker first identifies the patient with cardiovascular disease while taking the medical or drug history. It is common for these patients to have several cardiovascular conditions such as HF, hypertension, and hypercholesterolemia. For each disease, a patient may take one or more medications. The importance of this group of drugs is demonstrated by the fact that about 25% of the top 200 drugs (see Appendix A) are from this group.

¼ of Top 200 are cardiovascular drugs.

Because cardiovascular medications are often given for the patient's lifetime, a knowledge of the actions, problems, and effects of these drugs on dental treatment is essential. Both the disease and the drugs used in their treatment can affect the management of a patient's dental care.

Before each group of drugs is discussed, the disease for which the drugs are used is briefly described, beginning with general considerations concerning the dental treatment of patients with cardiovascular disease.

DENTAL IMPLICATIONS OF CARDIOVASCULAR DISEASE

Contraindications to Treatment

Although most patients with cardiovascular disease can be safely treated in the dental office, circumstances may arise in which dental treatment should be delayed until the patient's disease is under better control.

Certain medical situations listed in Box 15-1 are absolute contraindications to dental treatment until a consultation with the patient's provider has determined any special treatment alterations that might be warranted. These absolute contraindications apply only to uncontrolled or severe cardiovascular diseases. Examples of absolute contraindications to elective dental treatment include very high blood pressure and approximately 6 months after the patient has experienced a myocardial infarction (MI). Most patients with cardiovascular disease can be treated in the dental office. The type of procedure anticipated, the stress of the procedure, and the fact that many procedures are elective must be considered. By obtaining a thorough health history, a determination can be made about whether the patient's provider should be consulted before beginning dental treatment. When the health care provider is contacted, it is important to explain the procedure(s) that is indicated for the patient.

Vasoconstrictor Limit

| Cardiovascular patients should receive epinephrine. |

When a local anesthetic containing a vasoconstrictor is used in the treatment of patients with cardiovascular disease, the severity of the patient's disease must be considered. The majority of cardiovascular patients should benefit from the use of epinephrine in the local anesthetic agent. The amount and effect of the epinephrine administered must be weighed against the fact that poor pain management can produce the release of endogenous epinephrine. Limiting the dose of epinephrine to the cardiac dose may be warranted in a few severely affected patients (see Chapter 9 for a detailed discussion of vasoconstrictor limits).

Using a slow rate of injection and appropriate aspiration techniques to avoid intravascular injection reduces the chance of vasoconstrictor adverse reactions. A "fight or flight" reaction related to the patient's anxiety also results in the release of endogenous epinephrine indistinguishable in effect from that of the exogenous epinephrine. (So, being really scared feels exactly like epinephrine because one is making epinephrine.)

Infective Endocarditis

As stated in Chapter 7, the clear-cut uses of antibiotics for prophylaxis before a dental procedure (recommended by the

---

BOX 15-1 CARDIOVASCULAR CONTRAINDICATIONS TO DENTAL TREATMENT

Acute or recent myocardial infarction (MI) within the preceding 3 to 6 months
Unstable or the recent onset of angina pectoris
Uncontrolled heart failure (HF)
Uncontrolled arrhythmias
Significant, uncontrolled hypertension

American Heart Association [AHA] and the American Dental Association [ADA]) are a history of infective endocarditis, presence of a heart valve prosthesis, or congenital heart disease. The most current guidelines regarding antibiotic prophylaxis are discussed in detail in Chapter 7.

Cardiac Pacemakers

| Patients with pacemakers do not require premedication. |

A cardiac pacemaker is an electrical device implanted in a patient's chest to regulate the heart rhythm. If not appropriately shielded, some electrical devices commonly used in dentistry may interfere with proper pacemaker activity. Consultation with the patient's provider may be appropriate before treating a patient with a pacemaker. These patients do not require antibiotic prophylaxis.

Periodontal Disease and Cardiovascular Disease

Research has discovered a relationship between periodontal disease and both cardiovascular disease and stroke. Persons with untreated cardiovascular disease are at increased risk for severe periodontal disease, insulin-dependent diabetes mellitus, atherosclerosis, and emboli production. Several studies correlate the patient's periodontal condition to cardiovascular disease over time. In general, the studies found that the presence of periodontal disease predicts an increase in morbidity and mortality resulting from cardiovascular disease.

CARDIAC GLYCOSIDES

Heart Failure

| Heart failure (HF): heart cannot meet needs |

The heart functions as a pump, ensuring adequate circulation of the blood to meet the oxygen needs of all the body's tissues. When oxygen needs are increased, as in exercise, the normal heart adjusts its output to meet the increased oxygen needs. If the heart is unable to keep up with the body's needs, it becomes a "failing" heart and the pumping mechanism becomes inefficient. This occurs because the heart muscle has suffered an injury and cannot keep up its work. Some enlargement of the heart produces a more efficient heartbeat and cardiac output (Starling's law). However, over time, additional cardiac enlargement occurs (cardiac muscle stretched past its maximum effectiveness by the presence of excess blood that it cannot pump out), and the patient becomes tachycardic. This inefficient pumping mechanism results in an inadequate cardiac output and unsatisfactory circulation. Various forms of injury to the heart, such as MI (heart attack), arrhythmias, and valvular abnormalities from rheumatic heart disease, can contribute to a failing heart.

The heart has two sides: the right and left sides (Figure 15-1). In heart failure (HF), the heart does not provide adequate cardiac output to provide for the oxygen needs of the body. Over time, the blood accumulates in the failing ventricle(s). The ventricle(s) enlarges and finally becomes ineffective as a pump.

One or both sides of the heart can fail. Usually, the left side fails first. If the left side of the heart fails, the blood backs up into the pulmonary circulation (lungs). Pulmonary edema results, producing dyspnea and orthopnea. Dental patients with left failure may need to have dental treatment performed with the patient in the semireclined position. If the right side

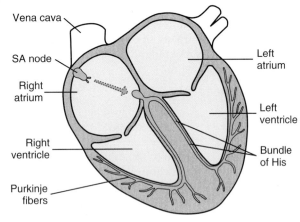

FIGURE 15-1
Cross-section of heart with conduction tissues.

of the heart fails, then the right ventricle is unable to remove all the blood from that side of the heart. Right-sided heart failure causes systemic congestion. Symptoms include peripheral edema with fluid accumulation evidenced by pitting edema (**pedal** edema). Over time, many patients experience failure of both sides of the heart, which causes symptoms from failure of both sides.

Digitalis Glycosides

Positive inotropic effect

The most common type of drug used in the treatment of HF was first described by William Withering in 1785. At first, he thought that these drugs affected the kidneys because they produced diuresis. Later, these substances were referred to as *cardiac* or *digitalis glycosides:* cardiac because they affect the heart and glycoside because of their chemical structure. Digoxin (di-JOX-in) (Lanoxin) is the most commonly used cardiac glycoside.

◆ PHARMACOLOGIC EFFECTS

The major effect of digoxin on the failing heart is to increase the force and strength of contraction of the **myocardium** (positive **inotropic** effect). It allows the heart to do more work without increasing its oxygen use. When the contractile force of the heart is improved, the heart becomes a more efficient pump and the cardiac output increases. After the patient takes digoxin, the heart is reduced to a more efficient size and can function more effectively.

Digoxin affects the heart rate in several ways. It has little effect on the heart rate of normal patients, but in HF the heart rate is first increased. This occurs because of increased sympathetic action resulting from decreased cardiac output. As digoxin increases the cardiac output, the sympathetic tone is decreased, with a decrease in heart rate (**bradycardia**) as the end result. Digoxin also reduces the edema that occurs with HF. As a result of the improved pumping action, more blood circulates through the kidneys (increase in glomerular filtration rate), which mobilizes the edema from the tissues, producing diuresis. The diuresis is not a result of an effect on the kidneys; it is a result of digoxin's indirect effect produced by the improving heart's function. The size of the heart is reduced as the excess blood volume that has collected there is removed via the kidneys.

Digoxin can affect automaticity, conduction velocity, and refractory periods of different parts of the heart in different ways. It slows atrioventricular (AV) conduction, prolongs the refractory period of the AV node, and decreases the rate of the sinoatrial (SA) node. By prolonging the refractory period of the AV node, fewer impulses will be transmitted to the ventricle and the heart rate will fall. These effects are useful in the treatment of certain arrhythmias.

◆ USES

The most common use of digoxin is in the treatment of HF. It is also used for atrial arrhythmias, including atrial fibrillation (AF) and **paroxysmal** atrial tachycardia (PAT). Patients with HF and normal sinus rhythm may not experience long-term benefit in reducing mortality from the use of digoxin. A recent large trial comparing the mortality of patients taking digoxin with placebo determined that digoxin did not reduce mortality. For this reason, the use of digoxin as first-line therapy is decreasing and other drugs such as angiotensin-converting enzyme inhibitors (ACEIs), angiotensin receptor blockers (ARBs), and β-adrenergic blockers are used more often. However, the results of a long-term clinical trial have found that addition of digoxin to other drugs decreases the rate of hospitalization, especially among sicker patients, but does not affect survival.

◆ ADVERSE REACTIONS

Because of digoxin's narrow therapeutic index (see Chapter 3), toxic effects are not uncommon. Even slight changes in dose, absorption, or metabolism can trigger toxic symptoms. In the elderly, toxicity is more likely to occur.

Gastrointestinal Effects. Early signs of digoxin toxicity include **anorexia**, nausea and vomiting, and copious salivation. A reduction in the dosage of digoxin usually alleviates these adverse reactions.

Arrhythmias. If a sufficient overdose is given, severe cardiac irregularities can develop. These arrhythmias can progress to ventricular fibrillation and death. Diuretics, often used in the treatment of HF, can produce hypokalemia, which can predispose a patient to serious arrhythmias. One should note that digitalis is used to treat arrhythmias and its toxicity can produce arrhythmias.

Neurologic Effects. The neurologic signs of toxicity include headache, drowsiness, and visual disturbances (green and yellow vision, halo around lights). A pain in the lower face resembling that of trigeminal neuralgia has been reported as a neurologic symptom of digitalis toxicity. Weakness, faintness, and mental confusion have also been reported.

Oral Effects. Increased salivation is associated with digoxin toxicity. Increase in gagging reflex has been produced, which may interfere with taking an impression.

Dental Drug Interactions. With either increased or decreased blood levels, serious problems can occur when digoxin interacts with other drugs. One drug interaction between digoxin and the sympathomimetics may result in an increase in the chance of arrhythmias. Because both drugs can produce ectopic pacemaker activity, their concomitant administration can increase the chance of arrhythmias.

For this reason, the vasoconstrictors added to local anesthetics, which are sympathomimetics, should be used with caution. In patients with severe cardiac disease, the epinephrine dose may be limited to the cardiac dose (see Chapter 9). Erythromycin and tetracycline can increase the toxicity of digoxin in some patients.

♦ MANAGEMENT OF THE DENTAL PATIENT TAKING DIGOXIN

Box 15-2 summarizes the management of the dental patient taking digoxin.

Gastrointestinal Effects. If a patient complains of nausea or vomiting, special care must be taken to prevent emesis. These symptoms may be associated with digitalis toxicity, and the patient's physician should be consulted if the nausea and vomiting have been protracted.

Epinephrine Administration. Because digoxin toxicity can sensitize the myocardium to arrhythmias, epinephrine should be used cautiously or limited to the cardiac dose in patients taking digitalis. Patients taking digitalis should be questioned about toxic symptoms before epinephrine is administered. Hypokalemia from diuretics can exacerbate this arrhythmogenic potential.

Pulse Monitoring. Because digitalis can cause bradycardia or arrhythmias, the patient's pulse should be checked before each dental appointment for a normal rate and a regular rhythm. An abnormally slow rate or an irregular rhythm should be reported to the patient's provider for evaluation.

♦ OTHER DRUGS

Angiotensin-Converting Enzyme Inhibitors. Current guidelines from the American College of Cardiology (ACC) and the AHA now recommend prescribing an ACEI for all patients with symptomatic (stage C) heart failure and asymptomatic patients with a decreased left ventricular ejection fraction (LVEF) or a history of MI. ACEIs improve symptoms in patients with heart failure within a period of 4 to 12 weeks, decrease the incidence of hospitalization and MI, and prolong survival. ACEIs are now considered first-line therapy and are the cornerstone of HF therapy.

Angiotensin Receptor Blockers. ARBs have also been shown to reduce mortality and symptoms. They are recommended for patients who cannot tolerate ACEIs and are also considered first-line therapy for HF. Candesartan and valsartan are the only ARBs currently approved by the Food and Drug Administration (FDA) for the treatment of heart failure.

β-Adrenergic Blockers. The ACC/AHA guidelines now recommend β-blockers for patients with symptoms of HF and asymptomatic patients with decreased LVEF or a history of an MI. Although it has been customary to start a β-blocker after an ACEI, the results of several clinical trials suggest that starting with a β-blocker may be equally, if not possibly more, effective.

Vasodilators. Hydralazine, an arterial vasodilator, reduces peripheral resistance by arterial vasodilation. With a reduction in the afterload, the work of the heart is reduced. Isosorbide dinitrate, a venous dilator, reduces the preload, which reduces the work of the heart. With this combination, the heart is pumping against less resistance and is getting less blood returned to it (some blood remains in the venous circulation). The heart's workload is reduced and symptoms of HF subside. The addition of hydralazine and isosorbide dinitrate to standard therapy in black patients with class III to IV heart failure significantly lowered mortality and the rate of hospitalization and improved quality-of-life scores. No data are available with this combination in addition to standard therapy in other populations.

Diuretics. Most patients with HF have edema or fluid retention. Diuretics are used in these patients to relieve the symptoms of HF. In clinical trials, patients taking a combination of a diuretic and other drugs used to treat HF showed an increase in survival. Loop diuretics, such as furosemide, appear to be more effective than thiazide diuretics.

Aldosterone Antagonists. In one clinical trial, the addition of spironolactone to standard therapy reduced the risk of mortality and hospitalization. In another clinical trial, the selective aldosterone antagonist eplerenone added to standard therapy reduced both all-cause and cardiovascular mortality in patients with an acute MI complicated by left ventricular systolic dysfunction and HF.

ANTIARRHYTHMIC AGENTS

The terms arrhythmia (*ar,* insensibility; *rhythmos,* rhythm) and dysrhythmia (*dys,* bad; *rhythmos,* rhythm) are used interchangeably to mean "abnormal rhythm." Arrhythmias may result from abnormal impulse generation or abnormal impulse conduction. Cardiac diseases, such as myocardial anoxia, arteriosclerosis, and heart block, can produce arrhythmias. The antiarrhythmic agents are drugs that are used to prevent arrhythmias.

Automaticity

> Cardiac tissue has inherent automaticity. (Each part has a different rate.)

The cells of the cardiac muscles, unlike those of skeletal muscles, have an intrinsic rhythm called *automaticity.* "Pacemaker" cells spontaneously produce action potentials as they undergo slow spontaneous depolarization during diastole (as they rest, they leak ions). If any heart muscle cell is left undisturbed and isolated from the rest of the heart with appropriate nutrients and oxygen, each cell will beat spontaneously at its own rate. Each type of cardiac cell differs in its automaticity depending on the function of the particular cell. The cells that specialize in conduction functions have a faster rate of automaticity than other cardiac cells. This design ensures that the heart will beat in a coordinated manner.

The SA node has the fastest rate of depolarization and therefore directs all the other cells in the heart. It normally fires impulses approximately 80 times/min. The SA node is innervated by both the parasympathetic nervous system (PNS) and the sympathetic nervous system (SNS). The SA node sends a message (action potential) to the AV node via the atrial muscle. When the impulse arrives at the AV node there is a slight delay because the muscles beyond the AV node are thinner. The AV node sends the message via the bundle of His to the Purkinje fibers. The Purkinje fibers then send the message to the cardiac

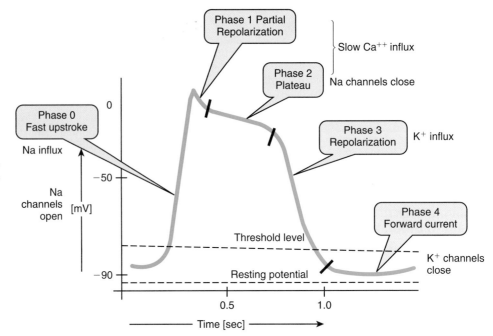

FIGURE 15-2
Electrical excitation from the nerve produces movement of ions across the membrane, generating an action potential.

muscle cells, to the apex of the ventricles, directing them all to contract as they get the message. This system is repeated with each heartbeat.

In the normal patient, this system functions seamlessly. In the patient with cardiac arrhythmias, diseased parts of the heart can produce abnormal conduction pathways, which may result in arrhythmias.

Action Potential

All action potentials have similar properties, but minor differences exist. During rest, the resting membrane potential varies but is −75 mV for some cardiac tissues. Electrical excitation from the nerve produces movement of ions across the membrane, generating an action potential (Figure 15-2). During each of these phases, there is a change in the ion flow that results in certain effects. These changes are seen in Figure 15-2.

Arrhythmias

There are many types of arrhythmias that produce various abnormalities of the heartbeat. These arrhythmias are usually divided into **supraventricular** (atrial) and ventricular types, depending on the location of the genesis of the arrhythmia. Abnormal arrhythmias may result in tachycardia or bradycardia of the supraventricular (atrial) or ventricular parts of the heart or from ectopic foci. The **ectopic** foci are "emergent leaders" that preempt the SA or AV nodal rate. The electrical impulses begin at the SA node and travel to the AV node. At the conduction level, different patterns of conduction include the normal pattern, bifurcation (conduction splits and goes two ways), reentry, unidirectional block (action potential is blocked from being stimulated from one side of the tissue but not from the other), and prolonged refractory period.

Several recent deaths of fit adolescents during athletic events have been linked to congenital presence of a prolonged QT interval (torsades de pointes, previously undiagnosed).

Antiarrhythmic Agents

♦ OVERVIEW

Long-term effects of drugs must be studied.

Antiarrhythmic agents are placed in groups designated by Roman numerals I to IV. Subsets of these Roman numerals use capital letters (A, B, C). The specific actions of the antiarrhythmics are complicated. The antiarrhythmic agents work by depressing parts of the heart that are beating abnormally. For example, if the Speaker of the House (an ectopic foci) attempts to take over the office of President (SA node) and send additional messages to the other officers, then the antiarrhythmic agents can "quiet" these foci.

Antiarrhythmics may change the slope of depolarization, raise the threshold for depolarization, and alter the conduction velocity in different parts of the heart. For example, by decreasing the slope of depolarization, there would be a decrease in the frequency of discharge and the rate would slow. By raising the threshold for producing an action potential, extra beats may be suppressed. Examples of specific actions of these drugs include decrease in the velocity of depolarization, decrease in impulse propagation, and inhibition of aberrant impulse propagation. Tables 15-1 and 15-2 describe the classification and mechanism of action of the antiarrhythmics, the dental-related adverse reactions, and the dental implications of the antiarrhythmias.

Conclusions drawn from data must be carefully analyzed to arrive at appropriate conclusions that can be applied clinically. One study demonstrated that IC antiarrhythmics can prevent post-MI arrhythmics. Although it would seem that this action would be beneficial, with additional data it was determined that although these drugs prevented arrhythmias, patient mortality doubled or tripled. Before this study was completed, these deaths were thought to be a result of fatal arrhythmias unrelated to the drug. It pays to look at future outcomes (e.g., death) to determine whether a drug is "beneficial."

TABLE 15-1   CLASSIFICATION AND MECHANISM OF ACTION OF THE ANTIARRHYTHMICS

Antiarrhythmic/Class		Mechanism	Effect	Comment
IA	Quinidine, procainamide, disopyramide	Na$^+$ channel blocker (medium)	Blocks conduction	Prolongs the duration of the AP
IB	Lidocaine	Na$^+$ channel blocker (fast)	Blocks conduction; decreases ERP	Shortens the AP
IC	Flecainide, encainide, propafenone	Na$^+$ channel blocker (slow)	Blocks conduction; little effect on ERP	Slows conduction without affecting the AP
II	Propranolol, esmolol, acebutolol, sotalol	β-blockers	Decreases SA node automaticity	Reduces sympathetic activity
III	Bretylium and *d*-sotalol (non-β–blocking enantiomer)	K$^+$ channel blockers	Prolongs the AP	Prolongs phase 3 repolarization
IV	Verapamil, diltiazem	CCBs	Slows conduction velocity at AV node	Decreases the firing rate of the SA and AV nodes

AP, action potential; *AV*, Atrioventricular; *CCBs*, calcium channel blockers; *ERP*, effective refractory period; K+, potassium; *Na+*, sodium; *SA*, sinoatrial.

TABLE 15-2   MANAGEMENT OF DENTAL PATIENTS TAKING ANTIARRHYTHMICS

Antiarrhythmics	Implications
All	Check for abnormal or extra beats when taking patient's blood pressure and pulse. Record the type of arrhythmia and the drug therapy.
Atrial fibrillation	Patient on warfarin—check INR.
Amiodarone	Liver toxicity, blue skin discoloration, photosensitivity—dental light
CCBs	Gingival enlargement (verapamil most reported)
Disopyramide	Anticholinergic xerostomia
Procainamide	Reversible lupus erythematosus–like syndrome, 25%-30%; CNS depression, xerostomia
Quinidine	Nausea, vomiting, diarrhea; cinchonism with large doses; atropine-like effect; xerostomia
Phenytoin	Gingival enlargement
β-Blockers, nonspecific	Drug interaction with epinephrine; limit to cardiac dose if patient's condition warrants

CCBs, Calcium channel blockers; *CNS*, central nervous system; *INR*, international normalized ratio.

◆ DIGOXIN

Although digoxin is not included in the other groups of antiarrhythmics, it is used to treat some arrhythmias. It shortens the refractory period of atrial and ventricular tissues while prolonging the refractory period and diminishing conduction velocity in the Purkinje fibers. Toxic doses of digoxin can result in ventricular arrhythmias.

Adverse Reactions

Because of their narrow therapeutic index, antiarrhythmic agents are difficult to manage. Therefore they are only used in patients with arrhythmias that prevent the proper functioning of the heart.

Dental Implications

The dental implications of the antiarrhythmic agents are summarized in Table 15-2.

ANTIANGINAL DRUGS

Angina Pectoris

> Angina: insufficient oxygen for body's demand

Angina pectoris is a common cardiovascular disease characterized by pain or discomfort in the chest radiating to the left arm and shoulder. Pain can also be reported radiating to the neck, back, and lower jaw. The lower jaw pain can be of such intensity that it may be confused with a toothache. Angina occurs when the coronary arteries do not supply a sufficient amount of oxygen to the myocardium for its current work. Anginal pain can be precipitated by the stress (increased workload on the heart) induced by physical exercise or emotional states such as the anxiety and apprehension generated by a dental appointment.

At one time, the nitroglycerin (NTG)-like compounds (Table 15-3) were the only class of drugs that could effectively relieve the symptoms of angina. More recently, the β-adrenergic blocking agents and the calcium channel blocking drugs have added a new dimension to drug therapy for angina.

The basic pharmacologic effect of drugs used to manage angina is reduction of the workload of the heart by decreasing the cardiac output, the peripheral vascular resistance, or both. The oxygen requirement of the myocardium is in turn reduced, which relieves the painful symptoms of angina. It is important, however, to keep in mind that these drugs are not curative, and the dental team should be alert to the fact that an anginal episode could occur at any time. Appropriate emergency procedures to manage an acute anginal attack should be reviewed before treating a patient with angina (see Chapter 23). Table 15-3 lists the major antianginal drugs and some of their more pertinent characteristics.

Nitroglycerin-Like Compounds

Nitroglycerin (nye-troe-GLI-ser-in) (NTG) is by far the most often used nitrate for the management of acute anginal episodes.

TABLE 15-3   ANTIANGINAL PREPARATIONS

Drugs	Route(s)	Onset (min)	Duration (min)
Acute Attacks			
Nitrates			
Amyl nitrite	Inhalation	0.5	3-5
Short-Acting Nitrates			
Nitroglycerin (NTG, Nitrostat) (Nitrolingual)	Sublingual	1-3	30-60
	Oral spray		30-60
Isosorbide dinitrate	Sublingual	1-2	180-300
Prophylactic Use			
Long-Acting Nitrates			
Nitroglycerin (Nitro-Bid)	Sustained-release oral tablets	20-45	3-8
(Nitro-Bid)	Ointment	30-60	2-12
(Nitro-Dur, Minitran)	Transdermal patches	30-60	to 24
Isosorbide dinitrate (Isordil, Sorbitrate-DSC)	Oral	20-40	4-6
Isosorbide mononitrate (Imdur, Ismo, Monoket)	Oral	30-60	6-8
Pentaerythritol tetranitrate (Peritrate)	Oral	30	to 12
β-Blockers*			
Propranolol	Oral	30	6-8
CCBs*			
Verapamil (Calan, Isoptin)	Oral	30	6-8
Nifedipine (Procardia)	Oral, sublingual	20	3-6

CCBs, Calcium channel blockers.
*For a more complete listing, see Box 15-4.

In addition to the long-acting nitrates, NTG is also used to prevent anginal attacks induced by stress or exercise. Box 15-3 provides guidelines for managing the patient taking NTG-like agents.

◆ MECHANISM

Releases nitric oxide (NO): vasodilator

NTG is a vasodilator. It releases free nitrite ion and nitric oxide (NO). NO, an even more potent vasodilator than nitrite, activates guanylyl cyclase and increases cyclic guanosine monophosphate (cGMP), producing relaxation of vascular smooth muscle throughout the body. Indirectly, there is a reduction in work of the heart produced by the effect on both the venous and the arterial sides of the circulation. The venous dilation reduces the amount of blood returning to the heart (preload) and thereby reduces the heart's workload. The arterial dilation reduces the resistance against which the heart must pump (afterload). By reducing workload on the heart, NTG decreases the oxygen demand with relief or reduction of angina pain (Figure 15-3). Tolerance to these effects occurs, unless a nitrate-free period is observed daily.

Amyl nitrite is the only NTG-like agent that is not a nitrate; it is a nitrite. It is a volatile agent in a closed container. It is administered by crushing the container and inhaling the volatile fumes in an emergency situation (similar to the aromatic ammonia spirit inhalant ampules sniffed when one faints). Because amyl nitrite has no advantage over sublingual

BOX 15-3   MANAGEMENT OF THE DENTAL PATIENT TAKING NITROGLYCERIN-LIKE AGENTS
Ensure availability before appointment begins.
Be seated before use.
Provide analgesic if headache occurs.
Watch for syncope, especially with rising.
Premedicate with anxiolytic or nitroglycerin (NTG).
Proper storage in dental office; avoid heat and moisture.
Watch expiration date.
Prepare office staff for an acute anginal attack.
Ensure that the patient has not taken a phosphodiesterase inhibitor within 24 hours of administering NTG.

(SL) NTG and it has unapproved recreational uses, it is not often used.

SL NTG is used to treat acute anginal attacks. It has a rapid onset (few minutes) by this route, and its effect can last up to 30 minutes. It is available as an SL tablet (Nitrostat) or spray used sublingually (Nitrolingual). SL isosorbide dinitrate is also effective for an acute anginal attack. The dental office emergency kit should contain one of these products to manage acute anginal attacks. Dental patients with a history of angina should be asked to bring their NTG to each dental appointment.

♦ ADVERSE REACTIONS

Most adverse reactions associated with NTG occur because of its effect on vascular smooth muscle. Severe headaches are often reported (vasodilation) after the use of NTG. Flushing, hypotension, lightheadedness, and syncope (fainting) can also result. Hypotension is enhanced by alcohol and hot weather. SL NTG can produce a localized burning or tingling at the site of administration. The presence of stinging is not indicative of the potency of the NTG.

♦ SIGNIFICANT DRUG INTERACTIONS AND CONTRAINDICATIONS

Phosphodiesterase 5 (PDE5) inhibitors are a class of drug used to treat erectile dysfunction. These drugs include sildenafil (Viagra), vardenafil (Levitra), and tadalafil (Cialis). The administration of any of these drugs with either daily or intermittent

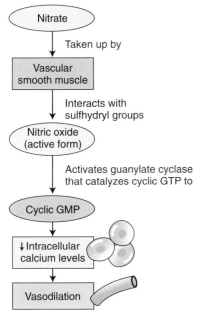

FIGURE 15-3
Pharmacologic action of nitrates. (From McKenry L, Tessier E, Hogman MA: *Mosby's pharmacology in nursing*, ed 22, St Louis, 2006, Mosby.)

doses of any nitrate is contraindicated. The combination of PDE5 inhibitors with any type of nitrate can cause dangerously low blood pressure.

♦ STORAGE

NTG is degraded by heat and moisture but not by light. NTG should be stored in its original brown glass container and tightly closed because it can be adsorbed by plastic. It should not be refrigerated because condensation of the moisture in the air produces moisture that can reduce its effectiveness.

If the original bottle is unopened, NTG is active until the expiration date printed on the bottle (assume average storage conditions). When the bottle is opened, the date opened should be written on the outside of the bottle. It should be discarded after 3 months or based on the expiration date printed on the bottle (whichever date is the earliest). The NTG spray is effective until its expiration date is reached because air does not enter the container with use.

Various long-acting NTG-like products (see Table 15-3), such as isosorbide dinitrate (eye-soe-SOR-bide dye-NYE-trate) and isosorbide mononitrate, are available for the long-term prophylaxis of anginal attacks. The dose forms available include tablets (swallowed) and topical (ointment and patch) products. With long-term, regular use, tolerance to this effect develops. In fact, no difference can be detected between a long-acting nitrate and placebo when taken without a daily "vacation." To prevent tolerance, prophylactic nitrates should be given with at least an 8- to 12-hour "vacation" every day (often during sleeping, depending on symptom pattern). The mononitrate dose form requires a 7-hour "vacation" daily; the first dose is given in the morning and the second dose is given 7 hours later.

Calcium Channel Blocking Agents

Another group of drugs approved for use in angina pectoris is the calcium channel blockers (CCBs) (see discussion in the section on hypertension). A few examples are verapamil (ver-AP-a-mil) (Calan, Isoptin), diltiazem (dil-TYE-a-zem) (Cardizem), and nifedipine (nye-FED-i-peen) (Procardia, Adalat) (Table 15-4).

> Vasodilation decreases the work of the heart.

The mechanism of action of CCBs for the treatment of angina pectoris is related to the inhibition of movement of calcium during the contraction of cardiac and vascular smooth muscle. Vasodilation and a decrease in peripheral resistance

Subgroups	Example	Mechanism	% AR	Comments
Diphenylalkylamines	Verapamil (only)	Least selective; affects both cardiac and vascular smooth muscle, vasodilator; direct effect on the myocardium (SA and AV nodes)	10	Inhibits P-450 enzymes
Benzothiazepines	Diltiazem (only)	Less selective; affects both cardiac and vascular smooth muscle, vasodilator; direct effect on myocardium (depresses SA and AV nodes); less negative inotropic effect and better side effect profile than verapamil	2	Inhibits P-450 enzymes
Dihydropyridines	Nifedipine and all others	Selective for vascular smooth muscle myocardium primarily vasodilation; reflex tachycardia	20	

TABLE 15-4 CALCIUM CHANNEL BLOCKER SUBGROUPS

AR, Autoregulation; *AV*, atrioventricular; *SA*, sinoatrial.

result, thereby decreasing the work of the heart. Some CCBs decrease myocardial contractility (negative inotropic effect), resulting in reduced cardiac output. Others increase coronary vasodilation. The choice of the specific CCB depends on the patient's cardiac disease.

In addition to their use in angina, these drugs are used in the treatment of cardiac arrhythmias and hypertension. Adverse effects include dizziness, weakness, constipation, and hypotension. Nifedipine has been associated with gingival enlargement and dysgeusia (altered sense of taste). The gingival enlargement is similar to that produced by phenytoin. Dental patients receiving these drugs should be given additional oral hygiene instructions, and frequent dental appointments should be planned.

β-Adrenergic Blocking Agents

β-Adrenergic blocking drugs such as propranolol (proe-PRAN-oh-lole) (Inderal), metoprolol (me-TOE-proe-lole) (Lopressor), and atenolol (a-TEN-oh-lole) (Tenormin), are used in the treatment of angina pectoris. These drugs block the β response to catecholamine stimulation, thereby reducing both the chronotropic and inotropic effects. The net result is a reduced myocardial oxygen demand. β-Adrenergic blockers are effective in reducing both exercise- and stress-induced anginal episodes. Adverse effects include bradycardia, HF, headache, dry mouth, blurred vision, and unpleasant dreams. β-Adrenergic blocking drugs are discussed in the section on hypertension and in Chapter 4 in the section on sympathetic blockers.

Ranolazine

In January 2006 the FDA announced the approval of ranolazine (Ranexa) for the treatment of chronic angina. In 2008 the FDA further approved the use of ranolazine for the treatment of chronic angina either alone or in combination with β-blockers, CCBs, and nitrates. It is a new molecular entity and is the first drug to be approved to treat chronic angina in more than 10 years. Although it has several pharmacologic activities, its exact mechanism of action is unknown. It does not significantly alter heart rate or blood pressure. It does prolong the QT interval, and caution should be used when it is used in combination with other drugs that increase the QT interval. Two major clinical trials found ranolazine to be more effective than placebo in treating chronic angina. In both studies, however, ranolazine appeared to be less effective in women than in men.

Dental Implications

♦ TREATMENT OF AN ACUTE ANGINAL ATTACK

The dental team should be prepared to treat an acute anginal attack before treating the patient with a history of angina. Before administering NTG the dental team should make sure that the patient has not used a PDE5 inhibitor within the past 24 hours. If the patient has used one of these drugs, then NTG cannot be given. The best course of action is to immediately contact 911. The patient's personal NTG tablets or spray should be available and placed on the bracket table in case of an acute attack. Long-acting nitrates and topical products are not useful for the treatment of an acute anginal attack. For acute emergencies, the dental office should have a supply of SL NTG (see discussion of storage). The patient should be in the seated position before ingesting the NTG. One tablet can be administered at once, followed in 5 minutes by another, and in another 5 minutes by

a third tablet. If these tablets do not stop the anginal attack, the patient should be taken to the emergency room. If using the spray, one should make sure that the patient does not inhale while spraying.

♦ PREVENTION OF ANGINAL ATTACK

Two methods to prevent an acute attack of angina include pretreatment with either an anxiolytic agent (e.g., benzodiazepine or nitrous oxide [N_2O]) or SL NTG. One should make sure that the patient has not used a PDE5 inhibitor within the past 24 hours. If he or she has, then SL NTG cannot be used as prophylaxis for an acute attack.

Anxiolytics. Because anxiety produces stress and causes the heart to work harder, an antianxiety agent, or anxiolytic (benzodiazepine), may be prescribed to allay anxiety and prevent an acute anginal attack. N_2O-oxygen (N_2O-O_2) can also relax an anxious dental patient, and N_2O itself produces vasodilation.

Nitroglycerin. Premedicating an anxious dental patient with SL NTG before an anxiety-provoking procedure can reduce the chance of an attack. For example, the patient can be given SL NTG a few minutes before a local anesthetic injection.

Because of NTG's instability, it must be properly stored in the dental office. One should check the expiration date on the office supply regularly.

♦ MYOCARDIAL INFARCTION

A patient with symptoms of an anginal attack that is not relieved by three doses of SL NTG (0.04 mg) may be experiencing an MI. If the patient who has not been previously diagnosed as having angina experiences chest pain, he or she should be taken to an emergency room for diagnosis. Occasionally, an anginal attack can proceed to an acute MI. For this reason, the dental team should make sure any patient with an attack that is not relieved by NTG is accompanied by an employee to the hospital emergency room.

ANTIHYPERTENSIVE AGENTS

> The silent killer: hypertension

Hypertension is the most common cardiovascular disease, affecting some 50 million Americans (28.6%) and 1 billion individuals worldwide. The most recent National Health and Nutrition Examinations Survey (NHANES) for 1999-2002 reported that the prevalence of hypertension increases with age and is higher among women than men (29% versus 27.8%). The age-adjusted prevalence of hypertension was 40.5% among non-Hispanic blacks, 27.4% in non-Hispanics, and 25.1% for Mexican Americans. Data from the recent Framingham Heart Study suggested that individuals with normal blood pressure at the age of 55 have a 90% lifetime risk for developing hypertension. Statistically, it is likely that many dental patients will be suffering from hypertension.

In 2003, the Seventh Report of the Joint National Committee on Prevention, Detection, Evaluation, and Treatment of High Blood Pressure (JNC 7) presented a new set of clear and concise guidelines that simplified the classification of blood pressure that was based on many new hypertension observational studies and clinical trials. Normal blood pressure is defined as a systolic pressure of less than 120 mm Hg and a diastolic pressure of less than 80 mm Hg. A new category designated prehypertension (120 to 139 mm Hg or 80 to 89 mm Hg) has been added, and people in the range of 130/80 to 139/89 mm Hg are at twice the risk of developing hypertension compared with those with lower values. Stages 2 and 3 were combined to form a new stage 2. Newer information suggests that even the blood pressure within the formerly "normal" blood pressure range is associated with an increase in morbidity and mortality. Most commonly, there are no symptoms associated with hypertension, which is why hypertension is called the "silent killer." Often, the use of the term *hypertension* gives patients the impression that it is related to stress or "tension." Patients need to be aware that high blood pressure occurs without regard to stress or tension. Complications of hypertension affect organs such as the heart, kidney, brain, and retina. After some damage has occurred, symptoms of malfunction become noticeable.

Eventually, a sustained elevated blood pressure damages the body's organs, so untreated hypertensive patients are more likely to have kidney and heart disease and cardiovascular problems (MI, CVA). These complications are greatly increased with concomitant smoking.

Fortunately, early detection and treatment with drug therapy (Box 15-4) reduces the possibility of damage to vital organs (reduced morbidity) and extends the patient's lifetime (reduced mortality). Only about 50% of those with known hypertension are properly treated. If hypertensive patients are properly treated (blood pressure is normalized), their risk of complications is equal to that of the patient without hypertension.

Hypertension is generally divided into the following categories based on the cause or progression of the disease:

* *Essential hypertension:* Approximately 85% to 90% of patients diagnosed with hypertension have essential, idiopathic, or primary hypertension. These terms all stand for hypertension from an unknown cause. Antihypertensive agents are used to control the hypertension in this group of patients. Essential hypertension is divided into stages, depending on the severity of the elevation of the blood pressure (Table 15-5). This is the form usually seen in the dental office.
* *Secondary hypertension (identifiable causes):* In approximately 10% of hypertensive patients, the cause can be identified and associated with (secondary to) a specific disease process involving the endocrine or renal systems. For example, renal hypertension can result from a narrowed renal artery. Drug therapy, such as steroids, nonsteroidal antiinflammatory drugs (NSAIDs), birth control pills, decongestants, and tricyclic antidepressants, can also produce secondary hypertension. Secondary hypertension can be eliminated by removing the cause, that is, by surgically correcting the renal artery narrowing or discontinuing the offending drug.
* *Malignant hypertension:* In the third group of hypertensive patients, those with malignant hypertension, blood pressures are very high or rapidly rising and there is usually evidence of retinal and renal damage. The small number of patients in this group must be treated aggressively with antihypertensive agents. Malignant hypertension can develop in about 5% of patients with primary or secondary hypertension.

Patient Evaluation

The evaluation of patients with hypertension has three objectives. They are to assess lifestyle and identify other cardiovascular risk factors or concomitant disorders that may affect prognosis and treatment, to reveal identifiable causes of hypertension, and to assess for the presence or absence of target-organ damage or cardiovascular disease.

Treatment of Hypertension

Pharmacologic management of hypertension involves the algorithm in Figure 15-4, as diastolic pressures become greater than 80 mm Hg. The principle of hypertension treatment is to treat blood pressures less than 140/90 mm Hg or less than 130/80 mm Hg in patients with diabetes or chronic kidney disease:

* *Lifestyle modifications* are the mainstay of prehypertension therapy and instituted for both stage 1 and stage 2 hypertension. Lifestyle modifications are encouraged even if the patient's blood pressure is normal. Lifestyle modifications include weight reduction; aerobic physical activity; a diet rich in fruits, vegetables, and low-fat dairy products with reduced content of saturated and total fats; dietary sodium restriction; moderate alcohol consumption; and smoking cessation. If patients with prehypertension present with compelling indications, these indications must be treated.
* *Initial drug choices:* Once the patient has been diagnosed with either stage 1 or stage 2 hypertension, he or she must be further evaluated for any compelling indications (Table 15-6). The choice of antihypertensive therapy is based on the stage of hypertension and the presence or absence of compelling indications (see Table 15-6 and Figure 15-4). Many people will require two drugs to control the blood pressure. By combining agents, the side effects of individual agents are less and the high blood pressure can be normalized. If compelling indications are present, the compelling indications must be treated and other antihypertensive drugs can be added as needed. Thiazide diuretics have been the basis of most antihypertensive clinical trials and have been virtually unsurpassed in preventing the cardiovascular complications of hypertension. Diuretics also enhance the antihypertensive efficacy of multidrug regimens, are useful in achieving blood pressure control, and are more affordable than other antihypertensive drugs.

Table 15-7 lists some common antihypertensive agents and their mechanisms of action and side effects, while Figure 15-5 reviews sites and mechanisms of action. The groups recommended for initial use include diuretics, β-blockers, ACEIs, CCBs, and ARBs (Box 15-5). Antihypertensive products may contain one drug or be combinations of more than one drug (see Box 15-4). If the patient is not at blood pressure goal, current drug dosages can be optimized or additional drugs can be added until goal pressure is achieved.

The control of blood pressure is an interplay of many factors, and treatment of hypertension is directed at some of the forces that alter blood pressure. The cardiac output and peripheral resistance determine blood pressure. Other changes that affect blood pressure produce changes in these two factors. Because the SNS can affect peripheral resistance, agents that block the SNS reduce blood pressure through their effect on peripheral resistance. Mechanisms of action of the antihypertensive agents attempt to lower blood pressure by their action on either cardiac output or total peripheral resistance.

Regardless of medication use, the blood pressure of each hypertensive patient seen in the dental office should be measured and recorded. Only by recording successive blood pressures for an individual patient can the patient's blood pressure control be

BOX 15-4   ANTIHYPERTENSIVE AGENTS

Diuretics
Thiazide
Chlorothiazide (Diuril)
Hydrochlorothiazide (HCTZ, Esidrix)

Thiazide-Like
Chlorthalidone (Hygroton)
Indapamide (Lozol)
Metolazone (Zaroxolyn, Mykrox)

Loop
Bumetanide (Bumex)
Furosemide (Lasix)
Torsemide (Demadex)

Potassium-Sparing
Amiloride (Midamor)
Spironolactone (Aldactone)
Triamterene (Dyrenium)
Eplerenone (Inspra)

β-Adrenergic Blockers
Atenolol (Tenormin)
Betaxolol (Kerlone)
Bisoprolol (Zebeta)
Metoprolol (Lopressor)
Metoprolol (Toprol-XL)
Nadolol (Corgard)
Propranolol (Inderal [LA])
Timolol (Blocadren)

β-Blockers with Intrinsic Sympathomimetic Activity
Acebutolol (Sectral)
Penbutolol (Levatol)
Pindolol (Visken)

β-Blockers with α-Blocking Activity
Carvedilol (Coreg)
Labetalol (Normodyne, Trandate)

Calcium Channel Blockers (CCBs)
Diltiazem (Cardizem [SR], Dilacor [XR])
Verapamil (Isoptin [SR], Calan [SR])

Dihydropyridines
Amlodipine (Norvasc)
Felodipine (Plendil)
Isradipine (DynaCirc)
Nicardipine (Cardene [SR])
Nifedipine (Procardia [XL], Adalat [CC])
Nisoldipine (Sular)

Angiotensin-Converting Enzyme Inhibitors (ACEIs)
Benazepril (Lotensin)
Captopril (Capoten)
Enalapril (Vasotec)
Fosinopril (Monopril)
Lisinopril (Zestril, Prinivil)
Moexipril (Univasc)
Perindopril (Aceon)
Quinapril (Accupril)
Ramipril (Altace)
Trandolapril (Mavik)

Angiotensin Receptor Blockers (ARBs)
Candesartan (Atacand)
Eprosartan (Teveten)
Irbesartan (Avapro)
Losartan (Cozaar)
Olmesartan (Benicar)
Telmisartan (Micardis)
Valsartan (Diovan)

α-Adrenergic Blockers
Doxazosin (Cardura)
Prazosin (Minipress)
Terazosin (Hytrin)

Central α-Adrenergic Agonists
Clonidine (Catapres [TTS])
Guanabenz (Wytensin)
Guanfacine (Tenex)
Methyldopa (Aldomet)

Peripheral Adrenergic Neuron Antagonists
Guanadrel (Hylorel)
Reserpine

Vasodilators (Direct)
Hydralazine (Apresoline)
Minoxidil (Loniten)

Selected Combinations
Thiazides + Potassium-Sparing Diuretics
Hydrochlorothiazide/spironolactone (Aldactazide)
Hydrochlorothiazide/triamterene (Dyazide, Maxzide)
Hydrochlorothiazide/amiloride (Moduretic)

β-Blockers + Diuretics
Propranolol/hydrochlorothiazide (Inderide)
Metoprolol/hydrochlorothiazide (Lopressor HCT)
Atenolol/chlorthalidone (Tenoretic)
Timolol/hydrochlorothiazide (Timolide)
Bisoprolol/hydrochlorothiazide (Ziac)

ACEIs + HCTZ
Benazepril/hydrochlorothiazide (Lotensin HCT)
Captopril/hydrochlorothiazide (Capozide)
Enalapril/hydrochlorothiazide (Vaseretic)
Lisinopril/hydrochlorothiazide (Prinzide, Zestoretic)
Moexipril/hydrochlorothiazide (Uniretic)

CCB + ACEIs
Felodipine/enalapril (Lexxel)
Amlodipine/benazepril (Lotrel)
Verapamil extended-release/trandolapril (Tarka)

evaluated and any abnormality for a particular patient noted. In addition, because control of blood pressure is so important to patient health, patients should be questioned about compliance with their antihypertensive medication. Abrupt discontinuation of some blood pressure medicines may result in rebound hypertension, which means that the blood pressure rises to a higher level than it was before treatment. Concern for patient total health is based on the fact that it is of little use for a patient to have clean and perfectly restored teeth if that patient has a fatal MI resulting from untreated hypertension.

Diuretic Agents

The three major types of diuretics are thiazides (-like), loop, and potassium (K) sparing (Figure 15-6).

TABLE 15-5   CLASSIFICATION OF BLOOD PRESSURE

Category	Systolic (mm Hg)		Diastolic (mm Hg)
Normal	<120	and	<80
Prehypertension	120-139	or	80-89
Hypertension			
Stage 1	140-159	or	90-99
Stage 2	≥160	or	≥100

◆ THIAZIDE DIURETICS

The thiazide diuretics are among the most commonly used agents for the treatment of hypertension. Hydrochlorothiazide (hye-droe-klor-oh-THYE-a-zide) (HCTZ) is the most commonly used thiazide. Many patients with stage 1 hypertension are treated solely with HCTZ. When other antihypertensive drugs are used, they are often combined with thiazides. Although a large number of thiazide and thiazide-like diuretics are currently available, these agents all have essentially the same pharmacologic effects. Even thiazide-like agents, such as chlorthalidone (klor-THAL-i-doan) (Hygroton), act by a similar mechanism by interfering with the sodium reabsorption in the distal tubule.

Mechanism of Action. The exact mechanism by which the thiazide diuretics lower blood pressure has not been determined (Table 15-8). The thiazides initially inhibit the reabsorption of sodium from the distal convoluted tubule and part of the ascending loop of Henle of the kidney. Water and chloride ions passively accompany the sodium, producing diuresis. Because more sodium is presented to the site of sodium-potassium exchange, there is also an increase in potassium excretion. If sodium intake is increased, the potassium loss is exacerbated.

The thiazides' effect on blood pressure may occur because of the following. Initially, thiazide diuretics reduce the extracellular fluid volume because of their natriuretic action. This volume

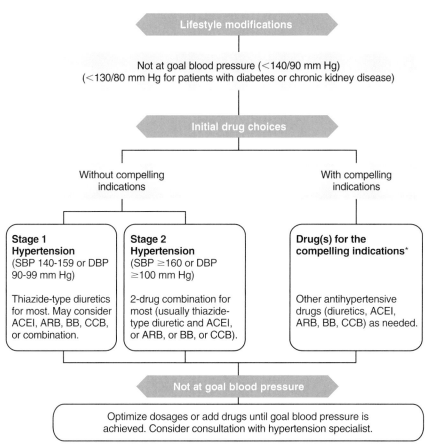

FIGURE 15-4

Algorithm for treatment of hypertension. *ACEI,* Angiotensin-converting enzyme inhibitor; *ARB,* angiotensin receptor blocker; *BB,* β-blocker; *CCB,* calcium channel blocker; *DBP,* diastolic blood pressure; *SBP,* systolic blood pressure. (From Chobanian AV, Bakris GL, Black HR, et al: Seventh Report of the Joint National Committee on Prevention, Detection, Evaluation, and Treatment of High Blood Pressure, *Hypertension* 42:1206-1252, 2003.)

* See Table 12, p. 1221, in Chobanian et al (2003) citation for additional information.

TABLE 15-6 COMPELLING INDICATIONS FOR DRUG CLASSES

Compelling Indication	ACEIs	Diuretics (Thiazide)	Angiotensin Receptor Blockers	Calcium Channel Blockers	β-Blockers	Aldosterone Antagonists
Heart failure	Y	Y	Y		Y	Y
Post-MI	Y				Y	Y
High cardiovascular risk	Y	Y		Y	Y	
Diabetes	Y	Y	Y	Y	Y	
Chronic kidney disease	Y		Y			
Recurrent stroke prevention	Y	Y				

ACEIs, Angiotensin-converting enzyme inhibitors; *MI,* myocardial infarction; *Y,* Yes.

TABLE 15-7 SELECTED ANTIHYPERTENSIVES, THEIR MECHANISMS, AND ADVERSE REACTIONS

Group	Examples	Mechanism	Important Dental Comments
Thiazides	Hydrochlorothiazide	Inhibit the reabsorption of Na in the distal convoluted tubules of the kidneys	Hypokalemia
β-Blockers	Atenolol Metoprolol	Reduce cardiac output, decreases sympathetic effect to blood vessels (blocks β stimulation), inhibits renin release	
ACEIs	Lisinopril	Block conversion of angiotensin I to II (inhibits ACEI activity)	Dry, hacking cough
Angiotensin receptor blockers	Candesartan Irbesartan	Lower blood pressure by blocking the angiotensin I receptor	Loss of taste
Calcium channel blockers	Verapamil Diltiazem Nifedipine	Inhibit calcium ion movement into the cell and lowers bp	Gingival enlargement

ACEIs, Angiotensin-converting enzyme inhibitors; *bp,* blood pressure.

FIGURE 15-5
Site and method of action of various antihypertensive drugs. (Modified from Lewis SM, Heitkemper MM, Dirksen SR: *Medical-surgical nursing: assessment and management of clinical problems,* ed 7, St Louis, 2007, Mosby.)

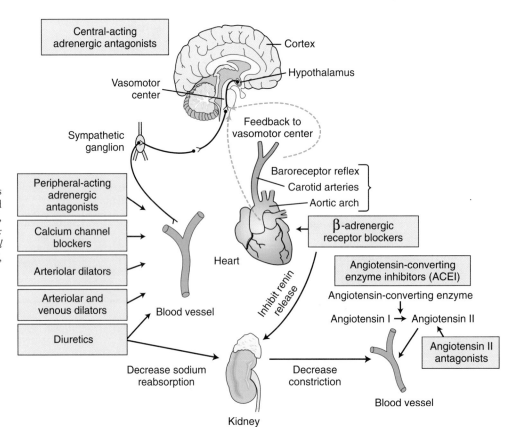

1. Diuretics
2. β-Blockers
3. Calcium channel blockers (CCBs)
4. Angiotensin-converting enzyme inhibitors (ACEIs)
5. Angiotensin receptor blockers (ARBs)

reduction returns to normal with continued therapy, but a slight decrease in interstitial volume may remain. Other effects of the thiazides that may contribute to their antihypertensive effects include changes in sodium and calcium concentrations or a reduced sensitivity to the sympathetic nervous system.

Adverse Reactions. Common adverse reactions associated with thiazides (Table 15-9) include hypokalemia (secondary to

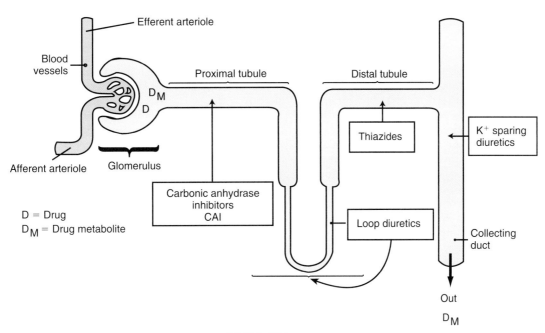

FIGURE 15-6
Location of action of diuretics.

TABLE 15-8   MECHANISM OF ACTION OF THE ANTIHYPERTENSIVE AGENTS

Group	Subgroup, Example	Mechanism	Comments	
Diuretics	Thiazide, loop	Decrease PVR	Counteract Na retention from other agents	
ANS	β-Blockers	↓CO, ↓sympathetic outflow from CNS, reduces renin release		
	α₁-Adrenergic blockers	Blocks α₁; decreases peripheral vascular resistance; relaxes arterial and venous smooth muscles	First-dose syncope; postural hypotension	
Calcium channel blockers		Vasodilators; ↓TPR		
ACEIs		Reduce PVR; decrease aldosterone secretion	Reduces rate of bradykinin (vasodilator) inactivation	
Angiotensin receptor blockers	Losartan	Vasodilation; decrease aldosterone secretion		
α₂-Adrenergic agonist, centrally acting	Clonidine α-Methyldopa	Reduces adrenergic outflow Reduces adrenergic outflow	Sedation, xerostomia	
Vasodilators	Hydralazine	Direct vasodilation, arteries, and arterioles	Headache, nausea, sweating, lupus-like syndrome	↓TPR, ↑HR and CO, use with β-blocker and diuretic
	Minoxidil	Arteriole dilation	Na/H₂O retention, reflex	

ACEIs, Angiotensin-converting enzyme inhibitors; *ANS,* autonomic nervous system; *CNS,* central nervous system; *CO,* cardiac output; *H₂O,* water; *HR,* heart rate; *NA,* sodium; *PVR,* peripheral vascular resistance; *TPR,* total peripheral resistance.

TABLE 15-9   ADVERSE REACTIONS OF THE THIAZIDES

Problem with	Adverse Reaction	Define
Potentiate arrhythmias	Hypokalemia	↓Potassium
Diabetes	Hyperglycemia	↑Glucose
Hyperlipidemia	Hyperlipidemia	↑Lipids
Gout	Hyperuricemia	↑Uric acid, ↑calcium, ↓magnesium, ↑sodium

sodium-potassium exchange) and hyperuricemia (inhibits uric acid secretion).

Hyperglycemia, hyperlipidemia, hypercalcemia (promote calcium reabsorption), and anorexia are other side effects. Hyperuricemia is of special concern when the patient has a history of gout. In the patient with diabetes, hyperglycemia, or impaired glucose tolerance, must be managed by diet or insulin alterations. There is a small chance of cross-hypersensitivity (allergy) between the sulfonamide oral medicine (antimicrobial agents) and the thiazides because of the similarity in their structures. The most common oral adverse reaction is xerostomia.

NSAIDs reduce the antihypertensive effect of HCTZ.

The most important dental drug interaction with the thiazides is inter-action with the NSAIDs. NSAIDs can reduce the antihypertensive effect of the thiazide diuretics. This interaction takes a few days to develop, and therefore a few doses of an NSAID can safely be used for acute pain control. A longer duration of use should be undertaken with blood pressure monitoring. Patients often have their own blood pressure monitoring systems at home. Patients are often taking thiazide diuretics for their blood pressure and NSAIDs for arthritis. With chronic use of both agents, their blood pressure medication is adjusted to account for the concurrent use of an NSAID.

Thiazides can cause hypokalemia and can therefore sensitize the myocardium to developing arrhythmias. The potential for arrhythmias is exacerbated in patients taking digoxin, especially if digitalis toxicity is present. Epinephrine, as contained in local anesthetic mixtures, also has arrhythmogenic potential. Therefore in a dental situation in which a patient is taking thiazide diuretics and digitalis toxicity may be present, the epinephrine dose should be limited to the cardiac dose (see Chapter 9). The thiazide diuretics potentiate the action of the other antihypertensives, increasing the potential for hypotension. This drug interaction is used to therapeutic advantage so that lower doses of each drug are needed to control the patient's blood pressure.

◆ LOOP DIURETICS

Loop diuretics can be considered the "strong cousins" of the thiazides. Furosemide (fur-OH-se-mide) (Lasix), the most commonly used loop diuretic, is the prototype drug. Furosemide acts on the ascending limb of the loop of Henle and has some effect on the distal tubule. Like thiazides, loop diuretics inhibit the reabsorption of sodium with a concurrent loss of fluids. Furosemide's side effects are similar to those of the thiazides and include hypokalemia and hyperuricemia. However, there is a higher risk of adverse reactions with furosemide because it is much more potent than the thiazide diuretics. Furosemide is used in management of hypertensive patients with HF. Loop diuretics can be used when rapid diuresis is required. As occurs with thiazides, NSAIDs can interfere with furosemide's antihypertensive action (see comments on HCTZ).

◆ POTASSIUM-SPARING DIURETICS

Potassium-sparing diuretics are "puny" diuretics with "potassium-catching" ability. Individual members of this group have different mechanisms of action, but all have weak diuretic action.

Spironolactone. Spironolactone (speer-on-oh-LAK-tone) (Aldactone) is chemically similar to aldosterone but competitively antagonizes its action (aldosterone antagonist). The result is sodium excretion through diuresis and loss of fluid volume. However, potassium ion is conserved because some of the potassium is reabsorbed at the expense of sodium in the sodium-potassium exchange system in the distal tubule.

Triamterene. Triamterene (trye-AM-ter-een) (Dyrenium), also a potassium-sparing diuretic, interferes with potassium-sodium exchange (active transport) in the distal and cortical collecting tubules and the collecting duct by inhibiting sodium-potassium-adenosine triphosphatase (Na-K$^+$-ATPase). The diuresis and potassium conservation that occurs resembles that of spironolactone.

The potassium-sparing diuretics act at different sites in the kidney than do the thiazide diuretics. These two types of diuretics have the opposite effect on potassium loss. A combination product is designed to reduce the amount of potassium loss and prevent hypokalemia. The combination of triamterene and HCTZ (Dyazide, Maxzide) is one of the most often used preparations.

◆ POTASSIUM SALTS

K$^+$: potassium

Although the potassium salts are not cardiac drugs, lack of potassium caused by the diuretics must be managed, often with potassium supplementation. Potassium is involved in many important physiologic processes such as nerve impulses; contraction of smooth, cardiac, and skeletal muscles; and maintenance of normal renal function. It is indicated in the treatment of hypokalemia produced by diuretics. It is relatively contraindicated in patients with severe renal impairment or those receiving potassium-sparing diuretics (a few exceptions to this statement exist). The most common adverse reaction of potassium relates to the gastrointestinal tract and includes nausea and abdominal discomfort caused by gastrointestinal irritation. Patients taking potassium supplements should be questioned about their use of diuretics, and the possibility of cardiovascular disease should be explored when a drug history is taken. ACEIs should not be given to persons taking potassium supplements because hyperkalemia occurs with ACEIs. Examples of potassium supplements are K-Dur, K-Tab, Micro-K, K-Lyte, K-Lor, and Klor-Con (K, the element symbol for potassium, is used in their names).

β-Adrenergic Blocking Agents

β-Adrenergic blockers, one group of adrenergic blocking agents, are used often to treat hypertension.

The adrenergic β-receptors are subtyped into β$_1$- and β$_2$-receptors (there also may be a β$_3$-receptor). They have been shown in clinical trials to decrease both the morbidity and mortality related to hypertension.

β_1-Receptor stimulation is associated with an increase in heart rate, cardiac contractility, and AV conduction. Stimulation of β_2-receptors produces vasodilation in skeletal muscles and bronchodilation in the pulmonary tissues. These receptors are initially described in Chapter 4, which discusses the autonomic nervous system drugs.

Many β-adrenergic blocking drugs are approved for use in the management of hypertension (see Box 15-4). Nonselective or nonspecific β-adrenergic receptor blocking drugs, such as propranolol (proe-PRAN-oh-lole), the prototype, block both β_1- and β_2-receptors. In usual doses, the selective, or specific, β-adrenergic receptor blocking drugs, such as metoprolol (me-toe-PROE-lole), block the β_1-receptors more than the β_2-receptors ($\beta_1 > \beta_2$). At larger doses, receptor selectivity disappears. Pindolol (PIN-doe-lole) and acebutolol (a-se-BYOO-toe-lole) have partial agonist activity and cause some β-stimulation while blocking catecholamine action. The selective β-blockers ($\beta_1 > \beta_2$) have some advantages in patients who may have preexisting bronchospastic disease, such as asthma, because they do not block the airway's bronchodilating action (not as likely to result in bronchoconstriction). They are less likely to produce a drug interaction with epinephrine.

β-Adrenergic blockers lower blood pressure primarily by decreasing cardiac output. Other effects that may contribute to their antihypertensive effect include a lowering of plasma renin levels, a reduction in plasma volume and venous return, a decrease in sympathetic outflow from the central nervous system (CNS), and a reduction in peripheral resistance. These drugs are often used as step 2 drugs, either as a single drug or in combination with other antihypertensive drugs.

Suffix: -olol

The side effects of the β-blocking agents include bradycardia, mental depression, and decreased sexual ability. HF and CNS effects, such as confusion, hallucinations, dizziness, and fatigue, have been reported. Gastrointestinal tract effects include diarrhea, nausea, and vomiting. β-Blockers can produce xerostomia (very mild) or worsen a patient's lipid profile. Exacerbations of asthma, angina, and peripheral vascular disease have been seen.

◆ DENTAL DRUG INTERACTIONS

Nonselective β-blockers can have a drug interaction with epinephrine. Patients pretreated with a nonspecific β-blocker, such as propranolol, and given epinephrine may have a twofold to fourfold increase in vasopressor response (blood pressure goes up more in patients pretreated with β-blockers than in untreated patients), resulting in hypertension. The increased blood pressure triggers, via the vagus nerve, a reflex bradycardia.

The amount of caution required with this drug interaction depends on the patient's underlying cardiovascular disease, if any increase in blood pressure, and the dose of the β-blocker the patient is taking. In patients with cardiovascular disease or higher blood pressure, the amount of epinephrine given to patients taking nonspecific β-blockers should be limited to the cardiac dose unless careful blood pressure monitoring accompanies the use of larger doses. Neither gingival retraction cord containing epinephrine nor 1:50,000 epinephrine should be used. Usual dental doses of epinephrine can be given to patients who are taking β-blockers provided that their blood pressure is under control. Box 15-4 separates the β-blockers into those without intrinsic sympathetic activity and those with intrinsic sympathetic intrinsic activity.

◆ α- AND β-ADRENERGIC BLOCKING DRUG

Labetalol (la-BET-a-lole) (Trandate, Normodyne) is a β-adrenergic receptor blocking drug that also has α-receptor blocking activity. In addition to the typical β-adrenoceptor blocking effects, labetalol also reduces peripheral resistance through its α-blocking action. Labetalol is used either alone or in combination with the diuretics. Side effects and drug interactions are similar to the α- and β-adrenergic blockers.

Calcium Channel Blocking Agents

Suffix: -dipine

The common CCBs include the drugs verapamil (ver-AP-a-mil) (Isoptin, Calan), nifedipine (nye-fed-i-peen) (Procardia, Adalat), and diltiazem (dil-TYE-a-zem) (Cardizem). Many CCBs (see Box 15-4) end in the suffix -dipine. These agents are used to treat hypertension and other cardiac conditions such as arrhythmias and angina.

◆ MECHANISM

CCBs inhibit the movement of extracellular calcium ions into cells, including those of the vascular smooth muscle and cardiac cells. The inhibition of calcium ion influx produces vasodilation, which produces coronary vasodilation and reverses vasospasms. By producing systemic vasodilation, the CCBs reduce the afterload on the heart (reduce the total peripheral resistance). These effects are useful in the treatment of both angina pectoris and hypertension.

Today, only long-acting CCBs are used. The short-acting channel blockers were associated with a higher risk of MIs and fatalities, when take at higher doses. This may have been a result of the short-acting CCBs' ability to suddenly and powerfully lower blood pressure. The heart would overcompensate for this sudden drop by dramatically increasing blood pressure. Long-acting CCBs have a gradual onset of action, which may allow time for the heart to adjust to the drop in blood pressure.

◆ PHARMACOLOGIC EFFECTS

Smooth Muscle Effects. Vascular smooth muscle is relaxed, and dilation of coronary and peripheral arteries and arterioles occur, reducing preload. Other smooth muscle is relaxed but to a lesser extent. Orthostatic hypotension is uncommon. Some CCBs, such as nifedipine and its relatives, are more specific for this effect.

Cardiac Muscle Effects. The effect of the CCBs on the heart may reduce its rate, decrease myocardial contractility (negative inotropic effect), and slow AV nodal conduction. Less specific CCBs have some of both effects.

◆ ADVERSE REACTIONS

Most side effects associated with the CCBs are merely extensions of their pharmacologic effects.

Central Nervous System Effects. CCBs can produce excessive hypotension, which can cause dizziness and lightheadedness. Dental patients should be warned to rise from the dental chair slowly. Headache can occur in up to 10% to 20% of patients taking CCBs.

Gastrointestinal Effects. Gastrointestinal side effects include nausea, vomiting, and constipation. Individual CCBs differ in the incidence of these various side effects.

Cardiovascular Effects. Because CCBs have a depressant effect on the heart, bradycardia and edema can result. Flushing as a result of vasodilation should not be confused with an allergic or adverse reaction. Peripheral edema has been reported.

Other Effects. Shortness of breath as a result of pulmonary edema has been reported. Nasal congestion and rhinitis may interfere with the administration of N_2O-O_2 for analgesia and anxiety relief.

♦ ORAL MANIFESTATIONS

Gingival enlargement

The oral manifestations of the CCBs include xerostomia, dysgeusia, and gingival enlargement (formerly called *gingival hyperplasia*). Gingival enlargement has been reported most often with nifedipine, but diltiazem, verapamil, and other CCBs have been implicated.

Nifedipine's manufacturer originally reported the incidence of gingival enlargement as less than 0.5%. Manufacturers of both diltiazem and verapamil have mentioned gingival enlargement as an infrequently reported postmarketing event. Other studies have found the incidence for nifedipine to be 15% to 80%, depending on the criteria used. In one study, diltiazem's incidence was determined to be 74%. These greatly varying rates of gingival enlargement may be the result of vastly differing criteria used in the studies (e.g., self-report by patients without prompting versus measuring gum changes in all patients). Studies with the highest rates evaluated the incidence of gingival enlargement versus a control group, prospectively.

The gingival enlargement can begin one to several months after starting therapy with a CCB. Some authors have found no relationship between the dose of the drug and the likelihood of a reaction occurring, whereas others indicate that higher doses produce more severe reactions. Like phenytoin enlargement, nifedipine enlargement begins as nodular and firm tissue that bleeds easily on probing. The enlargement begins in the anterior labial dental papillae and can proceed eventually to include the lingual and palatal gingiva. The hyperplastic interdental papillae can eventually extend onto crown surfaces, interfering with the ability to chew.

Detailed oral hygiene instructions and more frequent recall appointments to reduce plaque load have been said to reduce this enlargement, but no well-controlled studies have confirmed this suspicion. The patient may be told to maintain scrupulous oral hygiene until more information is available.

On discontinuation of the CCB or switching to a drug outside the CCB group, the gingival enlargement usually reverts to normal tissue and does not reappear. This may take weeks to months. If drug therapy cannot be discontinued because of the severity of the patient's cardiac condition, a gingivectomy or gingivoplasty may be required. Changing to another CCB does not appear to result in reversal of the enlargement.

♦ DENTAL DRUG INTERACTIONS

The CCBs are one of the few antihypertensive groups whose effect is not reduced by the NSAIDs. Both nausea and constipation, side effects of the CCBs, could be additive with the side effects produced by NSAIDs (e.g., ibuprofen) (nausea) and the opioids (e.g., codeine) (constipation).

Angiotensin-Related Agents

♦ ANGIOTENSIN-CONVERTING ENZYME INHIBITORS

Suffix: -pril

ACEIs prevent the conversion of angiotensin I to angiotensin II. ACEI drugs are commonly used as antihypertensives. Examples include captopril (KAP-toe-pril) (Capoten), enalapril (e-NAL-a-pril) (Vasotec), and lisinopril (lyse-IN-oh-pril) (Prinivil, Zestril). Many ACEIs (see Box 15-4) end in the suffix *-pril*.

Mechanism. A complex but important homeostatic mechanism involved in maintaining blood pressure is the renin-angiotensin-aldosterone system. This system adjusts the quantity of sodium and water retained (circulatory volume) and the peripheral resistance (blood vessels). When the kidney senses a decrease in blood pressure or flow, it releases renin, which catalyzes the conversion of angiotensinogen (inactive precursor) to angiotensin I. A second enzyme, ACE, converts angiotensin I to angiotensin II. This is the enzyme that is blocked by ACEIs (Figure 15-7). Angiotensin II produces vasoconstriction (increasing peripheral vascular resistance) and stimulates the adrenal cortex to release aldosterone, facilitating water retention. By blocking these events, the blood pressure is lowered. Cardiac output and heart rate are relatively unaffected. ACEIs retard the progression of diabetic nephropathy whether hypertension is present or not.

Adverse Reactions. The two most common kinds of adverse reactions associated with the ACEIs are those related to the cardiovascular system and CNS (Box 15-6).

Cardiovascular Effects. Hypotension has produced dizziness, lightheadedness, and fainting. Tachycardia and chest pain have been noted.

Central Nervous System Effects. CNS side effects may include dizziness, insomnia, fatigue, and headache.

Gastrointestinal Effects. Nausea, vomiting, and diarrhea can occur.

Respiratory Effects. An increase in upper respiratory symptoms, including a dry, hacking cough can occur. ACEIs can produce a dry cough, in up to 10% of patients, and this cough can occur within the first week of therapy and disappears after withdrawal of the drug. The cough begins as a tickle in the throat, leading to a dry, nonproductive, and persistent cough that may be worse at night or in the supine position. It occurs because the ACE also inactivates bradykinin, a potent stimulator of allergic reactions, including cough. The blood levels of bradykinin rise because the ACEIs are blocking the enzyme that normally destroys bradykinin.

Hyperkalemia. ACEIs can cause hyperkalemia, and potassium supplements and potassium-sparing diuretics should not be used with these drugs.

Allergic-Like Reactions. Allergic-like reactions including the following:
- Angioedema: Swelling of the extremities, face, lips, mucous membranes, tongue, glottis, or larynx can occur, especially after the initial dose. If airway obstruction is severe, it can impair breathing or swallowing and could be fatal.
- Rash

Other Effects: ACEIs should not be given to women who could be pregnant or become pregnant because of the risk of teratogenicity. Rarely, pancreatitis, with symptoms of abdominal pain, and abdominal distention have occurred. Proteinuria is more common in patients taking higher doses or who have renal impairment.

Oral Adverse Reactions. Dysgeusia, an altered sense of taste, is most commonly reported in patients taking captopril (6%). The loss of taste is usually reversible after a few months, even with continued drug treatment.

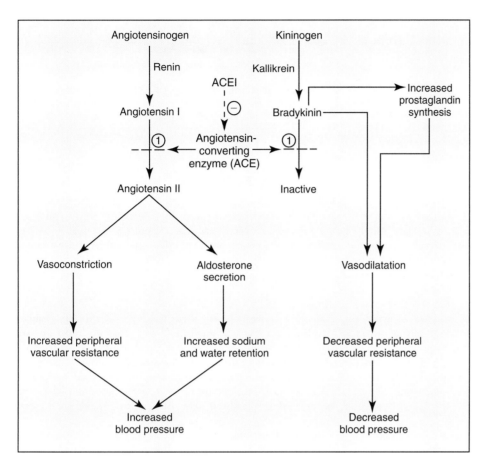

FIGURE 15-7
Site of action of angiotensin-converting enzyme (ACE) inhibitors (ACEIs).

| BOX 15-6 | ADVERSE REACTIONS OF ANGIOTENSIN-CONVERTING ENZYME INHIBITORS |

Hypotension
Allergic reactions
Neutropenia
Dry cough
Diabetic neuropathy

Autoimmune oral lesions, such as lichenoid or pemphigoid reactions, may produce oral manifestations. This reaction may have a photosensitivity factor.

Dental Drug Interactions. The antihypertensive effectiveness of ACEIs is reduced by administration of the NSAIDs. A few doses of an NSAID are of little concern, but chronic administration for several days might result in an increase in the patient's blood pressure. The ACEIs may be used alone or in combination with a β-blocker, thiazide diuretic, or CCB. These drugs are commonly prescribed, and the dental team will treat many patients taking one or more of these agents.

◆ ANGIOTENSIN RECEPTOR BLOCKERS

The ARBs act by attaching to the angiotensin II receptor and blocking the effect of angiotensin II. ARBs end with the suffix *–artan.* Losartan (loe-SAR-tan) (Cozaar), is the prototype. Losartan has a high affinity and selectivity for the type 1 angiotensin II receptor. It blocks the vasoconstrictor and aldosterone-secreting effects of angiotensin II. An increase in plasma renin level follows, thus causing vasodilation, decreased sodium and water retention, and reduction in blood pressure.

Adverse Reactions. Because ARBs work by blocking angiotensin II at its receptor, they are more specific than ACEIs and may be expected to have fewer adverse reactions.

Central Nervous System Effects. CNS effects can include dizziness, fatigue, insomnia, and headache.

Upper Respiratory Infections. Upper respiratory infections occur more often in patients taking losartan. A dry cough and nasal congestion can also occur.

Gastrointestinal Effects. Losartan can produce diarrhea.

Pain. Both muscle cramps and leg and back pain have been reported with losartan.

Angioedema. Rarely, angioedema can occur.

Teratogenicity. Fetal and neonatal morbidity and mortality can occur if losartan is administered to a pregnant woman.

Dental Drug Interactions. NSAIDs may antagonize the antihypertensive effect of losartan by inhibiting renal prostaglandin synthesis or by causing sodium and fluid retention.

Renin Inhibitors

Aliskiren (Tekturna) is the first of a new class of drugs approved by the FDA for the treatment of hypertension. It is indicated for oral use as either monotherapy or in combination with other antihypertensive drugs. Aliskiren is a renin inhibitor that works by binding to renin which then reduces the levels of angiotensin I, angiotensin I, and aldosterone. Unlike ACEIs and ARBs, aliskiren does not appear to increase plasma renin activity. The most commonly reported adverse reactions include headache, dizziness, fatigue, cough, and upper respiratory tract infections. There have been reports of angioedema of the head and neck and hypotension.

α_1-Adrenergic Blocking Agents

The adrenergic blockers include the α-blockers and β-blockers, which were discussed earlier. Two α-receptor subtypes, α_1 and α_2, have been identified (see Box 15-4). Doxazosin (doks-AYE-zoe-sin) (Cardura) and terazosin (ter-AY-zoe-sin) (Hytrin) are examples of selective α_1-adrenergic blocking drugs.

♦ MECHANISM

The α_1-receptors, located on postsynaptic receptor tissues, produce vasoconstriction and increase peripheral resistance when stimulated. The α_1-blocking agents produce peripheral vasodilation in the arterioles and venules that decreases peripheral vascular resistance. They have little effect on cardiac output or renal blood flow. They are more effective when combined with diuretics or β-blockers.

α_1-Adrenergic blockers result in a reduction in urethral resistance and pressure, bladder outlet resistance, and urinary symptoms. This effect accounts for their use in management of older males who have an enlarged prostate gland. Surgery can often be avoided in those patients who are managed by drug therapy. If a man has both hypertension and benign prostatic hypertrophy (BPH), then one can "kill two birds with one stone."

♦ ADVERSE REACTIONS

Orthostatic Hypotension. Orthostatic hypotension can result in dizziness or syncope. A "first-dose orthostatic hypotensive reaction" sometimes occurs with the initial dose or with changes in the dose of doxazosin. Syncope is more likely to occur when the patient is volume depleted or sodium restricted. Both exercise and alcohol may exaggerate the effect.

Central Nervous System Effects. α_1-Adrenergic blockers can cause CNS depression, producing either drowsiness or excitation and headache. Caution should be exercised when doing anything requiring alertness until the patient's response can be evaluated.

Cardiovascular Effects. Tachycardia, arrhythmias, and palpitations can occur. Peripheral edema is another side effect related to the cardiovascular system.

♦ DENTAL DRUG INTERACTIONS

Nonsteroidal Antiinflammatory Drugs. NSAIDs, especially indomethacin, can reduce the antihypertensive effect of the α_1-blockers (Box 15-7). They produce this effect by inhibiting renal prostaglandin synthesis or causing sodium and fluid retention.

Epinephrine. The sympathomimetics can increase the antihypertensive effects of doxazosin. The α_1-blockers prevent the α_1-agonist effects (vasoconstriction) of epinephrine, leaving the β_1- and β_2-agonist effects (vasodilation) to predominate. The combined vasodilation can result in severe hypotension and reflex tachycardia.

♦ USES

In addition to being indicated for the treatment of hypertension, both doxazosin and terazosin are indicated for the management of BPH. Difficulty in urination is reduced by taking these agents.

BOX 15-7 MANAGEMENT OF DENTAL PATIENTS TAKING α_1-BLOCKING AGENTS

Orthostatic hypotension dizziness, lightheadedness, or syncope
Drowsiness or nervousness
Nonsteroidal antiinflammatory drugs (NSAIDs) interfere with the antihypertensive effect of α_1-blockers
Epinephrine (sympathomimetics): do not use to treat hypotension

---

Other Antihypertensive Agents

These other antihypertensive agents are used less than those previously described because they generally have more or less tolerated adverse reactions. Clonidine is used in some patients in whom the previously discussed antihypertensives are ineffective.

♦ CLONIDINE

Clonidine (KLON-i-deen) (Catapres) is a CNS-mediated (centrally acting) antihypertensive drug. Clonidine reduces peripheral resistance through a CNS-mediated action on the α-receptor. Stimulation of presynaptic central α_2-adrenergic receptors results in decreased sympathetic outflow. Thus clonidine reduces heart rate, cardiac output, and total peripheral resistance. It is indicated for the management of essential hypertension and can be administered orally or by a transdermal patch (Catapres-TTS).

Adverse Reactions. Adverse effects include a high incidence of sedation and dizziness. Rapid elevation of blood pressure has occurred with abrupt discontinuation. CNS depressants used in dental conscious-sedation techniques may contribute to postural hypotension when used in a patient taking clonidine.

Oral Effects. The oral effects of clonidine include a high incidence of xerostomia (40%), parotid gland swelling, and pain. Another side effect is dysgeusia (unpleasant taste), whose mechanism is unknown but may be related to xerostomia.

♦ OTHER CENTRALLY ACTING ANTIHYPERTENSIVE AGENTS

Two other centrally acting antihypertensive drugs, methyldopa (meth-ill-DOE-pa) (Aldomet) and guanabenz (GWAHN-a-benz) (Wytensin), are also available. Adverse effects and indications for use are similar to those of clonidine. The centrally acting antihypertensive drugs may be combined with diuretics in essential hypertension management.

♦ GUANETHIDINE

Guanethidine's (gwahn-ETH-i-deen) (Ismelin) severe adverse reactions severely limit its use. It acts by blocking the release of norepinephrine from the sympathetic nerve endings. It also depletes the amount of norepinephrine stored in synaptic vesicles. Both actions decrease the amount of norepinephrine that can be released with sympathetic stimulation, thereby reducing SNS tone and decreasing blood pressure (see Figure 15-5). Guanethidine has a delayed onset of action, and its effects can persist for at least 2 weeks after it is discontinued.

Guanethidine causes severe postural and exertional hypotension, which is exacerbated by anything that causes vasodilation, such as warm weather, ingestion of alcohol, or exercise. Hypotension is most severe after the patient has spent several hours in a supine position, such as in the dental chair. Other adverse reactions include diarrhea, interference with ejaculation, and cardiac problems. Muscle weakness has also been reported.

◆ RESERPINE

Originally used as a tranquilizer, reserpine (re-SER-peen) is currently used in low doses as an antihypertensive agent. Like guanethidine, reserpine depletes norepinephrine from the sympathetic nerve endings and can accumulate in the body. Adverse reactions include diarrhea, bad dreams, sedation, and even psychic depression leading to suicide. Reserpine increases the production of stomach acid and aggravates peptic ulcers. It can also produce galactorrhea, breast engorgement, and gynecomastia.

◆ HYDRALAZINE

Hydralazine (hye-DRAL-a-zeen) (Apresoline) exerts its antihypertensive effect by acting directly on the arterioles to reduce peripheral resistance (vasodilation). At the same time, a rise in heart rate and output occurs. Propranolol is often administered concurrently to reduce the reflex tachycardia and increase cardiac output. Hydralazine is often used in combination with the thiazides or other antihypertensive agents. Both diastolic and systolic blood pressures are reduced proportionately, and there is little orthostatic hypotension. The most commonly reported side effects associated with hydralazine are cardiac arrhythmias, angina, headache, and dizziness. A serious toxic reaction produces symptoms like those of systemic lupus erythematosus (lupus-like reaction).

Management of the Dental Patient Taking Antihypertensive Agents

Although the antihypertensive drugs cause a variety of adverse reactions, many of them exert similar actions that can alter dental treatment (Box 15-8). Because the hypertension of patients taking antihypertensive medications may or may not be controlled, the blood pressure of each patient should be measured on each visit to the dental office. Not uncommonly, a patient whose blood pressure is "normal" on one visit might be found to be hypotensive or hypertensive on a subsequent visit.

◆ ADVERSE REACTIONS

Xerostomia. Dry mouth is an adverse reaction associated with several of the antihypertensives. If the dental health care worker notices this effect, it is imperative to discuss with the patient methods used to alleviate this discomfort.

Dysgeusia. With some antihypertensives, an altered sense of taste may occur, which may be related to xerostomia.

Gingival Enlargement. CCBs have the ability to produce gingival enlargement. Meticulous oral hygiene and frequent recall appointments may minimize this effect.

Orthostatic Hypotension. When a patient has been in a supine position and suddenly rises to an upright position, a sudden fall in blood pressure may occur. This side effect is called *orthostatic hypotension.* Patients taking antihypertensive agents who have been supine for some time should be slowly raised from that position. They should dangle their legs over the side of the chair or bed and wiggle them before rising to the standing position. The patient should be supported for a few steps to prevent syncope. Guanethidine causes this problem often; other agents produce variable amounts of orthostatic hypotension.

Constipation. Some antihypertensive agents (verapamil) can cause constipation, which could be additive with the constipation produced by the opioids. An increase in dietary fiber, a bulk laxative, or a stool softener may be considered if an opioid is prescribed for a patient receiving a constipation-producing antihypertensive medication.

Central Nervous System Sedation. Several antihypertensives (β-blockers, methyldopa) can produce sedation, which is additive with other CNS depressants such as opioids or benzodiazepines.

ANTIHYPERLIPIDEMIC AGENTS

| LDL: bad cholesterol |
| HDL: good cholesterol |

Hyperlipidemia and hyperlipoproteinemia are elevations of plasma lipid concentrations above accepted normal values. These metabolic disorders include elevations in cholesterol and/or triglycerides and are associated with the development of arteriosclerosis, although the exact correlation is unknown. There are many different types of hyperlipoproteinemias that result in elevations of chylomicrons, very-low-density lipoproteins (VLDLs), low-density lipoproteins (LDLs), or combinations of these.

Foam cells in the actual blood vessel, which are more prevalent in uncontrolled diabetes, become filled with cholesterol esters. Accumulation of these esters leads to deposition of lipids in the arteries. Collagen and fibrin also accumulate, occluding the vessels. Atherosclerosis can lead to coronary artery disease, MI, and cerebral arterial disease. The endothelium over the plaques activates platelets, leading to the formation of thrombi and clinical symptoms. Additional risk factors for development of complications include untreated hypertension, smoking, obesity, and alcohol use.

Cholesterol and other plasma lipids are transported in the blood in the form of protein complexes (lipoproteins) to make them more soluble in plasma. LDLs are referred to as "bad cholesterol" because they deposit excess cholesterol in artery walls and are considered to be the most dangerous. High-density lipoproteins (HDLs) are referred to as "good cholesterol" because they have the lowest cholesterol content and are considered to be beneficial (they carry cholesterol away from the blood vessels).

The first line of treatment of hyperlipoproteinemia is increasing exercise and decreasing saturated fat and cholesterol from the diet. Depending on the severity of the condition and the

---

BOX 15-8   MANAGEMENT OF THE DENTAL PATIENT TAKING ANTIHYPERTENSIVES

Check for xerostomia and its management.
If taking a calcium channel blocker (CCB), check for gingival enlargement.
Check blood pressure before each appointment.
Avoid dental agents that add to side effects, such as opioids (sedation and constipation).
If on diuretics, check for symptoms of hypokalemia, which may exacerbate arrhythmias from epinephrine.
If taking an angiotensin-converting enzyme inhibitor (ACEI), check for symptoms of neutropenia.

TABLE 15-10 EFFECT OF ANTIHYPERLIPIDEMIC AGENTS ON SERUM LIPIDS					
Type of Agent	Chol	TGD	VLDL	LDL	HDL
HMG Co-A Reductase Inhibitors ("Statins")					
Atorvastatin (Lipitor)	—	—	—	—	+
Fluvastatin (Lescol)	—	—	—	—	+
Lovastatin (Mevacor)	—	—	—	—	+
Pravastatin (Pravachol)	—	—	—	—	+
Simvastatin (Zocor)	—	—	—	—	+
Bile Acid Sequestrants					
Cholestyramine (Questran, Prevalite)	—	±	±	—	±
Colestipol (Colestid)	—	±	±	—	±
Miscellaneous					
Clofibrate (Atromid-S)	—	—	—	=,—	±
Ezetimibe (Zetia)	—	—	—	—	=
Ezetimibe/simvastatin (Vytorin)	—	—	—	—	+
Nicotinic acid (Niacin)	—	—	—	—	+
Fibrates					
Fenofibrate (Lipidil-DSC, TriCor)	—	—	—	=,—	+
Gemfibrozil (Lopid)	—	—	—	=,—	+

Chol, Cholesterol; *HDL,* high-density lipoproteins; *HMG Co-A,* 3-hydroxy-3-methylglutaryl coenzyme A; *LDL,* low-density lipoproteins; *TGD,* triglycerides; *VLDL,* very-low-density lipoproteins.

success of the patient in making permanent lifestyle changes, drug therapy may be considered.

Therapy of hyperlipoproteinemia is directed at lowering the level of LDL-cholesterol (LDL-C). Drugs are available that reduce hyperlipoproteinemias: some more specific for cholesterol and some more specific for the triglycerides. Antihyperlipidemic drugs include the bile acid–binding resins, niacin, gemfibrozil, and 3-hydroxy-3-methylglutaryl coenzyme A (HMG Co-A) reductase inhibitors (Table 15-10). The HMG Co-A reductase inhibitors are the most commonly used antihyperlipidemics.

3-Hydroxy-3-Methylglutaryl Coenzyme A Reductase Inhibitors

Suffix: -statins

The HMG Co-A reductase inhibitors are often referred to as the "statins" because their generic names end in that suffix. Their side effect profile is more desirable than any of the other drugs used to treat hyperlipidemias. However, their use is contraindicated in women who are pregnant or nursing. They have a Pregnancy Risk Factor of X.

Lovastatin (LOE-va-sta-tin) (Mevacor) was the first of the statins. The statins lower cholesterol levels by inhibiting HMG-CoA reductase, the rate-limiting enzyme in cholesterol synthesis. They may work because they are structural analogs of HMG Co-A reductase and thereby inhibit that enzyme. Another possible mechanism of the HMG Co-A reductase inhibitors may relate to the increase in the number of LDL receptors that occurs. The effectiveness of the HMG Co-A reductase inhibitors should be monitored by a lipid panel repeated once or twice a year.

◆ ADVERSE EFFECTS

Adverse effects of HMG Co-A reductase inhibitors include gastrointestinal complaints such as stomachache, constipation, diarrhea, and gas. Other side effects are myositis, skin rash, impotence, hepatotoxicity, blurred vision, and lens (in the eye) opacities. Myositis results in complaints of muscle pain. Liver function tests should be performed because of the small potential for hepatotoxicity. These agents can increase the anticoagulant effect of warfarin.

◆ INHIBITORS OF INTESTINAL ABSORPTION OF CHOLESTEROL

Ezetimibe (Zetia) was most recently approved to treat elevated cholesterol levels and low HDL-cholesterol (HDL-C) levels. This drug works by inhibiting the intestinal absorption of cholesterol. This drug can be used alone or in combination with an HMG-CoA reductase inhibitor. It currently comes in combination with simvastatin (HMG-CoA reductase inhibitor) to treat cholesterol from two different mechanisms of action. This drug decreases total cholesterol, LDL-C, and increases HDL-C levels. Side effects include fatigue, abdominal pain, and diarrhea.

Most recently, the ENHANCE trial has shown that there is little difference in the cholesterol lowering abilities of Vytorin (ezetimibe/simvastatin) and simvastatin alone. Vytorin was found to lower LDL-C, but it had little effect on plaque buildup in the arteries. The researchers went on to recommend that

Vytorin and Zetia should only be used if a person fails to achieve adequate cholesterol control with a statin or cannot tolerate the adverse reactions of statins.

Niacin

♦ OVERVIEW

Niacin (NYE-a-sin) (nicotinic acid) is a B vitamin (see Chapter 12). In larger doses, niacin produces a therapeutic effect. It lowers cholesterol levels by inhibiting the secretion of VLDLs without accumulation of triglycerides in the liver. This reduces LDL synthesis. At these larger doses, niacin commonly produces cutaneous flushing (especially the face and neck) and a sensation of warmth after each dose. The prostaglandin-mediated flushing is blocked by pretreatment with 0.3 gm of aspirin taken one-half hour before taking niacin or by taking one tablet of ibuprofen daily. This side effect can be minimized by beginning with low doses of niacin and slowly increasing the dose over a period of weeks. Increasing the dose of niacin enough to produce a decrease in lipids without having intolerable adverse effects is challenging. Hyperuricemia can occur and can be treated with allopurinol. Allergic reactions, cholestasis, and hepatotoxicity have been reported.

♦ DENTAL IMPLICATIONS

Hypotension may occur as a result of the vasodilation, especially in patients taking antihypertensives. Rising from the dental chair should be attempted slowly to prevent orthostatic hypotension.

Cholestyramine

The bile acid–binding resins, cholestyramine (koe-less-TIR-a-meen) (Questran) and colestipol (koe-LES-ti-pole) (Colestid), lower cholesterol concentrations because cholesterol is a precursor that is required for the synthesis of the new bile acids. When the resins bind with the bile acids, they produce an insoluble product that is lost through the gastrointestinal tract. The bile acids, which must be replaced, use up cholesterol, thereby reducing cholesterol levels. Adverse reactions relate to the gastrointestinal tract and include constipation and bloating, but serious side effects are infrequent. These drugs are poorly tolerated because of their effects on the gastrointestinal tract and poor taste. Patients often abandon their use.

Gemfibrozil

Gemfibrozil (gem-FI-broe-zil) (Lopid) is used to treat hyperlipidemias, especially when triglycerides are elevated. It works by increasing lipolysis of triglycerides, decreasing lipolysis in adipose tissue, and inhibiting secretion of VLDLs from the liver. This drug causes fewer gastrointestinal complaints than the bile acid–binding drugs, but it can promote gallstone formation (cholelithiasis). An altered sense of taste and hyperglycemia have been reported. Hematologic and liver function should be monitored routinely. This drug should not be given with statins because of the increased risk for muscle cramping, myopathy, and rhabdomyolysis.

Dental Implications

> Take blood pressure (BP) and heart rate (HR) at each appointment.

Patients who take antihyperlipidemic agents are at a higher risk for developing hypertension and coronary artery disease. These patients are at increased risk for MIs and cardiac arrest. Dental health care workers should be prepared to handle such emergencies. The patient's blood pressure and pulse rate should be taken before each appointment and recorded in the dental chart. If an emergency occurs, it is important to know the pre-emergency blood pressure and heart rate so that these can be compared with the current measurements. Because gastrointestinal and liver abnormalities are side effects associated with many of these drugs, their tolerance to the agents taken should be determined before dental drugs are prescribed or suggested. The small possibility of liver abnormalities requires laboratory testing for abnormal liver function.

DRUGS THAT AFFECT BLOOD COAGULATION

Anticoagulants

Anticoagulants are drugs that in some way interfere with coagulation. The first anticoagulant was discovered when cows that ingested spoiled sweet clover silage became hemorrhagic. The toxic agent in the clover was found to be dicumarol, and warfarin is a close relative. Warfarin has been used as a rodenticide. When the rats eat the warfarin, they begin to bleed and eventually die. Therapeutically, anticoagulants are administered in an attempt to prevent clotting. Examples of indications for warfarin are after an MI, thrombophlebitis, or to prevent a stroke. Warfarin (Coumadin) is the most important oral anticoagulant and is the one used almost exclusively in therapy.

♦ HEMOSTASIS

Hemostasis is a normal mechanism in the body that is designed to prevent the loss of blood after injury to a blood vessel. The leaking vessel is plugged by a complicated process of clot formation. In the presence of a vascular injury, the entire clotting mechanism is initiated. Thromboplastin; factors V, VII, and X; and calcium ions form prothrombin, thrombin, and finally fibrinogen and fibrin (Figure 15-8). The fibrin, along with

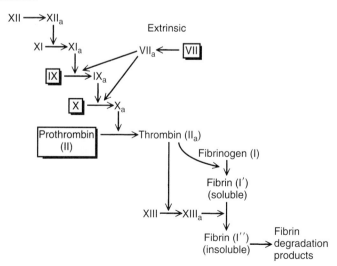

FIGURE 15-8

Intrinsic and extrinsic systems of blood coagulation. The boxed clotting factors (II [prothrombin], VII [extrinsic], IX [intrinsic], and X) depend on vitamin K for their synthesis. Warfarin inhibits these four clotting factors.

vascular spasms, platelets, and red blood cells, quickly forms the clot.

If the blood vessel's interior remains smooth, circulating blood does not clot. However, if internal injury to the vessel occurs and a roughened surface develops, intravascular clotting will take place. This process involves an intrinsic prothrombin activator that includes a platelet factor, factor V, factors VIII through XII, and calcium ions. The prothrombin activator, which was formerly called *thromboplastin,* converts prothrombin to thrombin. Thrombin then converts fibrinogen to fibrin, and clot formation occurs.

Many of the factors required in the clotting process are synthesized in the liver. Prothrombin (II) and factors VII, IX, and X require vitamin K for synthesis. Because warfarin antagonizes vitamin K, it interferes with the synthesis of four clotting factors to produce an anticoagulant effect.

In certain diseases, intravascular clots can form. These clots, or thrombi, may break off, forming emboli that lodge in the smaller vessels of major organs, such as the heart, brain, and lungs, producing severe and even fatal thromboembolic disease. Anticoagulant therapy attempts to reduce intravascular clotting and prevent life-threatening situations. Each person's anticoagulant therapy must be adjusted to suit his or her needs. If the dose of the anticoagulant is too large, hemorrhage may occur. If the dose is too small, the danger of embolism remains.

♦ WARFARIN

Warfarin (WAR-far-in) (Coumadin) is an oral anticoagulant (interferes with coagulation). It blocks γ-carboxylation of glutamate residues in the synthesis of factors VII, IX, and X; prothrombin (II); and endogenous anticoagulant protein C. Instead of forming the factors, incomplete and inactive molecules are formed that do not function properly. Warfarin also prevents the metabolism of the inactive vitamin K epoxide back to its active form.

Warfarin's pharmacologic effect is delayed when therapy begins and ends. This latent period in the onset of action of warfarin occurs for the following two reasons:

1. The blood level of the warfarin accumulates over time until it plateaus or reaches steady state. The maximum effect for one dose occurs after five half-lives = 5 = 42 hours = 210 hours (9 days).
2. Endogenous clotting factors II, VII, IX, and X have half-lives that are 60, 6, 24, and 40 hours, respectively. They must become depleted before the anticoagulant effect is maximized.

When reducing the dose of warfarin or discontinuing it, there will be a delay in the change in the effect because the drug must be metabolized to inactivate it and the clotting factors must be synthesized again.

Monitoring. Warfarin's effect is monitored using the international normalized ratio (INR). The INR is a function of the prothrombin time (PT) of the patient, PT of control, and the international sensitivity index (ISI). The ISI is a number that is a function of the potency of the specific (human or rabbit) thromboplastin used in the particular laboratory. The advantage of the INR over the PT ratio is that the INR value from any laboratory in the world can be compared, whereas the PT ratio varies among laboratories. The formula for the INR is seen in Figure 15-9.

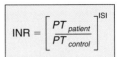

$$INR = \left[\frac{PT_{patient}}{PT_{control}} \right]^{ISI}$$

FIGURE 15-9
The formula for the international normalized ratio (INR).

TABLE 15-11 DRUG INTERACTIONS BETWEEN NONSTEROIDAL ANTIINFLAMMATORY AGENTS AND WARFARIN

Severity	Drug Examples
Major	Aspirin
Moderate	Indomethacin
	Meclofenamate
	Piroxicam
	Sulindac
Minor	Diclofenac
	Fenoprofen
	Ibuprofen
	Naproxen
	Acetaminophen (small)
None	Nonacetylated salicylates

The therapeutic target INR (number at which the provider is trying to keep the patient's INR) for most indications, such as thrombophlebitis or AF, is between 2 and 3. For patients with a prosthetic heart valve, the target INR is between 2.5 and 3.5. The INR can range from 1 (INR without drug effect) to 4, although with overdose it can reach higher levels.

In the past, the laboratory test that was used to monitor warfarin was the PT ratio. The prothrombin time ratio (PT$_r$) is the ratio of the PT$_{patient}$/PT$_{control}$. Some laboratories are still reporting the PT$_r$. PT$_r$ ranges from 1 (PT$_r$ without drug) to 2.5 or higher. The target numbers for the PT$_r$ and the INR are not interchangeable.

Because warfarin is orally effective and less expensive than heparin, it is used in long-term treatment of thromboembolic diseases such as thrombophlebitis and MI.

Adverse Reactions. The most common adverse effects associated with the oral anticoagulants are various forms of bleeding, including hemorrhage. Because of its narrow therapeutic index and because of numerous drug interactions, serious reactions can easily occur. One should look for petechial hemorrhages in the oral cavity. Ecchymoses can occur, even without concomitant trauma. With mild trauma, these effects may be seen in the oral cavity. Studies compared effects of lower and higher doses of warfarin in clot prevention. They found no advantage in use of higher doses but found an increase in adverse reactions. Dosing of warfarin is now titrated to a lower INR than in the past.

Aspirin. The most serious drug interaction of warfarin is with aspirin (Table 15-11). Patients taking warfarin should not be given aspirin or aspirin-containing products ("cold preparations") because bleeding episodes or fatal hemorrhages can result. Aspirin interacts with warfarin in several ways. First, aspirin causes hypoprothrombinemia and alters platelet adhesiveness (see Chapter 5). These effects in themselves reduce clotting ability. Aspirin can also irritate the gastrointestinal tract, which might bleed more in a patient taking warfarin.

Another factor in the aspirin-warfarin interaction is related to protein binding of drugs. Warfarin is more than 99% bound to plasma proteins and about 1% free drug. Only the free drug (<1%) exerts the pharmacologic effect of decreased clotting. Because warfarin and aspirin compete for the same plasma protein–binding site, aspirin displaces the bound warfarin, thereby increasing the proportion of free (unbound) warfarin and hence potentiating its activity. Only the free drug in the blood exerts a pharmacologic effect. The bound drug is merely a reservoir for the drug. Even a small increase in free warfarin can lead to a large increase in effect, leading to dire consequences, including hemorrhage. If an NSAID is to be used in a patient taking warfarin, ibuprofen or naproxen should be prescribed. These agents have only a minor interaction with warfarin, and a few doses can be given in the patient with an INR within the therapeutic target.

Acetaminophen. Acetaminophen and its effect on warfarin were prospectively analyzed. Hylek and colleagues studied patients taking warfarin in an attempt to identify factors that were associated with an INR above 6 (therapeutic INR = 2 to 3.5). A statistically significant association was found between acetaminophen use and the abnormal elevation of the INR. With higher doses of acetaminophen (9 gm/wk) there was a tenfold increase in the likelihood of presenting with an abnormal INR. Whether there is a causal relationship between acetaminophen use and warfarin, toxicity has not been proved. Managing patients taking warfarin who need analgesics may require more frequent monitoring of the INR, especially with intermittent use.

Antibiotics. Antibiotics can also potentiate the effect of warfarin. Antibiotics reduce the bacterial flora in the gastrointestinal tract that normally synthesize vitamin K. This results in a decrease in vitamin K absorbed. Because warfarin also inhibits vitamin K–dependent factors, there is an added anticoagulant effect. If an antibiotic is to be used with warfarin (Table 15-12), clindamycin has no effect; doxycycline, tetracycline, and amoxicillin have small effect; and erythromycin and metronidazole have the greatest effect on altering warfarin's anticoagulant action. If the antibiotic is used for prophylaxis before a dental procedure (one dose), the interaction would not have a chance to develop.

Induction of the microsomal enzymes increases warfarin's metabolism and reduces its effect. Phenobarbital induces the liver microsomal enzymes that would normally destroy the anticoagulant. Alcohol's effect on warfarin depends on the pattern of alcohol use. With chronic alcohol ingestion, the metabolism of warfarin is stimulated. Acute alcohol intoxication inhibits the metabolism of warfarin. Other agents that inhibit the metabolism of warfarin include cimetidine, disulfiram, and metronidazole.

Management of the Dental Patient Taking Warfarin. Box 15-9 summarizes the management of dental patients taking warfarin.

> Most dental procedures require no change in dose of warfarin.

Bleeding. Before any dental procedure is begun, the patient should be interviewed to determine whether any symptoms relating to bleeding have been noted. Many surgical procedures can be carried out on a patient receiving therapeutic doses of anticoagulants (Table 15-13). One should check with the prescribing physician to obtain the patient's INR or PT, and the date the blood for the test was drawn. A higher INR can be tolerated if local measures are added. When a decision is made to change the dose of warfarin, the risk of lowering the dose of warfarin must be weighed against the benefit of lowering the dose of warfarin (Box 15-10). Discontinuing warfarin for a few days without knowledge of the patient's INR could expose the patient to an increased risk of clotting. If the patient does not need the anticoagulant, then it can be permanently discontinued. If the patient needs anticoagulation, then the risk of intravascular clotting in these patients should not be underestimated.

Analgesics. Aspirin and aspirin-containing products are absolutely contraindicated in patients taking warfarin unless the patient is taking one aspirin tablet daily for its anticoagulant effect. In this case, the monitoring of warfarin effect is done while the patient is taking aspirin. Acetaminophen or any opioid alone or together may be substituted if analgesia is desired. A few doses of ibuprofen or naproxen may be safely used if there is no other contraindication to their use.

◆ HEPARIN

Heparin (HEP-a-rin) is one of the most commonly used anticoagulant agents in hospitalized patients. Because it must be given by injection and cannot be used orally, its outpatient use is essentially nonexistent. Newer heparins, termed *low-molecular-weight heparins,* are being used, but until an oral dose form is developed, use of these heparins will be limited. Because its effect begins quickly, heparin is the first anticoagulant given to hospitalized patients with excessive clotting. Patients who

TABLE 15-12	**WARFARIN AND ANTIINFECTIVE DRUG INTERACTIONS**	
Most	Some	Least
Metronidazole	Tetracycline	Clindamycin
Erythromycin	Doxycycline	
Ketoconazole (-azole antifungals)	Penicillin, ampicillin, amoxicillin, dicloxacillin	
Cephalosporins	Quinolones	

BOX 15-9 MANAGEMENT OF THE DENTAL PATIENT TAKING WARFARIN (COUMADIN)

Obtain prothrombin time (PT) or international normalized ratio (INR) and history to establish bleeding potential.
For PT or INR greater than two times normal, request reduction in dose.
Because of latent time to onset and recovery, allow several days for change in effect if dose of warfarin changed.
Check with physician regarding resuming dose.
Avoid aspirin and aspirin-containing compounds.
Acetaminophen and opioids OK.
Oral hygiene with subgingival calculus removal can produce bleeding (oozing); use local pressure.
Determine underlying disease of patient.
May have atrial fibrillation.
Patient should be free of infection before scaling/root planing.
Some suggest prophylactic antibiotics after surgery.
Check with patient regarding healing.

TABLE 15-13 SAFETY OF OUTPATIENT DENTAL TREATMENT FOR PATIENTS RECEIVING WARFARIN (COUMADIN) ANTICOAGULANT THERAPY

Dental Treatment	INTERNATIONAL NORMALIZED RATIO (INR)[a]					
	Suboptimal Range		Normal Target INR[c]		Mechanical Heart Valves[b]	Out of Range
	<1.5	1.5 to <2.0	2.0 < 2.5	2.5 to 3.0	>3.0 to 3.5	>3.5
Examinations, radiographs, study models	d					
Simple restorative dentistry, supragingival prophylaxis						e
Complex restorative dentistry, scaling and root planing, endodontics					Probably safe[f]	
Simple extraction, curettage, gingivoplasty				Local measures[g]	Local measures[g]	
Multiple extractions, removal of single bony impaction			Local measures[g]	Local measures[g]	Local measures[g]	
Gingivectomy, apicoectomy, minor periodontal flap surgery, placement of single implant	Probably safe (IR)[h]	Probably safe[f]	Probably safe[f]			
Full-mouth/full-arch extractions	Probably safe[f]	Local measures[g]				
Extension flap surgery, extraction of multiple bony impactions, multiple implant placement	Probably safe[f]					
Open-fracture reduction, orthognathic surgery						

From Hermann WW, Konzelman JL Jr, Sutley SH: Current perspectives on dental patients receiving coumarin anticoagulant therapy, *J Am Dent Assoc* 128(3):327, 1997. Copyright © 1997 American Dental Association. All rights reserved. Adapted 2009 with permission.

[a]INR is this ratio: [PT (patient)/PT (control)]^ISA.

[b]INR 2.5 to 3.5 = therapeutic range for mechanical prosthetic heart valves.

[c]INR 2 to 3 = therapeutic range for venous thrombosis, pulmonary embolism, systemic embolism (myocardial infarction, valvular, atrial fibrillation).

[d]White boxes indicate that it is safe to proceed in a routine manner (local factors, such as periodontitis or gingival inflammation, can increase the severity of bleeding; the clinician should consider all factors when making a risk assessment).

[e]Diagonal shading indicates procedure not advised at current INR level; refer to physician for adjustment.

[f]Probably safe, can perform procedure with care.

[g]Use local measures: increased need for sutures, oxidized cellulose hemostat, topical thrombin and tranexamic acid.

[h]*IR*, Insufficient research, but research data available for other similar procedures.

BOX 15-10 WARFARIN—TO CLOT OR BLEED: THAT IS THE QUESTION

Point-Counterpoint: The **risk** of clotting if the dose of warfarin is reduced must be weighed against the **benefit** of reduced oral cavity bleeding from lowering the dose of warfarin. *Perspective makes the difference.*

From the dental health care worker's perspective, the important risk is related to excessive bleeding. From the provider's viewpoint, the important risk is intravascular clotting. The international normalized ratio (INR) value and the indication for the use of warfarin will determine what would be best for the patient. Often, patients will be subtherapeutic and may have even taken the warfarin for the necessary time, but it had not been discontinued.

might receive heparin are those with MI, stroke (embolism), or thrombophlebitis. When the heparin is started (as soon as possible), warfarin is also begun. Because warfarin's effect has a latent period, the heparin can provide immediate anticoagulant effect while the warfarin is building up. The effect of an overdose of heparin is antagonized by protamine sulfate, which immediately reverses its anticoagulant effects.

◆ CLOPIDOGREL

The drug clopidogrel (Plavix) is an inhibitor of adenosine diphosphate (ADP)–induced platelet aggregation, which results in prolonged bleeding time. Clopidogrel is indicated for patients with recent history of MI or stroke, established peripheral arterial disease, and for those patients with acute coronary artery syndrome. Its major side effects include thrombotic thrombocytopenic purpura (TTP) and increased bleeding. TTP can occur within as little as 2 weeks of beginning therapy. TTP is characterized by thrombocytopenia seen on peripheral smear, neurologic findings, renal dysfunction, and fever. It does not alter PT or INR values.

Clopidogrel can be taken with or without food. Patients taking this drug should be carefully managed in the dental office because of the risk for increased bleeding. NSAIDs should be avoided because of the risk for gastrointestinal bleeding. Aspirin use should also be avoided. Patients may be taking a combination of clopidogrel and aspirin to treat acute coronary syndrome. This should only be done under a doctor's supervision. NSAID use should especially be avoided in these patients.

◆ TICLOPIDINE

The drug ticlopidine (tye-KLOE-pi-deen) (Ticlid) is an irreversible inhibitor of ADP-induced platelet aggregation, which results in prolonged bleeding time. Ticlopidine is indicated to decrease thrombotic stroke in patients with previous stroke. It is used in patients who are intolerant of aspirin. Its major side effect, neutropenia, is monitored by appropriate blood tests. An increase in infections could signal neutropenia. It does not alter the PT or INR.

Ticlopidine is taken with food because it can produce diarrhea, nausea, and vomiting. Patients taking ticlopidine have increased bleeding after trauma or surgery. It takes 10 to 14 days to eliminate the bleeding effect. Bleeding can lead to ecchymoses, epistaxis, and perioperative bleed. For emergency surgery, injectable methylprednisolone can reverse the prolonged bleeding to normal in a few hours. NSAIDs should be avoided because gastrointestinal bleeding can result. Patients taking this drug should be carefully managed in the dental office, but no laboratory tests are used to monitor ticlopidine.

◆ STREPTOKINASE AND ALTEPLASE

Enzymes, called *clot busters,* such as streptokinase (strep-toe-KYE-nase) (Streptase, Kabikinase) and the recombinant tissue-type plasminogen activator alteplase (AL-ti-plase) (tPA, Activase), are sometimes used in the therapy of deep vein thrombosis, arterial thrombosis, pulmonary embolism, and acute coronary artery thrombosis associated with MI. These may appropriately be termed *thrombolytic drugs* because they promote the conversion of plasminogen to plasmin, the natural clot-resolving enzyme. They are usually administered by direct vessel perfusion to the clot site. Considerable technical skill and immediate treatment of the thrombus is required for satisfactory results, within 3 hours of the onset of symptoms. Because streptokinase is a foreign protein, allergic reactions can occur. Hemorrhage may result from the use of any of these drugs and they are contraindicated in patients at risk for hemorrhage.

◆ DIPYRIDAMOLE

The drug dipyridamole (dye-peer-ID-a-mole) (Persantine) is used to prolong the life of platelets in patients with prosthetic heart valves. The artificial valves cause premature death of the platelets because of their mechanical effect (trauma) on the blood cells passing through the valves. Dipyridamole does not add any additional anticlotting benefit over the use of aspirin and/or warfarin. It does not affect bleeding related to dental treatment.

◆ PENTOXIFYLLINE

Pentoxifylline (pen-tox-IF-i-lin) (Trental) is a dimethylxanthine that improves blood flow by its hemorheologic effects, which include lowering blood viscosity and improving the flexibility of red blood cells. It is indicated for intermittent claudication produced by chronic occlusive artery disease of the limbs. Side effects associated with pentoxifylline include cardiovascular and gastric symptoms. Dry mouth, bad taste, excessive salivation, and swollen neck glands have infrequently been reported. Pentoxifylline does not alter blood clotting.

Drugs That Increase Blood Clotting

◆ HEMOSTATIC AGENTS (FIBRINOLYTIC INHIBITORS)

Aminocaproic acid (EACA) and its analog, tranexamic acid (Cyklokapron), are similar to the amino acid lysine, and they inhibit plasminogen activation (synthetic inhibitor of fibrinolysis).

Aminocaproic acid and tranexamic acid are used intravenously, orally, or topically. Adverse effects include intravascular thrombosis, hypotension, and abdominal discomfort. Some literature recommends the use of topical tranexamic acid before dental procedures in patients taking warfarin who are at risk of bleeding. It is indicated in the treatment of hemorrhage after dental surgery.

BIBLIOGRAPHY

Hylek EM, Heiman H, Skates SJ, et al: Acetaminophen and other risk factors for excessive warfarin anticoagulation, *JAMA* 279:657-662, 1998.

DENTAL HYGIENE CONSIDERATIONS

1. Measure the patient's blood pressure and pulse at every visit.
2. Make sure that the patient is experiencing a minimal amount of stress and maintain adequate pain control during each visit. Stress and pain can elevate blood pressure.
3. Conduct a thorough medication/health history in order to avoid drug interactions.
4. Evaluate the patient for adverse effects that may affect oral health care.
5. If a local anesthetic with a vasoconstrictor is required, make sure that the patient can receive it. If the patient can, make sure the patient receives the lowest dose possible.
6. Be careful when raising patients to the supine position. Raise the chair slowly.
7. Review Boxes 15-2, 15-3, 15-7, 15-8, and 15-9 and Table 15-2.
8. Although elevated cholesterol levels do not impact on oral health care, they often go hand in hand with high blood pressure. Always check the blood pressure and heart rate of patients with elevated cholesterol levels.
9. Antiarrhythmic medicines can cause arrhythmias. Always check the blood pressure and heart rate of patients with elevated cholesterol levels.
10. Patients with heart failure may have breathing difficulties when in the supine position. Work with the patient to find the most comfortable chair position. A semisupine position may be necessary.
11. Some medicines may cause GI adverse effects. Nonsteroidal antiinflammatory drugs should be avoided. Recommend acetaminophen for pain instead.
12. Make sure that patients with angina have brought their nitroglycerin with them. Have them place the nitroglycerin on the tray where it is easily accessed.
13. Patients taking warfarin should be monitored for INR levels.
14. Lower dose aspirin does not normally cause excess bleeding but it may take a little longer for blood to clot.
15. Anticoagulants should only be temporarily stopped prior to an appointment after the medical physician has been consulted and agrees with the decision. This should only happen if there is excessive bleeding.

CLINICAL SKILLS ASSESSMENT

1. What is angina and what are some of its causes?
2. What is the mechanism of action of nitroglycerin in treating angina and what are its adverse reactions?
3. Describe the role of nitrates in the treatment of angina.
4. Describe the interaction between nitrates and drugs used to treat erectile dysfunction.
5. What is hypertension and what is its prevalence in the United States?
6. Explain the pharmacologic effects of ACEIs for the treatment of hypertension.
7. Describe the current algorithm for treating hypertension. State the individual drug classes for treating compelling indications in patients with hypertension.
8. State the individual drug classes for treating hypertension and include pharmacologic effects, adverse effects, and any dental concerns.
9. What is the role of aspirin in anticoagulation therapy? List the other classes of anticoagulant drugs and include mechanism of action, adverse effects, and dental concerns.
10. What is the relationship between elevated cholesterol levels and heart disease?
11. Compare and contrast the classes of medication used to treat elevated cholesterol levels and include adverse effects and dental concerns.
12. Compare and contrast the classes of medication used to treat arrhythmias.
13. Compare and contrast the classes of medications used to treat HF and include adverse effects and dental concerns.

⊖volve _____

Please visit http://evolve.elsevier.com/Haveles/pharmacology for review questions and additional practice and reference materials.

16 Anticonvulsants

LEARNING OBJECTIVES

1. Define *epilepsy* and briefly summarize the various types of seizures.
2. List and describe general adverse reactions to anticonvulsants.
3. Summarize the pharmacologic effects, adverse reactions, and drug interactions of the main anticonvulsants—carbamazepine, valproate, phenobarbital, and phenytoin.
4. Name two miscellaneous anticonvulsants and describe the workings of each.
5. Provide several examples of new types of anticonvulsants, including the mechanism of action, indications, and adverse reactions of each.
6. Outline the dental treatment of patients with epilepsy.

EPILEPSY

Epilepsy comprises a group of disorders that involve a chronic stereotyped recurrent attack of involuntary behavior or experience or changes in neurologic function caused by electrical activity in the brain that can be recorded via an electroencephalogram (EEG). This activity can be localized or generalized. Each episode is termed a *seizure.* The seizure may be accompanied by motor activity, such as convulsions, or by other neurologic changes (e.g., sensory or emotional).

Because seizure disorders are estimated to affect approximately 1% of the population, the dental team is likely to encounter a patient with epilepsy. Because these anticonvulsant agents are used chronically, one must consider potential adverse reactions that might alter dental treatment.

| Idiopathic epilepsy (cause unknown) |

There are many etiologies for epilepsy, including infection, trauma, toxicity to exogenous agents, genetic or birth influences, circulatory disturbances, metabolic or nutritional alterations, neoplasms, hereditary factors, fevers, and degenerative diseases. The majority of epileptic patients have *idiopathic epilepsy;* this term is used when the cause is unknown.

Epilepsy has been classified based on causes, symptoms, duration, precipitating factors, postictal state (postseizure), and aura. Currently, The International Classification of Epileptic Seizures (Figure 16-1) divides seizures into two major groups and a miscellaneous group. The two major groups are partial and generalized seizures. Partial seizures are divided into simple and complex attacks. The most common generalized seizures are (1) tonic-clonic and (2) absence seizures (Box 16-1).

Generalized Seizures

Generalized seizures are divided into two large groups: (1) absence and (2) tonic-clonic types. Consciousness is lost in both types. Whereas little movement occurs in absence seizures, in tonic-clonic seizures, major movement of large muscle groups occurs. Management of seizures is discussed at the end of this chapter. Often, the patient may experience an aura (a brief period of heightened sensory activity) before the onset of the seizure. It may be characterized by numbness, nausea, or unusual sensitivity to light, odor, or sound.

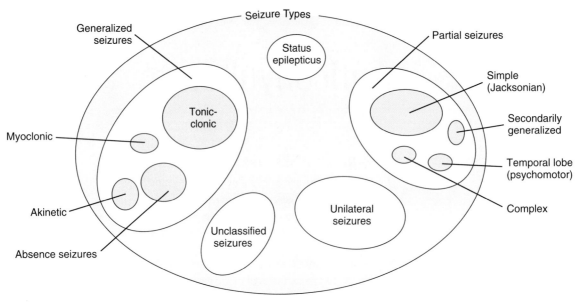

FIGURE 16-1

The International Classification of Epileptic Seizures: status epilepticus, elementary motor (Jacksonian) autonomic seizures, temporal lobe (psychomotor) seizures, secondarily generalized seizures, partial seizures, unilateral seizures, generalized seizures, tonic-clonic seizures, myoclonic seizures, akinetic seizures, and unclassified seizures. Seizure type patterns: same pattern indicates that same group of drugs are usually effective.

BOX 16-1   SEIZURE TYPES
Partial
Simple
Complex
Secondarily generalized
Psychomotor
Temporal lobe
Generalized
Tonic-clonic (grand mal)
Absence (petit mal)
Tonic
Atonic
Clonic/myoclonic

◆ ABSENCE SEIZURES (PETIT MAL)

> Absence: petit mal

The symptoms of absence (petit mal) seizures include a brief (few seconds) loss of consciousness with characteristic EEG waves and little movement. Absence seizures usually begin during childhood and disappear in middle age. The patient is usually unaware that these seizures are occurring and body tone is not lost. There is no aura or postictal state, and the patient quickly returns to normal activity. The drug of choice in the treatment of typical absence seizures is either ethosuximide, valproate, or lamotrigine (Table 16-1).

Management of absence seizures poses no problems for the dental team. The team's main concern when treating patients with absence seizures is the adverse reactions that can occur from long-term administration of the drugs used to treat the disease.

◆ TONIC-CLONIC SEIZURES

> Tonic-clonic: grand mal

The generalized tonic-clonic (grand mal) seizures include longer periods of loss of consciousness and major motor activity of the large muscles of the body. The seizure begins by the body becoming rigid and the patient falling to the floor. Urination, apnea, and a cry may be present. Tonic rigidity is followed by clonic jerking of the face, limbs, and body. The patient may bite the cheek or tongue. Finally, the patient becomes limp and comatose. Consciousness returns gradually, with postictal confusion, headache, and drowsiness. Some patients experience prodromal periods of varying durations, but a true aura does not occur. Because this seizure type involves the violent movement of major muscle groups, it is more likely to result in serious injury to the patient. Valproic acid, phenytoin, and carbamazepine are used to treat tonic-clonic seizures.

◆ STATUS EPILEPTICUS

Status epilepticus seizures are continuous tonic-clonic seizures that last longer than 30 minutes or recur before the end of the postictal period of the previous seizure. This is an emergency situation, and rapid therapy is required, especially if the seizure activity has produced hypoxia. Parenteral benzodiazepines, such as diazepam (Valium), are the drugs of choice to control this seizure type (see Chapter 11).

Partial (Focal) Epilepsies

Partial epilepsies involve activation of only part of the brain, and the location of the activity determines the clinical manifestation. When consciousness is not impaired, the attack is called an *elementary (simple) partial attack.* When consciousness is impaired, the attack is termed a *complex partial attack.* Complex seizures are also called *psychomotor* or *temporal-lobe seizures.* In contrast to absence seizures that last a few seconds, these complex

TABLE 16-1 ANTICONVULSANT DRUGS OF CHOICE

Seizure Disorder	DRUGS	
	First Choice	Alternatives
Generalized Seizures		
Tonic-clonic (grand mal)	Valproate* or phenytoin or carbamazepine	Lamotrigine† Topiramate Zonisamide‡ Oxcarbazepine‡ Levetiracetam‡ Primidone Phenobarbital
Absence (petit mal)	Ethosuximide or divalproex	Lamotrigine‡ Clonazepam Zonisamide‡ Levetiracetam‡
Atypical absence, atonic, myoclonic	Valproate* Lamotrigine†	Topiramate‡ Zonisamide‡ Clonazepam Felbamate§ Levetiracetam‡
Status epilepticus	Diazepam (Valium) IV Phenytoin (Dilantin) IV Phenobarbital (Luminal) IV	
Partial Seizures		
Simple Complex Secondarily generalized	Carbamazepine or phenytoin or lamotrigine† or oxcarbazepine	Valproate Gabapentin‖ Topiramate Tiagabine‖ Zonisamide‖ Levetiracetam‖ Primidone Phenobarbital Pregabalin‖ Felbamate

IV, Intravenous.
*Not Food and Drug Administration (FDA) approved unless absence is involved.
†FDA approved for adjunctive therapy in adults and children older than 2 years with partial seizures or with Lennox-Gastaut syndrome, and as monotherapy in adults with partial seizures as a substitute for carbamazepine, phenytoin, phenobarbital, or valproate as the single antiepileptic drug.
‡Not FDA approved for this indication.
§FDA approved as adjunctive therapy for patients with Lennox-Gastaut syndrome.
‖Only FDA approved for adjunctive therapy.

partial seizures last several minutes. Some patients with complex partial seizures have an aura, and full consciousness is slow to return. For the partial epilepsies, carbamazepine, phenytoin, phenobarbital, and primidone are used.

DRUG THERAPY OF PATIENTS WITH EPILEPSY

Dosing anticonvulsants is difficult.

Drug therapy of the patient with epilepsy has variable efficacy, from complete control of all seizures to reducing the frequency of seizures. Anticonvulsant agents may be used singly or in combination. The goal is to control seizures and

BOX 16-2 DENTAL MANAGEMENT OF PATIENTS TAKING ANTICONVULSANT AGENTS

- Review emergency management of epileptic patients (remove hands and dental instruments from mouth, turn head to side)
- Take a thorough medical and drug history including medications and frequency of seizures
- Additive CNS depression—use additional CNS depressants cautiously
- Additive gastrointestinal adverse reactions—use drugs that are gastric irritants cautiously (e.g., NSAIDs)
- Drug interactions—induction of hepatic microsomal enzymes, metabolizes certain drugs more quickly (lowers blood level and effect)
- Dental drugs affected—propoxyphene, doxycycline

CNS, Central nervous system; *NSAIDs*, nonsteroidal antiinflammatory drugs.

minimize potential adverse reactions. Some newer anticonvulsants are able to treat previously untreatable seizures, but more serious side effects can accompany them. General principles on the management of the dental patient taking any anticonvulsant agents are listed in Box 16-2.

Anticonvulsant agents are central nervous system (CNS) depressants that attempt to prevent epileptic seizures without causing excessive drowsiness. Although their exact mechanisms of action are unknown, these agents prevent the spread of abnormal electric discharges in the brain (Figure 16-2).

The anticonvulsant drug used to treat a specific patient depends on the type of seizures the patient has. Because these agents are usually taken for life, their chronic toxicity becomes an important consideration in choosing a particular anticonvulsant agent and determining the drug's dental implications.

General Adverse Reactions to Anticonvulsant Agents

Several factors make dosing with anticonvulsants more difficult than with other drugs. First, the anticonvulsants have a narrow therapeutic index, so the dose must be carefully titrated to obtain the desired blood levels. It cannot be too low or too high. Second, most anticonvulsants stimulate liver microsomal enzymes that metabolize both themselves, other anticonvulsants, and other drugs that the patient may be taking. When a second anticonvulsant is added to the first, it changes the metabolism of both anticonvulsants. The third effect, which may be even more important than the others, is that the metabolism of the anticonvulsants can saturate the liver microsomal enzymes. With low doses, the metabolism is first order and the drug is removed from the body. At some point, when the enzymes become saturated, the metabolism converts to zero-order kinetics and the drug level can increase abruptly. At the point of saturation, a small change in the dose can lead to a large increase in the blood level of the drug. The dental team must be aware of the side effects of the anticonvulsant agents that might influence dental treatment.

The anticonvulsant drugs possess a unique set of adverse reactions. Adverse reactions that the anticonvulsants have in common are discussed first.

◆ CENTRAL NERVOUS SYSTEM DEPRESSION

Depressed CNS function is a common side effect of the anticonvulsant agents. Tolerance often develops to these sedative

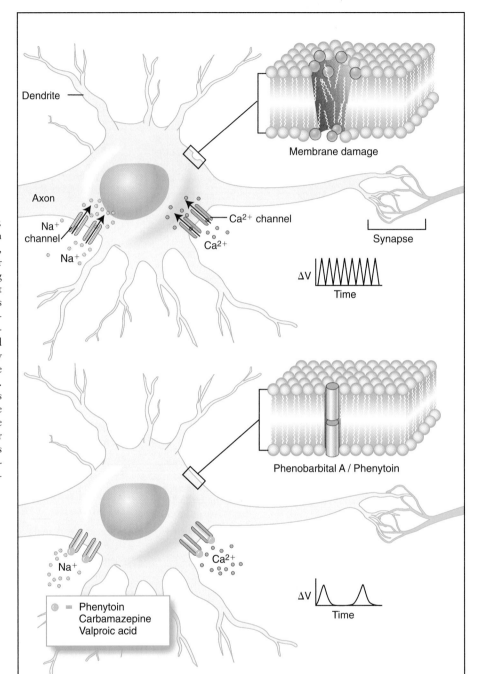

FIGURE 16-2

Effects of anticonvulsants on neurons. *Upper,* Damaged neuronal membranes, as shown in the section on the upper right of the figure, result in sodium and calcium influxes via their respective channels that cause repeated firing shown in the voltage-time curve to the right of the figure. *Lower,* Anticonvulsants, such as phenytoin (Dilantin), carbamazepine (Tegretol), and valproic acid (Depakote), represented by the small circles, block sodium and calcium channels, resulting in a substantially diminished rate of firing as shown in the voltage-time curve to the right of the figure. Both phenytoin and phenobarbital, shown as cylinders, are also thought to stabilize the damaged neuronal membrane as shown in the membrane section schematized in the upper right drawing. (From McPherson RA, Pincus MR: *Henry's clinical diagnosis and management by laboratory methods,* ed 21, Philadelphia, 2007, Saunders.)

effects while the anticonvulsant effect persists. Impaired learning and cognitive abilities occur in some patients. Behavior alterations reported include both hyperactivity and sedation. Another CNS side effect is exacerbation of a seizure type that is not being treated. This CNS depression is additive with other CNS depressants such as the opioids. If another CNS drug is given to the patient, the dose should be reduced.

♦ GASTROINTESTINAL DISTRESS

Gastrointestinal distress, including anorexia, nausea, and vomiting, can occur with most anticonvulsants. These effects can be minimized by taking the drug with food. Agents with adverse reactions related to the gastrointestinal tract, for example, nonsteroidal antiinflammatory drugs (NSAIDs) or opioids, should be prescribed cautiously.

♦ DRUG INTERACTIONS

Anticonvulsant drug interactions

Many drug interactions can occur with the anticonvulsants. They may interact with themselves, with each other, or with other drugs. The mechanisms of drug interactions include altering absorption or renal excretion and inducing or inhibiting metabolism. The outcome may alter the levels of the inducing drug itself, another concomitant anticonvulsant, or some other drug that is extensively metabolized by the liver microsomal enzymes.

The most important drug interaction of the anticonvulsants involves stimulation of the hepatic microsomal enzymes. Inducing these enzymes results in a reduction in the blood level of the affected drugs (those metabolized by the liver enzymes). Figure 2-13, *A*, shows the normal, unaffected enzyme situations. When the enzymes are stimulated (Figure 2-13, *B*), the level of the affected drug *(D)* is reduced because it is being metabolized more quickly, producing its metabolite *(D$_M$)*.

Drug interactions with the anticonvulsants are more significant than with other drug groups because of their narrow therapeutic indexes. If the level of an anticonvulsant is altered sufficiently by a drug interaction, either toxicity (level too high) or loss of seizure control (level too low) can result. Before any changes or additions are made to a patient's therapy, the possibility of drug interactions should be considered.

Idiosyncratic Reactions. A wide range of idiosyncratic reactions occurs with the anticonvulsants. Dermatologic side effects include rash, Stevens-Johnson syndrome, exfoliative dermatitis, and erythema multiforme. Drug-induced systemic lupus erythematosus and hematologic effects have also been reported with most of these agents.

Teratogenicity/Growth. Reports have associated the anticonvulsant agents with alteration in growth, with profound effects on fetal development and children receiving anticonvulsant medications during growth and development. The teratogenic potential of the anticonvulsants has been documented. Several have been implicated in the production of fetal anomalies. However, antiseizure therapy may be necessary. In some instances the mother's seizures may be more damaging to fetal development than the drug itself. In this case, the risk:benefit factor must be considered.

Withdrawal. Abrupt withdrawal of any anticonvulsant medication can precipitate seizures. Although many patients require medication for life, certain seizure types tend to disappear as the patient grows older. In these patients, gradual withdrawal of their seizure medication under controlled conditions can be undertaken after an appropriate interval of drug use.

Other Interactions. Another adverse reaction resulting from suppression of antidiuretic hormone (ADH) is dilutional hyponatremia. Renal toxicity or failure, paresthesias, and thrombophlebitis have also been recorded.

Carbamazepine

| Carbamazepine for trigeminal neuralgia |

Structurally related to the tricyclic antidepressants, carbamazepine (kar-ba-MAZ-e-peen) (Tegretol) is used to treat convulsions. It is of special interest in dentistry because of its use in the treatment of trigeminal neuralgia (tic douloureux). It is also indicated in the treatment of bipolar depression. In fact, several anticonvulsants are used to manage chronic pain syndromes.

◆ PHARMACOLOGIC EFFECTS

Carbamazepine has the following properties: anticonvulsant, anticholinergic, antidepressant, sedative, and muscle relaxant. It also has antiarrhythmic, antidiuretic, and neuromuscular transmission-inhibitory actions. Its mechanism of action involves blocking sodium channels, which block the propagation of nerve impulses. Other effects of carbamazepine include inhibition of high-frequency repetitive firing in neurons and decrease in synaptic transmission presynaptically.

◆ ADVERSE REACTIONS

Carbamazepine can have many types of adverse reactions; some are serious, but most patients seem to tolerate the medication well. CNS depression and gastrointestinal tract problems are most common.

Central Nervous System Effects. Carbamazepine can produce dizziness, vertigo, drowsiness, fatigue, ataxia, confusion, headache, nystagmus, and visual (diplopia) and speech disturbances. Activation of a latent psychosis, abnormal involuntary movements, depression, and peripheral neuritis occur rarely.

Gastrointestinal Effects. Gastrointestinal side effects include nausea, vomiting, and gastric distress. Abdominal pain, diarrhea, constipation, and anorexia have also been noted. Taking carbamazepine with food can reduce its chance of producing nausea and vomiting.

Hematologic Effects. Fatal blood dyscrasias, including aplastic anemia and agranulocytosis, have been reported related to carbamazepine therapy. These effects usually occur within 4 months and have been reported in elderly patients taking carbamazepine for trigeminal neuralgia (may be caused by the higher doses used). Thrombocytopenia and leukopenia have also been reported. Because of the hematologic adverse effects, it is necessary to perform laboratory tests to follow these patients. Patients should be made aware of the symptoms of blood dyscrasias and warned to stop the drug and report any of the symptoms immediately. The dental team should observe the oral cavity of patients taking carbamazepine with these side effects in mind (look for petechiae or signs of infection).

Dermatologic Effects. Rashes, urticaria, photosensitivity reactions, and altered skin pigmentation can occur. Erythema multiforme, erythema nodosum, and aggravation of systemic lupus erythematosus have been reported. Alopecia can also occur.

Oral Effects. Dry mouth, glossitis, and stomatitis can sometimes be seen in patients taking carbamazepine. A child who is taking chewable carbamazepine, often four times daily, will be exposed to a sugar for an extended period of time (sticks to teeth). The pediatric dose form of carbamazepine contains 63% sugar in its chewable tablet. The parents should be questioned about the child's medication use and the oral hygiene methods being used.

Other Effects. Cardiovascular side effects include congestive heart failure and alterations in blood pressure. Abnormal liver function tests and cholestatic jaundice have been reported. Urinary frequency and retention, oliguria, and impotence have been reported with carbamazepine use. Elevated blood urea nitrogen levels, albuminuria, and glycosuria have been seen. Lymphadenopathy, aching joints, and punctate lens opacities have occurred rarely.

◆ DRUG INTERACTIONS

Carbamazepine has many drug interactions. Like many of the other anticonvulsants, it can induce liver microsomal enzymes, altering the metabolism of many drugs, including carbamazepine itself. Carbamazepine can decrease the effect of doxycycline, warfarin, theophylline, and oral contraceptives. Carbamazepine's effects may be increased by erythromycin, isoniazid, propoxyphene, and calcium channel blockers. The dental

---

BOX 16-3   DENTAL MANAGEMENT OF PATIENTS TAKING CARBAMAZEPINE (TEGRETOL)

- Check for dry mouth, glossitis, and stomatitis.
- Additive bleeding—use drugs that can alter coagulation cautiously.
- Look for symptoms of blood dyscrasias.
- Check for flu-like symptoms.
- Monitor white blood cell counts.
- Consider drug interactions—doxycycline (reduced doxycycline effect) and erythromycin (increased carbamazepine).
- Perform appropriate laboratory testing (if being prescribed by dentist for trigeminal neuralgia):
  - Hematologic tests
  - Ophthalmologic examination
  - Complete urinalysis
  - Liver function tests
- Emphasize oral hygiene; for a child using chewable carbamazepine tablets, the large amount of sugar could predispose the child to a higher caries rate.

---

management of patients taking carbamazepine is discussed in Box 16-3.

Valproate

Valproate used: divalproex (Depakote)

A group of anticonvulsant agents that are not structurally related to any other anticonvulsants are the valproates, which include valproic (val-PRO-ik) acid, valproate (val-PRO-ate) sodium, and divalproex (dye-VAL-pro-ex) sodium. The term *valproate* is used here to refer to all of these agents. Divalproex sodium is a 1:1 ratio of valproic acid and valproate sodium. The mechanism of action of valproate may be its effect on sodium or potassium channels, a reduction in aspartate levels, or an increase in the inhibitory neurotransmitter γ-aminobutyric acid (GABA) (evidence is mounting against this as the only mechanism).

◆ ADVERSE REACTIONS

Gastrointestinal Effects. Indigestion, nausea, and vomiting are the most frequent adverse effects associated with valproate. These can be minimized by giving the drug with meals or increasing the dose very gradually. Divalproex sodium may have fewer adverse gastrointestinal effects than its components. Other gastrointestinal side effects include hypersalivation, anorexia, increased appetite, cramping, diarrhea, and constipation.

Central Nervous System Effects. Sedation and drowsiness have been reported with valproate. Rarely, ataxia, headache, and nystagmus have been noted. Some children exhibit hyperactivity, aggression, and other behavioral disturbances. Weight gain and an increase in appetite have been reported.

Hepatotoxicity. The idiosyncratic toxicity of valproate is hepatotoxicity. Dose-related changes in liver enzymes often occur in these patients. Deaths caused by hepatic failure have also been reported. Because valproic acid can produce serious hepatotoxicity, hepatic function tests should be performed. Signs of hepatotoxicity include nausea, vomiting, abdominal pain, loss of appetite, and diarrhea.

Bleeding. Valproate inhibits the second phase of platelet

Platelet aggregation inhibited

aggregation; therefore bleeding time may be prolonged. Thrombocytopenia, petechiae, bruising, and hematoma

---

BOX 16-4   DENTAL MANAGEMENT OF PATIENTS TAKING VALPROIC ACID (DEPAKOTE)

- Additive bleeding—use drugs that can alter coagulation cautiously.
- Look for signs of hepatotoxicity.

---

have been reported. Platelet counts, bleeding time, and coagulation studies should be performed before surgical procedures.

Teratogenicity. Several reports suggest an association between the use of valproate in pregnant women and an increase in birth defects (particularly neural tube defects).

◆ DRUG INTERACTIONS

Other drugs that are CNS depressants can have an additive CNS depressant effect when used with valproate. Valproate inhibits the metabolism of phenobarbital, producing excessive sedation. Valproate has also been associated with drug interactions with phenytoin resulting in decreased action of valproate and increased phenytoin action. Because valproate can affect bleeding, other drugs that affect bleeding should be used cautiously. Box 16-4 summarizes the management of dental patients taking valproic acid.

Phenobarbital

The most common barbiturate used in the treatment of epilepsy is phenobarbital (fee-noe-BAR-bi-tal). The barbiturates are discussed in detail in Chapter 11. Primidone (PRYE-mih-done) (Mysoline) differs from phenobarbital by one functional group, and mephobarbital (me-foe-BAR-bi-tal) (Mebaral) is metabolized to phenobarbital in the body, so both have actions similar to phenobarbital. Because these agents are similar in their action, phenobarbital is discussed as the prototype for this group.

Phenobarbital is used alone and in combination with other anticonvulsants such as phenytoin. It is used to treat tonic-clonic and partial seizure types (see Table 16-1). Other anticonvulsants are often used first.

The most common side effect associated with phenobarbital is sedation. With continued use, tolerance to the drowsiness but not the anticonvulsant effect often develops. In children, excitement and hyperactivity are often produced. The elderly sometimes exhibit confusion, excitement, or depression.

Skin reactions occur in 1% to 3% of patients. Rarely, exfoliative dermatitis, erythema multiforme, or Stevens-Johnson syndrome has been reported. Stomatitis may herald the onset of cutaneous reactions, some of which have been fatal. The barbiturates should be discontinued if any skin reactions occur.

Phenytoin

Because phenytoin (FEN-i-toyn) (Dilantin), formerly called *diphenylhydantoin,* is the most commonly used hydantoin, it is discussed as the prototype for the hydantoin group. Because phenytoin is associated with gingival enlargement, the dental team plays an integral role in the management of these patients.

Phenytoin is used to treat both tonic-clonic and partial seizures with complex symptomatology. It is not useful in the treatment of pure absence seizures but may be used in combination with other agents indicated for absence seizures to control combined seizure types. It has also been used to treat trigeminal neuralgia. In addition to its anticonvulsant properties, phenytoin has quinidine-like antiarrhythmic properties.

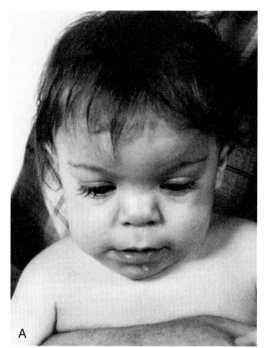
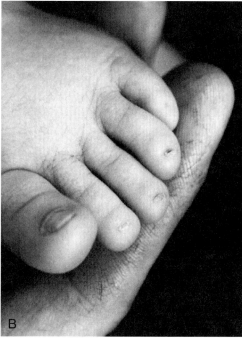

FIGURE 16-3
Infant with fetal hydantoin syndrome. **A,** Typical facial appearance with broad, depressed nasal bridge and widely spaced eyes. **B,** Hypoplasia of nails and distal phalanges. (From Bradley WG, Daroff RB, Fenichel GM, et al: *Neurology in clinical practice,* ed 5, Philadelphia, 2008, Butterworth-Heinemann.)

◆ ADVERSE REACTIONS

The adverse reactions associated with phenytoin are frequent, affect many body systems, and may be serious (rare). Because of phenytoin's narrow therapeutic index, adverse reactions associated with elevated blood levels can occur. The chance for toxicity is also increased because phenytoin's metabolism is a saturable process. Phenytoin has a propensity for drug interactions because of its enzyme-stimulating property.

Gastrointestinal Effects. Gastrointestinal adverse reactions are not uncommon. Taking the medication with food can reduce these side effects. Other drugs with the potential for adverse gastrointestinal tract effects, such as NSAIDs or opioids, should be used carefully.

Central Nervous System Effects. The CNS effects that can occur with phenytoin include mental confusion, nystagmus, ataxia, slurred speech, blurred vision, diplopia, amblyopia, dizziness, and insomnia. Because these effects are dose related, they can often be controlled by reducing the dose of phenytoin.

Dermatologic Effects. Skin reactions to phenytoin range from rash to (rarely) exfoliative dermatitis, lupus erythematosus, or Stevens-Johnson syndrome. Some patients experience irreversible hypertrichosis or hirsutism (excessive hairiness) on the trunk and face. This is one reason why alternative drugs are often selected, especially in the young female patient.

Vitamin Deficiency. Deficiency produced by phenytoin may involve vitamin D and folate. Osteomalacia may result from phenytoin's interference with vitamin D metabolism. The first symptoms of folate deficiency may be oral mucosal changes such as ulcerations or glossitis. Treatment involves administering folic acid.

Teratogenicity/Growth. *Fetal hydantoin syndrome* is the term given to the congenital abnormality associated with maternal ingestion of phenytoin (Figure 16-3). It includes craniofacial anomalies, microcephaly, nail/digit hypoplasia, limb defects, growth deficiency, and mental retardation. Thickening of facial structures and coarsening of facial features have been noted.

Gingival Enlargement. Another adverse reaction to phenytoin, gingival enlargement (previously referred to as *gingival hyperplasia*), occurs in approximately 50% of all chronic users (see Color Plates 16 and 17). The name change is the result of an increased understanding of the nature of the enlargement. In approximately 30% of affected patients, gingival enlargement is severe enough to require surgical intervention.

Gingival enlargement

Symptoms. The clinical symptoms that occur with gingival enlargement may appear as little as a few weeks or as long as a few years after initial drug therapy. It often begins as a painless enlargement of the gingival margin. The gingiva is pink and does not bleed easily unless other factors are present. With time, the interproximal papillae become involved and finally coalesce to cover even the occlusal surfaces of the teeth. The hyperplasia is more commonly located in the anterior rather than the posterior surfaces, and the buccal rather than the lingual surfaces. The affected areas of the mouth in order of severity are the maxillary anterior facial, mandibular anterior facial, maxillary posterior facial, and mandibular posterior facial areas. In the affected patient, both normal and abnormal tissue may be found. Edentulous areas are rarely involved.

The better the patient's oral hygiene, the less likely the lesions are to occur or the less severe they will be if they do occur.

Younger patients are more likely to experience this adverse reaction. Controversy exists on the contribution of dose and duration of therapy to the risk for the development of gingival enlargement.

Etiology. The cause of phenytoin gingival enlargement is unknown. Many causes have been investigated, including alteration in the function of the adrenal gland, hypersensitivity or allergic reaction, immunologic reaction, and vitamin C or folate deficiency. Because it is known that phenytoin may be found in the saliva, some investigators suggest a local etiology.

Management. The management of phenytoin-induced gingival enlargement requires consultation between dental personnel and the patient's physician. Some possible alternatives are as follows:

- *Choose another antiepileptic drug.* Choosing another effective antiepileptic drug is one method of handling the gingival enlargement produced by phenytoin.
- *Discontinue phenytoin.* Patients who have discontinued phenytoin will experience a decrease in gingival enlargement over a 1-year period. Surgical intervention should wait until at least 18 months after cessation of therapy because some patients experience additional reduction in the enlargement after the 1-year period.
- *Improve oral hygiene.* Scrupulous oral hygiene may delay the onset or reduce the rate of formation of enlargement. Avoiding irritating restorations may also reduce enlargement. Even with ideal oral hygiene, enlargement is not always totally preventable, and once it has formed is not easily reversed.
- *Consider gingivectomy.* When gingival enlargement interferes with plaque control, esthetics, or mastication and when oral hygiene has not been successful in controlling enlargement, surgical elimination is indicated. It is not a permanent solution because if the patient continues on phenytoin, enlargement quickly returns in most cases and can progress to the presurgical level in a short period.
- *Consider other drugs.* Although many types of drugs, such as diuretics, corticosteroids, mouthwashes, vitamin C, folic acid, and antihistamines, have been tried in the treatment of this condition, none has been shown to be effective in controlled trials.

Box 16-5 summarizes the management of dental patients taking phenytoin.

Miscellaneous Anticonvulsant Agents

♦ ETHOSUXIMIDE

The drug of choice for the treatment of absence seizures (see Table 16-1) is ethosuximide (eth-oh-SUX-i-mide) (Zarontin). Its mechanism of action may involve inhibiting the T-type calcium channels. It is ineffective in partial seizures with complex symptoms or in tonic-clonic seizures. In the treatment of mixed seizures, agents effective against tonic-clonic seizures must be used in addition to ethosuximide.

Gastrointestinal adverse effects include anorexia, gastric upset, cramps, pain, diarrhea, and nausea and vomiting. CNS adverse effects include drowsiness, hyperactivity, headache, and hiccups. Ethosuximide has been associated with blood dyscrasias, a positive direct Coombs' test, systemic lupus erythematosus, Stevens-Johnson syndrome, and hirsutism. Oral effects reported with ethosuximide include gingival enlargement and swelling of the tongue.

♦ BENZODIAZEPINES

Benzodiazepines, such as clonazepam (kloe-NA-ze-pam) (Klonopin) and clorazepate (klor-AZ-e-pate) (Tranxene), are used orally as anticonvulsant adjuvants. Diazepam (Valium), lorazepam (Ativan), and midazolam (Versed) are used parenterally to treat recurrent tonic-clonic seizures or status epilepticus.

Clonazepam is used as an adjunct to treat absence seizures not responsive to ethosuximide. Drowsiness and ataxia occur often. Behavioral disturbances and adverse neurologic effects can occur. Other side effects reported relate to the gastrointestinal tract and to the dermatologic and hematologic systems. Oral manifestations include increased salivation, coated tongue, dry mouth, and sore gums. It is also used as an adjunct in the treatment of certain mental illnesses.

New Anticonvulsant Agents

The newer anticonvulsants are listed in Table 16-2. Because gabapentin is gaining in popularity, it is discussed in more depth.

♦ FELBAMATE

Felbamate (fel-BA-mate) (Felbatol) is a newer anticonvulsant that has been associated with serious toxicities. Aplastic anemia and acute hepatic failure have been reported. The risk of death as a result of aplastic anemia depends on the severity and etiology of the anemia, with an estimated fatality rate of 20% to 30%. This agent should be reserved for use only if the seizures are refractory to other anticonvulsant agents. Prescribers are aware of these risks and patients must sign a patient information/consent form before they can receive the medication.

♦ GABAPENTIN

Gabapentin (GA-ba-pen-tin) (Neurontin), an analog of GABA, is effective as an adjunct against partial and generalized tonic-clonic seizures. Its mechanism of action is unknown, but it is not a GABA agonist. Like other anticonvulsants, it can cause CNS effects such as somnolence, dizziness, tremor, and ataxia. Gastric complaints include dyspepsia, nausea, and vomiting. It can increase the blood pressure and produce edema. There is an increase in rhinitis, pharyngitis, and cough. Ophthalmic adverse reactions include diplopia (6%) and amblyopia (4%). Myalgia and back pain have been reported. Hypersensitivity reactions have included skin rash and pruritus. Oral manifestations of gabapentin include mucositis, hiccups, and nasal obstruction.

One major advantage of gabapentin over the other anticonvulsant agents is that it is not metabolized. Because it does not affect the hepatic microsomal enzymes, it lacks significant drug interactions, which gives it a distinct advantage over the other anticonvulsants.

BOX 16-5   DENTAL MANAGEMENT OF PATIENTS TAKING PHENYTOIN (DILANTIN)

- If patient has nausea, avoid drugs that are gastric irritants.
- Monitor for gingival enlargement.
- Provide extensive oral hygiene instruction.
- Schedule more frequent oral prophylaxis.

TABLE 16-2 NEWER ANTICONVULSANTS

Drug	Mechanism	Indications	Adverse Reactions
Gabapentin (Neurontin)	GABA analog but does not interact with GABA receptor	Partial/generalized tonic-clonic seizures	Somnolence, dizziness, tremor, ataxia; good effect; may increase norethindrone level not metabolized and does not affect liver enzymes; antacids reduce effect, cimetidine increases gabapentin levels
Topiramate (Topamax)	Blocks Na channels, potentiates GABA at different site from other drugs	Partial/generalized tonic-clonic seizures	No effect on metabolism, some DI, BCP less effective
Tiagabine (Gabitril)	Inhibitor of GABA uptake	Adjunct, partial seizures	Dizziness, nervousness, tremor, depression; rash idiosyncratic
Lamotrigine (Lamictal)	Inactivates sodium channels	Partial/secondary generalized seizures; adjunct or monotherapy for several types of convulsions	Dizziness, headache, nausea, somnolence, diplopia, headache; rash/hypersensitivity
Felbamate (Felbatol)	Antagonist to glycine (stimulant neurotransmitter)	Adjunct for partial seizures	Bone marrow depression (agranulocytosis, aplastic anemia), severe hepatitis, monitor LFTs, third-line drug
Fosphenytoin (Cerebyx)	Stabilizes neuronal membranes	Acute seizures, status epilepticus	Parenteral use
Levetiracetam (Keppra)	Exact mechanism of action is unknown	Adjunct therapy for partial and myoclonic seizures	Dizziness, somnolence, weakness, irritability, behavioral changes, hallucinations, psychosis. No clinically significant pharmacokinetic drug-drug interactions
Oxcarbazepine (Trileptal)	Exact mechanism of action is unknown	Monotherapy and adjunct therapy for partial seizures	Somnolence, dizziness, diplopia, ataxia, nausea, vomiting, Stevens-Johnson syndrome reported. Does not cause induction of its own metabolism
Pregabalin (Lyrica)	In vitro, pregabalin reduces the calcium-dependent release of several neurotransmitters	Adjunct therapy for partial seizures in adults	Somnolence, dizziness, ataxia, weight gain, dry mouth, blurred vision, peripheral edema, abnormal thinking. Schedule V controlled substance because it caused euphoria in some clinical trials
Zonisamide (Zonegran)	In vitro trials suggest a blockade of sodium channels	Adjunct therapy for partial seizures in adults	Somnolence, dizziness, confusion, anorexia, nausea, diarrhea, weight loss, Stevens-Johnson syndrome, agranulocytosis, psychosis

BCP, Birth control pill; *DI,* drug interaction; *GABA,* γ-aminobutyric acid; *GE,* gingival enlargement; *LFTs,* liver function tests; *Na,* sodium.

DENTAL TREATMENT OF THE PATIENT WITH EPILEPSY

The dental team should not treat a patient who has a history of seizure disorders without reviewing the management of the patient with epilepsy, including the procedures for handling a patient experiencing tonic-clonic seizures. Preventive measures include a detailed seizure history, treatment planning to avoid excessive stress and missed medications, and education of the entire dental office staff. The management of the patient experiencing tonic-clonic seizures should include moving the patient to the floor if possible, tilting the patient's head to one side to prevent aspiration, and removing objects from the patient's mouth before the seizure to prevent fractured teeth. The use of tongue blades is not recommended because the blades may split and produce additional trauma in the oral cavity.

NONSEIZURE USES OF ANTICONVULSANTS

Neurologic Pain

Several anticonvulsants are used to manage chronic pain syndromes. An example is carbamazepine, which is used to treat trigeminal neuralgia and atypical facial pain. Phenytoin has also been used to treat neurologic pain. Valproic acid has been used for migraine headache prophylaxis.

Psychiatric Use

Anticonvulsants for bipolar disorder

Carbamazepine, valproic acid, clonazepam, and gabapentin have been used in the treatment of certain mental disorders (see Chapter 17). They are sometimes called *mood stabilizers* in this context. They can be used to "level out," or stabilize, the mood in patients with bipolar disorder. Thus a patient taking an anticonvulsant drug may or may not have a seizure disorder.

DENTAL HYGIENE CONSIDERATIONS

1. Conduct a thorough health history in order to determine the type, duration, and frequency of seizures.
2. Determine when the client had his or her last seizure.
3. Conduct a detailed medication history in order to avoid drug interactions and adverse effects.
4. Determine if the patient is experiencing any adverse effects from antiseizure medications.
5. Find out how often the patient takes his or her medication and if it was taken on the day of the appointment.
6. Several antiseizure medications can impact on oral health care. Always examine the patient for gingival enlargement or overgrowth.
7. Have the patient describe his or her seizure symptoms to you and how the seizure resolves itself.
8. Review the information in Boxes 16-2, 16-3, 16-4, and 16-5.

CLINICAL SKILLS ASSESSMENT

1. What is gingival hyperplasia and how can it be treated?
2. Discuss methods to minimize gingival hyperplasia.
3. What is the mechanism of action of phenytoin and what are its clinical uses?
4. What is hirsutism? Why would this be a concern among young women?
5. What are some of the gastrointestinal adverse reactions associated with phenytoin?
6. What should a patient be told about the use of an NSAID and phenytoin?
7. What are the dental concerns associated with the CNS adverse reactions of phenytoin?
8. What is carbamazepine and what is its role in treating seizure disorders?
9. What are the major classes of adverse reactions associated with carbamazepine therapy?
10. Can any of the CNS adverse reactions affect oral health care?
11. Why should a parent be concerned about the pediatric dose form of carbamazepine?
12. What would you tell a parent about the pediatric dose form of carbamazepine?
13. What are the dental concerns associated with carbamazepine and what should a parent be told about them?

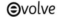volve

Please visit http://evolve.elsevier.com/Haveles/pharmacology for review questions and additional practice and reference materials.

Psychotherapeutic Agents

LEARNING OBJECTIVES

1. Name and describe the three categories of functional disorders discussed in this chapter.
2. Outline some basic precautions that the dental health care professional should keep in mind when treating patients with psychiatric disorders.
3. Summarize the basic mechanism of action, pharmacologic effects, adverse reactions, drug interactions, and uses of the antipsychotic agents.
4. Describe the mechanism of action, pharmacologic effects, adverse reactions, drug interactions, uses, and dental implications of the tricyclic antidepressants.
5. Describe the mechanism of action, pharmacologic effects, adverse reactions, drug interactions, uses, and dental implications of the selective serotonin reuptake inhibitors.
6. Name several other types of antidepressants.
7. List several drugs used to treat bipolar disorder.

Many drugs have the ability to affect mental activity. Some of these drugs are used in the treatment of psychiatric disorders. The dental health care worker is most likely to encounter the use of these agents in dental patients who have had them prescribed by psychiatrists or other physicians. Because these agents are so widely prescribed and can alter the patient's dental treatment, the dental health care worker must understand their pharmacologic effects, adverse reactions, and dental implications.

Agents used in the treatment of the major psychiatric disorders are discussed in this chapter. Those used to treat anxiety are discussed in Chapter 11. The anticonvulsants used as "mood stabilizers" are discussed in Chapter 16. Because the psychotherapeutic drugs are classified by their therapeutic use, a brief discussion of the common psychiatric illnesses follows.

PSYCHIATRIC DISORDERS

There are many psychiatric disorders. They may be divided into types such as organic and functional or primary and secondary, depending on their suspected cause. Organic illness is congenital or caused by an injury or a disease. Functional disorders are partially of psychogenic origin, without evidence (yet) of structural or biochemical abnormality (Figure 17-1). The naming and categorization of different mental disorders changes as more information becomes available. Functional disorders include the following categories:

1. Psychoses
2. Affective disorder
3. Neuroses (anxiety)

The psychoses are discussed first. Schizophrenia, the most common type of psychosis, is an extensive disturbance of the patient's personality function with a loss of perception of reality. Schizophrenia is derived from the word meaning "splitting," and in context it refers to patients splitting from reality (not into multiple personalities). The patient's

> Loss of reality

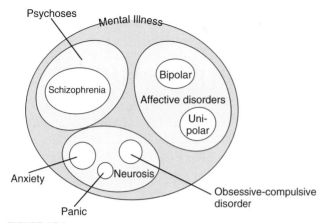

FIGURE 17-1
Classification of common mental illnesses.

BOX 17-1 SYMPTOMS OF PSYCHOSES
Positive
Hallucinations, auditory
Delusions
Unwanted thoughts
Disorganized behavior
Agitation
Distorted speech, communication
Negative
Flat affect
Unemotional
Apathetic, passivity
Abstract thinking difficult
Spontaneity and goals lacking
Thought and speech impaired
Lack of pleasure
Social withdrawal

ability to function in society is impaired because of altered thinking. The impaired thinking of these patients may be so detached from reality and their delusions or paranoia (e.g., someone is out to get me) so severe that their illness could lead to committing serious crimes, including assassination attempts or murders. Patients may suffer from hallucinations, delusions, or agitation. The positive symptoms of psychosis include agitation, extrapyramidal symptoms, and auditory hallucinations. Other patients may be introspective and uninvolved. The negative effects of psychosis include flat affect and apathy (Box 17-1).

The etiology of schizophrenia is not specifically known, but a familial pattern is often seen. The biochemical actions of the brain and even brain anatomy have been demonstrated to be different from findings in normal individuals in some patients with schizophrenia.

Affective disorders include endogenous and exogenous unipolar depression and bipolar depression (mania). The condition in patients who exhibit only depression is termed *unipolar depression*. Endogenous (involutional) depression seems to be unrelated to external events, whereas exogenous (reactive) depression appears to be related to specific external events. Whether there are actually two types of depression separated by circumstances of occurrence is questionable. Theories for several different types of depression based on the biochemical situation in the brain have been hypothesized, but no one has been able to show different groups. Patients who exhibit alternating periods of depression and excitation (mania, elation) have bipolar (*bi*, two) depression, also known as manic-depressive disorder.

Neuroses are less severe than psychoses but can also be helped by drug therapy. Examples include anxiety, panic disorder, phobias, and obsessive-compulsive disorder. Psychophysiologic (somatic) disorders are those that have an emotional origin but manifest by physiologic symptoms. Personality disorders include sexual deviation, alcoholism, and drug dependence. Although many of these conditions are managed using the antidepressants and/or antipsychotics, the anxiety-related problems sometimes require the use of the benzodiazepines. Divisions of these different mental disorders have been and are continually changing to reflect either an increased knowledge or a political or "fad" perspective. (What is "normal" anyway?)

This presentation is an oversimplification of the classifications of psychiatric disorders. The drug groups discussed in this chapter include antipsychotic agents, used to treat psychoses; antidepressant agents, used to treat affective disorders; and lithium, used to treat bipolar disorder. The benzodiazepines, used to treat anxiety and panic disorders, are discussed in Chapter 11.

Before the antipsychotic drugs were introduced into the management of psychiatric disorders, many physical methods were used to treat patients. Only electroconvulsive therapy (ECT, shock therapy) is still used in the treatment of depression. With the use of neuromuscular blocking agents, the use of ECT therapy has become much safer. ECT produces the fastest results of any treatment for depression. It is reserved for patients who are refractive to antidepressants. Some memory loss occurs during the treatment (several sessions).

Watch verbal interaction with patient.

When treating patients with mental disorders, the following general precautions should be observed by the dental health care worker:

- *Communication:* Patients with various mental disorders may perceive comments or movement from dental health care workers as threatening. Even normal office discussions may be perceived differently than they are intended. For example, small talk with a peer may be interpreted as a conspiracy by the patient. What you say around and to the patient should be carefully monitored. (I once asked a patient "How are you?" and the patient replied with a loud and angry voice, "Why are you asking me that question?")

- *Compliance:* Patients undergoing drug therapy for the treatment of psychoses often do not take their medication as prescribed. A thorough health history including the patient's medication and its dosage should be obtained.

- *Suicide:* Depressed patients may attempt suicide. Therefore the amount of any drug prescribed at one time should not exceed the amount required for a lethal dose (usually a 1-week supply). When patients are severely depressed, they have no motivation and usually do not act on any irrational thoughts of suicide. After beginning to take an antidepressant, partial improvement gives them the motivation to attempt suicide before the full antidepressant effects have developed. Children and teens appear to be at a higher risk for suicide with antidepressant therapy, especially with the newer class of drugs. In a suicide attempt, drugs are often combined. For example, a patient may mix an opioid analgesic given for the relief of a toothache, a sedative-hypnotic prescribed for dental anxiety, and an antidepressant medication prescribed by the patient's physician.

ANTIPSYCHOTIC AGENTS

The antipsychotic agents are divided into two major groups depending on their ability to target both the positive and negative symptoms of schizophrenia. Until the past few years, the conventional antipsychotics were the most often used group of antipsychotics. Table 17-1 lists the conventional antipsychotics and their usual adult daily dose for outpatient treatment. More patients are now being treated with the newer antipsychotics referred to as the "atypical" antipsychotics.

The atypical antipsychotics—so named because they were unlike the conventional antipsychotics—have different receptor activities and adverse reaction profiles. As a group, these agents have more nausea and less anticholinergic and sedative effects than occur with the conventional antipsychotics.

The actions of the antipsychotic agents are diverse. Of the conventional antipsychotics, no single agent is clearly superior in its antipsychotic action. However, with the advent of the atypical antipsychotics, patients who were previously resistant to conventional antipsychotic agents have been adequately managed with these new drugs. Antipsychotics that act on several receptors have a broader range of action and can be used in more difficult cases. Clinical judgment and the drug's side effect profile in a particular patient determine which agent is used. In general, the lower potency agents such as chlorpromazine (klor-PROE-ma-zeen) (Thorazine) have more sedation, more peripheral side effects, and more autonomic effects (e.g., dry mouth), whereas the higher-potency agents such as haloperidol (ha-loe-PER-i-dol) have more extrapyramidal effects and less sedation. Other common phenothiazines include thioridazine (thye-oh-RID-a-zeen) (Mellaril) and trifluoperazine (trye-floo-oh-PAIR-a-zeen) (Stelazine).

Pharmacologic Effects

◆ CONVENTIONAL ANTIPSYCHOTICS

When conventional antipsychotics are used for treatment of psychoses, any effects other than the antipsychotic effect could

TABLE 17-1 ANTIPSYCHOTIC AGENTS

Drug Group	Drug Name Generic (Trade)	Daily Dose (mg)*	SIDE EFFECTS			
			Sed	EP	AC	OH
Conventional Antipsychotics						
High Potency						
	Fluphenazine (Prolixin)	0.5-40	1	3	1	1
	Haloperidol (Haldol)	1-15	1	3	1	1
Medium Potency						
	Loxapine (Loxitane)	20-250	1	2	1	1
	Molindone (Moban)	15-225	2	2	1	1
	Perphenazine (Trilafon)	8-64	2	2	1	1
	Trifluoperazine (Stelazine)	2-40	1		1	1
	Thiothixene (Navane)	8-30	1	3	1	2
Low Potency						
	Chlorpromazine (Thorazine)	30-2000	3	2	3	3
	Chlorprothixene (Taractan)	75-600	3	2	2	2
	Mesoridazine (Serentil)	75-400	3	1	3	2
	Thioridazine (Mellaril)	150-800	3	1	3	3
Atypical Antipsychotics						
	Aripiprazole (Abilify)	10-30	1	2	1	2
	Clozapine (Clozaril)†	12.5-900	4	1	4	4
	Olanzapine (Zyprexa)	5-20	2	2	3	2
	Quetiapine (Seroquel)	50-800	3	2	0	2
	Risperidone (Risperdal)	1-16	1	2	1	2
	Ziprasidone (Geodon)	20-160	2	2	1	2

AC, Anticholinergic; *EP*, extrapyramidal; *OH*, orthostatic hypotension; *Sed*, sedation; *O*, nonexistent; *1*, very low; *2*, low; *3*, moderate; *4*, high.
*Usual oral dose for outpatient treatment in milligrams/day.
†Agranulocytosis; weekly white blood cell (WBC) count needed.

be considered an adverse reaction. When used as an antiemetic, other actions would be adverse reactions such as sedation. The pharmacologic effects of the conventional antipsychotic agents include the following.

Antipsychotic Effect. All conventional antipsychotics possess antipsychotic effects associated with slowing of the psychomotor activity in an agitated patient and calming of emotion with suppression of hallucinations and delusions. These agents are active against the positive effects of psychosis but have little effect on the negative effects. Atypical antipsychotics differ in that they are effective against both the positive and negative symptoms of schizophrenia.

Antiemetic Effect. The conventional antipsychotic's antiemetic effect is a result of depression of the chemoreceptor trigger zone, an area in the brain that causes nausea and vomiting. These agents are useful in the symptomatic treatment of certain types of nausea and vomiting. Historically, prochlorperazine (Compazine) has been used for this effect.

Potentiation of Opioids. When conventional antipsychotics are combined with central nervous system (CNS) depressants, such as opioids, they potentiate the action of the depressants. When conventional antipsychotics are added to opioids, the dose of the opioid used should be decreased by half.

◆ ATYPICAL ANTIPSYCHOTIC AGENTS

There are several differences between the conventional antipsychotic agents and the newest, or atypical, antipsychotic agents. The conventional antipsychotic agents were primarily dopamine antagonists (Figure 17-2). The atypical agents have action at more than one receptor, for example, the dopamine, serotonin (5-HT), and norepinephrine (NE) receptors, which results in the improved efficacy of these agents. The side effects of the atypical antipsychotics are less than the conventional antipsychotics. Like the conventional antipsychotics, the atypical antipsychotics are effective against the positive effects associated with psychoses. However, unlike the conventional antipsychot-

ics, the atypical antipsychotic agents are effective against the negative effects. Table 17-1 lists the conventional and atypical antipsychotics.

Adverse Reactions

Table 17-1 lists the side effects of the conventional and atypical antipsychotic agents, and Figure 17-3 demonstrates the relative side effects of several conventional antipsychotic agents. Management of patients taking these agents involves minimizing the troubling side effects in each patient.

◆ SEDATION

Conventional antipsychotics differ in the degree of sedation and drowsiness they produce. The degree of sedation is one factor that determines which antipsychotic agent is prescribed. In contrast to the sedative-hypnotic agents, with higher doses the conventional antipsychotics do not produce anesthesia and the patient is easily aroused. Tolerance develops to the sedative effect but not to the antipsychotic effect.

◆ EXTRAPYRAMIDAL EFFECTS

The most common type of adverse reactions associated with these agents results from stimulation of the extrapyramidal system. All conventional antipsychotics produce this effect, although the incidence of the reaction varies. The following types of extrapyramidal effects can occur:
- Acute dystonia consisting of muscle spasms of the face, tongue, neck, and back
- Parkinsonism with symptoms of resting tremor, rigidity, and akinesia
- Akathisia, or increased compulsive motor activity
- Tardive dyskinesia, an irreversible dyskinesia involving the tongue, lips, face, and jaw

Tardive dyskinesia is typically seen in women patients who are older than 40 years and have been taking large doses of the phenothiazines for a minimum of 6 months to 2 years or as long as 20 years. The onset is gradual and the movements are coordinated and rhythmic. This effect is exacerbated by drug withdrawal. The involuntary movements, especially those involving the face, jaw, and tongue, can make home care difficult if not impossible. Performing oral prophylaxis is difficult because of the strength of the oral facial and tongue muscles.

The dental health care worker should discuss the patient's side effects with his or her physician if oral prophylaxis cannot be performed. A dosage or drug change may be instituted by the

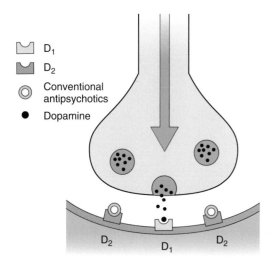

FIGURE 17-2
Conventional antipsychotics act to block postsynaptic dopamine receptors. Conventional antipsychotics have a greater affinity to D_2 receptors than to D_1 receptors. (From McKenry L, Tessier E, Hogan MA: *Mosby's pharmacology in nursing*, ed 22, St Louis, 2006, Mosby.)

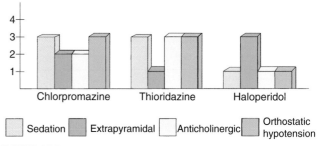

FIGURE 17-3
Comparison of selected antipsychotic adverse reactions.

patient's psychiatrist. With the availability of the atypical agents, extrapyramidal side effects can be greatly minimized.

The extrapyramidal side effects of conventional antipsychotics can cause severe intermittent pain in the region of the temporomandibular joint (TMJ). This pain is produced by a spasm of the muscles of mastication. In an acute attack, it becomes difficult or impossible to open or close the jaw. Should muscle spasm be present, force should not be exerted to open the patient's mouth for dental treatment because dislocations of the mandible can occur.

Treatment of an acute spasm of the mandible must be undertaken after consultation with the patient's prescribing physician. Alternatives may include decreasing the dose of the patient's medication, adding an anticholinergic medication to counteract the spasm, or changing the patient's antipsychotic medication to one that produces fewer extrapyramidal effects. The anticholinergics used to counteract the extrapyramidal side effects of the antipsychotics include benztropine (Cogentin) and trihexyphenidyl (Artane).

♦ ORTHOSTATIC HYPOTENSION

Because these agents depress the central sympathetic outflow and block the peripheral adrenergic receptors (α-sympathetic blockers), they can produce orthostatic hypotension that is additive with other CNS depressants. When a patient rises rapidly from the supine position, a compensatory tachycardia can accompany the orthostatic hypotension.

♦ OTHER CARDIOVASCULAR EFFECTS

These agents have also been reported to cause tachycardia. Ziprasidone significantly prolongs the QT/QTc interval. Periodic electrocardiograms (ECGs) should be performed on patients receiving ziprasidone.

♦ SEIZURES

Because conventional antipsychotics lower the convulsion threshold, seizures may be more easily precipitated in a patient taking these agents, especially if a previous history of epilepsy exists. Bupropion (Wellbutrin, Zyban) can produce seizures, and therefore patients on conventional antipsychotics may not be candidates for its use. Consultation with the patient's psychiatrist would be warranted.

♦ ANTICHOLINERGIC EFFECTS

Xerostomia with older antipsychotics

The anticholinergic effects of conventional antipsychotics produce blurred vision, xerostomia, and constipation. This is especially significant because the anticholinergic effects of other medications the patient may be taking are additive. The anticholinergics, such as benztropine, used to treat the extrapyramidal symptoms are additive, too. The dental health care worker should be aware of the presence of xerostomia and question patients regarding their method of managing this problem.

♦ OTHER EFFECTS

As previously mentioned, conventional antipsychotics have many adverse effects, including blood dyscrasias, cholestatic jaundice, skin eruptions, and photosensitivity reactions that are exaggerated by sunlight or even by the light from the dental unit.

♦ AGRANULOCYTOSIS

The atypical antipsychotic, clozapine (KLOE-za-peen) (Clozaril), is useful in treating patients with treatment-resistant schizophrenia. Because it produces potentially life-threatening agranulocytosis, clozapine should be tried only after several trials of other agents have failed. Frequent white blood cell counts with differential are required during therapy. With the release of newer atypical antipsychotic agents, use of this agent has decreased.

♦ METABOLIC EFFECTS

The atypical antipsychotics have been associated with a higher risk of hyperglycemia, diabetes, and metabolic syndrome. It is important to monitor patient plasma glucose and cholesterol levels. Patients should be encouraged to maintain a healthy diet and lifestyle.

Drug Interactions

♦ CENTRAL NERVOUS SYSTEM DEPRESSANTS

Conventional antipsychotics interact in an additive or even potentiating fashion with all CNS depressants, including barbiturates, alcohol, general anesthetics, and opioid analgesics. Sedation and respiratory depression can occur.

♦ EPINEPHRINE

Epinephrine, used as a vasoconstrictor in local anesthetic solutions, can be safely used in patients taking conventional antipsychotics. However, because the conventional antipsychotics are α-adrenergic blockers, epinephrine should not be used to treat vasomotor collapse (acute drop in blood pressure) because it could cause a further decrease in blood pressure. This occurs because of the predominant β-agonist (vasodilating) activity of epinephrine in the presence of the conventional antipsychotics (α-blockers). However, using epinephrine-containing local anesthetics in patients taking antipsychotics is acceptable in dentistry.

♦ ANTICHOLINERGIC AGENTS

To control excessive extrapyramidal stimulation, conventional antipsychotic therapy often must be combined with antiparkinson medication of the anticholinergic type, for example, benztropine (Cogentin). This combination is bound to exacerbate antimuscarinic peripheral effects such as xerostomia, urinary retention, constipation, blurred vision, and inhibition of sweating.

Uses

♦ ANTIPSYCHOTIC EFFECTS

Antipsychotics are the drugs of choice for treatment of schizophrenia. Long-acting injectable conventional antipsychotics, such as fluphenazine (Prolixin) and haloperidol (Haldol), are available for patients with schizophrenia who fail to take their oral medication.

♦ ANTIEMETIC EFFECTS

Because conventional antipsychotics prevent or inhibit vomiting, they are useful in the treatment of some types of nausea and

BOX 17-2	MANAGEMENT OF THE DENTAL PATIENT TAKING ANTIPSYCHOTIC AGENTS

- Use caution with patient interactions (patient may misinterpret your verbal or nonverbal actions).
- Check for xerostomia and its management.
- Emphasize oral hygiene instruction.
- Extrapyramidal dyskinesia may make oral hygiene more difficult.
- Check the TMJ for extrapyramidal side effects (mouth may be difficult to open, do not force).
- Sedation is additive with other agents with sedative effects.
- Epinephrine can be safely used in a dental local anesthetic.
- Encourage patient to rise slowly from the dental chair to minimize orthostatic hypotension.
- Disease may cause difficulty in following an oral care program (depends on disease severity).

TMJ, Temporomandibular joint.

vomiting. The drug prochlorperazine (proe-klor-PAIR-a-zeen) (Compazine) has traditionally been used.

◆ OTHER EFFECTS

Intractable hiccups and certain drug withdrawals have been successfully treated with conventional antipsychotics. Use of these agents as chemical restraints in nursing homes is unethical.

Dental Implications

The dental management of patients taking antipsychotics is summarized in Box 17-2.

◆ SEDATION

Sedation, an adverse reaction of the conventional antipsychotics, is additive with that of other sedating agents.

◆ ANTICHOLINERGIC EFFECTS

Conventional antipsychotics are additive with other agents with atropine-like effects; this combination can lead to toxic reactions, including tachycardia, urinary retention, blurred vision, constipation, and xerostomia. The dental health care worker should be aware that patients may use sugar-containing candy to counteract xerostomia. Use of sugarless products or artificial saliva (Orex, Xero-Lube, Moi-Stir) should be encouraged. Patients should be encouraged to stay away from caffeine-containing beverages because they can exacerbate dry mouth. They should also avoid alcohol-containing mouth rinses because alcohol can also exacerbate dry mouth.

◆ ORTHOSTATIC HYPOTENSION

Orthostatic hypotension effect can be minimized by raising the dental chair slowly and assisting the patient's first few steps.

◆ EPINEPHRINE

Epinephrine can be used with antipsychotics.

Epinephrine should be avoided in the management of an acute hypotensive crisis in patients taking antipsychotics. It may be safely used in local anesthetic solutions for dental patients.

◆ TEMPOROMANDIBULAR JOINT PAIN

As a result of the conventional antipsychotics' extrapyramidal effects, the muscles of mastication may be in spasm.

◆ TARDIVE DYSKINESIA

Tardive dyskinesia is irreversible and should be reported to the patient's physician.

ANTIDEPRESSANT AGENTS

Antidepressant agents are used not only to manage depression but also for a variety of other uses such as chronic pain adjuvant or migraine headache prophylaxis. One should question the patient to determine the indication for which a tricyclic antidepressant is being prescribed. The dental professional should not assume that the patient is being treated for depression. Until the late 1950s, there was no widely accepted pharmacologic treatment for depression. Forms of mild depression were treated with psychotherapy, and severe depression was treated with ECT. Several classes of antidepressants are currently available, including tricyclic antidepressants (TCAs) and selective serotonin reuptake inhibitors (SSRIs). Several new, atypical antidepressants, some with unique properties, have been recently released. ECT is still used in the treatment of severely suicidal patients and those resistant to antidepressants. In the case of suicidal thoughts, ECT works faster than any antidepressant drug.

The antidepressants may block NE and/or serotonin (5-HT) reuptake (Table 17-2 and Figure 17-4), produce sedation, and have anticholinergic side effects. One theory of their mechanism of action involves blocking reuptake of NE and/or 5-HT. Another involves downregulation of the β-adrenergic receptors.

Tricyclic Antidepressants

The TCAs are sometimes referred to as the first-generation antidepressants because they were developed and marketed before the second-generation agents. Table 17-2 lists the antidepressants with their usual adult outpatient daily dose in milligrams. All TCAs are similar in their antidepressant effectiveness, differing only in their side effect profile.

◆ PHARMACOLOGIC EFFECTS

The action of TCAs on normal and depressed patients is somewhat different. In the normal patient, an undesirable sedation and fatigue and strong atropine-like side effects are noted. In the depressed patient, a feeling of well-being, elevation of mood, and a dulling of depressive ideation are noted. Sedation occurs often, but tolerance to this effect often develops. Increased ability to concentrate and improvement in sleep is seen with the TCAs. It can take up to 6 weeks for the patient to experience the full pharmacologic effects of the antidepressant.

◆ ADVERSE REACTIONS

Some of the widely diverse adverse reactions associated with the TCAs resemble those of the antipsychotic agents (Figure 17-5; see Table 17-2).

Central Nervous System Effects. Almost all of the TCAs induce some degree of sedation. Patients should develop tolerance to this sedation.

Autonomic Nervous System Effects. The peripheral effects of TCAs are primarily on the autonomic nervous system. These agents possess distinct anticholinergic effects resulting in xerostomia, blurred vision, tachycardia, constipation, and

TABLE 17-2   COMMONLY USED ANTIDEPRESSANTS

Drug Name Generic (Trade)	Dose* Range (mg)	SIDE EFFECTS					BLOCKS REUPTAKE	
		AC	SED	OH	Wt+	N, D	NE	SERT
Tricyclic—Tertiary Amines								
Amitriptyline (Elavil)	50-300	4	4	2	4	0	2	4
Clomipramine (Anafranil)†	25-250	3	3	2	4	1	2	5
Desipramine (Norpramin, Pertofrane)	25-300	1	1	1	1	0	3	2
Doxepin (Adapin, Sinequan)	25-300	2	3	2	4	0	1	2
Imipramine (Tofranil)	30-300	2	2	3	4	1	2	4
Nortriptyline (Pamelor, Aventyl)	50-150	2	2	1	1	0	2	3
Protriptyline (Vivactil)	15-60	3	1	1	0	0	4	2
Tetracyclic Antidepressants								
Amoxapine (Asendin)	50-600	3	2	1	2	0	3	2
Maprotiline (Ludiomil)	50-225	2	2	1	2	0	3	0-1
Selective Serotonin Reuptake Inhibitors (SSRIs)								
Citalopram (Celexa)	20-60	0	0	0	3	0	0	5
Duloxetine (Cymbalta)	20-60	0-1	0-1	0-1	0-1	3	0-1	5
Escitalopram (Lexapro)	10-20	0	0	0	3	0	0	5
Fluoxetine (Prozac)	20-80	0-1	0-1	0-1	0	3	0-1	5
Fluvoxamine (Luvox)‡	50-300	0-1	0-1	0	1	3	0-1	5
Sertraline (Zoloft)	50-200	0	0-1	0	0	3	0-1	5
Paroxetine (Paxil)	20-60	0	0-1	0	1	3	0-1	5
Dopamine-Norepinephrine Reuptake Inhibitors								
Bupropion (Wellbutrin, Zyban)	100-450	2	2	1	0	1	0-1	0-1
Bupropion, sustained released (Wellbutrin SR)	150-400	2	2	1	0	1	0-1	0-1
Bupropion, extended release (Wellbutrin ER)	150-450	2	2	1	0	1	0-1	0-1
Serotonin-Norepinephrine Reuptake Inhibitors								
Venlafaxine (Effexor)§	75-225	1	0	0	0	3	3	3
Venlafaxine, extended release (Effexor XR)	75-225	1	0	0	0	3	3	3
Serotonin Modulators								
Nefazodone (Serzone)‖	200-600	1	2	1	0	1	0-1	3
Trazodone (Desyrel)	75-600	1	4	2	2	1	0	3
Norepinephrine-Serotonin Modulators								
Mirtazapine (Remeron)‖	15-45	2	3	2	0	3	3	3
Monoamine Oxidase Inhibitors								
Phenelzine (Nardil)	15-90	1	2	2	1	0	NA	NA
Tranylcypromine (Parnate)	30-60	1	1	2	1	0	NA	NA

0, Nonexistent; *1*, very low; *2*, low; *3*, moderate; *4*, high; *AC*, anticholinergic; *NA*, not applicable; *N, D*, nausea and diarrhea; *NE*, norepinephrine reuptake inhibitors; *OH*, orthostatic hypotension; *SED*, sedation; *SERT*, serotonin reuptake inhibitors; *Wt+*, weight gain.

*Usual adult daily dose (mg).

†Used for obsessive-compulsive disorder (OCD).

‡Used primarily for OCD.

§In divided doses.

‖Antagonizes α_2-adrenergic receptors.

NE neuron

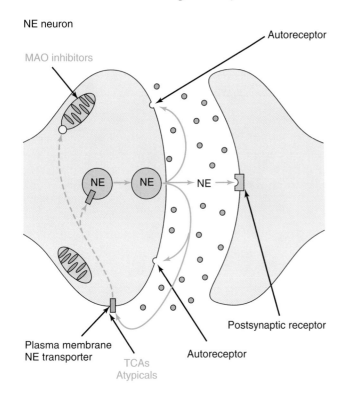

5-HT neuron

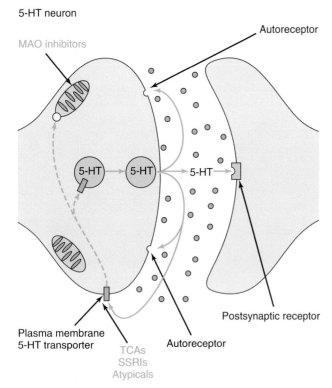

FIGURE 17-4
A noradrenergic and serotonergic synapse and sites at which antidepressants may exert their actions. TCAs, SSRIs, and some atypical antidepressants inhibit the reuptake transporter for NE and/or 5-HT. Monoamine oxidase, which is targeted by MAO inhibitors, is localized at the outer mitochondrial membrane. (From Minneman KP, Wecker L: *Brody's human pharmacology: molecular to clinical,* ed 4, Philadelphia, 2005, Mosby.)

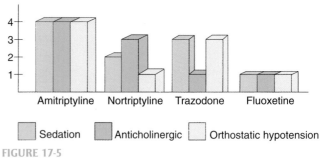

FIGURE 17-5
Relative side effects of antidepressants.

urinary retention. Some tolerance can develop with continued use. Although TCAs initially produce orthostatic hypotension like the conventional antipsychotics, tolerance to this effect occurs.

Cardiac Effects. The most serious peripheral side effect associated with the TCAs is cardiac toxicity. Myocardial infarction and congestive heart failure have occurred during the course of treatment. Arrhythmias and episodes of tachycardia can be caused by the antimuscarinic (anticholinergic, atropine-like) effects of the TCAs. New antidepressants do not cause this reaction.

Dependence or Withdrawal. Rarely, TCAs have been found to produce psychic or physical dependence. Slight withdrawal effects after abrupt discontinuation have been reported. Tolerance develops to many of the side effects, although not to the antidepressant effect.

♦ DRUG INTERACTIONS

TCAs potentiate the behavioral actions of the amphetamines and other CNS stimulants. TCAs potentiate the pressor effect of injected sympathomimetics. These agents also interact with monoamine oxidase inhibitors, resulting in severe toxic reactions. TCAs may be displaced from plasma protein binding sites by phenytoin. TCAs may be metabolized more quickly because of induction of hepatic microsomal enzymes by barbiturates, carbamazepine, and cigarette smoking. They may interfere with the antihypertensive effects of guanethidine and clonidine. Additive anticholinergic effects are seen if they are administered with other agents with anticholinergic action.

♦ POISONING

Accidental poisoning with TCAs has become more common, and such an overdose can be lethal. The effects of acute poisoning are severe hypertension, cardiac arrhythmias, hyperpyrexia, convulsions, coma, and respiratory failure. Survivors may have permanent myocardial damage. The treatment is symptomatic and should be conservative in view of the interactions with other CNS vasopressor agents. Activated charcoal or gastric lavage may be helpful. Physostigmine has been reported to be effective in treating mild poisoning by tricyclic antidepressants.

♦ USES

TCAs can be used alone or in combination with antipsychotics or ECT in the treatment of depression. In patients who are suicide risks, the long onset of action of the TCAs (several weeks) requires the use of ECT during the initial phase of drug treatment. These agents, which are allowed after several weeks for the development of their effects, can prevent relapse and thus provide long-term control of depression.

When sedation is desired, amitriptyline (a-mee-TRIP-ti-leen) (Elavil) is used. When less sedation is needed, nortriptyline (nor-TRIP-ti-leen) (Pamelor, Aventyl) or protriptyline (proe-TRIP-ti-leen) (Vivactil) can be tried. However, the use of TCAs has decreased because of their less than desirable adverse effect profile and because of the continuing development of newer antidepressants.

TCAs are often combined with one of the antipsychotics (usually an atypical because of the more tolerable side effect profile) in the treatment of patients with both psychoses and depression. Comments relating to the dental implications of both TCAs and antipsychotics apply to patients taking this type of product. Certain antidepressants are used for specific indications. For example, imipramine (im-IP-ra-meen) (Tofranil) is used to control nocturnal enuresis (incontinence) in children. Clomipramine (cloe-MIP-ra-meen) (Anafranil) is used only in the treatment of obsessive-compulsive disorder. Patients with obsessive-compulsive disorder repeatedly perform certain rituals such as hand washing. Doxepin (DOX-e-pin) (Adapin, Sinequan) is used when an antianxiety effect is desired.

◆ DENTAL IMPLICATIONS

The management of dental patients taking antidepressants is summarized in Box 17-3.

Sympathomimetic Amines. Vasoconstricting drugs (sympathomimetic amines) in the local anesthetic solution must be administered with caution to patients taking TCAs. They may potentiate vasopressor (increased blood pressure) response to epinephrine. In the usual cardiac dose (0.04 mg), the sympathomimetic amines present in a local anesthetic solution can be safely administered to patients without preexisting arrhythmias.

Xerostomia. The anticholinergic effect of sympathomimetic amines is additive with that of other agents that produce dry mouth. The dental health care worker should question patients about the products used to alleviate this troublesome side effect and suggest alternatives such as artificial saliva or sugarless gum.

Second-Generation Antidepressants

◆ OVERVIEW

Second-generation antidepressants (see Table 17-2) are newer antidepressants that possess fewer side effects than the tricyclic

---

antidepressants. For example, they have fewer anticholinergic effects and less cardiotoxicity, and some have less sedation effect. The choice of antidepressant is based on the adverse reaction profile and the individual patient's response to the agent.

◆ TRAZODONE

Trazodone (TRAZ-oh-done) (Desyrel) is a serotonin modulator antidepressant unrelated chemically to TCAs. It appears to have antidepressant effects equivalent to those of TCAs. Its advantages include that it has fewer anticholinergic effects (e.g., xerostomia) and is less cardiotoxic even in toxic doses. Its disadvantages include that it is highly sedative and has been associated with painful priapism requiring surgical intervention and leaving some patients permanently impotent.

Selective Serotonin Reuptake Inhibitors

A newer group of antidepressants, the SSRIs, have specific action on inhibiting the reuptake of 5-HT. Fluoxetine (floo-OX-uh-teen) (Prozac) was the first member of this group, and others have followed. Sertraline (SER-tral-leen) (Zoloft), paroxetine (pa-ROKS-e-teen) (Paxil), and fluvoxamine (floo-VOX-a-meen) (Luvox) are other members of this group. Their antidepressant action is equivalent to that of TCAs. Their advantage lies in their adverse reaction profile, which differs from that of TCAs (see Table 17-2).

◆ ADVERSE REACTIONS

Central Nervous System Effects. Unlike many of the TCAs, the SSRIs tend to produce CNS stimulation (activation) rather than CNS depression. Headache, dizziness, tremor, agitation, sweating, and insomnia are side effects associated with stimulation. Weight loss or weight stabilization occurs more often than the weight gain that occurs with TCAs. Somnolence and fatigue have also been reported.

Gastrointestinal Effects. Nausea and diarrhea occur in about 15% to 30% of patients. Anorexia, dyspepsia, and constipation have been reported.

Oral Effects. Oral side effects include xerostomia (10% to 15%); taste changes; aphthous stomatitis; glossitis; and rarely, increased salivation, salivary gland enlargement, and tongue discoloration or edema. The SSRIs have fewer differences in the incidence of the side effects.

Other Effects. The SSRIs often produce sexual dysfunction. The incidence varies but may be more than 75% with some agents. Excessive sweating is another common side effect. Palpitations have been reported.

Bupropion

Bupropion (byoo-PROE-pee-on) (Wellbutrin [SR]) is a dopamine-NE reuptake inhibitor that has been on the market and then off the market; in 1993 it was back on the market with increased warnings. About 0.4% of patients treated with bupropion have experienced seizures. This incidence may be 4 times greater than with the TCAs and as much as 10 times greater with TCAs at higher doses. Because of its seizure potential, it is reserved for patients who are not responsive to other agents. Gastrointestinal effects, such as constipation, nausea, and vomiting, occur in about 20% of patients. Neurologic effects, such as

---

> **BOX 17-3   MANAGEMENT OF THE DENTAL PATIENT TAKING ANTIDEPRESSANT AGENTS**
>
> - Use caution in patient interactions.
> - Drug used for other than depression; ask patient why he or she is taking the drug.
> - Check for xerostomia and its management.
> - Epinephrine may cause an increased vasopressor response (blood pressure response). Limit dose of epinephrine to 0.04 mg if blood pressure is a concern.
> - Limit total amount of any potentially lethal drugs prescribed if patient is depressed.
> - Increase motivation for good oral hygiene (usually improves with treatment of depression).

dry mouth (28%), headache (25%), excessive sweating, and tremors, have been reported. Agitation (32%) and dizziness (22%) occur often. Divided doses, slow titration of doses, and careful patient selection can minimize seizure risk.

Other Antidepressant Agents

Nefazodone (nef-AY-zoe-done) (Serzone), venlafaxine (Effexor), and mirtazapine (Remeron) are examples of newer antidepressants. They are indicated for the treatment of depression. Nefazodone, like trazodone, is a 5-HT modulator, and venlafaxine is a 5-HT-NE reuptake inhibitor. Mirtazapine is a NE-5-HT modulator. The incidence of xerostomia is greater than 10%, and sexual dysfunction often occurs with nefazodone and venlafaxine. Venlafaxine is a weak inhibitor of cytochrome P-450 2D6 isoenzymes. Nefazodone increases the serum levels of alprazolam, triazolam, and digoxin. Nefazodone carries a black box warning regarding its potential to cause life-threatening hepatic failure. Mirtazapine causes somnolence, weight gain, constipation, and dry mouth.

Monoamine Oxidase Inhibitors

MAOI: many drug interactions

Monoamine oxidase inhibitors (MAOIs) include a large variety of drugs that have the ability to inhibit monoamine oxidase. MAOIs possess many adverse effects, and an overdose can lead to a severe toxic reaction. MAOIs interact with many drugs, such as amphetamines, and with foods, such as cheeses, wines, and fish, precipitating a hypertensive crisis and even death. Patients taking MAOIs have detailed food prohibitions because of the chance of drug-food interactions. Because of the potential for life-threatening situations, MAOIs are used as drugs of last choice. Patients taking MAOIs should not be given any drug unless the prescriber has first consulted a reference source on drug interactions.

DRUGS FOR TREATMENT OF BIPOLAR DEPRESSION

Until fairly recently, lithium was the major drug used in the treatment of bipolar depression. Other agents commonly used today include a variety of anticonvulsants, including carbamazepine, valproate, and gabapentin. These agents are often referred to as "mood stabilizers."

Lithium

Lithium (LITH-ee-um) (Eskalith, Lithobid) is used in the treatment of bipolar (manic) depression, which is characterized by cyclic recurrence of mania alternating with depression. The side effects, which can be minimized by monitoring serum lithium levels, include polyuria; fine hand tremor; thirst; and in more severe cases, slurred speech, ataxia, nausea, vomiting, and diarrhea. Patients undergoing lithium therapy should be observed for signs of overdose toxicity, which may be exhibited by CNS symptoms, including muscle rigidity, hyperactive deep reflexes, excessive tremor, and muscle fasciculations. Because lithium is handled in the body like sodium, changes in sodium levels can affect lithium levels. Salt intake and sweating can also change lithium levels. Some nonsteroidal antiinflammatory drugs (NSAIDs) can decrease lithium clearance, leading to an increase in lithium levels (Box 17-4). A patient's serum lithium levels

---

BOX 17-4	MANAGEMENT OF THE DENTAL PATIENT TAKING LITHIUM

- Monitor toxicity related to lithium levels; sweating and salt intake can alter levels.
- Tremors may interfere with oral hygiene.
- Drowsiness additive with other CNS depressants.
- Xerostomia or excessive salivation reported.
- Naproxen (other NSAIDs) can produce lithium toxicity.

CNS, Central nervous system; *NSAIDs,* nonsteroidal antiinflammatory drugs.

---

before, during, and after taking naproxen are illustrated in Figure 5-10.

Anticonvulsants

In the treatment of bipolar depression (mania), several anticonvulsant agents have been used. The manic phase has been treated with anticonvulsants such as carbamazepine, valproate, and gabapentin. Valproate and carbamazepine are approved by the Food and Drug Administration (FDA) for treating bipolar disorder. Valproate is used more often than lithium because of its more tolerable side effect profile.

Atypical Antipsychotics

Most recently, all of the atypical antipsychotics have been approved for the treatment of bipolar disorder, as well as for the acute treatment of bipolar disorder. Olanzapine and aripiprazole are approved for relapse prevention of bipolar disorder.

DENTAL HYGIENE CONSIDERATIONS

1. Some patients are still reluctant to state that they have a mental health illness.
2. Ask questions pertaining to mental health in a nonthreatening manner.
3. Remind the patient that all information is confidential and the intent of gathering information is to ensure that the patient receives the necessary oral health care.
4. Determine which medications the patient is taking. Many medications used to treat psychiatric disorders can affect oral health care. There are also many drug interactions that could occur with medications prescribed in a dental practice.
5. Check the patient's blood pressure and pulse at each office visit because many of the medications can cause orthostatic hypotension or tachycardia.
6. Review Boxes 17-2, 17-3, and 17-4.

CLINICAL SKILLS ASSESSMENT

1. State the major pharmacologic effect of the conventional antipsychotics.
2. State the adverse reactions attributable to the conventional antipsychotics.
3. Explain the drug interactions between epinephrine and the conventional antipsychotics and epinephrine and the tricyclic antidepressants. State which is clinically significant.

4. Describe two advantages of the atypical antipsychotics.

5. List three adverse reactions associated with the tricyclic antidepressants.

6. State the agent used in the treatment of poisoning by tricyclic antidepressants.

7. Name a second-generation antidepressant and describe two advantages and two disadvantages.

8. State the advantages and disadvantages of the SSRIs over the TCAs.

9. Describe two advantages of the atypical antidepressants over the TCAs.

10. Name the agent used to treat bipolar affective disorders and describe its effect on saliva.

11. Describe the effect of the NSAIDs on lithium.

⊝volve

18 Autocoids and Antihistamines

LEARNING OBJECTIVES

1. Define *histamine* and discuss its pharmacologic effects, adverse reactions, and uses.
2. Describe the dental implications, pharmacologic effects, adverse reactions, toxicity, and uses of the antihistamines.
3. Name and discuss the mechanism of action of nonsedating H_1-receptor antagonists.
4. Categorize the prostaglandins and thromboxanes and outline their pharmacologic effects, uses, and dental implications.
5. List several other types of autocoids and describe how they work.

The term **autocoids** is derived from the Greek *autos* (self) and *akos* (remedy). Although the agents in this class possess widely differing pharmacologic actions, they all occur naturally in the body, are produced by many tissues, and are formed by the tissues on which they act.

The autocoid agonists or antagonists include the H_1- and H_2-receptor antagonists (H_1-RA) or blockers, the eicosanoids (prostaglandins [PGs], thromboxanes [TXs], and leukotrienes [LTs]), serotonin agonists, angiotensin inhibitors, and cytokinins. As research on these agents continues, the agonists and their potential antagonists hold great promise for future therapy in many different areas. In fact, LT antagonists (see Chapter 22) are new drugs used for the management of asthma.

HISTAMINE

Histamine is a ubiquitous biogenic amine. Although many of its peripheral actions are well known, its precise physiologic function, particularly in the central nervous system (CNS), is not clear. The structure of histamine is seen in Figure 18-1.

Almost all mammalian tissues contain or can synthesize histamine. In humans, histamine is stored in the mast cells in the intestinal mucosa and in the CNS. When an allergic reaction occurs, the **mast cells** degranulate and histamine is released.

Histamine is released from the tissues in the body by normal reactions, abnormal reactions, or the administration of certain drugs. The amount of histamine released in these reactions determines the effects seen in the patient.

Pharmacologic Effects

In humans, histamine causes the following effects:
    H_1-agonist effects
- Vasodilation
- Increased capillary permeability
- Bronchoconstriction
- Pain or itching in cutaneous nerve endings

    H_2-agonist effects
- Increased gastric acid secretion

With the synthesis of agents that can block some of the effects of histamine, new pharmacologic agents have been developed. The histamine receptors are

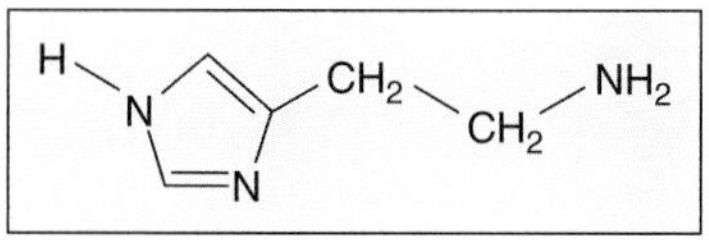

FIGURE 18-1
The structure of histamine.

termed H_1 and H_2. Some evidence of an H_3-receptor exists. The H_1-receptors are primarily related to vasodilation, increased capillary permeability, bronchoconstriction, and pain or itching at the nerve endings (the first four items on the preceding list). The H_2-receptors are responsible for stimulating gastric acid secretion (the last item on the preceding list) and will be reviewed in Chapter 22. The action of the H_3-receptor is unknown.

Histamine's actions are mediated by activation of H_1-receptors, H_2-receptors, or other receptors. Agents that block or antagonize the effects of histamine at the H_1-receptors are referred to as *H_1-blockers* or *H_1-receptor antagonists* (H_1-RA), and at the H_2-receptors they are H_2-blockers or *H_2-receptor antagonists* (H_2-RA).

Adverse Reactions

When an allergic reaction occurs, an antigen-antibody reaction causes the release of histamine and other autocoids. Anaphylaxis is a serious and sometimes fatal reaction to a foreign protein or drug introduced into the body. Difficulty in breathing, convulsions, lapses into unconsciousness, and death can ensue. The predominant feature in this syndrome is bronchoconstriction.

In addition to bronchoconstriction, the action of histamine during an anaphylactic reaction includes vasodilation and increased capillary permeability, both of which lead to decreased blood pressure followed by shock and cardiovascular collapse. Other symptoms of anaphylaxis include apprehension, paresthesia, urticaria, edema, choking, cyanosis, coughing, and wheezing. Fever, shock, loss of consciousness, coma, convulsions, and death may result.

Although the treatment of anaphylaxis is described in Chapter 23, it is discussed here in relation to its cause. The drug of choice for anaphylaxis is parenteral epinephrine, a physiologic antagonist (epinephrine dilates bronchioles via the β_2-receptors) rather than an antihistamine, which is a pharmacologic antagonist (antihistamine blocks the bronchoconstriction produced by histamine at the same H_1-receptor). The reason for this is that antihistamines antagonize only some of the effects of histamine, and they work competitively, whereas epinephrine acts as a direct β_2-agonist.

Uses

There are no established clinical uses for histamine.

ANTIHISTAMINES (H_1-RECEPTOR ANTAGONISTS)

The common term *antihistamine* refers to agents that are H_1-receptor antagonists or H_1-blockers. They are widely used drugs, and dental practitioners should be familiar with them for the following reasons:

- Many patients have seasonal allergic reactions (e.g., hay fever) that make dental treatment difficult. The dentist may prescribe, or the patient may self-medicate with antihistamines

before a dental procedure to reduce the symptoms of hay fever and make it easier for the patient to breathe.
- A mild allergic reaction to a drug may be treated with antihistamines in the dental office. If the allergic reaction is severe, epinephrine is the drug of choice.
- Patients taking antihistamines may experience side effects, such as xerostomia, but the newer nonsedating antihistamines have less anticholinergic effect.
- Antihistamines interact with many other drug groups and are additive with other CNS depressants.

Pharmacologic Effects

The older H_1-receptor antagonists, also called *H_1-blockers,* have several pharmacologic effects, including antihistaminic, anticholinergic, antiserotonergic, and sedative effects. Because they have a chemical structure similar to that of histamine, they can bind with the H_1-receptor and prevent or block the action of histamine (if it is released). Table 18-1 gives the chemical groups of various antihistamines, some examples of each group, and the properties of each group.

Figure 18-2 compares the relative sedative, antihistaminic, and anticholinergic effects of five common antihistamines: brompheniramine (brome-fen-EER-a meen) (Dimetane), chlorpheniramine (klor-fen-EER-a-meen) (Chlor-Trimeton), diphenhydramine (dye-fen-HYE-dra-meen) (Benadryl), fexofenadine (feks-oh-FEN-a-deen) (Allegra), and loratadine (lor-A-ti-deen) (Claritin). One should note that some antihistamines are effective for nausea and that some have more anticholinergic effects (more xerostomia).

The pharmacologic effects of antihistamines can be divided into those caused by blocking histamine at the H_1-receptor and those independent of this effect.

◆ H_1-RECEPTOR BLOCKING EFFECTS

Counteracts histamine's effects

Antihistamines, which are H_1-antagonists, competitively block or antagonize histamine's effect at the following sites:

- *Capillary permeability:* By blocking capillary permeability produced by histamine, less tissue edema occurs from the transport of the serum into the intracellular spaces.
- *Vascular smooth muscle (vessels):* The antihistamines block the dilation of the vascular smooth muscle that histamine produces.
- *Nonvascular (bronchial) smooth muscle:* Because other autocoids are also released in an anaphylactic reaction, antihistamines are not effective in counteracting all the bronchoconstriction present during that reaction.
- *Nerve endings:* Antihistamines can suppress the itching and pain associated with this histamine-mediated reaction at the cutaneous nerve endings.

◆ OTHER EFFECTS (UNRELATED TO H_1-BLOCKING EFFECTS)

Central Nervous System Effects. The antihistamines produce varying degrees of CNS depression. Because diphenhydramine produces a high degree of sedation, it is the principal agent used in over-the-counter (OTC) sleep aids (Sominex, Nytol). It is less expensive as an antihistamine than as a sleep aid.

Anticholinergic Effects. An anticholinergic effect (cholinergic blockade), weaker than but similar to that of atropine, can be

TABLE 18-1   ANTIHISTAMINES

Drug Name	Single Adult Dose	Dosing Interval (hr)	Sedative Effects*	Antihistamine Activity*	Anticholinergic Activity*	Antiemetic Effects*
Ethanolamines						
Diphenhydramine (Benadryl)†	25-50 mg	6-8	+++	+/++	+++	++/+++
Clemastine (Tavist)	1 mg	12	++	+/++	+++	++/+++
Ethylenediamines						
Tripelennamine (PBZ)	25-50 mg	4-6	++	+/++	+	−
Alkylamines						
Chlorpheniramine† (Chlor-Trimeton)	4 mg	4-6	+	++	++	−
Brompheniramine (Dimetane)†	4-8 mg	4-6	+	+++	++	−
Piperidines						
Cyproheptadine (Periactin)	4 mg	8	+	++	++	−
Piperazines						
Hydroxyzine (Vistaril, Atarax)	25-100 mg	4-8	++/+++	++	+++	−
Nonsedating Antihistamines						
Acrivastine	8 mg	4-6	±	++/+++	±	−
Azelastine (Astelin) Nasal Spray	137 µg	12	−	++/+++	−	−
Cetirizine (Zyrtec)‡	5-10 mg	24	++	++/+++	±	−
Desloratadine (Clarinex)	5	24	±	++/+++	±	−
Fexofenadine (Allegra)‡	120 mg	12	±	++/+++	±	−
	180 mg	24				
Loratadine (Claritin)‡	10 mg	24	±	++/+++	±	

*++++, Very high; +++, high; ++, moderate; +, low; ±, may have some effect; −, no effect.
†Available over-the-counter.
‡Also available in combination with pseudoephedrine.

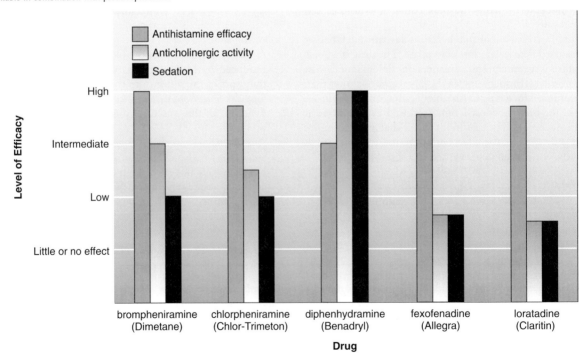

FIGURE 18-2
Comparison of efficacy and adverse effects of selected antihistamines. (From Lilley LL, Harrington S, Snyder JS: *Pharmacology and the nursing process,* ed 5, St Louis, 2007, Mosby.)

used to "dry up" secretions when treating the symptoms of certain upper respiratory diseases (allergies, "cold"). A potential disadvantage with the anticholinergic effect is that secretions may be "dried up" and more difficult to clear.

Antiemetic Effects. Some antihistamines, such as meclizine (Dramamine, Bonine), have pronounced antiemetic or anti–motion sickness activity. These agents are also effective in controlling the dizziness, nausea, and vomiting that occurs with vertigo.

Antihistamines with antiemetic effects may be useful in dentistry to manage postoperative nausea and vomiting, especially when opioid agents have been used. The antihistamines that have phenothiazine-like action, such as promethazine, are the most effective antiemetics.

Local Anesthesia. Although antihistamines are not as effective as the other local anesthetics, they can be administered topically or by injection to provide some local anesthesia.

Adverse Reactions

Like the pharmacologic effects of the antihistamines, the adverse reactions vary in relative amounts among the different agents. Figure 18-2 shows how adverse reactions and pharmacologic effects vary among antihistamines.

◆ CENTRAL NERVOUS SYSTEM DEPRESSION

CNS depression can be either a pharmacologic effect (the wanted effect) or an adverse reaction (the unwanted effect), depending on the use. Sedation is the most common side effect associated with the older antihistamines, and it may be accompanied by dizziness, tinnitus, incoordination, blurred vision, and fatigue. Patients who are given antihistamines should be warned against operating a motor vehicle or signing important documents. Sedation with antihistamines is additive with that caused by other CNS depressant drugs.

As with all drugs that depress the CNS, stimulation or excitation can occur in a few cases. Symptoms include restlessness, excitation, and, in severe cases, convulsions. It is more common in children, elderly patients, and those who use a larger dose than prescribed. The newer nonsedating H_1-blockers, such as loratadine (Claritin), produce less sedation because they do not penetrate the brain as easily.

When antihistamines are combined with decongestants (adrenergic agents), the antihistamine-related CNS depression is counteracted by the CNS stimulation of the decongestants. The planned result is for each agent's CNS effects to cancel out the other's effects.

Many antihistamine-decongestant combinations are marketed for treatment of colds or sinus problems. They are available OTC and by prescription

◆ GASTROINTESTINAL EFFECTS

The gastrointestinal complaints commonly associated with the antihistamines include anorexia, nausea, vomiting, and constipation. Xerostomia is categorized as an anticholinergic adverse reaction. The H_2-blockers (see Chapter 22), not the H_1-blockers, antagonize histamine's effect on the secretion of stomach acid.

◆ ANTICHOLINERGIC EFFECTS

Anticholinergic: xerostomia

The H_1-receptor antagonists have varying anticholinergic effects. The importance to the dental health care worker is that anticholinergic effects lead to xerostomia and xerostomia leads to numerous dental problems. Xerostomia can cause an increased caries rate in patients taking antihistamines on a long-term basis. In patients taking chronic antihistamines, the mouth should be observed for symptoms of xerostomia and counseling about techniques to manage it should be presented.

The nonsedating antihistamines have much less anticholinergic effect and are less likely to produce xerostomia. Loratadine (Claritin) is a heavily advertised nonsedating antihistamine.

Toxicity

Antihistamine poisoning has become more common in recent years because of the easy accessibility of the agents in OTC preparations promoted as sleep aids. Excitation predominates in small children, and sedation can occur in adults. Death usually results from coma with cardiovascular and respiratory collapse. The treatment is directed at specific symptoms.

Uses

◆ ALLERGIC REACTIONS

Certain allergic reactions, such as allergic rhinitis and seasonal hay fever, can be controlled by antihistamines. With continued use, tolerance can develop to the effects of a particular antihistamine. Changing to an agent in another chemical group can often restore the effects desired. These agents are less useful in the treatment of the common cold. Some people like the anticholinergic effect on secretions and want all their secretions to stop.

Acute urticarial attacks can be treated with antihistamines to relieve itching, edema, and erythema. In the treatment of anaphylaxis, the physiologic antagonist epinephrine rather than the antihistamines is indicated first. The xanthines (aminophylline) are also more effective than the antihistamines in producing bronchodilation in acute anaphylaxis. Because antihistamines produce some local anesthetic effect when applied topically, certain painful oral lesions can be treated with topical antihistamines. For example, with discomfort, the patient may swish and swirl diphenhydramine liquid inside the mouth.

◆ NAUSEA AND VOMITING

Because of the antiemetic action of some antihistamines, they are used to prevent and treat motion sickness and to control postoperative vomiting and vomiting induced by radiation therapy. The nausea and vomiting associated with pregnancy should not be treated with antihistamines because of these agents' alleged potential for fetal harm.

◆ PREOPERATIVE SEDATION

The use of the older H_1-antihistamines in dentistry is primarily based on their CNS effects. They are used for preoperative sedation because of their sedative and antiemetic effects. Hydroxyzine and promethazine are useful for this purpose (see Table 18-1). Their antiemetic actions can be helpful to counteract the adverse effect of the opioids.

◆ OVER-THE-COUNTER SLEEP AIDS

Diphenhydramine (Nytol) is used in products that are sold as OTC sleep aids.

◆ LOCAL ANESTHESIA

Although not as effective as the local anesthetics usually used, an antihistamine such as diphenhydramine (Benadryl) can be used by injection to provide some local anesthesia. This may be necessary when patients have exhibited allergies to the normally used local anesthetic agents.

PERIPHERAL (NONSEDATING) H₁-RECEPTOR ANTAGONISTS

Chemically, members of the nonsedating H₁-receptor antagonists do not have any common denominator. They are different in origin, chemical structure, solubility, and metabolic effects. They all share the specific blocking action of peripheral H₁-receptors. Because they do not cross the blood-brain barrier in usual therapeutic doses, they do not produce sedation (really, they are less likely to produce sedation). Table 18-1 lists the nonsedating antihistamines. Often, both sedating and nonsedating antihistamines are combined with a decongestant to treat nasal congestion along with the signs and symptoms of allergic response.

Peripheral (nonsedating) antihistamines have become valuable adjuncts in the therapy of seasonal and perennial rhinitis and certain forms of urticaria. It is likely that these agents will eventually replace the older H₁-receptor antagonists for these conditions. In the treatment of dental patients, however, the place of the older H₁-receptor blockers is ensured because these compounds are used as much for their side effects (sedation, potentiation of opioids, reduced nausea) as for their antihistaminic action. Many of them also come as a combination product with a decongestant.

Fexofenadine

Fexofenadine (Allegra) is an active metabolite of terfenadine (Seldane) and was developed by the manufacturer of terfenadine (Seldane) to replace it. Terfenadine was found to be responsible for cardiac arrhythmias and changes in the electrocardiogram (ECG) secondary to other drugs that inhibited its metabolism, and as a result, it was withdrawn from the market.

Because fexofenadine does not cross the blood-brain barrier to any appreciable degree, the potential for sedation is greatly reduced. Side effects include drowsiness and viral infections. It has little of the anticholinergic effects exhibited by the traditional H₁-blockers. Both erythromycin and ketoconazole increase the level of fexofenadine (by inhibiting its metabolism), but no clinical manifestations have been noted. Whether interactions will occur with other imidazoles or macrolides (clarithromycin, azithromycin) must be determined. Its onset of action is about 1 hour, and its time to peak serum concentration is 2.6 hours. Its duration of action is at least 12 hours, and its half-life is 14.4 hours. About 20% is metabolized in the liver and excreted in the urine, and 80% is excreted in the feces. Its dose is 60 mg twice a day.

Loratadine

Loratadine (lor-AT-i-deen) (Claritin), another nonsedating antihistamine, has similar action to the other drugs in this group. Its onset is 1 to 3 hours, its peak effect is 8.4 to 28 hours, its duration of action is 24 hours, and its half-life is 12 to 15 hours.

It is extensively metabolized to an active metabolite. Adverse reactions include headache, somnolence (less than 10%), fatigue, and xerostomia.

Desloratadine

Desloratadine (Clarinex) is the active metabolite of loratadine and is a nonsedating H₁-receptor blocker. It is also dosed once daily. Side effects include fatigue, dry mouth, headache, and gastrointestinal disturbances.

Cetirizine

Cetirizine (se-TI-ra-zeen) (Zyrtec) is another nonsedating H₁-receptor blocker. Its onset of action is usually less than ½ hour, and it peaks in about 1 hour. Its half-life is 8 hours. The intense competition among the companies selling nonsedating antihistamines is brutal. It is also available without a prescription.

Acrivastine

Acrivastine (Semprex) is another nonsedating antihistamine that has similar actions to the other drugs in this group. Its onset of action is less than 30 minutes. It is dosed twice a day. Adverse effects are minimal.

Azelastine

Azelastine (Astelin) is a nonsedating antihistamine and mast cell stabilizer that is available as a nasal spray and as eye drops. Adverse effects include bitter taste, headache, rhinitis, nose bleeds, and nasal burning.

OTHER AUTOCOIDS

Prostaglandins and Thromboxanes

The prostaglandins (PGs) and thromboxanes (TXs) are members of a group of biologically active agents termed *eicosanoids*.

Other members of this group include the leukotrienes (LTs), lipoxins, hydroperoxyeicosatetraenoic acids (HPETEs), hydroxyeicosatetraenoic acids (HETEs), and epoxyeicosatetraenoic acids (EETEs). The PGs and TXs have been found in most body tissues and fluids. They are produced in the body in response to many different stimuli, and small quantities produce a large spectrum of effects on many different body systems.

The family of PGs is divided into six main series of agents: A, B, C, D, E, and F, of which the last two (E and F) are predominant. These main groups are further subdivided and give rise to an extensive and complicated series of compounds. The subscript numbers (1, 2, and 3) following the letters indicate the degree of unsaturation. The α or β refers to the spatial configuration of the carbon 9 hydroxyl group (e.g., PGF₂α).

Until recently, PGEs and PGFs were the most abundant and most intensively studied PGs. Now, many new PGs (e.g., PGG and PGH), TXs (e.g., TXA and TXB), and prostacyclin (PGI) have become the central interest.

Because the individual PGs have many activities, it is unlikely that they have a single receptor. They are released by mechanical, thermal, chemical, bacterial, or traumatic injuries.

◆ PHARMACOLOGIC EFFECTS

The pharmacologic effects of the PGs encompass many diverse actions. Not only is there a wide spectrum of action, but different PGs have different activities in different tissue. As PG agonists or antagonists are identified, the number and range of actions in the body will be increased. Some currently known effects of the PGs include the following.

Smooth Muscle Effects. Vascular smooth muscle may be either relaxed (vasodilation) or stimulated (vasoconstriction) depending on the specific PGs. The effect of PGs on the gastrointestinal tract is to produce cramping (increased motility). Their effect on the uterus is to cause contraction, especially in the near-term uterus.

Platelets. Another example of the opposing actions of different PGs is TX and PGI. TX, produced by platelets, stimulates platelet aggregation and is a vasoconstrictor, whereas PGI, produced by the vessel walls, inhibits platelet aggregation and is a vasodilator. Fine gradations of action in the body can be elicited using this mechanism in which two different chemicals produce the opposite effect. If secretion of one of the paired autocoids is increased, then the desired action is produced. Conversely, secretion of the other autocoid produces the opposite effect. In addition, antagonists to these autocoids block their normal effects. For adjusting one particular effect, there may be both agonist and antagonist effects for each autocoid. This "system" to modulate adequate coagulation can be modified by adding a drug. Adding of aspirin can alter the clinical outcome. Even altering the dose of aspirin can produce different effects (low dose and high dose).

Effects on Reproductive Organs. PGs are abundant in the semen, but their role is unknown. Both PGE and PGF have oxytocic (uterine contraction) action, making them useful as abortifacients in the second trimester and as inducers of labor at full term.

Central Nervous System Effects. PGs increase body temperature by releasing interleukin-1, which promotes the release and synthesis of PGE. PGEs stimulate the release of hormones such as growth hormone, prolactin, thyroid-stimulating hormone (TSH), adrenocorticotropic hormone (ACTH), follicle-stimulating hormone (FSH), and luteinizing hormone (LH).

Other Effects. These include increased heart rate and cardiac output, increased capillary permeability, increased renal blood flow, sedation, and stimulation of pain fibers.

◆ DENTAL IMPLICATIONS

Prostaglandins are related to periodontal disease.

The PGs are important in dentistry because they have been implicated in periodontal disease. At least two stages of periodontal disease may involve PGs. The first is the inflammation of the gingiva with its resultant erythema, edema, and increase in gingival exudate. PGs, thought to be mediators of the inflammatory response in oral soft tissues, may be involved in this initial stage of periodontal disease. The second is the resorption of alveolar bone with tooth loss. PGs also prevent the synthesis of new bone by inhibiting osteoblastic activity. This explains the reason the use of nonsteroidal antiinflammatory drugs (NSAIDs) in the management of periodontal disease is being explored.

Newer research concerning the etiology of periodontal disease has discovered more correlations among different factors. Certainly, several autocoids, such as PGs, LTs, and cytokines, have been found to be involved in the production of periodontal disease.

◆ USES

One therapeutic use of the PGs is inducing midtrimester abortions. PGs are administered by intraamniotic injection (a salt of PGF) or vaginal suppository (PGE analog). For very early abortions, PGE analogs are combined with antiprogestins (mifepristone [Mifeprex] or RU-486) in an oral dose form currently available in France and the United States. A PG agonist (misoprostol [Cytotec]) is available for the prevention of NSAID-induced ulcers. PGE is cytoprotective at low doses. Currently, PGs are being studied in the treatment of bronchial asthma and hypertension.

◆ PROSTAGLANDIN ANTAGONISTS

The administration of PG antagonists may prove useful in the treatment of certain pathologic conditions. This seems reasonable in view of the many effects of the PGs in the body. For example, aspirin can inhibit platelet aggregation by blocking TX (which promotes aggregation). Indomethacin, an NSAID, blocks the effect of the PGs on the ductus arteriosus (PGs keep the ductus arteriosus open). After birth, if the ductus arteriosus does not close, indomethacin given intravenously can close the ductus, thereby making open heart surgery unnecessary. There is also some evidence that certain phenolic compounds, such as eugenol (clove oil), dentistry's poultice, inhibit PG. Because PGs are involved in inflammation, agents that inhibit the PGs may be useful in the treatment of inflammation.

Leukotrienes

Leukotrienes have a role in allergy and inflammation.

LTs are another complex group of autocoids that are also derived from arachidonic acid. They were formerly called *slow-reacting substance(s) of anaphylaxis* (SRS-A). Although they show considerable species variation, their dominant action in humans is powerful bronchoconstriction. In that effect, LTs are far more potent than histamines. They also contract other smooth muscle such as the uterus and gastrointestinal tract. Extensive research is devoted to these substances, and great progress can be expected, potentially in the treatment of asthma and other forms of bronchoconstriction.

Kinins

Kinins are polypeptides that are distributed in a great variety of body tissues. Two members of this group, kallidin and bradykinin, are found in plasma and may play a role in dental diseases. These agents are formed by the action of certain proteolytic enzymes (kininogenases), such as kallikrein, on their common precursor, kininogen. Other kininogenases include trypsin, plasmin, and certain snake venoms. There are at least two receptors for bradykinin: the B_1-receptor and the B_2-receptor. The "B" in these receptors stands for bradykinin; they are not to be confused with the β-adrenergic receptors present in the sympathetic autonomic nervous system.

The plasma kinins may be involved in shock and acute or chronic allergic or inflammatory conditions such as anaphylaxis and arthritis. Their effects on the body include vasodilation, increased capillary permeability, edema, pain resulting from action on nerve endings, and contraction or relaxation of nonvascular smooth muscles. The kinins apparently mediate pulpal pain and are implicated in the control of the synthesis of endogenous analgesics, particularly the endorphins, during caries formation. It is possible that inhibitors of kinins may be useful dental therapeutic aids in the future.

Although no specific antagonists of the kinins are yet available, some drugs are known to inhibit kinin-evoked responses. For example, salicylates (aspirin) and glucocorticoids (steroids) inhibit kallikrein activation and may play a role in future therapy.

The synthesis of antagonists to the autocoid kinins and their possible clinical use are currently being investigated.

Substance P

Substance P is a peptide thought to function as a neurotransmitter in the CNS and a local hormone in the gastrointestinal tract. It is a vasodilator and produces hypotension. It increases the action of the intestinal and bronchial smooth muscle. It also causes secretion in the salivary glands and an increase in sodium and water excretion from the kidney. Substance P may be a transmitter that is released from unmyelinated fibers that respond to pain. It is also involved in many other functions because it is present in areas of the brain that are not involved in pain.

DENTAL HYGIENE CONSIDERATIONS

1. Obtain a detailed medication history in order to avoid drug interactions.
2. First-generation, and to a lesser extent second-generation, antihistamines can cause sedation.
3. The combination of sedating antihistamines with opioid analgesics or antianxiety drugs can increase the patient's risk for sedation.
4. Instruct the patient to avoid driving or any other task that requires thought or concentration if a sedating antihistamine is necessary.
5. First-generation antihistamines can cause significant xerostomia.
6. Instruct the patient to drink plenty of water and to chew tart, sugarless gum or candy in order to avoid or minimize xerostomia.
7. Remind the patient that caffeinated beverages and alcohol can exacerbate xerostomia.
8. Remind the patient that even though fruit juices may help with xerostomia, they put the patient at increased risk for caries.

CLINICAL SKILLS ASSESSMENT

1. What are first-generation antihistamines and how do they work?
2. What are the pharmacologic effects of first-generation antihistamines?
3. What are the adverse reactions associated with first-generation antihistamines? Can they lead to toxicity?
4. What would the dental practitioner tell a patient about adverse reactions with a special emphasis on those with dental implications?
5. What are the drug interactions associated with first-generation antihistamines that are of dental concern?
6. What is the mechanism of action of second-generation antihistamines?
7. What are the adverse reactions of second-generation antihistamines?
8. What are the advantages of second-generation antihistamines over first-generation antihistamines?

⊖volve

Please visit http://evolve.elsevier.com/Haveles/pharmacology for review questions and additional practice and reference materials.

19 Adrenocorticosteroids

LEARNING OBJECTIVES

1. Define adrenocorticosteroids and describe how the body releases them.
2. Summarize the classification, administration, mechanism of action, and pharmacologic effects of adrenocorticosteroids.
3. Describes the various adverse reactions and uses of adrenocorticosteroids, including their application to dentistry.
4. Differentiate several examples of corticosteroids.
5. List several dental implications to the use of steroids.

The term *adrenocorticosteroids* (a-dree-noe-KOR-ti-KO-ster-oids) (adrenal cortico-steroids, adrenocorticoids, corticosteroids, or steroids) refers to a group of agents secreted by the adrenal cortex. The dental team should be aware of the effects, adverse reactions, and dental implications of these agents for at least the following reasons:

- *Use in dentistry:* These compounds are used topically or systemically for the treatment of oral lesions associated with inflammatory diseases.
- *Long-term therapy:* The adrenocorticosteroids, or *steroids* as they are commonly called, are prescribed for many patients with chronic systemic diseases such as asthma or arthritis. If taken chronically in high enough doses, these agents can cause a variety of adverse reactions that may influence the patient's dental treatment.

MECHANISM OF RELEASE

| Negative feedback mechanism |

The adrenocorticosteroids are naturally occurring compounds secreted by the adrenal cortex. Their release is triggered by a series of events (Figure 19-1). First, a stimulus such as stress (1) causes the hypothalamus (2) to release corticotropin-releasing hormone (CRH) (3), which acts on the pituitary gland (4). Under the influence of CRH, the pituitary gland secretes adrenocorticotropic hormone (ACTH) (5), which stimulates the adrenal cortex (6) to release hydrocortisone (7). Hydrocortisone then acts on both the pituitary (8) and the hypothalamus (9) to inhibit the release of CRH and ACTH, respectively. This mechanism is called negative feedback. Exogenous steroids act in the same way as hydrocortisone (10); that is, they inhibit the release of CRH and ACTH. With long-term administration of steroids, ACTH release is suppressed and the adrenal gland atrophies. If the administration of the exogenous steroid is then abruptly stopped, a relative steroid deficiency results. This can cause severe problems, including adrenal crisis.

CLASSIFICATION

| Glucocorticoids, mineralocorticoids |

The adrenocorticosteroids can be divided into two major groups: the glucocorticoids, which affect intermediate carbohydrate metabolism, and the mineralocorticoids, which affect the water and electrolyte composition of the body. The major glucocorticoid present in the body is cortisol (hydrocortisone). Without stress, the normal adult secretes about 20 mg of hydrocortisone daily. A tenfold increase can occur with stress. Maximal secretion occurs between 4 AM and 8 AM in people with a normal schedule. The chemical structures of the synthetic agents and the naturally occurring adrenocorticosteroids, such as hydrocortisone, are similar. Many chemical modifications have been made in an attempt to produce synthetic glucocorticoids with fewer adverse reactions and more specific activity.

Although the term *adrenocorticosteroids* refers to those steroids secreted by the adrenal cortex and includes both the glucocorticoids and the mineralocorticoids, this chapter discusses primarily the action of glucocorticoids because of their more frequent use.

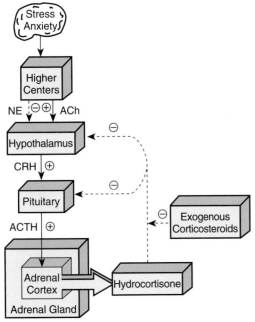

FIGURE 19-1

The body's release of adrenocorticoids. *ACh,* Acetylcholine pathways; *ACTH,* adrenocorticotropic hormone; *CRH,* corticotropin-releasing hormone; *NE,* norepinephrine pathways.

DEFINITIONS

The following terms are used in this chapter:
- *Addison's disease:* Disease/condition produced by a deficiency of adrenocorticosteroids
- *Adrenocorticosteroids/corticosteroids/steroids:* Steroidal components released from the adrenal cortex, including glucocorticoids and mineralocorticoids
- *Adrenocorticotropic hormone (ACTH):* Agent secreted by the pituitary that causes the release of hormones from the adrenal cortex
- *Cushing's syndrome:* Disease/condition produced by an excess of adrenocorticosteroids
- *Glucocorticoids:* Adrenocorticosteroids that primarily affect carbohydrate metabolism
- *Mineralocorticoids:* Adrenocorticosteroids that affect the body's sodium and water balance (fluid levels)

ROUTES OF ADMINISTRATION

Glucocorticoids are available in a wide variety of dose forms. They are routinely used topically, orally, intramuscularly, and intravenously. Systemic effects are commonly obtained when the drug is administered orally or parenterally, but topical administration may rarely cause systemic effects. If a large quantity of a steroid is applied topically, especially if the skin is denuded or an occlusive dressing such as plastic wrap is applied, systemic effects can occur. Table 19-1 shows the relative potency of selected topical corticosteroid products.

MECHANISM OF ACTION

| Effect has lag time. | The mechanism of action of the steroids involves binding to a specific receptor and forming a steroid-receptor complex. The complex then translocates into the nucleus and alters gene expression (turns genes on or off), resulting in the regulation of many cel-

TABLE 19-1	RELATIVE POTENCY OF SELECTED TOPICAL CORTICOSTEROID PRODUCTS		
Potency	Drug Generic (Trade)	Dose Form	Strength (%)
Super high	Clobetasol propionate (Temovate)	Cream, ointment	0.05
High	Fluocinolone acetonide (Lidex)	Cream	0.2
Medium	Triamcinolone acetonide (Aristocort, Flutex, Kenalog)	Ointment	0.1
Medium	Betamethasone valerate (Valisone)	Cream	0.1
Low	Fluocinolone acetonide (Synalar)	Cream, ointment	0.025
Low	Triamcinolone acetonide (Aristocort)	Cream, ointment, lotion	0.025
		Cream, ointment, lotion	0.1
		Cream, ointment	0.5
Low	Hydrocortisone (Cortaid, Anusol, Hytone, Dermacort, Penecort, Cetacort)	Lotion	0.25
		Cream, ointment, lotion, aerosol	0.5
		Solution	0.5
		Aerosol	1
		Cream, ointment, lotion	2.5

lular processes. Because of the mechanism, a lag time exists in the action of the steroids and the relationship between their effects and blood level is poor. Other effects of glucocorticoids are mediated by catecholamines producing vasodilation or bronchodilation.

Many effects

The antiinflammatory action of glucocorticoids results from their profound effects on the number, distribution, and function of peripheral leukocytes and to their inhibition of phospholipase A. The use of steroids results in an increase in the concentration of neutrophils and a decrease in the lymphocytes (T and B cells), monocytes, eosinophils, and basophils. Steroids induce the synthesis of a protein that inhibits phospholipase A, decreasing the production of both prostaglandins and leukotrienes from arachidonic acid.

These agents, responsible for the delayed phase of acute inflammation, act synergistically. Steroids also inhibit interleukin-2, migration inhibition factor, and macrophage inhibition factor.

PHARMACOLOGIC EFFECTS

The pharmacologic effects and the adverse reactions of corticosteroids are closely related (Figure 19-2). The effects for which they are used include their antiinflammatory action and suppression of allergic reactions. They also suppress the immune response. Corticosteroids are palliative rather than curative. The glucocorticoid effects and the mineralocorticoid effects are listed in Box 19-1. Many of these effects produce adverse reactions and are discussed in the following section.

ADVERSE REACTIONS

The adverse reactions of corticosteroids are proportional to the dose, frequency and time of administration, and duration of treatment. With prolonged therapy and sufficiently high doses, the following side effects occur.

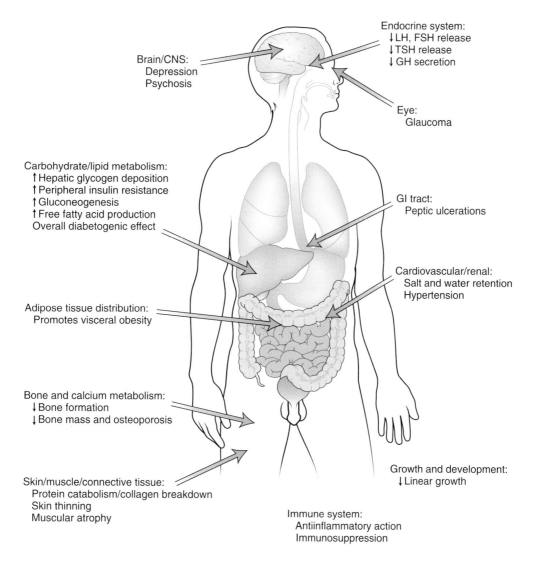

FIGURE 19-2

The principal sites of action of glucocorticoids in humans highlighting some of the consequences of glucocorticoid excess. *CNS,* Central nervous system; *GI,* gastrointestinal; *FSH,* follicle-stimulating hormone; *GH,* growth hormone; *LH,* luteinizing hormone; *TSH,* thyroid-stimulating hormone. (From Kronenberg HM, Melmed S, Polonsky KS, et al: *Williams' textbook of endocrinology,* ed 11, Philadelphia, 2008, Saunders.)

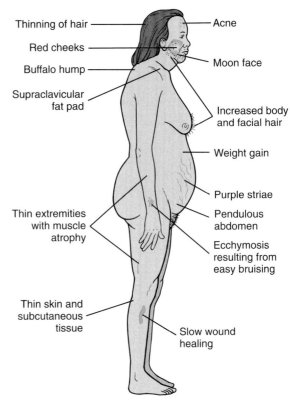

FIGURE 19-3

Body image alterations with glucocorticoid therapy. (From Lewis SM, Heitkemper MM, Dirksen SR: *Medical-surgical nursing: assessment and management of clinical problems,* ed 7, St Louis, 2007, Mosby.)

Metabolic Changes

Moon face (round), buffalo hump (fat deposited on back of the neck), truncal obesity, weight gain, and muscle wasting give patients the Cushing's syndrome appearance (Figure 19-3). Hyperglycemia (diabetes-like) may be aggravated or initiated, especially in prediabetic patients. More antidiabetic medication may be required.

Infections

Corticosteroids decrease resistance to infection. Because of their antiinflammatory action, they may also mask its symptoms. Patients taking long-term glucocorticoid therapy are given isoniazid, an antituberculosis agent, to prevent tuberculosis.

Central Nervous System Effects

Changes in behavior and personality, including euphoria (with increasing dose), agitation, psychoses, and depression (with decreasing dose), can occur.

Peptic Ulcer

Because corticosteroids stimulate an increase in production of stomach acid and pepsin, they may exacerbate peptic ulcers. Healing is impaired, and the ulcer may perforate.

Impaired Wound Healing and Osteoporosis

The catabolic effects of steroids that result from impaired synthesis of collagen can impair wound healing. This same process can cause osteoporosis or impair growth in children. If the osteoporosis affects alveolar bone, it could result in tooth loss. Thinning bones can also result in fractures in patients on chronic steroids without trauma. Muscle wasting, bruising, and abdominal striae are other symptoms associated with catabolism.

Ophthalmic Effects

Because corticosteroids can increase intraocular pressure, glaucoma may be exacerbated. Cataracts are also associated with steroids.

Electrolyte and Fluid Balance

Glucocorticoids that possess some mineralocorticoid action can produce sodium and water retention. Hypertension or congestive heart failure may be exacerbated. Hypokalemia may also result.

Adrenal Crisis

With prolonged use, adrenal suppression can occur. If a stressful situation arises, the adrenal gland cannot respond adequately. Symptoms of adrenal crisis include weakness, syncope, cardiovascular collapse, and death.

Dental Effects

Oral tissue changes may occur in patients taking corticosteroids. Their mucosal surfaces heal more slowly, are more likely to have infection, and are more friable. With the use of oral steroid inhalers for asthma, oral candidiasis may result. This may be prevented by rinsing the mouth after inhaler use.

USES

Medical Uses

There are many conditions for which corticosteroids may be administered (Box 19-2). Patients with these conditions should be questioned about past use of systemic steroids.

♦ REPLACEMENT

Patients with hypofunction of the adrenal cortex (Addison's disease) need replacement of glucocorticoid and mineralocorticoid activity. Usually, hydrocortisone is used to restore glucocorticoid activity and desoxycorticosterone is used to restore mineralocorticoid activity. Patients with a hyperfunctioning adrenal cortex (Cushing's syndrome) may have a majority of the gland removed surgically. In this case, replacement therapy is needed.

♦ EMERGENCIES

Corticosteroids are used in emergency situations for the treatment of shock or adrenal crisis, as discussed in Chapter 23.

♦ INFLAMMATION/ALLERGY

The most extensive use of the corticosteroids in both medicine and dentistry is in the treatment of a wide variety of inflammatory and allergic conditions. These agents are not curative but merely ameliorate symptoms because of their antiinflammatory activity. Some conditions that have been treated with corticosteroids are rheumatoid arthritis, rheumatic fever, systemic lupus erythematosus, scleroderma, inflammation of the joints and soft tissues, acute bronchial asthma, severe and acute allergic reactions, and severe allergic dermatoses. Prednisone (PRED-ni-sone) is the most common corticosteroid used orally.

Topical corticosteroids are used for
a variety of skin conditions, which

| Topical steroids |

involve various dermatoses or "irritations." The steroids can be divided into several classes depending on their relative maximum potency*: the least efficacious to the most efficacious and in between. An example of the weakest is hydrocortisone (hye-droe-KOR-ti-sone), an example of an "in between" is triamcinolone (trye-am-SIN-oh-lone) acetonide, and an example of the most potent is augmented betamethasone (bay-ta-METH-a-sone) dipropionate.

Dental Uses

Because of the adrenocorticosteroids' antiinflammatory action, they are administered topically, intraarticularly, or orally in several dental situations. The use of steroids in dentistry has had mixed success and double-blind controlled studies are needed to determine unequivocally their proper place in the therapeutic armamentarium.

♦ ORAL LESIONS

Systemically administered steroids are often effective in the treatment of oral lesions associated with noninfectious inflammatory diseases, including erythema multiforme, lichen planus, pemphigus, desquamative gingivitis, and benign mucous membrane pemphigoid. It is imperative that an infectious etiology, such as herpes, be ruled out.

♦ APHTHOUS STOMATITIS

The evidence for the benefit of adrenocorticosteroids in the treatment of aphthous stomatitis seems clear. Triamcinolone acetonide (Kenalog in Orabase) has been advocated. Orabase is a mineral oil gel base that sticks to the oral mucosa, forming a plasticlike surface. Other topical steroids, such as fluocinonide and fluocinolone (floo-oh-SIN-oh-lone), can be used topically.

♦ TEMPOROMANDIBULAR JOINT

The temporomandibular joint (TMJ) affected with arthritis (inflammation) also responds to the systemic administration of steroids. If only this joint is affected, an intraarticular injection can often decrease the pain and improve the joint movement.

♦ USES IN ORAL SURGERY

| Weigh pro versus con |

The adrenocorticosteroids have been used in oral surgery to reduce postoperative edema, trismus, and pain. Although the decrease in edema with steroid use can be easily documented, the magnitude of the benefit must be weighed against the potential risk of infection and decreased healing. The safety and effectiveness of these agents have not been proved in controlled double-blind studies.

♦ PULP PROCEDURES

The adrenocorticosteroids have been used in pulp capping, pulpotomy procedures, and the control of hypersensitive cervical dentin. Their use in these situations is currently empirical or experimental.

---

*Using the strict definition of potency and efficacy, the term *potency* as used to refer to topical steroids is really efficacy.

TABLE 19-2 SELECTED CORTICOSTEROIDS, ORAL

Group	Drug Name	ACTIVITY: Antiinflammatory	ACTIVITY: Retention	Equivalent Oral Dose (mg)
Short acting	Hydrocortisone (Cortisol)	1	1	20
	Prednisone (Deltasone)	4	0.3-0.5	5
	Methylprednisolone (Medrol)	5	0.3-0.5	4
Intermediate acting	Triamcinolone	5	0	4
	Prednisolone	4	0	5
Long acting	Dexamethasone	30	0	0.75
	Betamethasone	25	0	0.6-0.75

CORTICOSTEROID PRODUCTS

Selected synthetic corticosteroids are arranged in Table 19-2 according to their duration of action: short, intermediate, and long. The relative antiinflammatory and salt-retaining activity and equivalent oral dose are given, with hydrocortisone arbitrarily assigned the value of 1 for each activity. The other agents are then given values in relation to those of hydrocortisone. For example, prednisone, with an antiinflammatory activity of 4, has 4 times as much antiinflammatory action as hydrocortisone. Therefore only one-fourth as much prednisone is required to produce the same effect produced by hydrocortisone. The mineralocorticoid, or salt-retaining, properties of the glucocorticoids are also compared with those of hydrocortisone. For example, triamcinolone does not increase salt retention, whereas hydrocortisone does.

Table 19-2 lists the equivalent oral dose in milligrams based on 20 mg of hydrocortisone, the amount normally secreted daily by an adult without stress. One can see that 0.75 mg of dexamethasone or 5 mg of prednisone is approximately equivalent to 20 mg of hydrocortisone.

DENTAL IMPLICATIONS

Box 19-3 summarizes the management of dental patients taking steroids. Because steroids suppress immune reaction, with chronic administration of steroids, infections are more likely to occur and healing is delayed. These factors are important in dental patients, especially if a surgical procedure is to be performed. Because the symptoms of infection may be masked, the wound site should be carefully examined.

BOX 19-3 MANAGEMENT OF DENTAL PATIENT TAKING/WHO HAS TAKEN CORTICOSTEROIDS

Most dental patients taking steroids who are having normal dental treatment rendered DO NOT need additional corticosteroids. Supplemental steroids may be required if patient has severe dental fears or for major surgical procedures.

Precautions to Avoid Stress

Obtain good anesthesia
Check blood pressure
Provide postoperative analgesics (prn)

No Supplementation

Stop using >1 year ago
Dose <20 mg/day HC or 5 mg/day prednisone
Dose >40 mg/day HC or 10 mg/day prednisone
Duration of therapy <1 month
Every other day therapy
Topical use—rash, asthma inhaler, nose spray

May Need Supplementation

Dose 20-40 mg HC or 5-10 mg prednisone/day
Duration >2 weeks
Topical (above) in very large doses or over entire body
If supplementing—different regimens

- Double normal dose morning of appointment
- Double normal dose the day before, the day of, and 2 days after (depends on stress/pain level) appointment

HC, Hydrocortisone; *prn,* as needed.

Adverse Reactions

♦ GASTROINTESTINAL EFFECTS

Adrenocorticosteroids stimulate acid secretion; patients taking these agents should be given other ulcerogenic medications, such as the salicylates or the nonsteroidal antiinflammatory agents, with caution.

♦ BLOOD PRESSURE CHANGES

The blood pressure of patients taking corticosteroids should be measured because these agents can exacerbate hypertension. The more mineralocorticoid action, the more likely the agent is to raise blood pressure.

♦ GLAUCOMA

Other agents that can induce or exacerbate glaucoma, such as the anticholinergics, should be used with caution in patients taking adrenocorticosteroids.

♦ BEHAVIORAL CHANGES

A patient's bizarre behavior may be explained by the presence of, or withdrawal from, adrenocorticosteroids. Psychosis, euphoria, or depression might be seen.

♦ OSTEOPOROSIS

Dental radiographs may demonstrate osteoporosis in patients taking long-term adrenocorticosteroids. More than 50% bone loss is required to observe osteoporosis (radiographically). These patients are more likely to suffer fractures either with or without trauma.

◆ INFECTION

Because of the antiinflammatory activity of the adrenocorticosteroids, they may mask the symptoms of an infection. They decrease a patient's ability to fight infection by suppression of migration of polymorphonuclear leukocytes, thus reducing lymph system action.

◆ DELAYED WOUND HEALING

Because the adrenocorticosteroids cause delayed wound healing, special precautions should be taken when surgical procedures are performed in the oral cavity. Friability of the tissue also requires special care when closing wounds and extra sutures may be required.

◆ ADRENAL CRISIS

| Only with severe stress | The body releases corticosteroids and epinephrine from the adrenal gland when a person experiences stress. Under normal conditions, when the body sends a message (ACTH) to the adrenal gland, it is stimulated and secretes hydrocortisone. Because the adrenal gland of a normal person is regularly stimulated when the person experiences stress, the adrenal gland stays ready for a message to put out hydrocortisone. The body does not differentiate between the hydrocortisone (endogenous) it secretes and the hydrocortisone or prednisone (exogenous) given to a patient by any route. When a patient is taking chronic prednisone, the steroid provides negative feedback to the hypothalamus (reduces release of CRH) and the pituitary (reduces release of ACTH).

With prolonged administration of steroids, suppression of the hypothalamic-pituitary-adrenal axis occurs. With suppression, the body does not quickly respond to stress with release of hydrocortisone. Suppression is proportional to the potency of the agent, the dose of the agent, and the duration of administration. The longer the duration, the higher the dose, and the greater the potency of the steroid, the quicker the suppression occurs. Once suppression occurs, it can take weeks or months for the adrenal gland to respond normally. Without the proper response to stress, adrenal crisis is possible. The crisis occurs because of a relative lack of corticosteroids during stress, such as a dental appointment for a patient with dental phobia. It may be necessary to administer adrenal steroids before a stressful dental procedure to prevent crisis. A consultation with the patient's physician is helpful. Generally, low and very high (mega) doses do not present problems; problems may occur with mid-range doses.

◆ PERIODONTAL DISEASE

Steroids have actions that can contribute to periodontal disease. First, they interfere with the body's response to infection (inflammatory mediators are inhibited). Second, steroids can produce osteoporosis, which may reduce the bony support for the teeth.

Steroid Supplementation

| Maybe 5 to 10 mg prednisone/day | There are many ways of using supplemental steroids in patients who use chronic steroids and are to undergo a stressful dental procedure. One approach to determine if additional steroids are needed is diagrammed in Figure 19-4. With

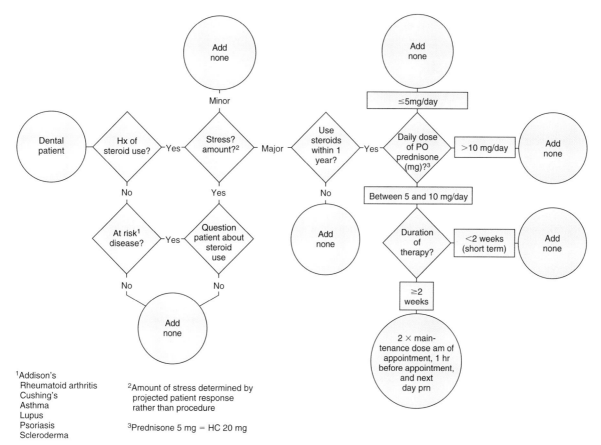

¹Addison's
  Rheumatoid arthritis
  Cushing's
  Asthma
  Lupus
  Psoriasis
  Scleroderma

²Amount of stress determined by
  projected patient response
  rather than procedure

³Prednisone 5 mg = HC 20 mg

FIGURE 19-4
Steroid decision tree. *PO,* Oral; *Hx,* history.

both low (<20 mg hydrocortisone or 5 mg prednisone) and very high doses (immunosuppressive; >40 to 60 mg hydrocortisone/day or 10 to 15 mg prednisone/day), no additional steroid supplementation is needed. With some intermediate doses of steroids (estimated to be between 20 and 40 mg/day hydrocortisone or 5 and 10 mg prednisone/day), additional steroids may be indicated if the procedure will produce severe stress.

After consultation with the patient's physician, one suggested regimen is to administer two to three times the patient's usual daily dose of steroids the day of the procedure and 1 hour before the surgery or procedure. If pain is expected to persist into the next day, then two times the usual daily dose of steroids should also be given the following day. Some authors state that steroid supplementation is only needed if severe stress is expected (evaluate dental anxiety and dental procedure severity). The patient should be evaluated for likelihood to experience stress based on the patient's degree of anxiety—not the specific procedure planned. Administering additional steroids for 1 or 2 days poses no additional risk above that produced by chronic use of steroids.

Topical Use

Steroids are used in dentistry to manage certain oral conditions, such as aphthous stomatitis, related to inflammatory or immune mechanisms. Both topical and systemic steroids are used in these instances. The relative potencies of selected topical glucocorticoids are listed in Table 19-1.

DENTAL HYGIENE CONSIDERATIONS

1. Obtain a detailed medication history in order to avoid drug interactions and adverse effects.
2. Obtain a detailed health history because corticosteroids can interfere with or exacerbate several medical illnesses.
3. Since corticosteroids can elevate blood pressure, it is important that the dental hygienist check the patient's blood pressure and pulse at each visit.
4. Encourage the patient to avoid the use of NSAIDs and aspirin since they can cause GI upset and ulcers. Corticosteroids also increase the risk for GI upset and ulcer.
5. Corticosteroids can cause behavioral changes that could interfere with the patient's ability to sit through an appointment. The appointment may need to be rescheduled if the patient can not cooperate.
6. Corticosteroids can mask the symptoms of infection and delay wound healing. Antibiotics may be necessary for patients using corticosteroids on a long-term basis.
7. Check for symptoms of osteoporosis of the jaw and bone because corticosteroids can increase the risk for osteoporosis.
8. Review the information in Box 19-3.

CLINICAL SKILLS ASSESSMENT

1. Compare and contrast the activity of the glucocorticoids and mineralocorticoids.
2. List the routes of administration for the steroids used in dentistry.
3. What are the dental concerns associated with steroids?
4. Are there any drug interactions to be aware of?
5. Describe the three major uses of the steroids in medicine.
6. Explain how to evaluate a patient undergoing therapy and how to determine whether the patient's physician should be consulted. State what problems could arise from dental treatment and how these adverse effects could be monitored.
7. Define the terms *Cushing's syndrome* and *Addison's disease*.
8. Both hypofunctioning and hyperfunctioning of the adrenal cortex require replacement therapy. What are the dental concerns regarding replacement therapy?

⊖volve

Please visit http://evolve.elsevier.com/Haveles/pharmacology for review questions and additional practice and reference materials.

20 Other Hormones

LEARNING OBJECTIVES

1. Outline the functions of the anterior and posterior glands.
2. Provide an overview of the thyroid hormones and the conditions known as *hypothyroidism* and *hyperthyroidism* and the antithyroid drugs.
3. Define diabetes mellitus, list and describe the two types of this disease, its complications, issues involving dentistry, cautions and contraindications in the treatment of patients with diabetes, and the effects of drugs on complications of diabetes.
4. Name and describe the types of drugs used to treat diabetes.
5. Summarize the major female and male sex hormones and name and describe several types of hormonal contraceptives.

Hormones are secreted by endocrine glands and transported by the blood to target organs, where they are biologically active. Endocrine glands include the pituitary, thyroid, parathyroids, pancreas, adrenals, gonads, and placenta (Figure 20-1). They help maintain homeostasis by regulating body functions and are controlled themselves by feedback systems. In most of these systems, the hormone released has a negative feedback effect on the secretion of the hormone stimulating substance. Patients being treated in the dental office may be taking these hormones to treat various diseases.

Drugs that affect the endocrine system include the hormones secreted by the endocrine glands, synthetic hormone agonists and antagonists, and substances that influence the synthesis and secretion of hormones. The most important clinical application of these drugs is their use in replacement therapy such as in the treatment of diabetes mellitus (DM) (insulin) and hypothyroidism (levothyroxine). Additional applications include diagnostic procedures, contraception, and the treatment of glandular hyperfunction, cancer, and other systemic disorders.

PITUITARY HORMONES

Pituitary: master gland

The pituitary gland (hypophysis) is a small endocrine organ located at the base of the brain. It has been called the *master gland* because of its regulatory effect on other endocrine glands and organs of the body. It secretes peptide hormones that regulate the thyroid, adrenal, and sex glands; the kidney and uterus; and growth.

In addition to their regulatory effect, the pituitary hormones have a trophic effect that is necessary for the maintenance of many systems. For example, without the gonadotropins, the entire reproductive system fails; without growth hormone and thyrotropin, normal growth and development are impossible.

The secretion of pituitary hormones is influenced by peripheral endocrine glands via hormonal feedback mechanisms and by neurohumoral substances from the hypothalamus. When the hypothalamus releases specific hormone-releasing substances, the specific pituitary hormone is released.

Pituitary deficiency (hypopituitarism) can produce a loss of secondary sex characteristics, decreased metabolism, dwarfism, diabetes insipidus, hypothyroidism, Addison's disease, loss of pigmentation, thinning and softening of the skin, decreased libido, and retarded dental development. Hypersecretion of pituitary hormones can produce sexual precocity, goiter, Cushing's disease, acromegaly, and giantism. There are two parts to the pituitary gland: the anterior lobe (adenohypophysis) and the posterior lobe (neurohypophysis).

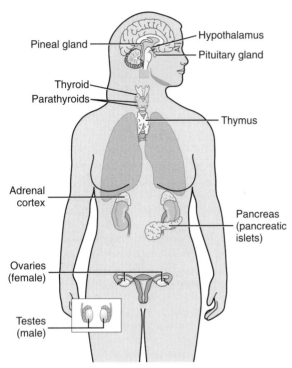

FIGURE 20-1
Locations of the major endocrine glands. (From McKenry L, Tessier E, Hogan MA: *Mosby's pharmacology in nursing,* ed 22, St Louis, 2006, Mosby.)

Anterior Pituitary

♦ OVERVIEW

> Anterior pituitary: gland-stimulating hormones

The anterior lobe of the pituitary gland secretes growth hormone, or somatotropin; luteinizing hormone (LH); follicle-stimulating hormone (FSH); thyroid-stimulating hormone (TSH), or thyrotropin; adrenocorticotropic hormone (ACTH), or corticotropin; and prolactin (Figure 20-2). β-Lipotropin, secreted by the pituitary, is a precursor to β-endorphin (see Chapter 6).

Genetic engineering has been able to produce human growth hormone since 1987. Human growth hormone is used medically to treat children who lack it and illicitly by body builders and weight lifters to develop muscles. (Some say that in athletic events at which the contestant's urine is tested, for example, the Olympics, growth hormone cannot be detected as easily as the androgenic steroids.)

Pharmaceutical gonadotropin-releasing hormone (GnRH) is a synthetic analog. One example, leuprolide, stimulates the pituitary function and is used to treat infertility. GnRH agonists are used to treat prostate cancer and endometriosis. The secretions from the anterior pituitary that stimulate other glands are used to test the function of the stimulated glands.

FSH-like products, which stimulate follicle growth, and LH-like products, which induce ovulation, are used in the treatment of infertility. Although LH itself is not available, human chorionic gonadotropin (hCG), which is almost identical in structure, can be used as an LH substitute for deficiency. Human menopausal gonadotropin (hMG) contains FSH and LH and is commercially available as menotropin (Pergonal). This preparation is used in infertility to stimulate ovarian follicle development. When follicular maturation has occurred, the hMG is discontinued and hCG is given to induce ovulation.

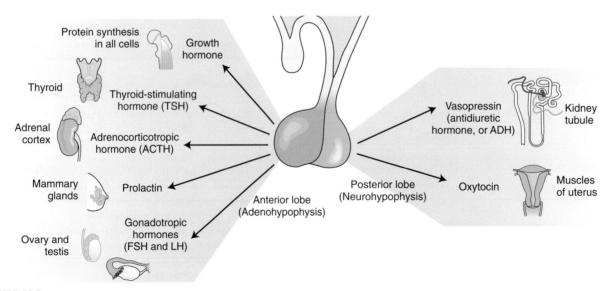

FIGURE 20-2
Pituitary hormones. Some of the major organs of the anterior and posterior lobes and their principal target organs. (From McKenry L, Tessier E, Hogan MA: *Mosby's pharmacology in nursing,* ed 22, St Louis, 2006, Mosby.)

♦ **BROMOCRIPTINE**

Bromocriptine (broe-moe-KRIP-teen) (Parlodel), an ergot derivative, inhibits pituitary function. Although not a hormone, it is a dopamine agonist that suppresses prolactin levels. It is used to treat prolactin-secreting adenomas (hyperprolactinemia), acromegaly, and Parkinson's disease. In the past, it was used to dry up the milk in a woman who did not want to nurse. It is no longer used for this purpose.

Posterior Pituitary

| Posterior: vasopressin and oxytocin |

The posterior pituitary gland secretes two hormones: vasopressin (antidiuretic hormone [ADH]) and oxytocin. Vasopressin (vay-soe-PRES-in) (Pitressin) has vasopressor and antidiuretic hormone activity and is used for treatment of transient diabetes insipidus. Synthetic analogs of vasopressin (desmopressin [DDAVP, Stimate] and lypressin [Diapid]) are used for chronic treatment of pituitary diabetes insipidus and to treat certain clotting disorders (hemophilia A and von Willebrand's disease). Available as nasal solutions, these two analogs have the same action as vasopressin but are longer acting.

Oxytocin (oks-i-TOE-sin) (Pitocin, Syntocinon), administered either by injection or intranasally, is used to induce labor, control postpartum hemorrhage, and induce postpartum lactation.

THYROID HORMONES

The thyroid gland secretes two iodine-containing thyroid hormones: triiodothyronine (T_3) and tetraiodothyronine (T_4, thyroxine). Calcitonin, another hormone secreted by the thyroid, regulates calcium metabolism. Thyroid hormones act on virtually every tissue and organ system of the body and are important for energy metabolism, growth, and development. Vulnerability to stress, altered drug response, and altered orofacial development are all possible manifestations of thyroid dysfunction. The head and neck examination performed by dental practitioners can identify some thyroid abnormalities. Swallowing can accentuate the thyroid to allow palpitation. The consistency of the gland varies with the abnormality.

Thyroid hormones are synthesized from iodine and tyrosine and stored as a complex protein until TSH stimulates their release. The actions of the thyroid hormones include those on growth and development, calorigenic effects, and metabolic effects. In frogs, thyroid hormone can transform a tadpole into a frog.

Iodine

| Iodine deficiency: goiter |

Normal function of the thyroid gland requires an adequate intake of iodine (approximately 50 to 125 mg per day). Without it, normal amounts of thyroid hormones cannot be made, TSH is secreted in excess, and the thyroid hypertrophies. This thyroid hypertrophy is called *simple* or *nontoxic goiter*. Because iodine is not abundant in most foods, simple goiter is prevalent in some areas of the world. Marine life is the only common food that is naturally rich in iodine. Use of iodized salt (contains potassium iodide [KI]) has decreased the incidence of simple goiter in many countries. Iodine is currently used in conjunction with

an antithyroid drug in hyperthyroid patients preparing for surgery.

Iodide in high concentrations suppresses the thyroid in a still poorly understood manner. It may produce gingival pain, excessive salivation, and sialadenitis as side effects.

Hypothyroidism

| ↓ Thyroid function in a child: cretinism |

In the small child, hypofunction of the thyroid is referred to as cretinism. In the adult, this condition is called myxedema or *simple hypothyroidism*. The main characteristics are mental and physical retardation. Such patients are usually drowsy, weak, and listless and exhibit an expressionless, puffy face with edematous tongue and lips. Oral findings in children usually include delayed tooth eruption, malocclusion, and increased tendency to develop periodontal disease. The teeth are usually poorly shaped and carious. The gingiva is either inflamed or pale and enlarged. The cretin is often uncooperative and difficult to motivate for plaque control. Diagnostic radiographs and routine dental prophylaxis in these patients may require special assistance.

Hypothyroid patients have difficulties withstanding stress and tend to be abnormally sensitive to all central nervous system (CNS) depressants, including the opioids and sedatives. If opioid analgesics are used, their doses should be reduced. Hypothyroid pregnant women tend to produce offspring with large teeth.

Thyroid hypofunction is rationally and effectively treated by oral administration of exogenous thyroid hormones. The most common thyroid hormone used for replacement therapy is levothyroxine (lee-voe-thye-ROX-een). Box 20-1 lists preparations used for thyroid hormone replacement therapy.

Hyperthyroidism

♦ **OVERVIEW**

| ↑ Thyroid function: Graves', Plummer's, or Hashimoto's disease |

Diffuse toxic goiter (Graves' disease) and toxic nodular goiter (Plummer's disease) are the two forms of thyroid hyperfunction. Diffuse toxic goiter is characterized by a diffusely enlarged, highly vascular thyroid gland. It is common in young adults and is considered to be a disorder of the immune response. Toxic nodular goiter is characterized by nodules within the gland that spontaneously secrete excessive amounts of hormone while the rest of the glandular tissue is atrophied. It occurs primarily in older patients and usually arises from long-standing nontoxic goiter.

Hashimoto's disease, a chronic inflammation of the thyroid associated with an autoimmune response, produces hyperthy-

---

BOX 20-1   THYROID AND ANTITHYROID AGENTS

Thyroid Replacements
- Levothyroxine sodium (L-T_4) (Synthroid)
- Liothyronine sodium (L-T_3) (Cytomel)
- Liotrix (T_3 + T_4) (Euthroid, Thyrolar)
- Thyroid (desiccated thyroid, Armour thyroid)

Antithyroid Drugs
- Propylthiouracil (PTU)
- Methimazole (Tapazole)

roidism. Antithyroglobulin antibody can be detected. It occurs in middle-aged women and often occurs concomitantly with other autoimmune diseases.

Excessive levels of circulating thyroid hormone produce thyrotoxicosis. The adverse effects include excessive production of heat, increased sympathetic activity, increased neuromuscular activity, increased sensitivity to pain, ophthalmopathy, exophthalmos (protruding eyes), and anxiety. Oral manifestations include accelerated tooth eruption, marked loss of the alveolar process, diffuse demineralization of the jawbone, and rapidly progressing periodontal destruction.

The cardiovascular system is especially hyperactive because of a direct inotropic effect, increased peripheral oxygen consumption, and increased sensitivity to catecholamines. Epinephrine is relatively contraindicated in these patients. The potentiating effects of excess thyroid hormone and epinephrine on each other could result in cardiovascular problems such as angina, arrhythmias, and hypertension. β-Blockers, such as propranolol, are used to counteract the tachycardia.

In addition to their increased sensitivity to pain, hyperthyroid persons have an increased tolerance to CNS depressants. They may require higher than usual doses of sedatives, analgesics, and local anesthetics.

No treatment should be begun for any patient with a visible goiter, exophthalmos, or a history of taking antithyroid drugs until approval is obtained from the patient's physician. Medical management of the condition is important before any elective surgery is performed. A surgical procedure or an acute oral infection could precipitate a crisis. Hydrocortisone should be administered intravenously, and cold towels should be placed on the patient. The use of epinephrine should be avoided in poorly treated or untreated thyrotoxic patients. The cardiac dose of epinephrine can be used carefully. Even in controlled patients who are considered to be euthyroid, stress should be kept at a minimum, preoperative sedation should be considered, and the dental team should be alert for signs of hypothyroidism or hyperthyroidism.

Treatment of hyperthyroidism usually includes one of the options highlighted in Box 20-2. The two most common treatments are radioactive iodine (^{131}I) and thyroidectomy. ^{131}I is usually the drug of choice for patients older than 21 years. It is taken internally and sequestered by the gland; localized destruction of thyroid tissue results. Thyroidectomy is the surgical approach to hyperthyroidism. Both radioactive iodine and thyroidectomy usually result in hypothyroidism because a dose that produces an inadequate effect would require repeating the procedure. If a patient has been adequately treated for hyperthyroidism with either radioactive iodine or thyroidectomy and is taking supplemental thyroid (as needed [prn]), then that patient may be treated like a euthyroid patient.

BOX 20-2   HYPERTHYROIDISM TREATMENT OPTIONS

Drugs
Iodide

Antithyroid Drugs
Radioactive iodine (iodine-131 [^{131}I])

Surgery
Partial thyroidectomy

◆ ANTITHYROID AGENTS

Antithyroid drugs, such as propylthiouracil (PTU) and methimazole (Tapazole), are used in patients who cannot tolerate surgery or treatment with ^{131}I. These drugs interfere directly with the synthesis of thyroid hormones by inhibiting the iodination of tyrosine moieties and the coupling of the iodotyrosines. Adverse reactions associated with PTU include fever, skin rash, and leukopenia. The most serious adverse reaction is agranulocytosis, which can lead to poor wound healing, oral ulcers or necrotic lesions, and oral infections. Paresthesia of facial areas and loss of taste are also seen. Not only are antithyroid drugs used over prolonged periods to bring a hyperactive thyroid to the euthyroid state but they are also given before thyroidectomy to reduce the possibility of thyroid storm, a life-threatening acute form of thyrotoxicosis.

Propranolol, a β-blocker, is often given concomitantly with antithyroid agents. The β-blocker prevents the tachycardia and tremors.

PANCREATIC HORMONES

Two primary hormones secreted by the islets of Langerhans of the pancreas are insulin and glucagon. Insulin promotes fuel storage (pack the bags: glucose out of blood), whereas glucagon promotes fuel mobilization (empty the bags: glucose into blood) in the body. Other hormones secreted by the pancreas are islet amyloid polypeptide (IAPP; amylin) and pancreatic peptide. Their functions have not yet been elucidated.

Diabetes Mellitus

Diabetes mellitus (DM) is a group of metabolic disorders characterized by persistent hyperglycemia. It is thought that the hyperglycemia leads to the many complications of diabetes. DM is currently classified as types I and II (Table 20-1).

Fasting blood sugar (FBS) > 126 mg/dl

Symptoms and complications result, usually from inadequate or poorly timed secretion of insulin from

---

TABLE 20-1   TYPES I AND II DIABETES

Properties	Type I	Type II
Age of onset	<30 years	>40 years
Onset of symptoms	Acute	Gradual
Incidence	10%	90%
Etiology	Autoimmune reaction	Insulin resistance, excess hepatic glucose production, diminished insulin secretion
Genetics	Just a little	Quite a bit
Receptors	Normal	Defective
Plasma insulin	No	Normal or elevated then over time reduced
Ketoacidosis	Yes	No

IDDM, Insulin-dependent diabetes mellitus; *NIDDM,* non–insulin-dependent diabetes mellitus.

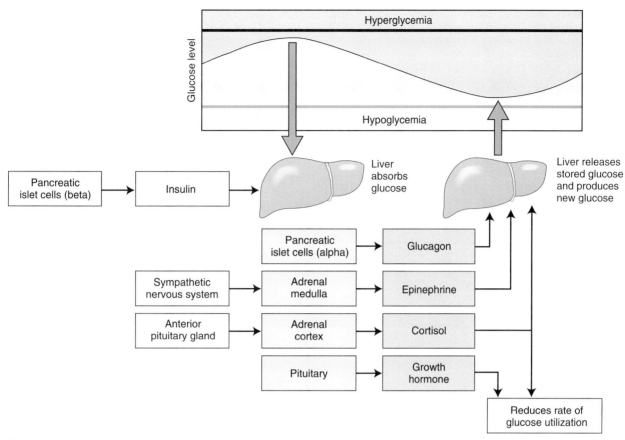

FIGURE 20-3
Physiologic response to changes in blood glucose levels. (From McKenry L, Tessier E, Hogan MA: *Mosby's pharmacology in nursing,* ed 22, St Louis, 2006, Mosby.)

the pancreas and/or insulin resistance of the cells. (Figure 20-3 outlines the body's physiologic response to changes in blood glucose levels.) The new criterion for the diagnosis of DM is two consecutive fasting blood sugars (FBS) of greater than 126 mg/dl. This will simplify the diagnosis of DM and add many patients to the ranks of people with diabetes.

Diabetes is primarily characterized by hyperglycemia and glycosuria. Other characteristics include hyperlipemia; azoturia; ketonemia; and, when the deficiency is severe, ketoacidosis. Patients usually experience general weakness, weight loss, polyphagia, polydipsia, and polyuria. Patients with type II diabetes often experience weight gain.

◆ TYPES OF DIABETES

Type I. Type I diabetes usually develops in persons younger than 30 years and results from an autoimmune destruction of the pancreatic β cells. The type I autoimmune response may be in response to an infection, a slow virus, environmental insults, or some as yet unknown factor. It is associated with a complete lack of insulin secretion, increased glucagon secretion, rapid onset of disease, ketosis, and severe symptoms. Without insulin, type I DM is fatal. Type I diabetes must be treated with injections of insulin because the pancreas does not produce any insulin.

Type II. Type II diabetes usually develops in persons older than 40 years. However, more and more cases of type II diabetes

are being reported in persons younger than 20 years. This is being attributed to a much more sedentary lifestyle and lack of exercise. Fast foods, video games, and television have replaced physical activity, and as a result, obesity is dramatically on the rise and obesity is a major risk factor for developing type II diabetes. Type II diabetes is associated with the ability of the pancreas to secrete enough insulin to prevent ketoacidosis but not enough to normalize plasma glucose. The insulin secreted does not reduce the glucose levels in the serum to normal levels and could be a result of a variety of reasons (Box 20-3).

Insulin resistance develops because of prolonged hyperglycemia and resulting hyperinsulinemia. Type II diabetes involves a slower onset of disease, less severe symptoms, and lack of ketoacidosis. Tissue insensitivity to insulin, a deficiency of the pancreas's response to glucose, and obesity results in impaired insulin action. In the presence of hyperglycemia, the resistance of the tissues to insulin and the impaired β cells' response are exaggerated. Normal serum glucose levels improve these parameters toward normal.

Type II diabetes is treated first with diet and exercise, then with orally acting agents, and if these modalities fail, with insulin. Therefore patients with type II diabetes may be taking insulin either with or without oral agents. Because of the etiology of the hyperglycemia in patients with type II diabetes, moderate improvement of the diet and/or an increase in exercise can produce a large improvement in the glucose levels. Exercise

1. β cells in the pancreas have a reduced or delayed response to glucose.
2. Secretion of insulin is delayed so that blood glucose levels are elevated.
3. Because cells in the body have insulin resistance (are not as sensitive to insulin as normal cells), more than the usual amount of insulin is required to produce a response. This leads to reduced insulin sensitivity; ultimately, insulin receptors do not respond to insulin.
4. "Pooped out" pancreas (P^3) (a euphemism). Because of the delay in insulin secretion and insulin resistance, the insulin released from the pancreas does not effectively lower the blood sugar. The pancreas is working overtime secreting a lot of insulin but without producing the desired results (decrease in blood sugar). Over time, the pancreas cannot continue to supply this increased production to keep up with the need for insulin. Either a relative (as a result of resistance) or absolute lack of insulin occurs.
5. Adipose tissue secretes a group of hormones called *adipokines* that may impair glucose tolerance.

increases the sensitivity of the cells to insulin. Unfortunately, these behavior modifications are difficult to carry out on a routine basis for almost all patients.

COMPLICATIONS OF DIABETES

Uncontrolled diabetes produces a pronounced susceptibility to dental caries. This is caused mainly by decreased salivary flow (xerostomia) related to fluid loss. The loss is secondary to an increase in urination that occurs because of poor use of carbohydrates and the glucose that is excreted via the kidneys (water follows glucose). The complications of xerostomia are a result of the lack of its normal functions: lubricating, cleansing, regulating pH, destroying microorganisms and their products, and maintaining the integrity of the oral structures.

A dry, cracking oral mucosa with the presence of mucositis, ulcers, infections, and an inflamed painful tongue may result. Any change in glucose in saliva probably contributes little to the increased caries rate.

Xerostomia. The small increase in parotid saliva glucose would appear to have little effect on the incidence of caries. In Finland, a recent study was conducted to determine the relationship between dental caries and NIDDM and its control. Over a 15-year period, 25 patients were monitored. The metabolic control of the diabetes was unrelated to dental caries. There was no increase in caries in type II diabetes over control patients. A relationship was found between a reduction in salivary flow and an increase in dental caries. DM can affect the dental development of children. Diabetic children have been shown to differ from normal children in the median ages at which they lose their deciduous teeth and gain their permanent teeth. Tooth eruption is accelerated in children with diabetes.

Periodontal Disease. Patients with uncontrolled or undiagnosed diabetes are more prone to periodontal disease. However, the periodontal status of the patient with well-controlled diabetes has been somewhat more controversial. Despite the fact that some investigators reported a lack of correlation between diabetes and increased periodontal disease, many other studies have resulted in the opposite conclusion. (It may be that if control is good, then there is hardly any effect, whereas if control is poor, then there is a greater effect.)

Periodontal findings include inflammatory and degenerative changes ranging from mild gingivitis to painful periodontitis with a widened periodontal ligament, multiple abscesses, putrescent exudates from periodontal pockets, and increased tooth mobility caused by destruction of supporting alveolar bone. Although it may be more severe, diabetic periodontal disease appears to be similar to that found in nondiabetics. The diabetic state probably serves as a predisposing factor that can accelerate the periodontal destruction originated by microbial agents. The proposed etiology for the periodontal changes seen in the patient with diabetes includes microangiopathy of the tissues, thickening of capillary basement membranes, changes in glucose tolerance factor (more glucose), altered polymorphonuclear leukocyte function, and enhanced collagenase activity.

DENTAL ISSUES

Dental appointments should not interfere with meals and should involve minimal stress. In patients with controlled diabetes, oral surgical procedures should be performed 1.5 to 2 hours after the patient has eaten normal breakfast and taken regular antidiabetes medication. Following surgery, the patient should receive an adequate caloric intake to prevent hypoglycemia. With general anesthesia, patients are often kept nothing by mouth (NPO) and should take half of their usual dose of insulin and receive intravenous 5% glucose in distilled water (D_5W).

Patients with diabetes have fragile blood vessels, delayed wound healing, and a tendency to develop infections; therefore surgical therapy should be approached with caution. Scaling and soft tissue curettage usually are tolerated well. The bulk of the literature suggests that prophylactic use of antibiotics should be avoided although many practitioners routinely use antibiotics. If infection is present or if infection ensues, it should be aggressively treated. Measures to reduce the possibility of infection should be used (sterilize instruments, rinse mouth before procedures). The oral complications of diabetes are summarized in Table 20-2.

CAUTIONS AND CONTRAINDICATIONS

Drugs that may decrease insulin release or increase insulin requirements, such as epinephrine, glucocorticoids, or opioid analgesics, should be used with caution in patients with diabetes. Caution should also be exercised with general anesthetics because of the possibility of acidosis. If diabetes is in good control, then these drugs can be used.

SYSTEMIC COMPLICATIONS OF DIABETES

The systemic complications of diabetes include actions affecting almost all the body tissues and organs.

Cardiovascular System Complications. The incidence of cardiovascular problems is higher in patients with diabetes. Macroangiopathy, microangiopathy, and hyperlipidemia are common. Atherosclerosis is also more common in these patients.

Retinopathy. Because microvascular disease affects the blood supply to the retina, the functioning of the retina is impaired. In fact, diabetes is the major cause of blindness in adults.

Neuropathy. Neuropathy is another complication of diabetes. It leads to reduced and sometimes absent feelings, especially in the lower extremities. A variety of sensations, including pain and burning, have been reported. The oral complaints of pain and discomfort related to the tongue and other oral structures are related to diabetic neuropathy. Drugs used to manage this

TABLE 20-2   ORAL COMPLICATIONS OF DIABETES MELLITUS

Manifestation	Comment	Outcome
Xerostomia	Increase in caries Problem with tasting Problem swallowing Wetting food difficult Problem with mastication Mucositis, ulcers, desquamation Painful tongue	Saliva lubricates, cleanses, regulates acidity; has electrolytes, glycoproteins, antimicrobial enzymes
Slightly elevated sugar	In parotid saliva	Not clinically significant
Caries rate	Some say less Some say more	Result of diabetic diet Glucose in saliva
Microvascular disease—small blood vessel disease	Less blood flow to oral cavity	Infection more difficult to treat (antibiotic cannot reach site)
Altered immunity/white blood cell abnormality	Less ability to fight microorganisms	Get infections more easily Periapical abscesses Periodontal abscesses
Regulate acidity	Oral infection reduces diabetes control, need more insulin Oral infection after surgery	Infection treated, better insulin control (need less)
Neuropathy	From diabetes	Numbness, burning, tingling, pain in nerves
Infections	Candidiasis Mucormycosis	Fungal infections more likely
Symptoms	Burning mouth syndrome	Unknown cause
Delayed, impaired healing	With oral trauma	Collagen poorly formed

All complications worsen with hyperglycemia, either acute or chronic. Acute fasting glucose (mg/dl) measured by glucose monitor are reflective of glucose at that moment, and chronic glucose levels measured by HgA$_{1c}$ are reflective of glucose control over the previous 2 to 3 months. Oral complications are xerostomia, infection, poor healing, increased caries, candidiasis, gingivitis, periodontal diseases, periapical abscess, and burning mouth syndrome.

problem include amitriptyline, carbamazepine, phenytoin, and capsaicin (made from hot peppers). The neurologic problems of diabetes can produce atony of the gastrointestinal (GI) tract (diabetic gastroparesis). Metoclopramide is used to manage this complication.

Infections. Gangrene can occur in the peripheral extremities, especially the feet and legs. This occurs because of the deficiencies of diabetes, depressed immunity, less effective white blood cells, microvascular changes (less blood), and neuropathy (cannot feel the problem).

Healing. Slower healing must be taken into account so that precautions during surgery are taken. Related to this problem is the likelihood of infection, which exacerbates the healing problem.

Summary of Complications. A patient with diabetes has reduced blood flow to the feet because of microvascular disease and reduced sensation because of peripheral neuropathy. The patient has reduced ability to fight infection as a result of altered leukocyte chemotactic properties. The blood does not get to the extremities as easily, so even when antiinfective agents are present in the blood the antibiotics have difficulty reaching the site of action. Neuropathy occurs in the extremities, and these patients cannot easily feel their feet. Because there is lack of feeling, trauma or infections of the feet go unnoticed. Poor circulation, lack of feeling, and inability to fight infection lead to infection of extremities. Couple that with the fact that the patient with diabetes cannot see as well, and the pathway to disaster becomes evident.

Amputations often begin with the toes, progress to ankles and knees, and finally result in amputation of the entire leg. At the same time, microvascular disease reduces the blood supply to the kidneys, producing an increase in protein loss in the urine. Additional reduction in renal function may require dialysis or a kidney transplant. Many of the dialysis beds are filled with patients with diabetes.

◆ EFFECT OF DRUGS ON COMPLICATIONS OF DIABETES

The Diabetes Control and Complications Trial (DCCT) was a randomized, controlled clinical trial conducted at 26 centers, primarily in the United States. The intensive intervention included additional interactions with a health care provider. Data were collected from patient notifications of events and from quarterly interviews. The 1441 volunteers had type I for 1 to 15 years. The average length of follow-up was 6.5 years. Subjects were randomly assigned to conventional or intensive diabetes treatment. Intensive therapy included three or more insulin injections daily or a continuous subcutaneous infusion of insulin (insulin pump) guided by four or more glucose tests per day.

Conventional therapy included one or two insulin injections daily. This study demonstrated that intensive treatment of patients with type I can substantially reduce the onset and progression of diabetic retinopathy, nephropathy, and neuropathy. The major risk associated with the intensive treatment is recurrent hypoglycemia that was three times higher than in those with conventional therapy.

Comparing the intensive therapy with traditional therapy resulted in both "good news" and "bad news":

- *Good news:* The complications of diabetes were decreased or delayed in onset of effect (60% reduction).
- *Bad news:* The risk of hypoglycemia increased three times, and the increase in weight gain tended to be greater.

♦ EVALUATION OF THE DENTAL PATIENT WITH DIABETES

Asking a patient "How well is your diabetes controlled?" does not often produce useable information. In my experience, the answer patients give to this question does not relate to the actual control of the patient's diabetes. Some questions for the patient that might provide useful information are "What numbers have you been getting for your blood sugar? What was your test this morning? When did you last test your blood glucose? What were the results?" No matter what the number is, one should not be judgmental.

Both the oral and systemic complications of diabetes are exacerbated by poor glucose control. There are two laboratory tests useful to evaluate a patient's glucose control: serum glucose and glycosylated hemoglobin (Table 20-3). Serum glucose is a measure of the patient's glucose control at the time that the blood is sampled. It does not reflect the patient's overall glucose control. The second test is the glycosylated hemoglobin (HbA_{1c}). Because this test reflects the glucose control over a 2- to 3-month period, it more accurately measures the patient's overall serum glucose control. Of course, a relationship exists between all the blood glucose levels and the glycosylated hemoglobin.

♦ TREATMENT OF HYPOGLYCEMIA

One can prevent hypoglycemia by remembering that "An ounce of prevention is worth a pound of cure." It is easy to question patients concerning their insulin use and dietary intake. The treatment of hypoglycemia depends on whether a patient retains the swallowing reflex. In the early stages, when the patient is awake, the treatment consists of any of the following: fruit juice, cake icing, glucose gel, or soluble carbohydrates. If the patient is unconscious and lacks a swallowing reflex, treatment consists of intravenous dextrose (50%). Intravenous glucose fluids and glucagon can be given. Because changes in behavior and in vital signs occur with hypoglycemia, dental teams should be able to use an oral product to manage their hypoglycemic patients. One of these items should be readily available in the dental office for emergencies.

Clinically, it is often difficult to distinguish an insulin reaction hypoglycemia (low glucose) from hyperglycemia (high glucose). It is useful to give a patient sugar for two reasons. First, the small amount of sugar used to treat hypoglycemia will produce little additional harm if hyperglycemia is present. Second, the dental office is not equipped to treat hyperglycemia. Insulin should not be administered in a dental office emergency; the patient should be immediately taken to a hospital emergency room.

♦ DRUGS USED TO MANAGE DIABETES

Insulins. Insulin (IN-su-lin) is usually administered by subcutaneous injection because its large molecular size prevents it from being absorbed from the GI tract. The major difference among the currently used types of insulin is their onset and duration of action. The older preparations were prepared from beef or pork pancreases, but human insulin is now used exclusively. Human insulin is produced by two different processes: through recombinant deoxyribonucleic acid (rDNA) synthesis and by modifying porcine (pig) insulin. Both compounds are identical to the human insulin secreted by people. rDNA synthesis produces human insulin by gene splicing carried out by *Escherichia coli.* The processing of pork insulin involves transpeptidation of the pork insulin until it is the same as human insulin. Pig insulin has only two amino acids that are different from those in human insulin.

Table 20-4 lists insulin preparations, their peak effect, and their duration of action. The most common insulins used in clinical practice are human regular and neutral protein Hagedorn (NPH) (isophane insulin suspension) insulin (Figure 20-4). Lispro is made by exchanging two amino acids in the structure of human insulin. This change results in an insulin with a faster onset of action. Lispro insulin is commonly used to obtain tighter control of blood glucose.

TABLE 20-3	TEST RESULTS FOR AVERAGE PATIENT AND PATIENT WITH DIABETES			
	Normal	Goal	Take Action
Fasting plasma glucose (mg/dl)	<110	80-120	<80 or >140
Glycosylated hemoglobin (HbA_{1c}) (%)	<6	<7	>8

TABLE 20-4	SELECTED INSULIN PREPARATIONS			
Action	Preparation	Onset	Peak	Duration
Rapid-acting	Insulin aspart (NovoLog) Insulin lispro (Humalog) Insulin glulisine (Apidra)	10-30 min	30-60 min	3-5 hr
Short-acting	Insulin regular (Novolin R, Humulin R)	30-60 min	1.5-2 hr	5-12 hr
Intermediate-acting	Insulin NPH (Humulin N, Novolin N) Humulin L Lente	1-2 hr	4-8 hr	10-20 hr
Long-acting	Insulin detemir (Levemir) Insulin glargine (Lantus)	1 hr 1-2 hr	No peak No peak	20 hr 24 hr

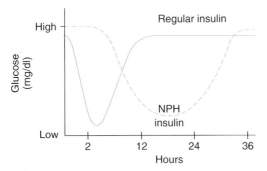

FIGURE 20-4
Serum levels of insulin and its effect on plasma glucose (milligrams per deciliter) levels. *NPH,* Neutral protein Hagedorn.

BOX 20-4 MANAGEMENT OF THE DENTAL PATIENT TAKING INSULIN OR ORAL HYPOGLYCEMICS

- Hypoglycemia—Question patient regarding last meal ingested.
- Infection more likely—Monitor closely and give antibiotics if needed (treat aggressively).
- Healing prolonged—Follow patient with any surgical procedure.
- Drug interactions—Large doses of salicylates may produce hypoglycemia.
- Give patient an appointment in morning after breakfast and insulin or oral hypoglycemic agent.
- Provide quick glucose source for hypoglycemia (cake icing, orange juice).
- Check for oral complications related to diabetes.
- Ask patient what the results of his or her blood glucose monitoring have been (if checked).

The most common adverse reaction associated with any insulin product is hypoglycemia. Besides hypoglycemia, inhaled insulin can cause shortness of breath, dry mouth, and cough.

The dental health care worker should be most concerned about a hypoglycemic reaction (Box 20-4) in the dental patient with diabetes who takes insulin. This can be caused by an unintentional insulin overdose (insulin shock), failure to eat, or increased exercise or stress. Symptoms that can be explained by an increased release of epinephrine from the adrenals include sweating, weakness, nausea, and tachycardia. Symptoms caused by glucose deprivation of the brain include headache; blurred vision; mental confusion; incoherent speech; and eventually, coma, convulsions, and death.

Another side effect associated with insulin is an allergic reaction, usually caused by noninsulin contaminants. Lipodystrophy at the injection site produces atrophy of the subcutaneous fatty tissue. The incidence of these reactions has decreased because the newer insulin preparations are purer and because patient education regarding changing the injection site has improved.

Oral Antidiabetic Agents. There are currently four groups of oral agents used to treat diabetes, referred to as *oral antidiabetics.* Each group works by a different mechanism and has a different adverse reaction profile. The oldest group of oral antidiabetic agents, the sulfonylureas, are also known as *oral hypoglycemic agents.* The other three groups are more precisely referred to as the *antihyperglycemic agents* because they lower an elevated blood sugar but do not produce hypoglycemia by themselves.

Figure 20-5 summarizes the mechanism of action of the various types of antidiabetic agents.

Biguanides. Metformin (met-FOR-min) (Glucophage) is a member of the biguanide group. It lowers blood glucose but, used alone, does not produce hypoglycemia. Metformin increases hepatic and peripheral insulin sensitivity, resulting in decreased hepatic glucose production (by reducing gluconeogenesis). It also increases peripheral skeletal muscle glucose uptake.

Metformin may be used alone, in combination with a sulfonylurea, or with insulin for management of type II diabetes.

Adverse reactions of metformin are primarily related to the GI tract (30%) and include anorexia, dyspepsia, flatulence, nausea, and vomiting. It can produce headache and interfere with vitamin B_{12} absorption. It accumulates in renal and hepatic impairment. Lactic acidosis, its most serious side effect, is rare. Predisposing factors to lactic acidosis include alcoholism, binge drinking, and renal or hepatic dysfunction. Metformin is contraindicated in patients with these conditions or patients who are fasting because metformin predisposes a patient to lactic acidosis. Oral manifestations include a metallic taste. The dose ranges from 1500 to 2550 mg divided into two or three daily doses.

Sulfonylureas. For many years, the sulfonylureas were the only orally active agents used to manage diabetes. There are two major groups: first-generation and second-generation sulfonylureas. Their actions are similar, but the second-generation agents are more potent than the first-generation agents so their doses are smaller. Second-generation sulfonylureas have replaced first-generation sulfonylureas because they are less toxic and easier to dose than first-generation sulfonylureas. Glyburide, one of the most commonly used oral sulfonylureas, is discussed as the prototype.

The mechanism of action of the sulfonylureas (Figure 20-6) includes stimulation of the release of insulin from the β cells of the pancreas, reduction of glucose from the liver, reduction in serum glucagon levels, and increase in the sensitivity of the target tissues to insulin (probably secondary to reduced hyperglycemia).

Sulfonylureas are indicated for the treatment of patients with type II diabetes who cannot be treated with diet and exercise alone. Adverse reactions of the sulfonylureas include blood dyscrasias, GI disturbances, cutaneous reactions, and liver damage. Aspirin can interact with the sulfonylureas, producing a decrease in serum glucose levels. This is not clinically significant unless the diabetic patient is especially brittle. Table 20-5 lists the first-generation and second-generation sulfonylureas, their average daily dose, and their duration of action. Tolbutamide (tole-BYOO-ta-mide) is an older first-generation sulfonylurea that was once popular, but most patients currently take a second-generation sulfonylurea.

The first line of treatment of type II diabetes usually involves a sulfonylurea and/or a biguanide. These two agents can be used together to lower the blood level more than either one individually.

In addition to the biguanides, there are two other new antihyperglycemic* drug groups that have become available for the

---

*Antihyperglycemic refers to agents that prevent an elevation in the blood glucose, whereas hypoglycemic refers to agents that lower blood glucose (sometimes grouped with sulfonylureas as oral hypoglycemic agents). One should note that the former does not produce hypoglycemia, whereas the latter may.

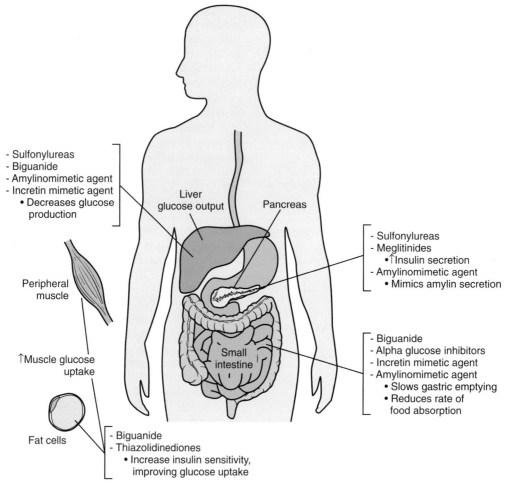

FIGURE 20-5
Mechanisms of action of antidiabetic agents. (From Clayton BD, Stock YN, Harroun RD: *Basic pharmacology for nurses,* ed 14, St Louis, 2007, Mosby.)

FIGURE 20-6
Mechanism of action of sulfonylureas. (From McKenry L, Tessier E, Hogan MA: *Mosby's pharmacology in nursing,* ed 22, St Louis, 2006, Mosby.)

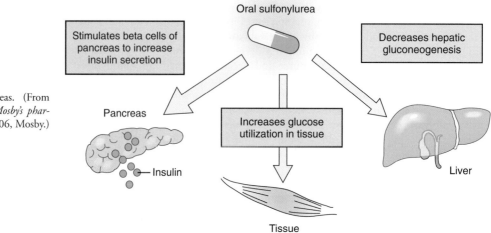

TABLE 20-5 ANTIDIABETIC AGENTS: SULFONYLUREAS

Drug	Total Daily Dose; How Divided (mg)	T ½ (hr)	Onset (hr)	Peak (hr)	Duration (hr)
First Generation					
Chlorpropamide (Diabinese)	250-750 qd	36	1	2-4	24-72
Tolazamide (Tolinase)	250-500 qd or bid (max: 1000 mg qd)	7	4-6	3-4	10-24
Tolbutamide (Orinase)	1000-2000 qd or bid (max: 3000 mg qd)	4.5-6.5	1	3-4	6-12
Second Generation					
Glimepiride (Amaryl)	1-4 qd (max: 8 mg qd)	5-9	0.5-1.5	2-3	12-24
Glipizide (Glucotrol)	5-20 qd or bid (max: 40 mg qd)	2-4	1-1.5	1-3	10-24
Glipizide (Glucotrol-XL)	5-20 qd	2-4	—	6-12	24
Glyburide (DiaBeta, Micronase) = nonmicronized	2.5-20 qd or bid (max: 20 mg qd)	6-10	2-4	3.4-4.5	12-24
Glyburide (Glynase PresTab) = micronized	1.5-12 qd or bid (max: 12 mg qd)	4	1	2.3-3.5	24

bid, Twice a day; *qd,* daily.

management of diabetes. It has been suggested that rather than being called *oral hypoglycemic agents* they should be called *euglycemic agents.* They work to lower blood glucose and glycosylated hemoglobin by different mechanisms. In some instances, combining agents from more than one group can produce a greater reduction in blood glucose than either agent used alone. Table 20-6 lists some properties of these three groups of antihyperglycemic agents.

Non-Sulfonylurea Secretagogues. Repaglinide (Prandin) and nateglinide (Starlix), although structurally different from the sulfonylureas, bind to adenosine triphosphate (ATP)–sensitive potassium channels on β cells and increase insulin release. These drugs stimulate the release of insulin from the pancreas. Insulin release is glucose-dependent and requires functioning β cells. These drugs are rapidly absorbed from the GI tract resulting in peak plasma levels of insulin within 30 to 60 minutes and return to baseline before the next meal. They must be taken with meals. If a meal is missed, then the drug should not be taken. Blood glucose control with these drugs is comparable to that of sulfonylureas. Repaglinide may be a useful alternative to a sulfonylurea in patients with renal impairment or in patients who eat sporadically. Both drugs are Food and Drug Administration (FDA) approved for combined use with metformin or a thiazolidinedione.

Hypoglycemia appears to occur less often with repaglinide and nateglinide than with sulfonylureas.

α-Glucosidase Inhibitors. Acarbose (Precose) is an α-glucosidase inhibitor. Simply, it slows the breakdown of ingested carbohydrates so that postprandial hyperglycemia is reduced. It is a competitive, reversible inhibitor of GI tract enzymes: intestinal α-glucosidase and pancreatic α-amylase. The intestinal glucosidases hydrolyze saccharides to glucose or other monosaccharides that can be absorbed. The pancreatic amylase hydrolyzes complex starches to oligosaccharides in the intestine. By inhibiting these enzymes, glucose availability and therefore absorption are delayed and postprandial hyperglycemia is lowered.

Acarbose can be used alone or with other agents, including insulin, sulfonylureas, and biguanides. Its major adverse effect is flatulence (77%), which is produced by bacteria acting on the undigested carbohydrates and producing gas. Other GI tract

adverse reactions include diarrhea, abdominal pain, and distention. These effects are often tolerated if the dose of the drug is increased slowly and after using the drug for some time. Anemia and elevated transaminase levels have been reported. The dose of acarbose is 25 to 100 mg two or three times daily, given with the first bite of food.

Thiazolidinediones. Pioglitazone (Actos) and rosiglitazone (Avandia) are the only two thiazolidinediones available in the United States. These drugs increase the insulin sensitivity of adipose tissue, skeletal muscle, and the liver. They can take up to 6 to 14 weeks to achieve maximum effect. Both are FDA approved as monotherapy or in combination with metformin, a sulfonylurea, or insulin. Rosiglitazone is also approved as a third drug with both metformin and a sulfonylurea. Thiazolidinediones have an additive blood glucose–lowering effect when used in combination with metformin, sulfonylureas, or insulin.

> Reduces insulin resistance

Troglitazone (Rezulin), the first thiazolidinedione, was removed from the U.S. market because of a rare, sometimes fatal, hepatic toxicity. Hepatotoxicity has rarely been reported with rosiglitazone and pioglitazone. The FDA recommends checking serum alanine aminotransferase (ALT) levels before starting therapy and periodically thereafter. These drugs should not be used in patients with underlying liver disease or with ALT levels greater than 2.5 times the upper limit of normal. Other common adverse effects include weight gain and fluid retention.

Other New Drugs
Exenatide. Exenatide (Byetta) is the first in a new class of drugs called *incretin mimetics* that has an amino acid sequence similar to human glucagon-like-peptide-1 (GLP-1) and in the presence of glucose acts to stimulate insulin secretion. Exenatide is indicated as an alternative to starting insulin in patients with type II diabetes who have not achieved adequate control with metformin, a sulfonylurea, or both. This drug is available as a subcutaneous injection.

The most commonly reported adverse effects include nausea, vomiting, and diarrhea. There have been postmarketing surveillance reports of acute pancreatitis in patients taking exenatide. The FDA is currently considering label changes. There is also a

TABLE 20-6 ORAL ANTIDIABETIC AGENTS

Drug	Dose	Mechanism	Adverse Reactions	Oral/DDI	Pharmacokinetics* (hr)	Comments
Biguanides						
Metformin (Glucophage)	1500-2550 mg in divided doses	Decreases hepatic production of glucose, ↑peripheral and hepatic insulin sensitivity and peripheral glucose uptake	Diarrhea, nausea, vomiting, lactic acidosis (serious)	Metallic taste DI-EtOH acute/chronic, elevates lactate concentration, especially without food	Peak: 2 hr t½: 18	Alone or in combination with a sulfonylurea
α-Glucosidase Inhibitors						
Acarbose (Precose)	25-100 mg tid with first bite of meal (max: 300 mg qd)	Delays digestion (breakdown) of ingested carbohydrate, so delays glucose absorption,† producing a smaller rise in BG	GI: abdominal pain, flatulence (77%), diarrhea, pain	None reported	Peak: 1 t½: 2; metabolized within the GI tract	Alone or in combination with a sulfonylurea
Miglitol (Glyset)	50-100 mg tid	Same as above	GI: flatulence (42%), diarrhea, abdominal pain, no hypoglycemia alone	No dental drug interactions	Peak: 2-3 t½: 2 No metabolites	Same as above
Thiazolidinediones						
Pioglitazone (Actos)	15-45 mg qd	Improve the action of insulin in muscle and fat tissue	Weight gain, fluid retention, reports of hepatotoxicity	None reported	Peak: 2 t½: 3-7 (parent drug), 16-24 (total)	Alone or in combination with metformin, a sulfonylurea, or insulin
Rosiglitazone (Avandia)	4-8 mg qd or divided	Same as above	Same as above	None reported	Peak: 1 t½: 3-4	Same as above
Non-Sulfonylurea Secretagogues						
Nateglinide (Starlix)	60-120 mg tid before meals	Bind to ATP-sensitive potassium channels on β cells, ↑insulin release	Hypoglycemia, weight gain	Clarithromycin, rifampin	t½: 1.5	Combined with metformin or a thiazolidinedione
Repaglinide (Prandin)	1-4 mg PO tid before meals	Bind to ATP-sensitive potassium channels on β cells, ↑insulin release	Hypoglycemia, weight gain	Clarithromycin, rifampin	t½: 1	Same as above

Other

	Dosage	Action	Side Effects	Drug Interactions	Pharmacokinetics	Use
Exenatide (Byetta)	5-10 μg SC bid before breakfast and dinner	Helps to stimulate insulin secretion in the presence of glucose, lowers serum glucagon levels, increases satiety	Nausea, vomiting, diarrhea, risk of hypoglycemia when used with a sulfonylurea	Avoid the use of anticholinergic drugs because of delayed gastric emptying	Peak: 2.1 t½: 2.4	Approved for use as an alternative to starting insulin in patients with type II diabetes who have not achieved adequate control with metformin, a sulfonylurea, or both
Pramlintide (Symlin)	60-120 μg tid before main meals	Modulation of gastric emptying, prevention of postprandial rise in plasma glucagon levels, increased satiety	Nausea, vomiting, diarrhea, risk of hypoglycemia when used with a sulfonylurea or insulin	Same as above	Peak: 20 min t½: 48 min	Type I diabetes: Adjunct therapy for patients who cannot achieve adequate glycemic control with mealtime insulin therapy Type II diabetes: Adjunct therapy for patients who cannot achieve adequate glycemic control with mealtime insulin therapy with or without concurrent sulfonylurea and/or metformin therapy
Colesevelam (Welchol)	3.8 gm qd or divided bid	Bile-acid sequestrant used to lower LDL cholesterol. Reduces HbA$_{1C}$ when given with metformin, sulfonylureas, or insulin.	Constipation, nausea, dyspepsia	Interferes with the absorption of other oral drugs	Not absorbed, not classified	Adjunct to diet and exercise in patients with type II diabetes

Dipeptidyl-Peptidase (DPP)-4 Inhibitors

	Dosage	Action	Side Effects	Drug Interactions	Pharmacokinetics	Use
Sitagliptin (Januvia)	100 mg PO qd	Inhibits DPP-4 enzyme responsible for the inactivation and degradation of the incretin hormones thereby lowering serum glucose concentrations	Weight gain	None	t½: 8-14	

BG, Blood glucose; *bid*, twice a day; *DDI*, dental drug interactions; *EtOH*, alcohol; *GI*, gastrointestinal; *LDL*, low density lipoprotein; *PO*, by mouth; *qd*, every day; *tid*, three times a day.

*t½, peak, duration (hr).

†Does not produce hypoglycemia alone; reduces the insulinotropic and weight-increasing effects of sulfonylureas.

risk for mild-to-moderate hypoglycemia when it is used in combination with a sulfonylurea. The dose of the sulfonylurea may have to be lowered if either of these drugs is started.

Pramlintide. Pramlintide (Symlin) is an amylinomimetic agent that is responsible for modulation of gastric emptying, prevention of the postprandial rise in plasma glucagon, and satiety, which leads to decreased caloric intake and potential weight loss.

It is approved for type I diabetes as an adjunct treatment in patients who use mealtime insulin therapy and who have failed to achieve desired glucose control despite optimal insulin therapy. It is also indicated for type II diabetes as an adjunct treatment in patients who use mealtime insulin therapy and who have failed to achieve desired glucose control despite optimal insulin therapy, with or without a concurrent sulfonylurea agent and/or metformin. Like exenatide, pramlintide is available as a subcutaneous injection and should be given immediately before major meals. The most commonly reported adverse effects include nausea, vomiting, and headache.

Colesevelam. Colesevelam (WelChol) is a bile-acid sequestrant that is used to lower low-density lipoprotein (LDL) cholesterol. Its mechanism of action in treating type II diabetes is unclear. It has been approved by the FDA as an adjunct to diet and exercise for the treatment of type II diabetes. Colesevelam can cause constipation, nausea, dyspepsia, and increase serum triglyceride concentrations. It can interfere with the absorption of other oral drugs.

Dipeptidyl-Peptidase-4 Inhibitors. Sitagliptin (Januvia) is an oral dipeptidyl-peptidase-4 (DPP-4) inhibitor that has been approved for use in the treatment of type II diabetes as monotherapy or in combination with metformin, a sulfonylurea, or a thiazolidinedione, but not with insulin. It inhibits the DPP-4 enzyme that is responsible for the inactivation and degradation of the incretin hormones GLP-1 and glucose-dependent insulinotropic polypeptide. These GI hormones potentiate insulin synthesis and release by pancreatic β cells and decrease glucagon production by pancreatic α cells, thereby lowering serum glucose concentration. Modest weight gain may occur with this drug. The incidence of hypoglycemia increases when used in combination with a sulfonylurea.

Glucagon. Glucagon is a polypeptide hormone produced by the α cells of the pancreas.

Glucagon's role is as an antagonist to insulin. Higher levels of glucagon are present in the blood of patients with diabetes, even when normal blood glucose levels are maintained. Glucagon may be used parenterally for the emergency treatment of hypoglycemia, but glucose is usually preferred.

FEMALE SEX HORMONES

There are both male and female sex hormones, and most sex hormones occur in both sexes but in different proportions.

The two major female sex hormones are the estrogens (ES-troe-jenz) and progestins (proe-JES-tins) (e.g., progesterone [proe-JES-te-rone]). Products containing these hormones are listed in Table 20-7. They are secreted primarily by the ovaries but also by the testes and placenta. They are largely responsible for producing the female sex characteristics, developing the reproductive system, and preparing the reproductive system for conception.

TABLE 20-7	SELECTED FEMALE HORMONE DOSE FORMS AND DOSES
Hormones	**Equivalent Dose**
Estrogens	
Conjugated estrogens (Premarin)	0.3-1.25 mg/day
Esterified estrogens (Estratab, Menest)	0.3-1.25 mg/day
Estradiol transdermal system (Estraderm)	0.05 mg patch applied twice weekly
Estradiol (Estrace)	0.5-2 mg/day (cyclic pattern)
Ethinyl estradiol (Estinyl)—DSC	0.025-0.05 mg/day
Estropipate (Ogen, Ortho-Est)	0.75 mg/day
Progestins	
Medroxyprogesterone (Provera)	2.5-10 mg for 5-10 days for amenorrhea
Contraceptive progestins	Miscellaneous
Parenteral	
Medroxyprogesterone (Depo-Provera): IM	150 mg q 3 months
Norplant: implant	36 mg
Minipills	0.35 mg/day
Norethindrone (Micronor)	0.075 mg
Norgestrel (Ovrette)—DSC	0.075 mg
Oral Estrogen-Progestin Combinations	
Estradiol/norgestimate (Prefest)	1 mg estradiol/day × 3 days, followed by 0.9 mg norgestimate—1 mg estradiol/day × 3 days, repeated
Estradiol/norethindrone acetate (Activella)	1 tablet (1 mg estradiol/0.5 mg norethindrone acetate) daily
Ethinyl estradiol/ norethindrone acetate (Femhrt)	1 tablet (2.5 μg ethinyl estradiol/0.5 mg norethindrone acetate) daily
Conjugated estrogen/ medroxyprogesterone Premphase	0.625 mg/day estrogen days 1-14, then 0.625-5 mg/day estrogen/ medroxyprogesterone for days 15-28
Prempro	0.3 estrogen/1.5 mg medroxyprogesterone per day for 28 days in one tablet

IM, Intramuscular.

Estrogen and progesterone levels vary daily. These changes are dependent on the pituitary gonadotropic hormones FSH and LH. The interrelationship among these hormones during the female sexual cycle is as follows: On day 1 of an average 28-day cycle, when the menstrual flow begins, the secretions of FSH and LH begin to increase. This release is caused by a reduction in the blood levels of estrogen and progesterone, which normally inhibit their release. In response to increased FSH, an ovarian egg matures, and the follicle in which it is contained grows in size and begins to produce and secrete estrogen. For reasons not entirely understood, on approximately day 12, the rate of secretion of FSH and LH increases markedly to cause a rapid swelling of the follicle that culminates in ovulation on day 14.

Following ovulation, LH causes the secretory cells of the follicle to develop into a corpus luteum that secretes large quantities of estrogen and progesterone. This causes a feedback decrease in the secretion of both FSH and LH. On approximately day 26, the corpus luteum completely degenerates. The resultant decrease in estrogen and progesterone leads to menstruation and increased release of FSH and LH. The FSH initiates growth of new follicles to begin a new cycle. Figure 20-7 illustrates the steps in the typical female menstrual cycle.

Estrogens

◆ OVERVIEW

In addition to their role in the female sexual cycle, estrogens are largely responsible for the changes that take place at puberty in girls. They promote the growth and development of the vagina, uterus, fallopian tubes, breasts, and axillary and pubic hair. They increase the deposition of fat in subcutaneous tissues and increase the retention of salt and water. They also cause increased osteoblastic activity and early fusion of the epiphyses.

The most potent endogenous estrogen is 17β-estradiol. The liver readily oxidizes it to estrone, which in turn can be hydrated to estriol. Because synthetic estrogens can be administered orally, they are used for therapy and contraception. Table 20-8 lists some estrogens and progestins used for birth control.

In addition to their presence in oral contraceptives, estrogens are used to treat menstrual disturbances (dysmenorrhea, dysfunctional uterine bleeding), osteoporosis, atrophic vaginitis, nondevelopment of the ovaries, hirsutism, cancer, and symptoms of menopause (particularly vasomotor instability [hot flashes and night sweats]). Estradiol transdermal system (Estraderm) is applied to the skin twice a week to treat the vasomotor symptoms of menopause.

The most common side effects of estrogen therapy are nausea and vomiting. With continued treatment, tolerance develops and these symptoms usually disappear. Other side effects include uterine bleeding, vaginal discharge, edema, thrombophlebitis, weight gain, and hypertension. Estrogen therapy may also promote endometrial carcinoma in postmenopausal women. This risk may be canceled out by administration of a progestin (e.g., medroxyprogesterone [Provera]) for the last 10 days of the cycle. A small increase in risk of breast cancer has been demonstrated, but the unusual form is more easily "cured" than the usual breast cancer. The incidence of vaginal and cervical

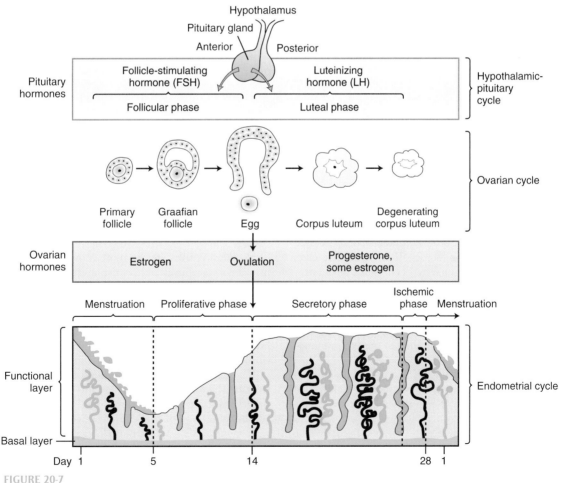

FIGURE 20-7

The menstrual cycle. (From McKenry L, Tessier E, Hogan MA: *Mosby's pharmacology in nursing,* ed 22, St Louis, 2006, Mosby.)

TABLE 20-8 SELECTED HORMONAL CONTRACEPTIVE DRUGS		
Oral Contraceptives	**Estrogen**	**Progestin**
Norinyl 1/50, Ortho-Novum 1/50	Mestranol	Norethindrone
Desogen, Ortho-Cept	Ethinyl estradiol	Desogestrel
Demulen 1/35, 1/50; Zovia 1/35	Ethinyl estradiol	Ethynodiol
Levlen, Tri-Levlen, Levora, Nordette, Triphasil	Ethinyl estradiol	Levonorgestrel
Brevicon; Loestrin 1/20, 1.5/30; Modicon; Ovcon 35/50; Tri-Norinyl; Norinyl 1/35; Ortho-Novum 1/35	Ethinyl estradiol	Norethindrone
Ortho-Cyclen, Ortho Tri-Cyclen	Ethinyl estradiol	Norgestimate
Lo/Ovral, Ovral	Ethinyl estradiol	Norgestrel
New Oral Contraceptives		
Seasonale (0.03 mg/0.15 mg)	Ethinyl estradiol	Levonorgestrel
YAZ	Ethinyl estradiol	Drospirenone
Contraceptive vaginal ring (Nuva Ring)	Ethinyl estradiol	Etonogestrel

carcinoma has been shown to increase in the female offspring of women given diethylstilbestrol (DES).

◆ EFFECT ON ORAL TISSUES

Estrogens influence the gingival tissues. For example, changes in sex hormone levels during the life of the female are related to the development of gingivitis at puberty (puberty gingivitis), during pregnancy (pregnancy gingivitis), and after menopause (chronic desquamative gingivitis). Conscientious plaque control helps to minimize these conditions. The increase in gingival inflammation may occur even with a decrease in the amount of plaque. This may be a result of increased levels of prostaglandin E (PGE), estradiol, and progesterone in the saliva.

Other side effects of estrogens are discussed in the section on oral contraceptives.

Progestins

The corpus luteum is the primary source of progesterone during the normal female sexual cycle. Progesterone promotes secretory changes in the endometrium and prepares the uterus for implantation of the fertilized ovum. If implantation does not occur by the end of the menstrual cycle, progesterone secretion declines, and the onset of menstruation occurs. If implantation takes place, the developing trophoblast secretes chorionic gonadotropin, which sustains the corpus luteum, thus maintaining progesterone and estrogen levels and preventing menstruation. Other effects of progesterone include suppression of uterine contractility, proliferation of the acini of the mammary gland, and alteration of transplantation immunity to prevent immunologic rejection of the fetus.

Medroxyprogesterone (me-DROKS-ee-proe-JESS-ter-one) (Provera), a progestin, is used orally by postmenopausal women in conjunction with estrogens. It prevents the increase in the risk of uterine cancer that can occur with unopposed estrogen. Women who have had a hysterectomy do not need to take medroxyprogesterone with estrogens.

Progestins alone are used in a variety of dose forms. Parenteral medroxyprogesterone (Depo-Provera) is administered every 3 months as a contraceptive. Progestin-only "minipills"

(see Table 20-7) are used orally for contraception in patients in whom estrogens are contraindicated. They must be taken each day of the month and are slightly less effective than the combination oral contraceptive products. They are very infrequently used.

A progestational agent can be administered in the form of an intrauterine device (IUD) impregnated with a progestational agent (Progestasert) or an implant placed under the skin on the arm (levonorgestrel [Norplant]). Norplant provides contraception for at least 5 years. These implants can produce prolonged, spotty, and irregular bleeding or amenorrhea; however, many women find them convenient and problem free. The problem with Norplant seems to be that removing the five containers in which the drug was contained has proved very difficult.

The primary use of the progestins is as one of the ingredients in almost all oral contraception combinations. The second most common use is in combination with estrogen for postmenopausal women. Other uses of the progestational agents include the treatment of endometriosis, dysmenorrhea, dysfunctional uterine bleeding, and premenstrual tension.

Hormonal Contraceptives

Oral contraceptives are the most common dose forms of hormonal contraceptives and consist of estrogens and progestins in various combinations. These are the most common birth control pills and are more than 99% effective (if patient compliance is perfect). Preparations that contain a progestin alone (the minipill) are slightly less effective and produce less regular menstrual cycles but do not have most of the side effects of the estrogen contained in the combination preparation (Box 20-5).

The compounds most commonly found in oral contraceptives are the estrogens, ethinyl estradiol and mestranol, and the progestins, norgestrel, norethindrone, and norethynodrel. The combination type of oral contraceptive is taken for 21 days of each month. With a 28-day pack, the seven pills in the fourth week contain no active ingredient but remind the patient to take a pill every day. After the third week, the menstrual cycle occurs. At least three different formulations exist: the fixed combination, the biphasic (two different strengths of tablets), and the

OCs, Oral contraceptives.

triphasic (three different types of tablets with varying amounts of the estrogenic and progestogenic component). The biphasic and triphasic agents are said to mimic the "natural" hormones more closely. No documented advantage has been demonstrated between these three combinations.

Seasonale (ethinyl estradiol/levonorgestrel) is the newest in combination oral contraceptives. Seasonale is different in that it is an extended-cycle oral contraceptive. Women take Seasonale for 3 months. Seasonale is taken once daily until the last tablet in the extended-cycle tablet dispenser is taken. The active tablets (n = 84) are pink, and the inactive tablets (n = 7) are white. The new dispenser is started the very next day. As a result, women only bleed once every 3 months (4 periods a year).

The contraceptive vaginal ring is a new dose form that introduces hormonal contraception into the body. NuvaRing is the only combination dose form in this group. It contains ethinyl estradiol and etonogestrel. The patient inserts the ring for 3 weeks during which the ring continuously releases low doses of ethinyl estradiol and etonogestrel. The ring is removed at the start of the fourth week, and the patient will then experience bleeding (their period). A new ring is inserted on day 29 of the patient's cycle after being ring-free for a week. Patients must insert the new ring on the same day each month.

An injectable hormonal contraceptive is also available. Lunelle is a monthly birth control shot that is 99% effective when given as prescribed. It contains the hormones ethinyl estradiol and drospirenone. The injection is given by a health professional on a monthly basis.

Hormonal contraceptives interfere with fertility by inhibiting the release of FSH and LH and therefore preventing ovulation. Early follicular FSH and midcycle FSH and LH increases are not seen. In addition, these contraceptive agents interfere with impregnation by altering the endometrium and the secretions of the cervix.

The side effects associated with hormonal contraceptives include increased tendency to clot (produces thrombophlebitis and thromboembolism) and carcinogenicity. The minor side effects of nausea, dizziness, headache, weight gain, and breast discomfort resemble those during early pregnancy and are mainly attributable to the estrogen in the preparation. These effects usually last only several weeks. Other side effects include blood pressure elevation and liver damage.

The hormones in contraceptives increase gingival fluid, stimulate gingivitis, and are associated with gingival inflammation similar to but not as prominent as that seen in pregnancy. Others have not shown any significant differences between the plaque scores, gingival scores, or loss of attachment when comparing users and nonusers of oral contraceptives. This discrepancy may be based partly on differences in dose between studies. In addition, this effect may not be evident in all users but may be of clinical significance only in those persons who are highly susceptible to oral soft tissue disorders. In any case, the dentist and dental hygienist should be aware that hormonal contraceptives do have the potential to cause or aggravate gingival inflammation.

Hormonal contraceptives are also associated with a significant increase in the frequency of dry socket after extractions. This risk can be minimized by performing extractions during days 23 through 28 of the tablet cycle. For patients taking Seasonale, extractions should be limited to the end of the extended-cycle tablet dispenser when the patient is taking the white tablets. Contraindications for the use of oral contraceptives include thromboembolic disorders, significant dysfunction of the liver, known or suspected carcinoma of the breast or other estrogen-dependent neoplasm, and undiagnosed genital bleeding.

In light of the increased use of antibiotics in periodontal therapy, the importance of the antibiotic hormonal contraceptive interaction must be mentioned (Table 20-9). Certain antibiotics have been said to reduce the effectiveness of hormonal contraceptives. They are thought to do so indirectly by suppressing the intestinal flora and thus diminishing the availability of hydrolytic enzymes to regenerate the parent steroid molecule. Consequently, plasma concentrations of the steroids are said to be abnormally low, and the steroid is cleared more rapidly from the body than under normal circumstances. Some recommend that the patient might want to use an additional method of contraception until the end of her cycle. Other suggestions include the substitution of topical for systemic antibiotics, if possible, and the use of hormonal contraceptives with higher levels of the estrogen component. The latter suggestion should only be undertaken by the patient's physician. Although all antibiotics have been implicated in this drug interaction, the incidence is indeed rare. If the patient is in the last week (week 3) or the placebo week (week 4), the chance of hormonal

TABLE 20-9   ORAL CONTRACEPTIVES: DENTAL DRUG INTERACTIONS

Drug	Interaction
Penicillin	Decreased effectiveness of OC
Tetracyclines	Decreased effectiveness of OC
Acetaminophen	OC increased hepatotoxicity of acetaminophen
Benzodiazepines	OC increased clearance of benzodiazepines

OC, Oral contraceptive.

contraceptive therapy failure is even slimmer. In our litigation-conscious society, there should be documentation in the dental chart that the patient was informed about the rare chance of a drug interaction between oral contraceptives and antibiotics (see Table 20-9).

MALE SEX HORMONES

Androgens

The main androgen, testosterone, has both androgenic and anabolic effects. Because there is overlap between androgens and anabolic steroids, separating them is difficult. Table 20-10 lists the male hormones and their antagonists and the female hormone antagonists. Androgens are responsible for the development of secondary male sex characteristics. Their anabolic action results in an increase in tissue protein and nitrogen retention in the body. Other actions of the androgens include increased osteoblastic activity, epiphyseal closure (cannot grow any taller), and an increase in sebaceous gland activity (increased acne).

Puberty gingivitis can occur related to hormonal changes. Androgenic steroids are used medically in the treatment of breast cancer or for replacement therapy. Treatment includes subgingival debridement and oral hygiene instructions (Box 20-6).

Androgens are used illicitly by body builders, weight lifters, and other athletes for muscle mass gain. Many athletic events now test the urine for the presence of anabolic steroids. Because of their abuse, androgenic steroids are Schedule III controlled substances (same category as Tylenol #3). The side effects of androgenic steroids include nausea, cholestatic jaundice, hepatocellular neoplasms, increased serum cholesterol, habituation, and depression and excitation. In females, virilization (acne, hirsutism, deepening voice, clitoral enlargement, malelike baldness) occurs. Considering the potential for side effects, the illicit use of these agents is difficult to understand.

OTHER AGENTS THAT AFFECT SEX HORMONE SYSTEMS

Other agents that affect sex hormones may either act like the hormones or inhibit the action of the naturally occurring sex hormones (Table 20-11). Hormones from the opposite sex are often used to manage prostate, breast, and uterine cancers because the cancer is often stimulated by the patient's own sex

TABLE 20-10 MALE HORMONES, AGONISTS, AND ANTAGONISTS; FEMALE HORMONE ANTAGONISTS

Drug Group	Examples	Indications
Male Reproductive System		
Androgens	Testosterone Methyltestosterone	Deficiency of testosterone, estrogen- dependent malignancy
Anabolic agents	Methandrostenolone (Dianabol) Nandrolone Stanozolol	Body builders use illicitly
Antiandrogens	Cyproterone acetate Flutamide (Eulexin) Nilutamide (Nilandron) Bicalutamide (Casodex)	Prostate cancer Advanced or metastatic prostate carcinoma in males
	Finasteride (Propecia, Proscar)	Inhibits 5-α-reductase; baldness, benign prostatic hypertrophy
Female Reproductive System		
Gonadotropin-releasing hormone	Gonadorelin (Factrel)	Stimulates release of FSH and LH; used to test hypothalamus and pituitary gland function
Nonpituitary chorionic gonadotropin	Gonadotropin, chorionic (A.P.L., Pregnyl)	Infertility
Menotropins	Menotropins (Pergonal)	Infertility; like FSH and LH
Antiestrogens	Danazol (Danocrine) Tamoxifen (Nolvadex) Fulvestrant (Faslodex) Toremifene (Fareston) Raloxifene (Evista)	Endometriosis Advanced breast cancer Advanced breast cancer Advanced breast cancer Prevents breast cancer in selected high-risk populations of women
	Clomiphene (Clomid, Serophene) Nafarelin (Synarel)	Infertility; increases FSH and LH Endometriosis; gonadotropin-releasing hormone agonist; stimulates LH and FSH
Aromatase inhibitors	Anastrozole (Arimidex) Exemestane (Aromasin) Letrozole (Femara)	Advanced breast cancer Advanced breast cancer Advanced breast cancer
Progestin antagonist	Mifepristone (RU-486)	Fetal abortion, used with prostaglandin E

FSH, Follicle-stimulating hormone; *LH*, luteinizing hormone.

Androgenic/Anabolic Steroid Indications

- Testosterone deficiency: androgen replacement therapy in the treatment of delayed male puberty, postpartum breast pain and engorgement, inoperable breast cancer, male hypogonadism
- Methyltestosterone (Metandren, Android): hypogonadism, delayed puberty, impotence, and climacteric symptoms
- Female: palliative treatment of metastatic breast cancer; postpartum breast pain and/or engorgement
- Used with estrogen in postmenopausal women
- Nandrolone (Androlone, Deca-Durabolin): metastatic breast cancer, anemia of renal insufficiency
- Oxymetholone (Anadrol): anemias caused by antineoplastics
- Danazol (Danocrine): endometriosis, hereditary angioedema
- Stanozolol (Winstrol): hereditary angioedema
- Fluoxymesterone (Halotestin)
- Methandrostenolone (Dianabol)

Antiandrogen Indications

- Bicalutamide (Casodex), nilutamide (Nilandron): in combination therapy with luteinizing hormone–releasing hormone (LH-RH) agonist analogs—prostatic carcinoma
- Finasteride (Proscar): benign prostatic hyperplasia (BPH), prostatic cancer; alopecia

TABLE 20-11 OTHER AGENTS THAT AFFECT SEX HORMONE SYSTEMS

Drug	Action	Indication
Clomiphene (Clomid, Serophene)	Estrogen antagonist and agonist	Infertility
Leuprolide injections (Lupron, Eligard)	Initially, increases LH and FSH; continuous administration results in reduced LH and FSH	Infertility
Tamoxifen (Nolvadex)	Estrogen agonist-antagonist Antiestrogen	Breast cancer
Toremifene (Fareston)	Estrogen agonist-antagonist	Breast cancer
Danazol (Danocrine)	Estrogen antagonist Antiestrogen	Endometriosis

hormones. For example, prostate cancer is often stimulated by testosterone, so men with prostate cancer are given estrogens to inhibit the cancer's growth.

Clomiphene

Clomiphene (KLOE-mi-feen) (Clomid, Serophene) has the ability to induce ovulation in some anovulatory women. Clomiphene reduces the number of estrogenic receptors (antiestrogen) by binding to them. The hypothalamus and pituitary then falsely interpret the situation as estrogen levels that are low and increase their secretion of LH, FSH, and gonadotropins. Because clomiphene is a partial estrogen agonist, it acts as a competitive inhibitor of endogenous estrogen. Ovarian stimulation then results. Its side effects include hot flashes, eye problems, headaches, and constipation. Other side effects result from the symptoms of ovulation. Clomiphene is used to treat infertility in females and has been used experimentally for males also. The

chance of multiple pregnancies increases about six times with clomiphene treatment. Female dental patients being treated with clomiphene should be considered to be pregnant, unless known to be not pregnant.

Leuprolide

Leuprolide (loo-PROE-lide) (Lupron) is a GnRH analog used intramuscularly in the management of endometriosis and to treat infertility. It suppresses production of male and female steroids as a result of a decreased level of LH and FSH.

Tamoxifen

Tamoxifen (ta-MOKS-i-fen) (Nolvadex) is a competitive inhibitor of estradiol at the receptor. It is indicated in the palliative treatment of advanced breast cancer in postmenopausal women. A large study recently published determined that the use of tamoxifen as a prophylactic (preventive) for primary breast cancer in women at increased risk reduced the risk by about 50%. A similar new drug is raloxifene (Evista).

Danazol

Danazol (DA-na-zole) (Danocrine) possesses weak progestational and androgenic action. It suppresses ovarian function and prevents LH and FSH midcycle surge. Its side effects include an increase in weight, decrease in breast size, acne, increased hair, lowered voice, headache, and hot flushes. It is used to treat endometriosis and fibrocystic breast disease in women.

Aromatase Inhibitors

Aromatase inhibitors are the newest in a group of drugs to help treat breast cancer. These drugs reduce almost the entire amount of estrogen made in the bodies of postmenopausal women. One of the advantages of aromatase inhibitors is that because they cut off the estrogen supply, they tend to cause fewer side effects than tamoxifen, especially stroke, blood clots, and uterine cancer. However, women taking aromatase inhibitors are at a higher risk for osteoporosis because they have less estrogen to protect bone density. They are indicated for the treatment of advanced breast cancer in postmenopausal women. Anastrozole is also FDA-approved for women with early-stage disease right after surgery, exemestane is FDA-approved for women with early-stage disease that have already received 2 to 3 years of tamoxifen therapy, and letrozole is FDA-approved for women with early-stage disease right after surgery and for women with early-stage disease who have completed 5 years of tamoxifen therapy.

BIBLIOGRAPHY

A new indication for Colesevelam (Welchol), *Med Lett Drugs Ther* 50:33, 2008.

Collin HL et al: Caries in patients with NIDDM, *Oral Surg Oral Med Oral Pathol Oral Radiol Endod* 85:680-685, 1998.

Crofford OB: Diabetes control and complications, *Annu Rev Med* 46:267-279, 1995.

Drugs for Type 2 Diabetes. Treatment Guidelines, *The Medical Letter* 47-54, 2008.

Eurich DT, et al: Improved clinical outcomes associated with metformin in patients with diabetes and heart failure, *Diabetes Care* 28:2345, 2005.

Nathan DM, et al: Management of hyperglycaemia in type 2 diabetes: a consensus algorithm for the initiation and adjustment of therapy: a consensus statement from the American Diabetes Association and the European Association for the Study of Diabetes, *Diabetologia* 49: 1711, 2006.

The ADVANCE Collaborative Group: Intensive blood glucose control and vascular outcomes in patients with type 2 diabetes, *N Engl J Med* 358:2560, 2008.

The Diabetes Control and Complications Trial Research Group: The effect of intensive treatment of diabetes on the development and progression of long-term complications in insulin-dependent diabetes mellitus, *N Engl J Med* 329:977-986, 1993.

DENTAL HYGIENE CONSIDERATIONS

1. Regardless of the disease state being treated, the dental hygienist should obtain a detailed medication/health history from the patient.
2. The patient's appointment time may depend on when the patient has taken his or her medication and when he or she has eaten.
3. The medication history will help to avoid drug interactions.
4. Patients who are hyperthyroid may require higher doses of local anesthetics or CNS depressant medications until they are considered euthyroid.
5. Epinephrine use should be avoided in patients who are hyperthyroid.
6. Patients who are hypothyroid may require lower doses of CNS depressant drugs. These patients should be counseled about the increased risk for sedation and the need to avoid driving or any activity that requires thought or concentration.
7. Patients with diabetes are at an increased risk for caries and other oral disorders. Encourage these patients to maintain excellent home oral health care.
8. Review the information in Box 20-4 and Table 20-2.
9. Patients with diabetes are at an increased risk for infection and delayed wound healing. Antibiotics may be necessary.
10. Hypoglycemia can occur if the patient has taken his or her medicine but has not eaten. Be prepared to treat hypoglycemia if it should occur.
11. The dental hygienist should review the importance of good home oral hygiene with all patients taking oral contraceptives because of the potential for gingivitis and gingival inflammation.
12. Extractions should be performed on days 23 to 28 of the oral contraceptive cycle in order to avoid dry socket.
13. Always check the patient's blood pressure because oral contraceptives and hormone replacement therapy can elevate blood pressure.
14. Have patients take a break and stretch their legs if the dental procedure is longer than 30 minutes. Oral contraceptives and hormone replacement therapy can cause thrombophlebitis.
15. Review the information in Table 20-5 for all patients taking oral contraceptives.
16. Patients taking anabolic steroids and male sex hormones can experience mood changes. Appointments may need to be rescheduled if patients become aggressive or psychotic.
17. These drugs can also elevate blood pressure, so always check the patient's blood pressure at each visit.

CLINICAL SKILLS ASSESSMENT

1. What is diabetes and what are its signs and symptoms?
2. Compare and contrast Type I and Type II diabetes.
3. What are some of the dental concerns associated with diabetes and how would the dental practitioner counsel a pediatric patient with diabetes?
4. When should a diabetic patient's dental appointment be scheduled and why?
5. Describe the commonly used types of insulin and state their most common usage pattern.
6. What are the adverse reactions associated with insulin?
7. Name the four oral hypoglycemic agents (from different groups) and state two side effects of this group of drugs.
8. How do oral contraceptives work and what are their clinical uses?
9. What are some of the adverse reactions associated with oral contraceptives?
10. What are the dental concerns associated with oral contraceptives?
11. Describe the dental effects of hypothyroidism and hyperthyroidism.
12. What is the difference between hypoglycemic agents and antihyperglycemic agents?

⊖volve

Please visit http://evolve.elsevier.com/Haveles/pharmacology for review questions and additional practice and reference materials.

21 Antineoplastic Drugs

LEARNING OBJECTIVES

1. Define antineoplastic agents.
2. Summarize the use, mechanisms of action, and classification of antineoplastic agents.
3. Describe several adverse drug effects associated with antineoplastic agents.
4. Discuss the dental implications of patients planning to take or actively taking antineoplastic drugs.

Antineoplastic agents were designed to treat malignancies. A relatively new use of these agents is in the management of diseases with an inflammatory component such as psoriasis, rheumatoid arthritis, and systemic lupus erythematosus. Depending on their use, these agents are prescribed by oncologists, rheumatologists, and oral pathologists (for oral conditions related to systemic autoimmune diseases). For treating malignancies, the dental health care worker should be aware of the relationship between the timing of the treatments and the effects on the bone marrow. The dental health care worker should be familiar with the side effects of these agents, especially their oral manifestations.

Current research is elucidating many different mechanisms involved in the etiology of cancer, including genetics, viruses, deleted or damaged tumor-suppressor genes, specific oncogenes, and changes in both ribonucleic acid (RNA) and deoxyribonucleic acid (DNA) that affect the growth of cells. Many animal carcinogens have been identified, but proving carcinogenic potential in humans is much more difficult.

Environmental carcinogens

Many human carcinogens are environmental carcinogens, for example, polychlorinated biphenyls (PCBs) from transformers. Other known carcinogens include tobacco smoke, aflatoxins (produced by moldy peanuts), sunlight (increase in malignant melanoma and squamous cell carcinoma), radiation, chemicals, dioxin, and benzene. Most believe that the herpes viruses and papillomaviruses have a potential for producing cancerous changes. Patients with a history of certain diseases, such as hepatitis, have a higher incidence of liver cancer than normal patients.

Normal cells have a mechanism to turn off cell growth under certain signals. With cancer, a change in the cells occurs so that they continue to grow. With a lack of control (switch does not turn off), the abnormal neoplastic cells continue to grow. The cell-surface antigens appear similar to the normal fetal types, so the body does not mount an immune response. The tumor stem cells have chromosomal abnormalities, repetitions, and select subclones. With repeated cycles the cells can migrate to distant sites and metastases form colonies. For example, cancer that begins in the breast may spread to the bone or liver.

USE OF ANTINEOPLASTIC AGENTS

Antineoplastic agents, sometimes called *cancer chemotherapeutic agents,* are used clinically to interfere with the neoplastic cells. The antineoplastic agents interfere with some function of the malignant cells. They suppress the growth of the cells and attempt to destroy and prevent the spread of malignant cells. (Figure 21-1 illustrates the way in which cancer cells respond to chemotherapy.) These agents

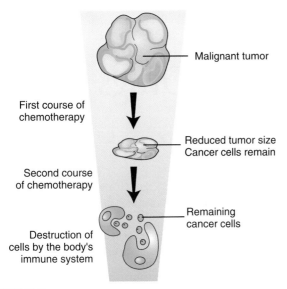

FIGURE 21-1
Cancer cell response to chemotherapy. (From McKenry L, Tessier E, Hogan MA: *Mosby's pharmacology for nursing*, ed 22, St Louis, 2006, Mosby.)

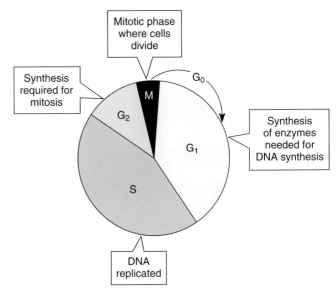

FIGURE 21-2
Cell cycle.

are used either alone or in combination or with radiation or surgery, depending on the type of malignancy being treated. Each type of malignancy may be sensitive to each of the three modalities: drugs, radiation, or surgery.

| Drugs effective for some cancers |

For treatment of certain malignancies, for example, the leukemias, choriocarcinoma, multiple myeloma, and Burkitt's lymphoma, drugs are considered the primary choice. Often, combinations of several antineoplastic agents, used in conjunction with surgery and/or irradiation, may effect a cure that each procedure alone could not. Certain cancers are relatively insensitive to antineoplastic agents. These cancers are treated with either radiation and/or surgery. Box 21-1 lists malignancies and their likelihood of sensitivity to cancer chemotherapy agents.

The current philosophy for the use of the antineoplastic agents involves treating the initial stages of disease very aggressively. This approach promises more chance of controlling and curing the disease but also involves many severe side effects, including some that affect the oral cavity. The treatment of some cancers involves the removal of cells from the bone marrow before administering the chemotherapy or radiation. In the past, the dose administered would have been fatal. However, after treatment is complete, the cells taken from the bone marrow are returned to the patient's body and they begin making the blood elements that are made in bone marrow. Gene therapy is being used, and many advances are continuing to be made. New research is attempting to use the body's immune system to fight the cancer cells.

MECHANISMS OF ACTION

The efficacy of antineoplastic agents is based primarily on their ability to interfere with the metabolism or reproductive cycle of the tumor cells, thereby destroying them. The reproductive cycle of a cell consists of the following four stages (Figure 21-2):

BOX 21-1   SENSITIVITY OF NEOPLASTIC DISEASES TO CHEMOTHERAPY

Highly Sensitive
Acute lymphocytic leukemia
Acute myelocytic leukemia
Breast cancer
Burkitt's lymphoma
Ewing's sarcoma
Hodgkin's disease
Oat cell
Wilms' tumor

Moderately Sensitive
Head and neck, squamous
Endometrial
Neuroblastoma
Prostate
Bladder
Chronic lymphocytic leukemia
Colorectal
Chronic myelocytic leukemia
Cervix
Kaposi's sarcoma (acquired immunodeficiency syndrome [AIDS])
Ovary

Little Sensitivity
Liver
Pancreatic
Lung
Renal
Melanoma

---

1. G_1 ("gap" 1), which is the postmitotic or pre-DNA synthesis phase
2. S, which is the period of DNA synthesis
3. G_2 ("gap" 2), which is the premitotic or post-DNA synthesis phase
4. M, which is the period of mitosis

Cells in a resting stage that are not in a process of cell division are described as being in the G_0 stage. Cells enter the cycle from the G_0 stage. In some tumors, a large proportion of the cells may be at the G_0 level. These cells are difficult to reach and destroy.

Cell-cycle—specific or nonspecific

Most of the antineoplastic agents are labeled as being either cell-cycle specific (Table 21-1 and Figure 21-3), indicating that they are effective only at specific phases of cellular growth, or cell-cycle nonspecific, indicating that they are effective at all levels of the cycle (effective both in the resting and the proliferating cells). For example, the alkylating agents interfere with the malignant cells during all phases of the reproductive cycle and the resting stage (G_0) and therefore are classified as cycle independent.

A major problem with treating neoplastic cells is that the cell growth is exponential. Before diagnosis is made, a large cell load must be present. If 10^{12} cells are present and 99.9% of the cells are killed, 10^9 cells would remain; if 99.9% of those cells were killed, 10^6 cells would still be present. Mixing several chemotherapeutic agents can increase the chance of killing more cells

because they work by different mechanisms and have different adverse reactions.

Resistance to chemotherapy occurs by either of the following methods:
- *De novo resistance:* The neoplasm was always resistant to the chemotherapeutic agents.
- *Acquired resistance:* Resistance occurs through the natural selection of mutations.

CLASSIFICATION

Groups divided by how they work

The antineoplastic agents are divided into groups depending on their mechanism and site of action (Figure 21-4). Box 21-2 lists some antineoplastic agents by classification.

The alkylating agents contain alkyl radicals that react with DNA in all cycles of the cell, preventing reproduction. The antimetabolites attack the cells in the S period of reproduction by interfering with purine or pyrimidine synthesis. They incorporate the drug into a compound or inhibit an enzyme from functioning and are more effective on rapidly proliferating neoplasms. Plant alkaloids are mitotic inhibitors and act by arresting cells in metaphase. Because of their low bone marrow toxicity, they are often used in combination with other agents with more bone marrow toxicity. Antibiotics are cell-cycle nonspecific and are effective for solid tumors. Other agents include hormones, such as prednisone, which interrupt the cell cycle at the G stage. Steroids are used to suppress lymphocytes in leukemias and lymphomas and in combination therapies. Estrogens are used for palliation in inoperable breast cancer. Tamoxifen, an

TABLE 21-1 CLASSIFICATION OF ANTINEOPLASTIC DRUGS	
Cell-Cycle Specific	Cell-Cycle Nonspecific
Antimetabolites	Alkylating agents
Bleomycin	Antibiotics
Vinca alkaloids	Cisplatin
Podophyllin	Nitrosoureas

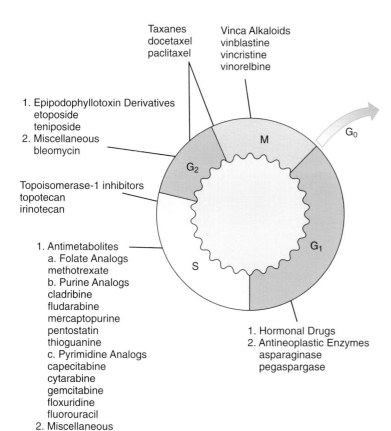

FIGURE 21-3
General phase of the cell cycle in which the various cell-cycle—specific chemotherapeutic drugs have their greatest proportionate kill of cancer cells. (From Lilley LL, Harrington S, Snyder JS: *Pharmacology and the nursing process,* ed 5, St Louis, 2007, Mosby.)

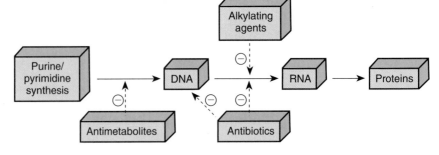

FIGURE 21-4
Location of action of some antineoplastic agents. The synthesis of proteins can be interfered with at the purine/pyrimidine, DNA, or RNA level.

BOX 21-2   ANTINEOPLASTIC AGENTS BY GROUP

Alkylating Agents
Nitrogen Mustard
Mechlorethamine (Mustargen)
Cyclophosphamide (Leukeran)
Chlorambucil (Leukeran)
Melphalan (Alkeran)
Uracil mustard
Ifosfamide (Ifex)

Nitrosoureas
Carmustine (BCNU, BiCNU)
Lomustine (CCNU, CeeNU)
Semustine (Methyl-Cee NU)
Streptozocin (Zanosar)
Estramustine (Emcyt)

Miscellaneous
Busulfan (Myleran)
Pipobroman (Vercyte)
Thiotepa
Cisplatin (Platinol)
Carboplatin (Paraplatin)

Antimetabolites
Folic Acid Analog
Methotrexate (Amethopterin)

Pyrimidine Analog
Fluorouracil (5-FU)
Floxuridine (FUDR)
Cytosine arabinoside (ARA-C, Cytosar-U)
Azacytidine

Purine Analog
Mercaptopurine (6-MP, Purinethol)
Thioguanine (6-TG)
Cladribine (Leustatin)
Fludarabine (Fludara)
Pentostatin (Nipent)

Miscellaneous Antineoplastics
Plant Alkaloids
Vinblastine (Velban)
Vincristine (Oncovin)

Antibiotics
Dactinomycin (Actinomycin-D, Cosmegen)
Doxorubicin (Adriamycin)
Bleomycin (Blenoxane)
Mitomycin-C (Mutamycin)
Plicamycin (Mithramycin, Mithracin)
Daunorubicin (Cerubidine)

Hormones
Adrenocorticosteroids (prednisone)
Androgen
   Testolactone (Teslac)
   Fluoxymesterone (Halotestin)
Antiandrogen
   Flutamide (Eulexin)
   Nilutamide (Nilandron)
   Bicalutamide (Casodex)
Estrogen
   Diethylstilbestrol
   Ethinyl estradiol (Estinyl)
Antiestrogen
   Tamoxifen (Nolvadex)
   Raloxifene (Evista)
   Fulvestrant (Faslodex)
   Toremifene (Fareston)
Aromatase inhibitors
   Anastrozole (Arimidex)
   Exemestane (Aromasin)
   Letrozole (Femara)
Progestin
   Medroxyprogesterone
   Megestrol (Megace)
Goserelin (Zoladex)
Leuprolide (Lupron)

Immune Modulators
Levamisole (Ergamisol)
Interferon α-n3 (Alferon N)
Interferon α-2b (Intron A)
Interferon α-2a (Roferon-a)

Podophyllotoxin Derivatives
Etoposide (VePesid)
Teniposide (Vumon)

Aminobisphosphonates
Alendronate (Fosamax)
Ibandronate (Boniva)
Pamidronate (Aredia)
Risedronate (Actonel)
Zoledronic acid (Zometa)

Other
L-Asparaginase (Elspar)
Hydroxyurea (Hydrea)
Procarbazine (Matulane)
Paclitaxel (Taxol)
Altretamine (Hexalen)
Trastuzumab (Herceptin)
Imatinib mesylate (Gleevec)

---

antiestrogenic substance, is used to manage breast cancer. It has also recently been shown to prevent breast cancer when used in women who have a high risk for breast cancer. Cisplatin, a heavy metal complex of platinum, is cell-cycle nonspecific. Hydroxyurea inhibits ribonucleoside diphosphate reductase, which interferes with the conversion of ribonucleoside diphosphates to deoxyribonucleoside diphosphates. Procarbazine produces chromosomal breakage.

ADVERSE DRUG EFFECTS

Rapidly growing cells, such as neoplastic cells, are more susceptible to inhibition or destruction by antineoplastic agents. The most serious difficulty encountered in antineoplastic therapy stems from the lack of selectivity between tumor tissue and normal tissue. Some normal cells exhibit a faster reproduction

TABLE 21-2 SELECTED ADVERSE REACTIONS OF SOME ANTINEOPLASTIC AGENTS

Drug	Uses/Adverse Reactions
Methotrexate (MTX)	GI, BMS, leucovorin rescue; used for severe arthritis and psoriasis
5-Fluorouracil	GI, BMS, topical for superficial basal cell carcinoma
Dactinomycin	GI, **BMS**
Doxorubicin	GI, BMS, **cardiotoxicity**
Mechlorethamine	Nitrogen mustard during WWI (chemical warfare); vomiting, BMS, bifunctional (binds at two sites)
Cyclophosphamide	BMS, **hemorrhagic cystitis** (Tx: ↑H$_2$O + mannitol + topical in bladder [mesna]), ↑ADH (Tx: furosemide)
Nitrosoureas	**Hematopoietic depression,** BMS
Vinblastine	**BMS,** peripheral neuropathy
Vincristine	**Peripheral neuropathy** (numbness and tingling of extremities; foot drop)
Tamoxifen	Increased bone and tumor pain
Cisplatin	Platin complex, persistent vomiting, **nephrotoxicity** (Tx: ↑H$_2$O + mannitol); electrolyte disturbances, ototoxicity, paresthesias, BMS
Procarbazine	**BMS,** psychic disturbances, procarbazine possesses MAO inhibitor activity and has potential for severe drug and food interactions
Asparaginase	**Hypersensitivity,** bleeding/clotting abnormalities, liver toxicity, pancreatitis, seizures

Boldface indicates that toxicity is usually dose limiting.
ADH, Antidiuretic hormone; *BMS,* bone marrow suppression; *GI,* gastrointestinal tract toxicity; *MAO,* monoamine oxidase; *Tx,* treatment; *WWI,* World War I.

cycle than do slowly growing tumor cells. In an effort to eradicate a malignancy, certain normal cells are also destroyed, resulting in adverse effects. Because the cells of the gastrointestinal tract, bone marrow, and hair follicles are among the faster growing normal cells, the early side effects are associated with these tissues.

Table 21-2 lists the most common adverse reactions associated with some antineoplastic agents. These are the more common or agent-specific reactions associated with the drugs listed. The principal adverse effects are as follows.

Bone Marrow Suppression

The bone marrow is suppressed because it is a tissue that is rapidly turning over. Inhibition of the bone marrow results in leukopenia or agranulocytosis, thrombocytopenia, and anemia. The degree of cytopenia that results depends on the drugs being used, the condition of the bone marrow at the time of administration, and other contributing factors. Symptoms of this adverse reaction may include susceptibility to infection, bleeding, and fatigue. The rise and fall in hematologic effects are related to location in the cycle of administering the drug.

Osteonecrosis

Osteonecrosis of the jaw bone is a recently recognized adverse effect of the bisphosphonates. About 94% of all cases of osteonecrosis have been reported in cancer patients receiving intravenous bisphosphonates, in particular pamidronate and zoledronic acid, for multiple myeloma or metastatic carcinoma. The incidence is much lower for patients taking oral bisphosphonates for osteoporosis with less than 1 case per 100,000 patients per year. It has been reported that bisphosphonates can produce microdamage because they alter bone deposition and the repair process. Prolonged use may suppress bone turnover to the point that microdamage persists and accumulates, which results in hypodynamic bone with decreased biomechanical competence. Most of the cases of osteonecrosis of the jaw occurred after tooth extractions and other dental procedures that traumatize the jaw. Unfortunately, osteonecrosis is very difficult to treat once it occurs. There are several means to help minimize or prevent it. The dental hygienist should ask if the patient is taking or receiving a bisphosphonate drug. Maintenance oral health examinations and any other dental procedure should be performed before starting bisphosphonate therapy or within 3 months of beginning therapy, if possible. Dental surgical procedures should be performed using minimal bone manipulation and supported with local and systemic antibiotic prophylaxis. Those with osteonecrosis of the jaw should have dead bone removed as necessary with minimal trauma to adjacent tissue. Chlorhexidine rinses, systemic antibiotics, and analgesics should be used if clinically necessary. Bisphosphonate-free holidays are not recommended before a dental procedure because these drugs stay in the bone for years. Bisphosphonate therapy is often stopped until the bone heals or the disease progresses to the point that bisphosphonate therapy is necessary.

Gastrointestinal Effects

Gastrointestinal problems are common because the gastrointestinal tract tissue is rapidly turning over. The sloughing of the gastrointestinal mucosa can produce many symptoms. Clinically, these disturbances are expressed as nausea, stomatitis, oral ulcerations, vomiting, and hemorrhagic diarrhea. Nausea and vomiting may be treated using phenothiazines (prochlorperazine [Compazine]), cannabinoids (dronabinol [Marinol] and nabilone [Cesamet]), metoclopramide (Reglan), and scopolamine.

Dermatologic Effects

Cutaneous reactions vary from mild erythema and maculopapular eruptions to exfoliative dermatitis and Stevens-Johnson syndrome. Alopecia is frequent, but the hair usually regrows when therapy is discontinued.

Hepatotoxicity

Liver problems occur principally with the antimetabolites (e.g., methotrexate [MTX]) but may occur with other agents as well.

Neurologic Effects

Neurotoxic effects, such as peripheral neuropathy, ileus, inappropriate antidiuretic hormone secretion, and convulsions, have been associated primarily with vincristine or vinblastine administration.

Nephrotoxicity

| Allopurinol prevents hyperuricemia. | The renal tubular impairment that occurs secondary to hyperuricemia is caused by rapid cell destruction and the

release of nucleotides. The treatment of leukemias and lymphomas often results in rapid tumor destruction with a consequent high uric acid level. Allopurinol (Zyloprim) is a xanthine oxidase inhibitor used in the management of gout. It blocks the production of uric acid by blocking its synthesis. Before the initiation of a regimen of antineoplastic agents that release purines and pyrimidines, allopurinol is administered to prevent hyperuricemia. Allopurinol can prolong the action and increase the toxicity of cyclophosphamide and the thiopurines (azathioprine and mercaptopurine).

Immunosuppression

Because the antineoplastic agents have an immunosuppressant effect, enhanced susceptibility to infection or a second malignancy may occur after treatment.

Germ Cells

Inhibition of spermatogenesis and oogenesis is frequent, at least temporarily. Mutations within the germ cells may occur. The menstrual cycle may also be inhibited. Recovery occurs after discontinuation of the drug.

Oral Effects

Adverse effects on the oral tissue are primarily those of discomfort, sensitivity of the teeth and gums, mucosal pain and ulceration, gingival hemorrhage, dryness, and impaired taste sensation. Infection of the oral mucosa from leukopenia and bleeding (petechiae on the hard palate) from thrombocytopenia can occur. Appropriate maintenance of the oral cavity (Box 21-3) should be undertaken even before and certainly during antineoplastic therapy.

Patients taking antineoplastic agents may experience inflammation of the mouth, xerostomia, or glossitis. In these cases, the dental health care worker should not recommend any products

containing alcohol (e.g., elixirs) because alcohol is drying to the oral mucosa.

COMBINATIONS

Agents of widely differing mechanisms of action are often used together to inhibit the reproduction of neoplastic cells in all phases and to gain therapeutic advantage for the host. Mixtures of these agents may act synergistically, leading to enhanced cytotoxicity with fewer side effects. This is the rationale for combination drug therapy.

Antineoplastic drugs are used in lower doses to manage diseases associated with inflammation or autoimmune conditions and transplants. Examples include azathioprine (Imuran), MTX (Rheumatrex), and cyclosporin (Sandimmune). Diseases that are treated with these agents include rheumatoid arthritis, systemic lupus erythematosus, pemphigus vulgaris, and psoriasis.

The doses of these agents used to treat diseases with an autoimmune component are often lower than the doses used to treat cancer. Some drug interactions that would be important with higher doses are often safe in the lower doses used for autoimmune diseases. With organ transplants, immunosuppressives are used to prevent rejection of the foreign tissue.

DENTAL IMPLICATIONS

Dental patients who are to take cancer chemotherapy agents should optimize their oral health before antineoplastic agents are begun (ideal conditions). However, often the dental health care worker has less than a day in which to attempt to attain this degree of dental health.

| Timing important: agranulocytosis— infections; thrombocytopenia— bleeding | If oral hygiene or dental procedures are to be performed on a patient who is taking antineoplastic agents, the procedures should be planned to coincide with the presence of the highest level of formed blood elements. That time

would be either just before treatment or on the first few days of treatment (drug does not immediately depress the bone marrow maximally).

After a cycle of drugs is completed, the effect on the bone marrow increases until the maximum effect is obtained. During this time, dental treatment should be avoided. The white blood cell count is often too low (agranulocytosis), and the chance of infection is great. The platelets may also be low (thrombocytopenia), and bleeding can occur. The optimal time for performing dental procedures will vary with each drug or drug regimen. Proper oral management of the patient receiving chemotherapy is given in Box 21-3. The general dental implications of the antineoplastic agents are listed in Box 21-4.

BOX 21-3   ORAL CARE FOR PATIENTS ON ANTINEOPLASTIC AGENTS

Before Chemotherapy
Eliminate and/or manage infection.
Control periodontal disease (include prophylaxis).
Provide oral hygiene instruction.

During Chemotherapy
Schedule appointment just before next chemotherapy.
Consult with oncologist before any procedure.
Document hematologic status (laboratory test).
Treat only if neutrophil count is >1000/mm.
Give endocarditis antibiotic prophylaxis if venous catheter present.
Institute oral hygiene program: brush properly, rinse with baking soda/ saline and/or chlorhexidine (avoid mouthwash), soda/saline after emesis, no dentures at night, topical fluoride if prolonged xerostomia.
Culture lesions for infection.

After Chemotherapy
Follow and maintain oral health.

BOX 21-4   MANAGEMENT OF THE DENTAL PATIENT TAKING ANTINEOPLASTIC AGENTS

- Maximize oral hygiene before chemotherapy
- Hygiene instructions to match patient's symptoms
- Potential for infection; watch for symptoms
- Check neutrophil count before treatment
- Check thrombocytes for adequate clotting
- Rinse with soda/saline and/or chlorhexidine

DENTAL HYGIENE CONSIDERATIONS

1. Patients receiving cancer chemotherapeutic drugs must be treated carefully.
2. The dental hygienist should meet with the patient prior to beginning chemotherapy in order to outline an optimal oral hygiene plan. The dental hygienist should then meet with the patient during and after chemotherapy in order to adjust the plan as necessary.
3. The best defense for the patient is to receive maximum oral hygiene and health care prior to chemotherapy.
4. Dental procedures should be avoided during chemotherapy because the patient is at high risk for infection as a result of low white blood cell counts.
5. Platelets may also be low, putting the patient at increased risk for bleeding.
6. Patients should come in just prior to beginning a chemotherapeutic regimen because this is when they are feeling their best and white blood cell counts are at their highest.
7. Review the information in Boxes 21-3 and 21-4.

CLINICAL SKILLS ASSESSMENT

1. Explain the adverse effects associated with the antineoplastic agents.
2. Explain oral care for patients receiving chemotherapy. Explain the importance of factors such as white blood cell count.
3. How would you counsel a patient on the appropriate oral hygiene program during chemotherapy?
4. Do GI adverse reactions affect oral hygiene? If so, how?

 Evolve ———————————————————————

Please visit http://evolve.elsevier.com/Haveles/pharmacology for review questions and additional practice and reference materials.

22 Respiratory and Gastrointestinal Drugs

LEARNING OBJECTIVES

1. Summarize the two groups of respiratory diseases.
2. Name and describe the mechanisms of action of several types of drugs used to treat respiratory diseases.
3. Discuss the types of drugs used to treat respiratory infections, including the implications to dentistry.
4. Summarize the most common types of gastrointestinal diseases.
5. Name and describe the types of drugs used to treat gastrointestinal diseases, including any implications to dentistry.

Diseases of the respiratory and gastrointestinal tracts are common, so dental health care workers are sure to encounter patients taking drugs for these diseases (Figure 22-1). Because the medications given to treat these diseases can affect dental treatment, the dental health care worker should be aware of the effects of these drugs on the patient and how these drugs can alter the dental treatment plan.

RESPIRATORY DRUGS

Diseases that are treated with respiratory drugs include asthma, chronic obstructive pulmonary disease (COPD), and upper respiratory tract infections (Figure 22-2). Respiratory drugs come from a wide range of drug groups, from adrenergic drugs for bronchodilation to corticosteroids for reducing inflammation. Drugs that increase expectoration and reduce coughs are also included in this discussion. Many drugs used to treat respiratory problems are administered topically via the lungs by the use of a metered-dose inhaler (MDI).

Respiratory Diseases

Noninfectious respiratory diseases are divided into two groups: (1) asthma and (2) COPD (see Figure 22-2). COPD is further divided into chronic bronchitis and emphysema. Other respiratory problems are related to respiratory infections, such as viral or bacterial.

♦ ASTHMA

Asthma: reversible airway obstruction with inflammation

One common respiratory disease is asthma. It is characterized by reversible airway obstruction and is associated with reduction in expiratory airflow. A few hours later, inflammation occurs, resulting in an increase in secretions in the lungs and swelling in the bronchioles. Asthma is classified as being either intermittent or persistent. Persistent asthma is further categorized as mild, moderate, or severe. Patients with intermittent asthma experience symptoms less than two times a month and the symptoms do not interfere with normal activity. Persistent asthma occurs anywhere from more than twice a week to all day long. Persistent asthma can cause minor limitation of normal activities, and severe persistent asthma can severely limit the patient's normal activities. When asthma is treated, both components of the disease must be addressed. The *National Asthma Education and Prevention Program Expert Panel Report 3,* published in October 2007, presents the latest recommendations of the National Heart Lung and Blood Institute regarding asthma therapy. Figure 22-3 reviews the stepwise approach for managing asthma in children older than 12 years of age and adults.

Asthma may be precipitated by allergens, pollution, exercise, stress, or upper respiratory infection (allergic reaction to viruses). In status asthmaticus, patients have persistent life-threatening bronchospasm despite drug therapy. Environmental pollution may also play an important role in the increase in asthma. The dental health care worker should treat dental patients with asthma so that minimal stress is induced. Patients should bring their fast-acting β₂-agonist inhalers to be used prophylactically or in the management of an acute asthmatic attack in the dental office. Signs of asthma include shortness of breath and wheezing. Observation and questioning of the patient for asthma control before the dental appointment by the dental health care worker can prevent an acute attack. β-Adrenergic agonists, xanthines, cromolyn, corticosteroids, leukotriene (LT)-altering agents, and anticholinergics are used to treat this disease (Figure 22-4).

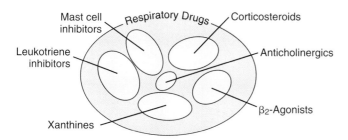

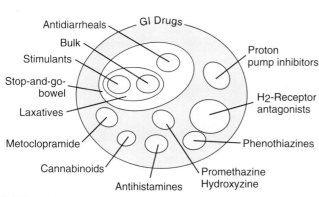

FIGURE 22-1
Respiratory and gastrointestinal drug groups. *GI*, Gastrointestinal.

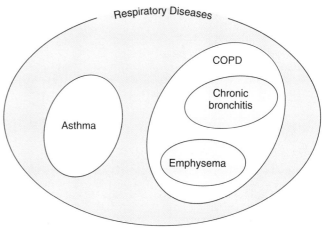

FIGURE 22-2
Respiratory diseases. *COPD*, Chronic obstructive pulmonary disease.

Intermittent asthma	Persistent asthma: Daily medication Consult with asthma specialist if step 4 care or higher is required Consider a consult with step 3

| **Step 1** Preferred: SABA, PRN | **Step 2** Preferred: Low-dose ICS Alternatives: Cromolyn, LTRA, nedocromil, or theophylline | **Step 3** Preferred: Low-dose ICS + LABA or medium-dose ICS Alternatives: Low-dose ICS + either LTRA, theophylline, or zileuton | **Step 4** Preferred: Medium-dose ICS + LABA Alternatives: Medium-dose ICS + either LTRA, theophylline, or zileuton | **Step 5** Preferred: High-dose ICS + LABA AND Consider omalizumab for patients who have allergies | **Step 6** Preferred: High-dose ICS + LABA + oral corticosteroids AND Consider omalizumab for patients who have allergies |

FIGURE 22-3
Stepwise approach for the management of asthma in persons 12 years of age or older. All patients require a rescue SABA inhaler whether they have intermittent or persistent asthma. *SABA,* Short-acting β₂-agonist; *ICS,* inhaled corticosteroid; *LABA,* long-acting β₂-agonist; *LTRA,* leukotriene receptor antagonist. (From National Asthma Education and Prevention Program Expert Panel 3: *Guidelines for the diagnosis and management of asthma,* Bethesda, Md, 2007 [October], National Heart Lung and Blood Institute, National Institutes of Health, U.S. Department of Health and Human Services.)

ALLERGENS such as dust, wool blankets, feather pillows, pollen, etc., in hypersensitive persons with IgE antibodies stimulate mast cells in lungs to release histamine (H) and slow-reacting substance of anaphylaxis (SRS-A).

HISTAMINE stimulates larger bronchi to cause smooth muscle spasms, inflammation, and edema.

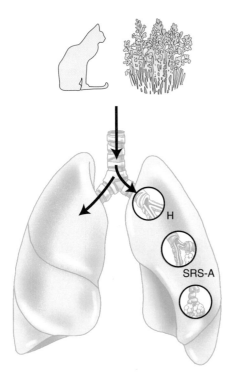

SRS-A stimulates small bronchi to cause smooth muscle swelling.

Result is spasms of smooth bronchial muscle, increased mucus secretions, swollen mucosa, hyperinflation of alveoli eventually leading to loss of elasticity and collapsed alveoli.

LEUKOTRIENE ANTAGONISTS block the release of leukotrienes in the lungs. Inflammation causes an increase in leukotrienes, substances that constitute the slow-reacting substance of anaphylaxis (SRS-A).

THEOPHYLLINE increases cyclic AMP to inhibit breakdown of sensitized mast cells that stimulate the release of histamine, serotonin, and SRS-A.

MAST CELL STABILIZERS inhibit the release of histamine from mast cells to reduce allergic effects.

SYMPATHETIC AGONISTS stimulate sympathetic systems to decrease mucus secretions and relax bronchial muscle spasms.

CORTICOSTEROIDS produce an antiinflammatory effect and reduce mucus secretions and tissue histamine.

FIGURE 22-4
Overview of the effects of various antiasthmatic medications. (From McKenry L, Tessier E, Hogan MA: *Mosby's pharmacology in nursing,* ed 22, St Louis, 2006, Mosby.)

♦ CHRONIC OBSTRUCTIVE PULMONARY DISEASE

> COPD: irreversible airway obstruction

COPD is characterized by irreversible airway obstruction, which occurs with either chronic bronchitis or emphysema. Smoking is associated with almost all COPD. Chronic bronchitis is a result of chronic inflammation of the airways and excessive sputum production. Emphysema is characterized by alveolar destruction with airspace enlargement and airway collapse. The anticholinergics are the first-line treatment, but β-adrenergic agonists and xanthines are also used to produce bronchodilation in these patients. In many instances patients receive a combination metered dose inhaler with an anticholinergic drug and a β₂ agonist. COPD and emphysema are associated with an increase in the incidence of bronchospasm and with fixed airway obstruction. Patients with upper respiratory tract infections often take adrenergic agonists for nasal congestion or bronchoconstriction, antihistamines to reduce secretions, expectorants to thin sputum, and antitussives to control coughing. Each drug group is discussed separately.

In the normal person, the drive for ventilation (breathing) is stimulated by an elevation in the partial pressure of carbon dioxide (Pa_{CO_2}). The partial pressure of oxygen (Pa_{O_2}) can vary widely without stimulating ventilation in the normal patient. Patients with COPD, because their ventilation is compromised, experience a gradual rise in Pa_{CO_2} over time. Because this mechanism becomes resistant to changes in Pa_{CO_2}, a new stimulus emerges, the partial pressure of Pa_{O_2}. The patient's ventilation is then driven by a decrease in Pa_{O_2}. If a patient with COPD is given oxygen and the Pa_{O_2} rises, the stimulant to breathing is removed, and there is the possibility of inducing apnea. For patients with severe COPD, it is suggested that oxygen be limited to less than 3 L/min. Other literature recommends that in severe COPD, oxygen by nasal cannula be used during a dental appointment, especially if pain or stress is expected (increased oxygen demand).

DRUGS USED TO TREAT RESPIRATORY DISEASES

Metered-Dose Inhalers

Inhalers: quick onset, low toxicity

The MDI (Figure 22-5), developed in the 1950s, provides a useful method to administer certain medications to the respiratory tree. It is the preferred route of delivery for most asthma drugs. Its advantages include the following:

- It delivers the medication directly into the bronchioles, thereby keeping the total dose low and side effects minimal.
- The bronchodilator effect is greater than a comparable oral dose.
- The inhaled dose can be accurately measured.
- The onset of action is rapid and predictable (versus unpredictable response with orally administered agents).
- MDIs are compact, portable, and sterile, making them ideal for the ambulatory patient.

Disadvantages of MDIs are that they are difficult to use properly (particularly for children) and they can be abused, with a resultant decrease in response. Additional patient education is required to get the most from this dose form. Often, a "spacer" is placed between the MDI and the mouth to increase the amount of drug delivered to the lungs (see Figure 22-5, *B*). Medications currently available in MDIs include β-agonists, both specific and nonspecific; corticosteroids; cromolyn; and anticholinergic drugs.

Chlorofluorocarbons (CFCs), which have ozone-depleting properties, have been phased out as propellants in MDIs. Non-chlorinated hydrofluoroalkane (HFA) propellants that do not deplete the ozone layer have replaced the CFCs.

Sympathomimetic Agents

Sympathomimetic or adrenergic agonists produce bronchodilation by stimulation of the β-receptors in the lungs. Chapter 4 discusses the presence of β-receptors in the heart (β_1) (tachycardia) and lungs (β_2) (bronchodilation). With the development of selective β_2-agonists ($\beta_2 > \beta_1$), bronchodilation with fewer cardiac side effects can be achieved. The selective β_2-agonists, used orally, by inhalation, and parenterally, are currently one of the mainstays of respiratory therapy.

◆ SHORT-ACTING β_2-AGONISTS

The short-acting β_2-agonists have specificity for the respiratory tree. Side effects include nervousness, tachycardia, and insomnia. Short-acting β_2-agonists, such as albuterol, may be administered by inhalation (metered dose

Albuterol: β_2-agonist

or nebulization with an air compressor) or orally (tablet or liquid). Table 22-1 lists some short- and long-acting β_2-agonists and their routes of administration. The first line of treatment for intermittent asthma is a short-acting β_2-agonist (see Figure 22-3). The short-acting β_2-agonists are the drugs of choice for the emergency treatment of an acute attack of asthma. Recent studies have found that the overuse of these agents results in airway hyperresponsiveness and a decrease in the lung's response to them. Therefore these agents should be used primarily for the treatment of acute problems, not for the management of normal breathing function. One major mistake that many asthmatics make is to rely on the albuterol inhaler and omit using the steroid inhaler. The reason this occurs is because the albuterol gives an immediate response.

◆ LONG-ACTING β_2-AGONISTS

Long-acting β_2-agonist inhalers (see Table 22-1 and Figure 22-1) are used in conjunction with low-dose corticosteroids, to treat patients with persistent asthma that are not well-controlled on low-dose inhaled corticosteroids. Long-acting β_2-agonists improve lung function, decrease symptoms, and reduce exacerbations and rescue use of short-acting β_2-agonists. They are *not* recommended as monotherapy for asthma. Long-acting

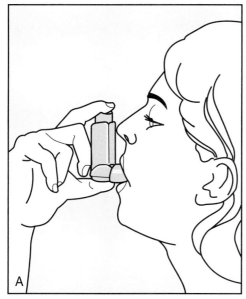
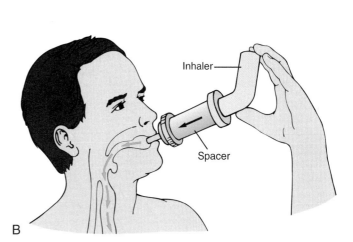

FIGURE 22-5

A, Metered-dose inhaler (MDI) for treatment of respiratory conditions. **B,** MDI with spacer. (**B** from Clayton BD, Stock YN, Harroun RD: *Basic pharmacology for nurses,* ed 14, St Louis, 2007, Mosby.)

TABLE 22-1	FDA-APPROVED DRUGS USED TO MANAGE ASTHMA				

	DRUG				
Group	Example(s)	Mechanism of Action	Adverse Reactions	Dental Drug Implications	
Adrenergic Agonists (Inhaler)					
β_2-Agonist					
Short-acting*	Albuterol (Proventil, Ventolin)* Metaproterenol (Alupent†, Metaprel) Levalbuterol (Xopenex HFA) Pirbuterol (Maxair Autohaler)	Stimulates β_2-receptors (bronchodilation)	Nervousness, dry mouth, throat irritation, fast or irregular heartbeat	Increased risk for dry mouth (rinse mouth to prevent) Can increase heart rate	
Long-acting	Salmeterol (Serevent Diskus)† Formoterol (Foradil Aerolizer)†	Stimulates β_2-receptors (bronchodilation)	Nervousness, dry mouth, throat irritation, fast or irregular heartbeat	Increased risk for dry mouth (rinse mouth to prevent) Can increase heart rate	
Corticosteroids					
Corticosteroids, inhaled	Beclomethasone (QVAR) Budesonide (Pulmicort) Ciclesonide (Alvesco) Flunisolide (AeroBid) Fluticasone (Flovent HFA) Mometasone furoate (Asmanex Twisthaler) Triamcinolone (Azmacort)	Reduces inflammation, inhibits release of inflammatory substances	Cough, dysphonia (hoarseness)	Oral candidiasis (rinse mouth to prevent), unpleasant taste, xerostomia	
Corticosteroids, oral	Prednisone (Deltasone, Meticorten) [PO]	Reduces or prevents inflammatory processes	Hyperglycemia, osteoporosis, fluid retention	Suppresses adrenal gland Healing slower Infection more likely, symptoms masked	
Inhaled Corticosteroids/Long-Acting β_2-Agonists					
Corticosteroid/β_2-agonist	Fluticasone/salmeterol (Advair HFA) Budesonide/formoterol (Symbicort HFA)	The steroids reduce airway inflammation and the β_2-agonists cause bronchodilation	Nervousness, dry mouth, throat irritation, fast or irregular heartbeat, cough, dysphonia (hoarseness)	Increased risk for dry mouth (rinse mouth to prevent) Can increase heart rate, oral candidiasis (rinse mouth to prevent), unpleasant taste	
LT Antagonists					
LT pathway antagonist	Zafirlukast (Accolate) [PO] Montelukast (Singulair) [PO]	Blocks the action of cysteinyl leukotrienes (LTRA)	Nausea, CNS depression, increase in LFTs, myalgia, headache	Erythromycin lowers zafirlukast levels (40%); inhibitor of CYP 3A 3/4 Aspirin raises zafirlukast levels (45%) [PO 20 bid]	
LT pathway synthesis inhibitor (LPI)	Zileuton (Zyflo) [PO]	Inhibits 5-lipoxygenase that catalyzes production of LT (LTD_4 and LTE_4)	Headache, dyspepsia, nausea, abdominal pain, asthenia		
Mast Cell Degranulation Inhibitors					
Mast cell stabilizers	Cromolyn (Intal) (NasalCrom) [IH] Nedocromil (Tilade) [IH—see benefit in 2 weeks]	Mast cell stabilizer (degranulation inhibitor); affects cells of inflammation	Nausea, headache, cough, epistaxis	Taste perversion (bad, unpleasant), burning mouth/throat; sputum increased; swollen parotid glands; dry throat	
Methylxanthines					
Methylxanthines	Theophylline‡ (Theo-Dur, Slo-Bid) [PO] Aminophylline-theophylline ethylene diamine	Direct smooth muscle relaxant	Gastric reflux, headache, tachycardia, insomnia, nausea, trembling, nervousness	Erythromycin may increase the levels of theophylline	

TABLE 22-1   FDA-APPROVED DRUGS USED TO MANAGE ASTHMA—cont'd

Group	DRUG Example(s)	Mechanism of Action	Adverse Reactions	Dental Drug Implications
Anti-IgE Antibody				
Anti-IgE antibodies	Omalizumab (Xolair)	Prevents IgE from binding to mast cells and basophils, which prevents an inflammatory response	Injection site pain and bruising	

Consideration for asthma patients: avoid morning appointments, more allergenic potential, hypersensitivity to aspirin, NSAIDs, sulfites; more common, especially with nasal polyps.

bid, Twice a day; *BP*, blood pressure; *CNS*, central nervous system; *IH*, inhalation; *LFTs*, liver function tests; *LT*, leukotriene; *PO*, by mouth.

*Use for an acute attack.

†Do not use in an emergency, delayed onset >1 hr, prolonged effect (12 hr).

‡Relative of caffeine found in coffee and cola beverages.

β_2-agonists carry a black box warning about a higher risk of asthma-related deaths because of a high number of asthma-related deaths reported with salmeterol therapy during a clinical trial. Long-acting β_2-agonists are best administered in a fixed-dose combination in the same inhaler with an inhaled corticosteroid (see Table 22-1). Long-acting β_2-agonists are combined with corticosteroid inhalers so that two different drugs, at lower doses, can be used to treat persistent asthma.

Corticosteroids

Steroid inhaler: for inflammation

Inhaled corticosteroids are the most effective long-term treatment for control of symptoms in all patients with mild, moderate, or severe persistent asthma (see Table 22-1). Randomized, controlled clinical trials have demonstrated that inhaled corticosteroids are more effective than LT modifiers, long-acting β_2-agonists, cromolyn, or theophylline in improving pulmonary function, preventing symptoms and exacerbations, reducing the need for emergency room visits, and decreasing the number of asthma-related deaths. Most patients experience a positive response at relatively low doses. The optimal dose may decrease or increase over time but it should always be tailored to the lowest possible dose. Doses depend on the inhaled corticosteroid and the inhaler device. Common inhalers contain beclomethasone (be-kloe-METH-a-sone), triamcinolone (trye-am-SIN-oh-lone), and fluticasone (Flovent) (see Table 22-1). Patients taking these corticosteroids have a significant improvement in pulmonary function with a decrease in wheezing, tightness, and cough. The orally inhaled corticosteroids are especially useful in reducing inflammation and therefore the secretions and swelling that occur within the lungs after an asthma attack occurs. Although the steroids produce no immediate benefit in an acute asthmatic attack, they hasten recovery and decrease morbidity in these patients. They also reduce hyperreactive airway.

The side effects of steroids vary, depending on the route of administration, frequency of intake, duration of intake, total dose, and preexisting diseases a patient may have.

Chronic oral corticosteroids, such as prednisone, may be necessary in some severely asthmatic patients and even in patients with moderate asthma, especially during respiratory infections. Prolonged systemic use can result in adrenal suppression, poor wound healing, and immunosuppression. Supplemental steroids may need to be considered if adrenal suppression has occurred (see Chapter 19).

Candidiasis of the oral cavity can result from the chronic use of an inhalation corticosteroid. When the dental health professional performs an oral examination of any patient using steroid inhalers, any symptoms of candidiasis should be noted and treated. Patients using oral corticosteroid inhalers should be advised to rinse the mouth and gargle with water after using the inhaler to minimize the chance of candidiasis.

Steroids are also available as sprays for allergies. An example is beclomethasone (Beconase, Vancenase). It reduces the stuffiness by reducing inflammation within the nasal canal.

Leukotriene Modifiers

♦ OVERVIEW

LTs are synthesized by the enzyme 5-lipoxygenase from arachidonic acid, which also produces prostaglandins (PGs). These LTs are produced by cells of inflammation and produce bronchoconstriction, increased mucus secretion, mucosal edema, and increased bronchial hyperreactivity. The LT pathway inhibitors block the effects of the release of LTs. They are used to manage patients with asthma that is not controlled by β_2-agonists and corticosteroid inhalers.

Zileuton (Zyflo) is a 5-lipoxygenase inhibitor that works by preventing the synthesis of the LTs. Zafirlukast (Accolate) and montelukast (Singulair) are LT receptor antagonists (LTRA). They are not as effective as the corticosteroid inhalers. Both are effective when taken orally. Some patients respond better than others, but who will respond cannot be predicted.

The adverse reactions of these agents include irritation of the stomach mucosa, headache, and alteration of liver function tests. Zafirlukast has a drug interaction with erythromycin and aspirin. Zafirlukast increases the effect of warfarin. Caution should be exercised when giving to patients taking drugs metabolized by 2C9 (tolbutamide, phenytoin, and carbamazepine) or 3A3/4 (dihydropyridines, cyclosporin, astemizole, and cisapride) cytochrome P-450 enzymes. Erythromycin lowers the level of zafirlukast by about 40%. Aspirin raises zafirlukast levels by about 50%. Zafirlukast has recently been found to increase the level of theophylline in the blood. This may be explained by the fact that zafirlukast is an inhibitor of cytochrome P-450 3A3/4 iso-enzymes and is a substrate for cytochrome P-450 isoenzyme 2C9. Both zafirlukast and zileuton have been reported to cause life-threatening hepatic injury. Alanine aminotransferase levels need to be monitored, and patients should discontinue the drug immediately if abdominal pain, nausea, jaundice, itching, or lethargy occurs. Also, there have been reports of mood changes in patients taking montelukast.

◆ CROMOLYN

Inhibits mast cell degranulation

An agent that is effective only for the prophylaxis of asthma and not for treatment of an acute attack is cromo-lyn (KROE-moe-lin) (Intal, Nasalcrom). It has no intrinsic bronchodilator, antihistaminic, or antiinflammatory action. Cromolyn prevents the antigen-induced release of histamine, LTs, and other substances from sensitized mast cells. It appears to do this by preventing the influx of calcium provoked by immunoglobulin E (IgE) antibody-antigen interaction on the mast cell. This effect accounts for the group name that these drugs have been given: mast cell degranulation inhibitors. Cro-molyn is the least toxic of all asthma medications. It is currently available in a metered-dose form like the other inhalation agents. Nedocromil (Tilade) is similar in action to cromolyn.

The advantage of cromolyn is its safety. It may be used pro-phylactically by patients with chronic asthma or taken before exercise-induced asthma. Intranasal cromolyn (Nasalcrom) is available over-the-counter (OTC) for allergic rhinitis.

Methylxanthines

The xanthines and methylxanthines consist of theophylline (thee-OFF-i-leen) (Theo-Dur, Slo-Bid), caffeine, and theobro-mine. Theophylline, used as a bronchodilator, can be combined with ethylenediamine to produce aminophylline (am-in-OFF-i-leen), which is more soluble. Theophylline is used to treat per-sistent asthma and the bronchospasm associated with chronic bronchitis and emphysema. Bronchodilation is the major thera-peutic effect desired.

Side effects associated with the methylxanthines include central nervous system (CNS) stimulation, cardiac stimulation, increased gastric secretion, and diuresis. Patients often complain of nervousness and insomnia. Erythromycin can increase the serum levels of theophylline, and toxicity may result.

Intravenous aminophylline and rapidly absorbed oral liquid preparations are used to manage acute asthmatic attacks and status asthmaticus. To manage persistent asthma, sustained-release preparations in tablet or capsule form are used. Patients on chronic theophylline may have blood levels drawn to deter-mine if the dose they are taking is appropriate. Current literature suggests that the use of theophylline should be limited to patients whose asthma is not controlled with other agents. When the chance of theophylline toxicity is weighed against the potential therapeutic benefit, theophylline is often omitted from an asth-matic's therapeutic regimen.

Anticholinergics

Ipratropium: first choice for COPD

Inhaled anticholinergic drugs appear to inhibit vagally mediated reflexes by antagonizing the action of ace-tylcholine. This then causes bronchodilation. Ipratropium

(i-pra-TROE-pee-um) bromide (Atrovent) is a short-acting anti-cholinergic available for oral inhalation for people with COPD. Tiotropium bromide (Spiriva) is an inhaled long-acting anticho-linergic drug used to treat COPD. Side effects, including dry mouth and bad taste, are minimized with administration by inhalation. Both drugs have a cross-hyperreactivity with peanut and soybean allergies. Ipratropium bromide's bronchodilating effect is additive with that of the β-agonists. It is available as in combination with albuterol sulfate (Combivent) and is used in patients with COPD on a regular aerosol inhalation bronchodi-lator who continue to have evidence of bronchospasm. Neither ipratropium bromide nor tiotropium bromide are approved by the Food and Drug Administration (FDA) for treating asthma.

Anti-Immunoglobulin E Antibodies

Omalizumab (Xolair) is the first in a new class of medications introduced to treat asthma due to allergens. It is a recombinant humanized monoclonal antibody that prevents IgE from binding to mast cells and basophils, thereby preventing the release of inflammatory mediators after allergen exposure (see Table 22-1 and Figure 22-3). This drug is FDA-approved for adjunctive use in patients at least 12 years of age, with well-documented specific allergies and moderate-to-severe persistent asthma that is not well-controlled on an inhaled corticosteroid with or without a long-acting β$_2$-agonist. Omalizumab is administered as a subcu-taneous injection every 2 to 4 weeks. It is expensive. Adverse effects include injection site pain and bruising. Anaphylaxis can occur within 2 hours of injection but sometimes 4 days later. It is advised that patients be kept under observation for 2 hours after the first 3 injections and for 30 minutes after subse-quent injections. Patients are educated about the signs and symptoms of anaphylaxis and when to self-administer injectable epinephrine.

Agents Used to Manage Upper Respiratory Infections

◆ NASAL DECONGESTANTS

Nasal decongestants are β-adrenergic agonists that act by con-stricting the blood vessels of the nasal mucous membranes (α effect). Some examples of these include pseudoephedrine (soo-doe-e-FED-rin) (Sudafed, Sucrets, in Actifed) and phenyleph-rine (fen-ill-EF-rin) (Neo-Synephrine, Sinex, Allerest). Many nasal decongestants are available OTC for both local and sys-temic use (see also Table 4-5). Chronic topical use of deconges-tants may result in rebound swelling and congestion. Therefore decongestant nose sprays should not be used for more than a few days. Unwanted side effects of adrenergic stimulation may occur. Phenylephrine (Neo-Synephrine) is used topically as a nasal spray, and phenylpropanolamine is used systemically as a decongestant (α-agonist action). Pseudoephedrine, both an α-adrenergic agonist and a β-adrenergic agonist, is used systemi-cally as a nasal decongestant.

◆ EXPECTORANTS AND MUCOLYTICS

Expectorants are drugs that promote the removal of exudate or mucus from the respiratory passages. Liquefying expectorants are drugs that promote the ejection of mucus by decreasing its viscosity. Mucolytics destroy or dissolve mucus.

Some expectorants act by their ability to cause reflex stimu-lation of the vagus, which increases bronchial secretions.

Guaifenesin (gwye-FEN-e-sin), the most popular expectorant, is contained in a variety of OTC products mixed with other active ingredients. Robitussin is available as guaifenesin alone (Robitussin plain) and mixed with an antitussive agent (Robitussin DM).

Mucolytics are enzymes that are able to digest mucus, decreasing its viscosity. Acetylcysteine (Mucomyst) is a mucolytic used to loosen secretions in pulmonary diseases, including cystic fibrosis. It is also used orally as an antidote for acetaminophen toxicity.

♦ ANTITUSSIVES

Antitussives may be opioids or related agents used for the symptomatic relief of nonproductive cough. Opioids are the most effective, but because of their addicting properties, other agents are often used. Codeine-containing cough preparations are commonly used, but their histamine-releasing properties may precipitate bronchospasm.

Dextromethorphan (dex-troe-meth-OR-fan) (the DM in cough medicines such as Robitussin DM), an opioid-like compound, suppresses the cough reflex by its direct effect on the cough center. It does not cause the release of histamine. It may potentiate the effects of CNS depressants. It is available both alone and in combination with other ingredients. By impairing coughing, dextromethorphan may not allow the secretions to be cleared from the lungs.

Dental Implications of the Respiratory Drugs

About 10% of the population has some pulmonary disease, so patients taking medications for asthma, emphysema, or chronic bronchitis are often encountered. With severe COPD, a patient can develop pulmonary hypertension, increasing the risk for cardiac arrhythmias. Stress should be minimized and adrenal supplementation instituted if the patients are taking certain doses of steroids and the procedure is likely to produce severe stress. Patients prone to developing respiratory failure, if given oxygen (either alone or with nitrous oxide) or CNS depressants, may manifest acute respiratory failure. Aspirin should be avoided in patients with asthma, and erythromycin may alter the metabolism of theophylline (Box 22-1). Emergency equipment and medications should be available when treating these patients (see Table 23-1 and Box 23-3).

BOX 22-1   MANAGEMENT OF THE DENTAL PATIENT WITH ASTHMA

- Watch analgesic use—avoid aspirin, nonsteroidal antiinflammatory drugs (NSAIDs), and strong opioids; weaker opioids, acetaminophen probably OK.
- Watch sulfiting agents in local anesthetic agents with vasoconstrictor → bronchoconstriction.
- Avoid erythromycin with theophylline → toxicity.
- Review emergency treatment of asthma with staff.
- Have patient's inhaler available for use—albuterol.
- Watch for oral candidiasis—inhaled steroid; rinse mouth to prevent.
- Patients on long-term oral (PO) steroids may need supplemental steroids for severe stress.
- Patient management—reduce stress.
- Use nitrous oxide (N_2O) with caution if needed for sedation.

GASTROINTESTINAL DRUGS

Many drugs, both OTC and on prescription, are used for gastrointestinal diseases. Some are used to treat specific gastrointestinal diseases, and others are used to provide symptomatic relief.

Gastrointestinal Diseases

Ulcers and gastroesophageal reflux disease are common gastrointestinal tract diseases. With the discovery of the etiology of ulcers, the incidence of ulcers in the population has decreased substantially. Nonspecific complaints of gastroesophageal reflux disease (GERD) include burping, cramps, flatulence, fullness, and congestion in the stomach. The gastrointestinal tract is highly susceptible to emotional changes because it is innervated by the vagus nerve associated with the autonomic nervous system.

♦ GASTROESOPHAGEAL REFLUX DISEASE

GERD: heartburn

GERD, or "heartburn," is the most prevalent gastrointestinal disease in the U.S. population. In this condition, the stomach contents, including the acid, reflux, or flow backward through the cardiac sphincter, up into the esophagus. Because the esophagus is not designed to endure the stomach's acid, irritation, inflammation, and erosion can occur. The pain from the inflamed esophagus may be severe and located in the middle of the chest, causing it to be interpreted as a heart attack and trigger an emergency room visit. The main problem is the lack of adequate function of the cardiac sphincter, allowing backflow to occur. The symptoms of GERD are exacerbated by eating large meals (blowing up a balloon [stomach] increases the back pressure) and by assuming the supine position (gravity no longer helping).

Lifestyle changes that can reduce symptoms include avoiding eating for 4 hours before bedtime, eating smaller meals more often, and raising the head of the bed with bricks or using several pillows. If untreated, some patients may have such severe symptoms that they cannot sleep lying down and must sit in a chair.

GERD is treated in two ways: one is to decrease the acid in the stomach and the other is to constrict the cardiac sphincter (the muscle between the stomach and the esophagus). If the sphincter is tighter, it is less likely that the contents will flow back into the esophagus. The H_2-blockers and the proton pump inhibitors (PPIs) reduce or eliminate the stomach's acid. The gastrointestinal stimulants act by increasing the tone in the cardiac sphincter. Sometimes both of these approaches are required to make the patient asymptomatic. Antacids are used for acute relief of symptoms.

♦ ULCERS

Ulcers may occur in the stomach or small intestine. In the past, it was thought that ulcers were caused by "too much acid." However, in the last decade it has been determined that most ulcers are related in some way to the presence of the organism *Helicobacter pylori*. Many ulcers can now be cured by using a combination of one or more antibiotics and an H_2-blocker or a PPI to reduce the acid in the stomach. Some ulcers, especially in the elderly, are secondary to the chronic use of the nonsteroidal antiinflammatory drugs (NSAIDs). NSAID-induced ulcers occur because NSAIDs inhibit synthesis of PGs, which are cytoprotective to the stomach.

Dental Implications

Box 22-2 summarizes the treatment of dental patients with peptic ulcer disease (PUD) and GERD.

BOX 22-2 MANAGEMENT OF DENTAL PATIENTS WITH PEPTIC ULCER DISEASE OR GASTROESOPHAGEAL REFLUX DISEASE

- Avoid the use of aspirin or NSAIDs because they can exacerbate an existing ulcer and further aggravate GERD.
- Patients with GERD may not be able to be in the supine position in the dental chair because of acid reflux.
- Work with patients to determine the best position for them.
- Some drugs may cause xerostomia. Encourage the patient to maintain good oral hygiene and drink plenty of water.
- Tart sugarless gum or candy can help with dry mouth.
- Avoid caffeinated and alcohol-containing beverages or mouth rinses because they can exacerbate dry mouth.

DRUGS USED TO TREAT GASTROINTESTINAL DISEASES

Histamine₂-Blocking Agents

Histamine$_2$ (H$_2$)-receptor antagonists block and inhibit basal and nocturnal gastric acid secretion by competitive inhibition of the action of histamine at the H$_2$-receptors of the parietal cells. They also inhibit gastric acid secretion stimulated by other agents such as food and caffeine. All the members of this group, which are now available OTC, are listed in Table 22-2. Cimetidine (sye-MET-i-deen) (Tagamet) is discussed as the prototype. However, it has largely been replaced by famotidine, ranitidine, and nizatidine because of their more tolerable side effect profiles.

♦ USES

This group is indicated for the treatment of ulcers and the management of the symptoms of ulcers and GERD. Combining H$_2$-blockers with antacids has no therapeutic advantage; in fact, antacids inhibit their absorption and should not be administered within 1 hour of H$_2$-blockers. H$_2$-blockers should be adminis-

---

TABLE 22-2 DRUGS USED TO TREAT PEPTIC ULCER DISEASE AND GASTROESOPHAGEAL REFLUX DISEASE		
Drug Group	Subgroup	Examples
Acid reducers	H$_2$-blockers	Cimetidine (Tagamet)
		Famotidine (Pepcid)
		Ranitidine (Zantac)
		Nizatidine (Axid)
	Proton pump inhibitors	Omeprazole (Prilosec)
		Lansoprazole (Prevacid)
		Esomeprazole (Nexium)
		Pantoprazole (Protonix)
		Rabeprazole (AcipHex)
GI stimulant	Dopamine antagonists	Metoclopramide (Reglan)
Antacids		Sodium bicarbonate
		Magnesium hydroxide
		Aluminum hydroxide
		Calcium carbonate
Laxatives	Bulk	Psyllium seed (Metamucil)
		Carboxymethylcellulose
		Methylcellulose (Citrucel)
		Polycarbophil (FiberCon)
	Stool softeners, emollient	Docusate (dioctyl sodium sulfosuccinate, DSS, Colace)
	Stimulants	Magnesium hydroxide (Milk of magnesia [MOM])
		Bisacodyl (Dulcolax)
		Cascara sagrada
		Senna
		Casanthranol
		Castor oil
		Phenolphthalein
	Hyperosmotic	Glycerin
		Lactulose
		Salts (magnesium citrate, hydroxide, oxide, or sulfate; sodium phosphate)
Prostaglandins		Misoprostol (Cytotec)
Antiflatulents		Simethicone (Mylicon, Gas-X)

GI, Gastrointestinal.

tered with meals and at bedtime. For maintenance, if only one dose is needed daily, the bedtime dose is most effective.

Because smoking increases acid production and reduces the effect of the H$_2$-blockers, smoking cessation assistance should be offered to dental patients who smoke. Cimetidine blocks H$_2$-receptors, which in part are responsible for the inflammatory response in the cutaneous blood vessels of humans.

◆ ADVERSE REACTIONS

The side effects of cimetidine include CNS effects such as slurred speech, delusions, confusion, and headache. Because cimetidine binds with the androgen receptors, it produces antiandrogenic effects such as gynecomastia, reduction in sperm count, and sexual dysfunction (e.g., impotence). Unlike cimetidine, neither ranitidine nor famotidine has been found to possess antiandrogenic activity. Famotidine has been associated with dry mouth and taste alterations. Cimetidine's hematologic effects include granulocytopenia, thrombocytopenia, and neutropenia. Reversible hepatitis and abnormal liver function tests have been reported with all of the H$_2$-blockers.

Cimetidine inhibits liver microsomal enzymes responsible for the hepatic metabolism of some drugs (cytochrome P-450 oxidase system), resulting in a delay in elimination and an increase in serum levels of some drugs, possibly producing toxicity. Ranitidine inhibits the P-450 enzymes much less than does cimetidine, and the other H$_2$-blockers have no effect on the P-450 enzymes. A few examples of drugs that are metabolized by the P-450 pathway include warfarin, metronidazole, lidocaine, phenytoin, theophylline, diazepam, and carbamazepine.

◆ DENTAL DRUG INTERACTIONS

The metabolism of the following drugs occasionally used in dentistry may be reduced by the administration of cimetidine:

- *Ketoconazole and itraconazole:* Toxic levels of these antifungal agents may be produced if they are used continuously for the management of chronic fungal infections. H$_2$-receptor antagonists may increase gastrointestinal pH. Concurrent administration with H$_2$-receptor antagonists may result in a marked reduction in absorption of itraconazole or ketoconazole. Patients taking itraconazole or ketoconazole should take H$_2$-receptor antagonists at a different time.
- *Alcohol:* The blood alcohol levels of persons who have ingested alcoholic beverages may be higher if the patient has been taking cimetidine.
- *Benzodiazepines:* The metabolism of the benzodiazepines, such as diazepam and midazolam, may be slower. The recovery from use of these drugs might be slower.

The other H$_2$-blockers are unlikely to produce important dental drug interactions.

Proton Pump Inhibitors

Proton pump inhibitors (PPIs) are potent inhibitors of gastric acid secretion that are effective (in combination with the antibiotics) in healing duodenal ulcers, and as monotherapy for the acute treatment and maintenance therapy of GERD. The mechanism of action involves the inhibition of the hydrogen/potassium adenosine triphosphatase (H$^+$/K$^+$ ATPase) enzyme system at the surface of the gastric parietal cell. Currently available PPIs are listed in Table 22-2. PPIs heal ulcers more rapidly than H$_2$-receptor blockers or any other drug. Tolerance does not occur

with PPIs because the increased gastric-mediated histamine release cannot overcome proton pump blockade.

Side effects include headache and abdominal pain. In rats, omeprazole produced an increase in gastric carcinoid tumors, but it has now been determined that this is unlikely to occur with use in humans. Therefore the original limit on the duration of use of omeprazole has been lifted. Although it is unknown whether a relationship exists between omeprazole and mucosal atrophy of the tongue and dry mouth, these side effects have been reported. Long-term use of PPIs, particularly at high doses, has been associated with an increased risk of osteoporotic fractures.

Mixed Antiinfective Therapy for Ulcer Treatment

Ulcers are closely related to the organism *H. pylori*. To treat ulcers, a combination of two antiinfective agents (tetracycline, metronidazole, clarithromycin, or amoxicillin), an H$_2$-blocker or a PPI, and bismuth subsalicylate (Pepto-Bismol) may be used. Common multidrug regimens are listed in Table 22-3. Newer combinations often use one antibiotic and a PPI such as esomeprazole and clarithromycin. These agents are used for 2 weeks and result in a cure in many patients.

Antacids

Antacids are used to treat a variety of gastric conditions, by both self-medication and recommendation of the patient's prescriber. Acute gastritis and symptoms of ulcers are sometimes managed with antacids. Acute gastritis, the most common type of gastric distress, is termed *heartburn* or *upset stomach*. The symptoms include epigastric discomfort or a burning feeling. The symptoms of gastric ulcers can be managed with antacids.

Antacids are drugs that partially neutralize hydrochloric acid in the stomach. By raising the pH to 3 or 4, the erosive effect of the acid is decreased and pepsin activity is reduced (see Table 22-2).

Sodium bicarbonate rapidly neutralizes gastric acid. Its major disadvantage is that alkalosis can occur. It also contains sodium and is contraindicated in cardiovascular patients who are to

TABLE 22-3	COMMON MULTI-DRUG REGIMENS FOR *HELICOBACTER PYLORI*	
Drug	Daily Dose	Duration
Triple Therapy		
Clarithromycin +	500 mg bid	10-14 days
amoxicillin	1 gm bid	10-14 days
or		
Metronidazole +	500 mg bid	10-14 days
a PPI	standard PPI dose	
Quadruple Therapy		
Bismuth subsalicylate (Pepto-Bismol) +	2 tablets bid or qid or 30 ml tid or qid	14 days
Metronidazole +	500 mg tid or qid	14 days
Tetracycline +	500 mg tid or qid	14 days
PPI or H$_2$-blocker	Standard dose	

PPI, Proton pump inhibitor; *bid*, twice a day; *tid*, three times a day; *qid*, four times a day.

minimize sodium intake. For these reasons, it is not recommended, although it is still used by the lay public.

Calcium carbonate, aluminum and magnesium salts, and magnesium-aluminum hydroxide gels are the active ingredients in all other antacids. Calcium salts may result in acid rebound, constipation, or hypercalcemia. Aluminum salts can produce constipation. Magnesium salts produce osmotic diarrhea. Hypermagnesemia has been reported in patients with renal disease. Drug interactions with the antacids include altering the absorption of other drugs from the gastrointestinal tract. Drugs whose absorption is inhibited include tetracyclines, digitalis, iron, chlorpromazine, and indomethacin. Conversely, levodopa's absorption is increased because stomach emptying time is shortened. By mixing aluminum and magnesium salts in a single preparation, the effects on the bowel can be balanced.

Miscellaneous Gastrointestinal Drugs

◆ MISOPROSTOL

Misoprostol (mye-soe-PROST-ole) (Cytotec) is $PGE_{2\alpha}$ and is indicated in the management of NSAID-induced ulcers. Both H_2-blockers and PPIs reduce the symptoms of NSAID-induced ulcers but do not prevent the ulcers. Misoprostol increases gastric mucus and inhibits gastric acid secretion. Its side effects include stomach distress and diarrhea (caused by PGs). Its FDA pregnancy category is X because it stimulates uterine contractions and will induce labor.

◆ SUCRALFATE

Sucralfate (soo-KRAL-fate) (Carafate), a complex of aluminum hydroxide and sulfated sucrose (a polysaccharide with antipeptic activity), is used to treat duodenal ulcers. In the stomach, the aluminum ion splits off, leaving an anion that is essentially nonabsorbable. Sucralfate combines with proteins, forming a complex that binds preferentially with the ulcer site. It can be thought of as a "bandage" for ulcers. It inhibits the action of pepsin and absorbs the bile salts. Its acid-neutralizing capacity does not contribute to its antiulcer action. Constipation is the most frequent side effect reported (2.2%). Other side effects (<0.3%) include dry mouth, nausea, rash, and dizziness. It must be taken on an empty stomach and can inhibit the absorption of tetracycline.

◆ METOCLOPRAMIDE

The drug metoclopramide (met-oh-KLOE-pra-mide) (Reglan) is a dopaminergic antagonist. It blocks the action of dopamine and that action facilitates cholinergic effects within the gastrointestinal tract. Metoclopramide stimulates the motility of the upper gastrointestinal tract without stimulating secretions and relaxes smooth muscle innervated by dopamine. It relaxes the pyloric sphincter and increases peristalsis in the duodenum. This results in an accelerated gastric emptying time. It also increases the tone of the lower esophageal sphincter. Its antiemetic property is the result of its antagonism of dopamine receptors both centrally and peripherally.

Metoclopramide is indicated for the relief of symptoms associated with diabetic gastroparesis (gastric stasis) and improves delayed gastric emptying time. Another indication is short-term therapy for gastroesophageal reflux with symptoms. The most common CNS side effects are restlessness, drowsiness, and fatigue, and these occur in 10% to 25% of patients. Parkinson-

like reactions can occur in up to 10% of patients. Gastrointestinal side effects include nausea and diarrhea. Additive CNS depression may occur when other CNS depressants are used concomitantly.

◆ SIMETHICONE

Simethicone (Mylicon, Gas-X) is an agent used to relieve flatulence (gas). It lowers the surface tension and breaks up gas pockets so they can be expelled.

Laxatives and Antidiarrheals

◆ LAXATIVES

Self-medication with laxatives is a common practice among the lay public. Although a few indications for the use of laxatives exist, overuse is common and habituation can result. The myth that "regular" bowel habits are essential has led to this practice. Abuse of these substances occurs in bulimic patients. Short-term, occasional use for constipation and use before diagnostic procedures (barium enema) are legitimate indications. The types of laxatives (Table 22-4) are as follows:

- *Bulk laxatives:* Bulk laxatives are preferred because they are the safest and act most like the normal physiology of humans. They contain polysaccharides or cellulose derivatives that combine with intestinal fluids to form gels. This increases peristalsis and facilitates movement through the intestine. Patients with problems with constipation can increase their intake of fiber or use any bulk laxative daily without problems.

TABLE 22-4	DRUGS USED TO TREAT OTHER GASTROINTESTINAL DISORDERS	
Drug Group	**Subgroup**	**Examples**
Antidiarrheals	Opioid-like agents	Loperamide (Imodium) Diphenoxylate (in Lomotil)
	Adsorbents	Kaolin and pectin (Kaopectate)
Antiemetics	Phenothiazines	Prochlorperazine (Compazine)
	Antihistamines	Meclizine (Bonine) Dimenhydrinate (Dramamine) Trimethobenzamide (Tigan)
	Cannabinoids	Dronabinol (Marinol) Nabilone (Cesamet)
Agents used in the treatment of IBD	Non-aspirin salicylates	Sulfasalazine (Azulfidine) Mesalamine (Rowasa, Pentasa, Asacol) Olsalazine (Dipentum)
	Adrenocorticosteroids	Prednisone
	Immune modifiers	Cyclosporine Azathioprine Mercaptopurine (6-MP, Purinethol)
	Antibiotics	Metronidazole (Flagyl)

IBD, Inflammatory bowel disease.

- *Lubricants:* Mineral oil, a lubricant that was previously often used, is no longer recommended. It can be absorbed if used over a long period and can interfere with the absorption of the fat-soluble vitamins (A, D, E, and K).
- *Stimulants:* Stimulant laxatives act by producing local irritation of the intestinal mucosa. Because of their potent effect, intestinal cramping can result. Bisacodyl, a member of this group, is often used before bowel surgery or radiologic examinations but should not be used for simple constipation.
- *Stool softeners (emollients):* Dioctyl sodium sulfosuccinate, an anionic detergent, wets and softens the stool by accumulating water in the intestine. These agents should be limited to short-term use, although they are nontoxic.
- *Osmotic (saline) laxatives:* Magnesium sulfate or phosphate produces its laxative effect by osmotically holding water. It should be used with caution in patients with renal impairment.

◆ ANTIDIARRHEALS

Drugs used to treat diarrhea are either adsorbents or opioid-like in action. Antidiarrheals are used to minimize fluid and electrolyte imbalances. In certain poisonings or infections, antidiarrheals are contraindicated. The most common adsorbent combination used to treat diarrhea is kaolin and pectin (Kaopectate). The opioids, such as diphenoxylate with atropine (Lomotil) and loperamide (OTC Imodium), are the most effective antidiarrheal agents. They decrease peristalsis by acting directly on the smooth muscle of the gastrointestinal tract.

Antiemetics

Drugs used to induce vomiting and to prevent vomiting are used for certain gastrointestinal tract problems. Vomiting may occur because of a variety of situations such as motion sickness, pregnancy, drugs, infections, or radiation therapy, and many sites within the body can activate the emetic center to produce vomiting (Figure 22-6). Choice of the drug to treat vomiting depends to some extent on the cause of the vomiting.

◆ PHENOTHIAZINES

Phenothiazines (e.g., prochlorperazine [Compazine]) are used to control severe nausea. Their side effects include sedation and extrapyramidal symptoms, including tardive dyskinesia (see Chapter 17). Promethazine (Phenergan), a phenothiazine with antihistaminic and anticholinergic properties, is used in dentistry to treat nausea and vomiting associated with surgery and anesthesia. It also has sedative and antisialagogue action. It is sometimes used concurrently with opioids to minimize the nausea they produce.

◆ ANTICHOLINERGICS

Anticholinergics can be used for the nausea and the vomiting associated with motion sickness and labyrinthitis. Both dimenhydrinate (Dramamine) and meclizine (Bonine) possess antiemetic, antivertigo, and antimotion sickness action. Because they have antihistaminic action, sedation is a side effect. A scopolamine transdermal patch (Transderm-Scop) is placed behind the ear and releases medication over a 3-day period. It is used for motion sickness on ships and boats. It is contraindicated whenever anticholinergics are used (see Chapter 4). Dry mouth, blurred vision, sedation, and dizziness have been reported.

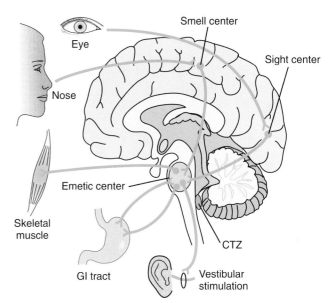

FIGURE 22-6
The chemoreceptor trigger zone (CTZ) and other sites that activate the emetic center. (From McKenry L, Tessier E, Hogan MA: *Mosby's pharmacology in nursing,* ed 22, St Louis, 2006, Mosby.)

◆ ANTIHISTAMINES

The agent diphenhydramine (Benadryl), an antihistamine with antiemetic properties, commonly produces sedation. Hydroxyzine (Atarax) is used in dentistry as an antiemetic or antianxiety agent.

◆ TRIMETHOBENZAMIDE

The drug trimethobenzamide (Tigan) has an antiemetic effect that is mediated through the chemoreceptor trigger zone. It produces sedation, agitation, headache, and dry mouth. It is available orally or as a suppository that contains 2% benzocaine (avoid in patients allergic to ester local anesthetics).

◆ METOCLOPRAMIDE

Metoclopramide (Reglan) can control the nausea and vomiting of patients receiving cancer chemotherapeutic agents. It acts both centrally (dopamine antagonist) and peripherally (stimulates release of acetylcholine). It is also indicated for the management of gastric motility disorders such as diabetic gastric stasis.

◆ CANNABINOIDS

Dronabinol (droe-NAB-i-nol) (Marinol) and nabilone (NAB-i-lone) (Cesamet) are psychoactive substances derived from *Cannabis sativa L.* (marijuana). They produce effects similar to those of marijuana. These agents are indicated to treat the nausea and vomiting associated with cancer chemotherapy in patients who have failed to respond to conventional antiemetic therapy. These agents can be abused. Tolerance and both physical and psychologic dependence can occur. Close supervision is required when these agents are administered. Side effects include drowsiness and dizziness. Perceptual difficulties, muddled thinking, and elevation of mood can also occur.

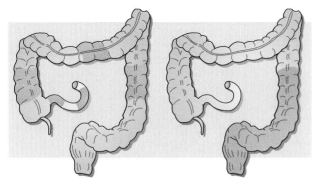

FIGURE 22-7
Crohn's disease *(left)* and ulcerative colitis *(right)*. (Modified from Cotran KS, Kumar V, Robbins SI: *Robbins and Cotran pathologic basis of disease*, ed 7, Philadelphia, 2005, Saunders.)

Agents Used to Manage Chronic Inflammatory Bowel Disease

Inflammatory bowel disease: IBD

Chronic inflammatory bowel disease (IBD) is divided into two subcategories: ulcerative colitis and Crohn's disease (Figure 22-7). Although probably multifactorial, an autoimmune response is thought to be associated with ulcerative colitis. Crohn's disease extends through all layers of the intestinal wall, whereas ulcerative colitis involves only the mucosa. Crohn's disease can involve the whole intestine, but the colon is most commonly affected. Ulcerative colitis involves the rectum and may involve the distal part of the colon but does not involve the small intestine. Smoking is protective against ulcerative colitis, and smoking cessation may exacerbate the disease. NSAIDs should be used with caution in patients with IBD.

The drugs used to treat IBD include laxatives, colonic stimulants, and osmotic agents and are indicated for patients that do not respond to fiber supplementation. Loperamide (Imodium) and atropine/diphenoxylate (Lomotil) are antidiarrheal agents that are also used to treat IBD in patients with diarrhea-predominant irritable bowel syndrome (IBS). Antispasmodics, such as hyoscyamine and dicyclomine, are best used on an as-needed basis for acute attacks of abdominal pain or before meals in patients with postprandial symptoms. The newer agents, tegaserod (Zelnorm) and alosetron (Lotronex), are serotonin 5-hydroxytryptamine modulators. They play a major role in the regulation of intestinal motility, secretion, and visceral sensitivity. Tricyclic antidepressants are used when diarrhea-persistent IBS is moderate to severe. These drugs modulate the perception of visceral pain, alter gastrointestinal transit, and treat psychiatric comorbidities.

Infliximab (Remicade) is the newest agent approved by the FDA to treat ulcerative colitis. It works by neutralizing tumor necrosis factor (TNF). Infliximab finds TNF in the bloodstream and removes it before it causes inflammation in the gastrointestinal tract. The drug has been linked to an increased risk of infection, especially tuberculosis, and may increase the risk of blood problems and cancer. Once started, infliximab is often continued as long-term therapy, although its effectiveness may wear off over time.

DENTAL HYGIENE CONSIDERATIONS

1. Always conduct a thorough medication/health history in order to avoid drug interactions or prescribing medications that could exacerbate a respiratory or gastrointestinal disorder.
2. Patients with emphysema or COPD should not receive nitrous oxide because of their diminished oxygen capacity.
3. NSAIDs can exacerbate an asthma attack and should be avoided. Acetaminophen can be used instead.
4. NSAIDs and aspirin can exacerbate peptic ulcer disease and GERD. Acetaminophen can be used instead.
5. Oral steroid inhalers can cause candidiasis and the patient should be examined at each visit.
6. Oral steroid inhalers, oral β_2-agonist inhalers, and oral anticholinergic inhalers can cause dry mouth.
7. Instruct patients on the importance of good oral health care after using their inhalers.
8. Patients with respiratory and gastrointestinal disorders may require a semi-supine position. Work with patients to determine what is best for them.
9. Review the information in Box 22-1 and Box 22-2.

CLINICAL SKILLS ASSESSMENT

1. What are some of the risk factors of GERD?
2. What is the role of antacids, H_2-receptor antagonists, and PPIs in the treatment of GERD?
3. What are the dental concerns associated with the medications used to treat GERD?
4. Compare and contrast the different antacids.
5. What is the role of sucralfate in the treatment of PUD?
6. What are some common adverse effects of antidiarrheals, antiemetics, and laxatives?
7. Discuss different methods of minimizing an asthma attack in the dental office.
8. What is the role of steroids in the treatment of asthma?
9. Why are oral, inhaled steroids the preferred dose form in the treatment of asthma?
10. What is the role of β_2-adrenergic agonists in the treatment of asthma?
11. What are the dental concerns associated with β_2-adrenergic agonists? What would the dental practitioner tell a patient about them?

ⓔvolve ───────────────────────

Please visit http://evolve.elsevier.com/Haveles/pharmacology for review questions and additional practice and reference materials.

SPECIAL SITUATIONS

23 Emergency Drugs

LEARNING OBJECTIVES

1. Summarize the general measures a dental professional should follow to train for an emergency and the preparation for treatment in the event of an emergency.
2. Name and describe several categories of emergencies and provide common examples within each category.
3. List the critical drugs to include in a dental office emergency kit and several examples of second- or third-level drugs that would be optional.
4. Name several pieces of equipment that would be included in the emergency kit.

An increasing number of older patients who are taking multiple drugs seek dental treatment each year. The demographics of our population, the use of fluorides, and management of periodontal disease has increased the age of the average dental patient. Dental offices are administering more complicated drug regimens; dental appointments are taking longer; and dental patients are on average getting sicker. With these changes, the chance of an emergency occurring in the dental office continues to increase. Both the dentist and the dental hygienist should become familiar with the most common emergency situations, their management, and the drugs used to treat these conditions. When an emergency occurs, working together can increase the chance of producing the best outcome. Many emergency situations can be handled correctly with adequate knowledge. Lack of this knowledge during an emergency may cause panic in a dental office. If the dental office and its personnel are prepared for an emergency, handling one will be easier. Before treating patients who might be at risk for an emergency, the treatment of a potential emergency related to their disease should be reviewed. It is the responsibility of each dental health care worker to make sure the members of the team can act in a coordinated manner.

GENERAL MEASURES

Steps Indicated

To prepare the dental office for an emergency, the following steps should be taken:

- *Training:* All office personnel should be trained and retrained in emergency procedures before an emergency occurs. They should practice for an emergency at least once every 6 months.
  Basic cardiac life support (cardiopulmonary resuscitation [CPR]) training (required)
  Advanced cardiac life support (ACLS) training (optional, unless performing conscious sedation)
- *Phone number:* One should post the telephone number of the closest physician, emergency room, and ambulance service (often 911). The number(s) should be programmed into the speed dial function of the phone.
- *Emergency kit:* One should select the items for the office's emergency kit, including the drugs and the devices (nondrug items) needed. The kit should be checked every 3 months to make sure that the drugs are not out of date. Some companies have this service by subscription.

BOX 23-1   METHODS OF MINIMIZING EMERGENCIES IN THE DENTAL OFFICE

- Observe the patient's stature, build, gait, coloring, age, facies, and respiration.
- Observe and record the amount of anxiety; use active listening to determine hidden nervousness.
- Take the patient's blood pressure and pulse rate, and perform any necessary laboratory examination.
- Take a complete patient history, including medication history, past dental and anesthetic experiences, restrictions on physical activity, diseases, and present condition.
- Request medical consultations as needed.
- Prescribe premedication, if appropriate, and avoid drug interactions.

BOX 23-2   TREATMENT OF AN EMERGENCY IN THE DENTAL OFFICE

- Recognize the abnormal occurrence.
- Make a proper diagnosis.
- Call 911 (or appropriate emergency number).
- Note the time.
- Position the patient properly.
- Maintain an airway.
- Administer oxygen.
- Monitor vital signs.
- Provide symptomatic treatment.
- Administer cardiopulmonary resuscitation (CPR) if there is no pulse.

To minimize the chances of an office emergency, the procedures listed in Box 23-1 should be performed on each new dental patient. It is easier to prevent rather than treat a dental emergency. If an emergency occurs in the dental office, the steps listed in Box 23-2 should be taken.

Preparation for Treatment

A: Airway
B: Breathing
C: Circulation

Before any emergency treatment can be administered, investigation of the patient's signs and symptoms must lead to a diagnosis of the problem. In most cases, the maintenance of the airway *(A)*, respiration (breathing, *B*), and circulation *(C)* are of primary importance. The use of drug therapy in these situations is only ancillary to the primary measures of maintaining adequate circulation and respiration. One should remember that drugs are not necessary for the proper management of most emergencies. Whenever there is doubt as to whether to give the drug, it should not be given.

In the dental office, each health care worker should be certified. The legal implications of lack of CPR training could be serious. ACLS training can be helpful in certain rural situations or if the technique of preoperative sedation or conscious sedation is used in the dental office.

The categories of emergencies are discussed in the next section. The most commonly used drugs and the choice of drugs and equipment for a dental office emergency kit are addressed.

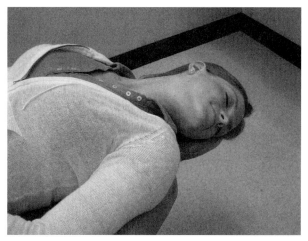

FIGURE 23-1
In the Trendelenburg position, the individual should be tilted back even further in the dental chair so that the head is below the level of the heart and turned to one side. (From Malamed SF: *Medical emergencies in the dental office,* ed 6, St Louis, 2007, Mosby.)

CATEGORIES OF EMERGENCIES

This section discusses the signs, symptoms, and treatment of the most common emergency situations, dividing them into changing consciousness; respiratory, cardiovascular, and other emergencies; and drug-related emergencies.

Lost or Altered Consciousness

Many common dental emergencies involve either unconsciousness or altered consciousness. Dental office personnel should be ready to handle these emergencies and determine the best course of treatment.

◆ SYNCOPE

Syncope most common

The emergency most often encountered in the dental office is simple syncope (fainting, also known as vasomotor collapse) or transient unconsciousness. The skin takes on an ashen-gray color, and diaphoresis occurs. The release of excessive epinephrine results in a pooling of the blood in the peripheral muscles (β effect, vasodilation), a decrease in total peripheral resistance, and a sudden fall in blood pressure. A reflex tachycardia follows, but soon, decompensation results in severe bradycardia. These effects are brought about by anxiety, fear, or apprehension, all of which are common in a dental situation. Treatment involves placing the patient in the Trendelenburg position (head down) (Figure 23-1), causing blood to rush to the head, which has the effect of giving the patient a transfusion of whole blood.

The most important component in the treatment of syncope is for the dental health care worker to exhibit confidence in action and voice. If the hygienist shows control over the situation, the patient will be less anxious and apprehensive and less likely to repeat the syncopal attack.

Spirits of ammonia can be administered by inhalation. The old practice of putting the head between the legs should be avoided because venous return is cut off by the slumped position.

◆ HYPOGLYCEMIA

The most common cause of hypoglycemia is an excessive dose of insulin in a patient with diabetes. The medical history in this case is important, so the dental health care worker can determine the dose and type of insulin and food intake before the appointment. Often, patients inject their usual daily dose of insulin but fail to eat before coming to the dental office. If this is the case, then patients should be asked to eat before any dental procedures are begun. The time of the hypoglycemia can be estimated by knowledge of the peak effect of the particular insulins used (see Chapter 20).

The patient with hypoglycemia has a rapid pulse and decreased respiration and is very talkative. Hunger, dizziness, weakness, and occasionally tremor of the hands can occur. Diaphoresis, nausea, and mental confusion are other signs of hypoglycemia. If the signs of hypoglycemia are recognized before they become severe, the patient can be given a sugary drink or oral glucose. If the patient lapses into unconsciousness and has no swallowing reflex, dextrose must be given intravenously.

◆ DIABETIC COMA

Less common than hypoglycemia, the diabetic coma is caused by elevated blood sugar. Symptoms of frequent urination, loss of appetite, nausea, vomiting, and thirst are seen. Acetone breath; hypercapnia; warm, dry skin; rapid pulse; and a decrease in blood pressure can occur. Treatment is undertaken only in a hospital setting and includes insulin after proper laboratory results are obtained (blood sugar).

◆ CONVULSIONS OR SEIZURES

Seizures/epilepsy

Convulsions are most commonly associated with epilepsy, especially the grand mal type (see Chapter 16), but can also result from a toxic reaction to a local anesthetic agent. Convulsions are abnormal movements of parts of the body in clonic and/or tonic contractions and relaxations. The patient may become unconscious. Generally, convulsions are self-limiting, and treatment should include protecting the patient from self-harm, moving any sharp objects out of the patient's reach, and turning the patient's head to the side to prevent aspiration. In some situations, diazepam may be administered intravenously, but observation of the patient is often sufficient.

Respiratory Emergencies

Respiratory emergencies involve difficulty in breathing and exchange of oxygen. They include hyperventilation, asthma, anaphylactic shock, apnea, and acute airway obstruction.

◆ HYPERVENTILATION

Hyperventilation is one of the most common dental emergency situations. The increased respiratory rate is often brought on by emotional upset associated with dental treatment. Tachypnea, tachycardia, and paresthesia (tingling of the fingers and around the mouth) have been reported. Nausea, faintness, perspiration, acute anxiety, lightheadedness, and shortness of breath can also occur. The treatment is calm reassurance. The dental professional should encourage patients to hold their breath or "rebreathe" into a paper bag or an unconnected face mask (occasionally portrayed in movies).

◆ ASTHMA

Normally, patients who have acute asthmatic attacks have a history of previous attacks and carry their own medication. The most common sign of an asthmatic attack is wheezing with prolonged expiration (squeak). The patient's own medication (multidose inhalers containing β_2-agonist such as albuterol) should be used first. The dose should be repeated several times. If there is no response to these, hospitalization for administration of aminophylline (parenteral or oral) and parenteral corticosteroids and epinephrine should be considered. Oxygen should also be administered.

◆ ANAPHYLACTIC SHOCK

Anaphylaxis: emergency; 4 minutes to treat

The most common cause of anaphylactic shock is an injection of penicillin, although anaphylactic reactions have also been caused by many other agents. Examples include eating peanuts or being exposed to latex rubber items. The reaction usually begins within 5 to 30 minutes after ingestion or administration of the antigen. Usually, a weak, rapid pulse and a profound decrease in blood pressure occur. There is dyspnea and severe bronchial constriction.

Parenteral epinephrine is the drug of choice and must be administered immediately in cases of severe anaphylactic shock. It may be given in the deltoid muscle or injected under the tongue. If bronchoconstriction is predominant, albuterol administered by inhalation or nebulization may suffice. After the life-threatening symptoms have been controlled, intravenous corticosteroids, intramuscular diphenhydramine, and aminophylline may also be used.

◆ ACUTE AIRWAY OBSTRUCTION

Acute airway obstruction or aspiration (e.g., aspiration of vomitus) is usually a result of a foreign body (e.g., a crown) in the pharynx or larynx; laryngospasm may be drug induced. Gasping for breath, coughing, gagging, acute anxiety, and cyanosis are signs and symptoms of acute airway obstruction. Treatment begins by placing the patient in a Trendelenburg position on the right side and encouraging coughing. One should not allow the patient to sit up. Clearing the pharynx and pulling the tongue forward before performing the Heimlich maneuver (external subdiaphragmatic compression) should be attempted next. Finally, the Heimlich maneuver should be performed and repeated if needed (Figure 23-2). A cricothyrotomy or tracheotomy, hardly dental office maneuvers, is indicated if the object cannot be dislodged by the other methods.

For aspiration, the use of suction, intubation, and ventilatory assistance is suggested. Steroids, antibiotics, and aminophylline are also administered. When drug-induced laryngospasm is present, succinylcholine, a neuromuscular blocking agent, and positive-pressure oxygen are the agents of choice. The operator must have training and equipment to artificially breathe for the patient before succinylcholine is administered. Prevention of swallowed objects can best be attained by the use of a rubber dam and throat packing, when appropriate.

Cardiovascular System Emergencies

Emergency situations involving the cardiovascular system include angina pectoris, myocardial infarction (MI), cardiac

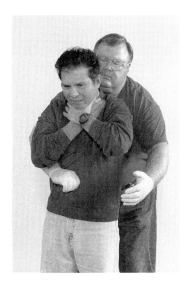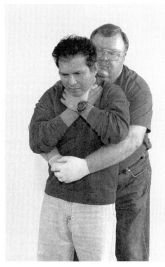

FIGURE 23-2
The proper technique for an abdominal thrust (Heimlich maneuver). (From Chapleau W: *Emergency first responder: making the difference,* St Louis, 2004, Mosby.)

arrest, acute congestive heart failure, arrhythmias, and hypertensive crisis. The primary concern in any cardiovascular emergency is the maintenance of adequate circulation. Administering CPR, calling emergency personnel, and administering oxygen are appropriate for most emergencies. The drugs used in cardiovascular emergencies are discussed individually later in the chapter.

◆ ANGINA PECTORIS

Without a previous history of angina, diagnosis of this condition can be difficult. It often begins as substernal chest pain that radiates across the chest, to the left arm, or to the mandible. It may also produce a feeling of heaviness in the chest. The pulse becomes rapid, and tachypnea can occur. An anginal attack can be brought on by stress from pain, trauma, or fear, especially in a dental situation.

Premedication with sublingual nitroglycerin before a stressful dental situation may prevent an acute anginal attack. Treatment of an acute anginal attack (see Chapter 15) is with sublingual nitroglycerin. Opioids or diazepam are used in hospitalized patients. One should always check and make sure that the patient has not taken a medication used to treat erectile dysfunction within 24 hours of receiving nitroglycerin. If the patient has taken a medication to treat erectile dysfunction, then he should not receive nitroglycerin but should be treated in a hospital for the acute angina attack. Nitroglycerin should not be used to prevent an acute attack if these drugs have been used within 24 hours of the scheduled appointment.

◆ ACUTE MYOCARDIAL INFARCTION

An acute MI (heart attack) often begins as severe pain, pressure, or heaviness in the chest that radiates to other parts of the body. Sweating, nausea, and vomiting can occur. The pain is persistent and unrelieved by rest or nitroglycerin (three doses). In this way, an MI can be differentiated from an anginal attack. An irregular rapid pulse, shortness of breath, diaphoresis, and indigestion can occur. Treatment includes administration of oxygen, an aspirin tablet, and an opioid analgesic agent and transfer to a hospital. The risk of death is greatest within the first 6 hours.

Hospitalized patients who have suffered an MI are given lidocaine for arrhythmias and vasopressor agents to maintain an adequate blood pressure. New drugs that can dissolve clots are administered soon after the event and may reverse the clot.

◆ CARDIAC ARREST

When cardiac arrest occurs, generally there is sudden circulatory and respiratory collapse. Without immediate therapy, cardiac arrest is fatal. Permanent brain damage occurs in 4 minutes. Pulse is absent, and blood pressure is unobtainable. After a few minutes, the patient becomes cyanotic and the pupils are fixed and dilated. The first and most important treatment is immediate, adequate CPR.

Today, dental practices should have an automated external defibrillator (AED). An AED, if administered within the first 5 minutes of cardiac arrest, can save up to 50% of those experiencing cardiac arrest. In March of 2002, the American Dental Association (ADA) Council on Scientific Affairs recommended that dentists consider purchasing an AED for their dental offices if emergency medical services personnel with defibrillation skills and equipment are not available within a reasonable period of time. In fact, most states require AEDs for dental practices that use general anesthesia and many require them for conscious sedation. Several states require AEDs, or full-function defibrillators, for all dental practices.

Other medications used in a hospital setting for cardiac arrest include epinephrine for cardiac stimulation and lidocaine for arrhythmias. Parenteral opioid analgesics are given for the pain. Defibrillation is used to treat asystole.

◆ OTHER CARDIOVASCULAR EMERGENCIES

Arrhythmias, another cardiovascular emergency, depend on an electrocardiogram for diagnosis before treatment. A cerebrovascular accident (CVA, stroke), resulting in weakness on one side of the body or speech defects, is treated with oxygen administration and immediate hospitalization so "clot busters" can be administered. Hypertensive crisis is treated with antihypertensive agents given intravenously (see Chapter 15). Treatment of these cardiovascular emergencies is undertaken in a hospital setting.

Other Emergency Situations

Some emergency situations involve symptoms that do not fit into the other categories.

◆ EXTRAPYRAMIDAL REACTIONS

The antipsychotic agents (see Chapter 17) can produce extrapyramidal reactions. Parkinson-like movements, such as uncoordinated tongue and muscular movements and grimacing, can occur. Prochlorperazine (Compazine), which is used for nausea and vomiting, can produce this type of reaction. Intravenous diphenhydramine (Benadryl) is the treatment of choice.

◆ ACUTE ADRENOCORTICAL INSUFFICIENCY

Adrenal crisis usually occurs in patients who are taking enough steroids to suppress the adrenal gland. When they are subjected to acute severe stress without increasing their steroid dose, a crisis may occur. Unable to respond to the stress, the patient has an adrenal crisis. Nausea, vomiting, abdominal pain, and confusion may result. Cardiovascular collapse and irreversible shock may result in a fatality. The treatment for adrenal crisis is parenteral hydrocortisone and oxygen by inhalation. After hospitalization, patients receive fluid replacement and vasopressor agents if symptoms dictate.

◆ THYROID STORM

Thyroid storm is a condition in which hyperthyroidism is out of control. Signs and symptoms include hyperpyrexia, increased sweating, hyperactivity, mental agitation, shaking, nervousness, and tachycardia. Congestive heart failure and cardiovascular collapse may follow. Temperature is controlled by tepid baths and aspirin. β-Blockers are given to control the cardiovascular symptoms. Another agent that may be used is hydrocortisone. Aspirin should be avoided in these patients (displaces thyroxine [T_4] from binding sites). Sodium iodide and propylthiouracil are given to inhibit the action of the thyroid gland. Untreated severely hyperthyroid patients should not be given atropine or epinephrine because these agents may precipitate a thyroid storm.

◆ MALIGNANT HYPERTHERMIA

Malignant hyperthermia is a genetically determined reaction that is triggered by inhalation general anesthetics or neuromuscular blocking agents such as succinylcholine. The most notable symptom is a rapidly rising temperature. Baths and aspirin are used to control the elevated temperature. Prompt treatment with dantrolene (Dantrium) can control acidosis and body temperature by reducing calcium released into the muscles during the contractile response. Before dantrolene, death was a common outcome. Fluid replacement, steroids, and sodium bicarbonate may be used.

Drug-Related Emergencies

◆ OPIOID OVERDOSE

Opioids, administered in the dental office or prescribed by the dentist, can produce overdose symptoms. Respiration can be depressed, or respiratory arrest may occur. Illegitimate use of street drugs (e.g., heroin) may also produce overdose symptoms. The most common symptoms of overdose from the opioids are shallow and slow respiration and pinpoint pupils. The drug of choice for opioid overdose is naloxone (Narcan), an opioid antagonist (see Chapter 6).

◆ REACTION TO LOCAL ANESTHETIC AGENTS

Toxic reactions to local anesthetic agents usually result from excessive plasma levels of the anesthetic. Both central nervous system (CNS) stimulation, and CNS depression can occur. The stimulation is exhibited as excitement or convulsions (see Chapter 9). Following stimulation, depression can occur with symptoms of drowsiness, unconsciousness, or cardiac and respiratory arrest. The treatment of this toxic reaction is symptomatic. If convulsions are a predominant feature, diazepam can be administered. If hypotension is predominant, a pressor agent can be given. In the presence of reflex bradycardia, atropine may be administered. Usually, patients who have a toxic reaction to local anesthetics must be watched closely, but drug administration is rarely necessary. This reaction requires a dose of local anesthetic above the maximum dental dose.

Epinephrine

Toxic reactions to epinephrine occur most often after the placement of a gingival retraction cord used before taking impressions. The symptoms range from nervousness to frank shaking and can also include tachycardia. Because epinephrine is quickly metabolized, the main treatment is to remove the cord and reassure the patient. Becoming panicky will cause the patient to release endogenous epinephrine, and the reaction will continue. Above all else, the dental health care worker must remain calm.

EMERGENCY KIT FOR THE DENTAL OFFICE

Although the choice of drugs for a dental office emergency kit will depend on individual circumstances, experience, and personal preference, the dental health care worker should make sure there is an emergency kit in the dental office (Figure 23-3). Table 23-1 lists some emergency drugs, their therapeutic uses, and their usual adult doses. Other drugs that may be included if the office personnel are trained in ACLS include level 2 drugs, atropine and lidocaine, and calcium chloride.

Drugs

Table 23-1 lists the drugs that should be considered for inclusion in a simple emergency dental kit. These may vary, depending on the preference and experience of the practitioner. Some equipment and drugs that are not used by dental office personnel are kept in the emergency kit for use by a physician or for those with ACLS training in an emergency.

Obtaining small quantities of these medications may be difficult because they are often sold in packages of 12. A hospital pharmacy may be able to help the practitioner because the pharmacy buys in large quantities and could sell the few ampules that are needed for the dental office emergency kit. The security of the kit should be ensured by the use of a "breakable" lock that can be used to determine whether tampering has occurred. The kit should be stored in a prominent place in the dental office, but control of the agents, such as the diazepam or an opioid, if included, should be ensured.

◆ LEVEL 1 (CRITICAL) DRUGS

Epinephrine. Epinephrine (Figure 23-4) must be included in the dental office emergency kit for treatment of cardiac arrest, anaphylaxis, or acute asthmatic attack. It should not be used in

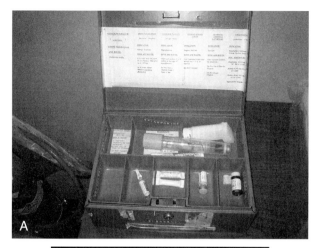

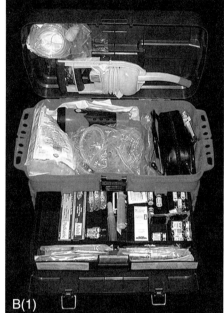

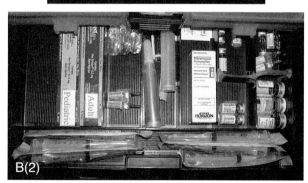

FIGURE 23-3
Examples of self-made emergency kits. **A,** Simple version with basic items only. **B,** Large version with many drugs and additional equipment. (From Malamed SF: *Medical emergencies in the dental office,* ed 6, St Louis, 2007, Mosby.)

TABLE 23-1	EMERGENCY DRUGS AND THEIR INDICATIONS
Drug	Indications
Level 1: Critical Drugs	
Albuterol (IH; Ventolin)	Treatment of an acute asthma attack
Diphenhydramine	Treatment of allergic reaction
Epinephrine	Treatment of cardiac arrest, anaphylaxis, or acute asthma attack
Glucose, oral (usually in the form of a tube of cake frosting)	Treatment of hypoglycemia
Nitroglycerin	Treatment of an acute anginal attack
Oxygen	Treatment of emergency situations in which the individual is having difficulty breathing
Level 2: Secondary Drugs	
Atropine	Increase in cardiac rate
β-Blockers	Reduction in blood pressure
Dextrose 50%	IV solution for hypoglycemic patients who cannot swallow
Diazepam/alprazolam	Initial treatment of status epilepticus
Glucagon	Management of severe hypoglycemic reactions
Hydrocortisone	Treatment of allergic reactions, anaphylaxis, or adrenal crisis
Morphine	Opioid analgesic used to treat the pain associated with MI
Spirits of ammonia	Treatment of syncope
Other Drugs	
Bretylium	Treatment of arrhythmias
Procainamide	Treatment of arrhythmias
Verapamil	Treatment of arrhythmias
Lidocaine	Treatment of arrhythmias
Flumazenil	Treatment of benzodiazepine overdose
Naloxone	Treatment of opioid overdose

IH, Inhaled; *IV,* intravenous; *MI,* myocardial infarction.

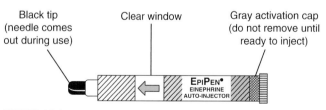

FIGURE 23-4
The EpiPen is an emergency preloaded supply of epinephrine. (From Lehne RA: *Pharmacology for nursing care,* ed 6, Philadelphia, 2007, Saunders.)

treatment of shock because it can cause decreased venous return with increased ischemia and can precipitate ventricular fibrillation. The rationale for the use of epinephrine for cardiac arrest is β-stimulation of the myocardium. In the treatment of severe anaphylaxis and acute asthmatic attacks, it acts as a physiologic antagonist to the massive release of mediators that occurs in these conditions. Without epinephrine, these chemicals lead to bronchoconstriction and decreased oxygen exchange. Because epinephrine's cardiac effects are diminished in the presence of acidosis, adequate mechanical resuscitation and external cardiac massage accompany its administration. Epinephrine may be administered by intravenous or intracardiac routes (by trained personnel). Dental personnel may find injection into the frenulum under the tongue more convenient.

Diphenhydramine. Diphenhydramine (Benadryl), an antihistamine, is used in the treatment of some allergic reactions. Because antihistamines compete with histamine for tissue receptor sites, a rapid reversal of allergic symptoms cannot be expected. For this reason, epinephrine and diphenhydramine are used together in severe allergic reactions or anaphylaxis.

Oxygen. Oxygen is indicated in most emergencies, especially if respiratory difficulty is a problem. Patients with chronic obstructive pulmonary disease (COPD) should be given oxygen with caution because apnea may result. All dental office personnel should know the procedure for administering inhalation oxygen. All potential members of the dental team should review the procedure on a regular basis.

Nitroglycerin. Sublingual nitroglycerin tablets or nitroglycerin spray (see Chapter 15) should be kept in the dental office emergency kit to manage an acute anginal attack. The sublingual spray may be used in place of the tablets (Figure 23-5).

Glucose. Oral glucose (Figure 23-6), or any available liquid carbohydrate, is used to manage hypoglycemia in the conscious or semiconscious patient with diabetes. If the patient can

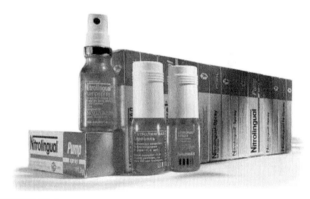

FIGURE 23-5
Nitrolingual spray. (From Malamed SF: *Medical emergencies in the dental office,* ed 6, St Louis, 2007, Mosby.)

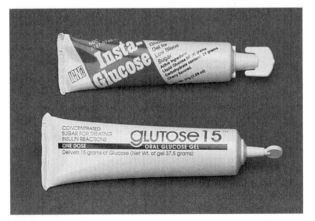

FIGURE 23-6
Oral glucose gels. (From McSwain N: *The basic EMT: comprehensive prehospital care,* St Louis, 2003, Mosby.)

swallow, then the oral route is preferable. A small amount may be placed in the buccal pouch, where it can be slowly swallowed. Tubes of glucose for this purpose are available, or cake frosting in tubes may be used.

Albuterol. Albuterol is a short-acting β_2-adrenergic agonist that produces bronchodilation. It is used in the management of an acute attack of asthma or respiratory distress accompanying anaphylaxis. If used properly, albuterol can produce bronchodilation in a few seconds.

◆ LEVEL 2 DRUGS

Benzodiazepines. Diazepam (Valium) and midazolam (Versed) are the drugs of choice for the treatment of most convulsions if a drug is needed. However, in the majority of cases, convulsive episodes are self-limiting and require only supportive care in the form of protecting the patient from physical harm and administering oxygen.

One cause of convulsions in the dental office is a toxic reaction to a local anesthetic from an overdose or an idiosyncrasy (see Chapter 9). Anticonvulsant drugs should be used conservatively because they may enhance CNS depression of the local anesthetic.

Aromatic Ammonia Spirits. Containers of aromatic ammonia spirits, designed to be crushed, can be used to treat syncope (Figure 23-7). Aromatic ammonia acts by irritating the membranes of the upper respiratory tract, resulting in stimulation of respiration and blood pressure. A dental office should have one (unexpired) container near each dental chair for easy access.

Morphine. Morphine and meperidine are opioid analgesics administered to a patient who has suffered an acute MI. These agents relieve pain and allay apprehension. They are used for cases of pulmonary embolism and angina for the same reasons.

Hydrocortisone. A corticosteroid used for allergic reactions, anaphylaxis, and adrenal crisis is hydrocortisone sodium. Even given intravenously, hydrocortisone has a slow onset of action. Epinephrine is still the drug of choice for anaphylaxis and serious allergic reactions because it acts immediately as a physiologic antagonist. Administration of hydrocortisone should follow the use of epinephrine, and it may be given intramuscularly or intravenously.

Dextrose. Intravenous dextrose is used to manage hypoglycemic episodes when a patient with diabetes is unconscious and cannot swallow. Hypoglycemia occurs most commonly when the patient's insulin, exercise, and food intake are out of balance. In the dental office, all patients with hypoglycemia should be recognized before unconsciousness occurs.

Glucagon. Glucagon is used for the management of severe hypoglycemic reactions. It can be given intramuscularly, intravenously, or subcutaneously. If the patient does not respond to the glucagon, intravenous glucose should be considered.

Atropine. Atropine is used as a preoperative antisialagogue and to increase the cardiac rate when it has been slowed by vagal stimulation. It is administered intramuscularly, intravenously, and subcutaneously.

β-Blockers. β-Blockers, such as esmolol or labetalol, are administered by intravenous infusion to manage intraoperative or postoperative tachycardia or hypertension.

◆ OTHER DRUGS

Naloxone. Naloxone (Narcan), a pure opioid antagonist, is the drug of choice for opioid-induced apnea. Its use is extremely

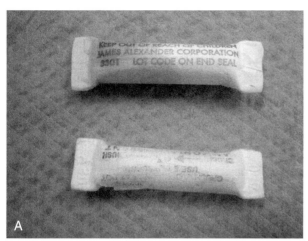

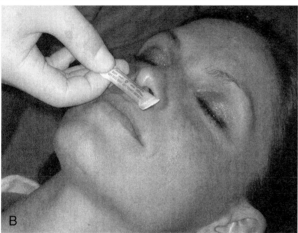

FIGURE 23-7
A, Ammonia Vaporole, used *(top)* and unused *(bottom).* **B,** Ammonia crushed and held under the nose. (From Malamed SF: *Medical emergencies in the dental office,* ed 6, St Louis, 2007, Mosby.)

safe, but more than one administration may be needed because of its short duration of action. The initial dose is 0.4 mg (1 ml) intravenously, but it can also be given subcutaneously or intramuscularly. The onset of action is approximately 2 minutes by the intravenous route. This dose should be repeated several times in case the dose of opioid was high (sometimes a combination of self-administered plus dentist-administered opioids).

Another potential problem with giving naloxone is precipitating withdrawal in an addict (see Chapter 6). Naloxone is effective in reversing the respiratory depression caused by opioid drugs; if no response occurs, other causes for the respiratory depression must be considered. Naloxone should be in a dental emergency kit if patients are given opioids preoperatively or intraoperatively.

Flumazenil. Flumazenil (Romazicon) is a benzodiazepine antagonist used for reversing most of the effects of the benzodiazepines. It may be used after conscious sedation with diazepam or lorazepam. It should be in the emergency kit only if parenteral benzodiazepines are administered in the dental office.

Antiarrhythmics. Procainamide, lidocaine, verapamil, and bretylium are used for their antiarrhythmic effect. The specific

arrhythmia should be identified before an antiarrhythmic agent is selected. Arrhythmias are not something that most dental offices are equipped to treat.

Equipment

An oxygen mask, a manual resuscitation bag, and an oxygen tank with a flow gauge are needed to administer positive pressure oxygen. A sphygmomanometer and stethoscope are used to take a patient's blood pressure. Disposable syringes, needles, and a tourniquet are used to administer medications. A laryngeal suction cannula is used to suction the throat if aspiration occurs. All dental practices should have an AED in case a patient goes into cardiac arrest. Box 23-3 lists essential equipment for a dental office emergency.

With ACLS training, a more advanced emergency kit can be prepared. Nasal and oral airways are used to maintain an unobstructed airway. Endotracheal tubes and a laryngoscope are required for intubation. Intravenous solutions, tubing, butterfly needles, and adhesive tape are used for intravenously administering drugs. A cricothyrotomy (incision through skin and cricothyroid membrane before performing a tracheotomy) kit can be used for acute airway obstruction when other measures fail.

Many dental offices will not have staff trained to use the more advanced equipment. Without training, attempts to use this equipment may be more harmful than using simple measures. If untrained, stick to CPR.

BOX 23-3   EMERGENCY DEVICES

Level 1 (Critical Devices)
- Syringes/needles
- Tourniquets
- System to administer oxygen*
- Automated external defibrillator (AED)

Level 2 (Secondary Devices)
- Cricothyrotomy device
- Endotracheal tube
- Laryngoscope
- System to administer intravenous (IV) infusions

*Oxygen and system (e.g., Ambu bag).

DENTAL HYGIENE CONSIDERATIONS

1. The best way to treat a medical emergency is to prevent one from occurring.
2. Well-trained dental hygienists can treat those that occur.
3. Make sure that patients have brought their rescue medication with them and have placed the medication within easy reach.
4. Monitor vital signs.
5. Always check and make sure that the drugs in the emergency kit are within their expiration dates.
6. Keep oxygen close by.
7. Be able to assess a patient should an emergency occur and relay that information to the dentist and emergency medical personnel.
8. Review Boxes 23-1 and 23-2.

CLINICAL SKILLS ASSESSMENT

1. State what general measures the dental health care worker should be familiar with to respond to any emergency situation.

2. For each of the following common emergencies, state the signs, symptoms, and treatment (including drugs):

    a. Cardiac arrest

    b. Angina pectoris

    c. Acute MI

    d. Convulsions

    e. Syncope

    f. Asthma

    g. Anaphylactic shock

    h. Hypoglycemia

3. List the equipment required to treat the emergencies in question 2 and explain the rationale for the inclusion of each item.

4. Give the names of the drugs required in an emergency kit for the dental office.

5. What drugs should be included in an ideal emergency kit?

6. What are the indications for the drugs most commonly found in an emergency kit for the dental office?

⊖volve

Please visit http://evolve.elsevier.com/Haveles/pharmacology for review questions and additional practice and reference materials.

24 Pregnancy and Breast Feeding

LEARNING OBJECTIVES

1. List the two main concerns in the administration of drugs during pregnancy.
2. Define *teratogenicity* and outline the Food and Drug Administration's categories of drugs for pregnancy.
3. Name several types of local anesthetic, antiinfective, and antianxiety agents and state their indications or contraindications for pregnant women.

Dental treatment of the pregnant or nursing woman is always of special concern to dental health care workers. Pregnant women often need additional dental treatment during their pregnancies, and in addition, that treatment must be carefully planned. Many questions about drug therapy for the pregnant or breast-feeding woman arise. The literature, unfortunately, does not provide all the answers. This chapter attempts to offer guidelines for determining the relative risk when prescribing drugs for the pregnant woman or nursing mother. No unnecessary drug should be administered to the pregnant woman. If a drug is to be administered, the risk to the fetus must be weighed against the benefit to the woman. An adequate health history, including whether a woman might be pregnant (puberty to menopause) should be taken at each dental appointment. Close coordination with the patient's obstetric health care professional is recommended when questions about her potential use of drugs arise. Consultations should be documented in the patient's chart. Box 24-1 lists the dental implications involved in managing a pregnant dental patient.

GENERAL PRINCIPLES

Two Main Concerns

> Teratogenic: produces abnormal fetus

Two main concerns must be addressed when considering whether to give a drug to a pregnant woman. The first is that the drug may be teratogenic. The term *teratogen* is derived from the Greek prefix *terato-*, meaning "monster," and the suffix *-gen,* meaning "producing." These two combine to give rise to the meaning of *teratogen*: "producing a monster." The second is that the drug can affect the near-term fetus, causing the newborn infant to have an adverse reaction, such as respiratory depression or jaundice. A relatively new concern is the long-term (physiologic and psychological) consequences of in utero exposure to agents not evident at birth.

History

In 1941, a relationship between getting German measles during pregnancy and blindness, deafness, and death of the offspring was noted. Scientists recognized that exogenous agents could affect the unborn fetus, producing congenital abnormalities. In 1961, a "harmless" sedative, thalidomide, available over the counter (OTC) in Europe, was taken by pregnant women. An increase in the rare birth defect phocomelia (short or absent limbs) occurred shortly thereafter. Thalidomide was later implicated in these birth defects. Environmental factors are also thought to contribute to birth defects.

BOX 24-1 **MANAGEMENT OF THE PREGNANT DENTAL PATIENT**

- Avoid elective dental treatment except in the second trimester.
- Avoid any unnecessary drugs, especially during the first trimester.
- If drugs are needed, check the FDA categories to choose the safest.
- Minimize periodontal problems; perform oral prophylaxis before pregnancy or during second trimester; monitor for periodontal conditions.
- Avoid radiographs unless absolutely necessary; use lead apron.
- Pay particular attention to periodontal disease because it has been associated with low-birth-weight newborns.
- Position patient in recumbent position in last trimester with right hip elevated (not Trendelenburg).
- If morning sickness is a problem, schedule an afternoon appointment.
- Give frequent breaks for urination, especially during the first trimester.

FDA, Food and Drug Administration.

PREGNANCY

Pregnancy Trimesters

Pregnancy involves three trimesters, each 3 months long. During the first trimester, the organs in the fetus are forming. This is considered the most critical time for teratogenicity. If abnormalities occur very early in development, spontaneous abortion is the usual outcome. With later exposure, abnormalities occur in the fetus. Often, a woman is unaware that she is pregnant for at least one-half of this trimester. Dental prophylaxis with detailed instructions and a visual examination of the oral cavity without x-rays should be performed if the patient is pregnant. Because this is the time when the woman may feel nauseated at any time during the day or night (often referred to as morning sickness), other elective dental treatment should be avoided during this time.

The second trimester is an excellent time for the patient to receive both oral health instructions and another dental prophylaxis, if needed. The patient's periodontal status should be carefully evaluated during this time. The patient is most comfortable during this trimester.

The third trimester is closest to delivery. The woman is beginning to feel uncomfortable, and it is difficult for her to lie prone for any length of time.

If dental treatment is needed, she may feel more comfortable sitting or with the right hip elevated. In addition, this is the time when premature labor is most likely to begin. Drugs that may affect the newborn child should not be given during this trimester.

Teratogenicity

Teratogenicity difficult to identify

It is difficult to prove that a drug is teratogenic in humans (Box 24-2).

Drugs that are known teratogens include drugs such as thalidomide, certain vitamin A analogs (isotretinoin), antineoplastic agents (busulfan, cyclophosphamide), oral anticoagulants (warfarin), lithium, methimazole, penicillamine, some antiepileptic agents (phenytoin, trimethadione, and valproic acid), the tetracyclines, certain steroids (diethylstilbestrol, androgens), and ethyl alcohol. Table 24-1 lists selected drugs with adverse effects on the fetus.

BOX 24-2 **REASONS IT IS DIFFICULT TO PROVE A DRUG IS TERATOGENIC**

- Different animal species and humans vary among themselves in their responses to drugs.
- Timing of the drug exposure varies with each drug.
- One drug can produce a variety of abnormalities, and different drugs can produce the same abnormality.
- Drugs that are teratogenic are not uniformly so.
- A drug's effect on the fetus may be different from its effect on the mother.
- The teratogenic effects of a certain drug on the fetus may not be evident for many years.

Food and Drug Administration Pregnancy Categories

FDA pregnancy "grades"

The U.S. Food and Drug Administration (FDA) has developed pregnancy categories A, B, C, D, and X. Each drug that is the subject of FDA regulation for pregnancy labeling is given a category based on its known potential for risk. Table 24-2 gives a summary of the criteria for the different categories. One should note that the availability of animal or human studies is a criterion. Category A is the safest, and category X should not be used in pregnant women. Categories B, C, and D fall in between these two criteria.

BREAST FEEDING

Questions about the safety of a certain drug given to a nursing mother are appearing more often because nursing is becoming more popular. As during pregnancy, the risk-to-benefit ratio should be carefully considered before drugs are given to the nursing mother. Drugs without strong indications for use should not be taken. Almost all drugs given to the mother can pass into the breast milk in varying concentrations. While nursing, the baby ingests the drug, which may produce an effect in the infant. The amount of drug that appears in the milk depends on the plasma concentration of the drug, lipid solubility, degree of ionization, and binding to plasma proteins.

For a few drugs, nursing is clearly contraindicated. If these drugs must be given, breast feeding should be discontinued or the milk expressed and discarded until the mother stops taking the contraindicated drug. For drugs that are not contraindicated, the timing of nursing can further reduce the dose to which an infant is exposed. Table 24-3 summarizes the available data on the use of dental drugs for nursing mothers.

DENTAL DRUGS

Questions relating to drug administration in conjunction with dental treatment refer to whether a specific drug may be safely given to the pregnant woman. In general, a drug should be used in a pregnant woman only if the benefits to the pregnant woman outweigh the risks to the fetus and a definite indication exists. Table 24-3 summarizes the information about which dental drugs can be used in pregnant women.

TABLE 24-1 SELECTED DRUGS WITH ADVERSE EFFECTS ON THE FETUS

Drug	Trimester	Effect
ACEIs	All	Renal damage, congenital malformations
Amphetamines	All	Abnormal development patterns, neonatal withdrawal symptoms
Androgens	All	Masculinization of female fetus
Antidepressants, tricyclic	Third	Neonatal withdrawal symptoms
Antineoplastics	All	Congenital malformation
Barbiturates	All	Neonatal dependence
Carbamazepine	All	Neural tube defects; congenital malformation
Chlorpropamide	All	Neonatal hypoglycemia, prolonged
Clomipramine	First, third	Neonatal lethargy, hypotonia, cyanosis, hypothermia
Cocaine	All	Increased spontaneous abortion, abruptio placentae, premature labor, abnormal development, decreased school performance, seizure
Diazepam	All	Neonatal dependence, sedation; congenital malformations during first trimester
Diethylstilbestrol	All	Vaginal adenosis, vaginal adenocarcinoma, genital abnormalities, testicular cancer
Ethanol	All	Fetal alcohol syndrome
Etretinate	All	Multiple congenital malformations
Heroin	All	Neonatal dependence
Iodide	All	Congenital goiter, hypothyroidism
Isotretinoin	All	Extremely high risk of congenital anomalies
Lithium	First	Ebstein's anomaly
Methadone	All	Neonatal dependence, neonatal withdrawal symptoms
Methylthiouracil	All	Hypothyroidism
Metronidazole	First	May be mutagenic
Penicillamine	All	Cutis laxa, connective tissue defects, other congenital malformations
Phencyclidine	All	Abnormal neurologic examination, poor suck reflex and feeding
Phenytoin	All	Fetal hydantoin syndrome
Propylthiouracil	All	Hypothyroidism
Smoking	All	Intrauterine growth retardation, sudden infant death syndrome
Streptomycin	All	Eighth nerve toxicity, fetal ototoxicity
Tamoxifen	All	Increased spontaneous abortion and fetal damage
Tetracycline	All	Discolored teeth/altered bone growth
Thalidomide	All	Phocomelia, severe birth defects
Valproic acid	All	Neural tube defects, congenital malformations
Warfarin	First	Hypoplastic nasal bridge, chondrodysplasia
	Second	CNS malformations
	Third	Risk of bleeding, D/C 1 month before delivery

Data from Katzung BG: *Basic & clinical pharmacology*, ed 7, Stamford, Conn, 1988, Appleton & Lange.
Boldface indicates dental drug.
ACEIs, Angiotensin-converting enzyme inhibitors; *CNS*, central nervous system; *D/C*, discontinue.

Local Anesthetic Agents

No drug is used more often in the dental office than a local anesthetic agent. Local anesthetic amides have been reported to produce fetal bradycardia and neonatal depression when given in very large doses near to term. High doses may produce uterine vascular constriction, leading to fetal heart rate changes. Lidocaine, prilocaine, and etidocaine have been tested in animals without teratogenic effects (category B). Bupivacaine has been shown to be teratogenic in rats and rabbits (category C), whereas mepivacaine has not been tested (category C). Small doses used by careful, slow injection have not been associated with any problems in the fetus. Lidocaine is the local anesthetic of choice for the pregnant woman because it is a category B drug and is not associated with methemoglobinemia (as is prilocaine) and not highly lipid soluble (as is etidocaine), prolonging its effect.

Epinephrine

Small doses of epinephrine, administered with appropriate care, are similar to those produced endogenously. Large doses could produce adverse effects in the fetus, including anoxia from vasoconstriction. If procedures are to be short, then local anesthetics

TABLE 24-2 FDA PREGNANCY CATEGORIES FOR DRUGS*

Category	Description	Examples
A	Adequate studies have failed to demonstrate a risk to fetus (in first trimester) and no evidence of risk in later trimesters; possibility of fetal harm appears remote.	Thyroid supplements (levothyroxine), vitamins (folic acid, riboflavin; vitamins A, D, and C†), potassium chloride
B	Animal studies have failed to demonstrate a risk to the fetus, and there are no adequate studies in pregnant women; or animal studies show an adverse effect on the fetus but well-controlled studies in pregnant women have failed to demonstrate a risk to the fetus.	Acetaminophen, acyclovir, opioids,‡ penicillins, cephalosporins, erythromycin,§ caffeine, cimetidine, insulin, NSAIDs‖
C	Animal studies have shown an adverse effect on the fetus and there are no adequate studies in humans, or no studies are available in either animals or women. Potential benefits may warrant its use.	Epinephrine, phenylpropanolamine, trimethobenzamide, aspirin,‖ atropine, promethazine, theophylline, lisinopril, disulfiram, propranolol, fluoxetine, amitriptyline, sulfonamides,¶ prednisone
D	Positive evidence of human fetal risk based on adverse reaction data, but potential benefits in serious situations may warrant its use.	Warfarin, tetracycline, phenytoin, diazepam, trimethadione, lorazepam
X	Studies in animals or humans have demonstrated fetal abnormalities and/or there is positive evidence of human fetal risk, and the risks clearly outweigh any potential benefits.	Isotretinoin, diethylstilbestrol, phencyclidine (PCP), triazolam

FDA, Food and Drug Administration; *NSAIDs,* nonsteroidal antiinflammatory drugs.
*Any unnecessary medication should be avoided in pregnant women.
†When used at recommended daily allowance (RDA) levels.
‡In usual therapeutic doses.
§Except erythromycin estolate.
‖Except near term, when dystocia and delayed parturition can be produced and then categorized as D.
¶Except near term, when kernicterus can be produced.

without epinephrine are preferred. These comments also apply to other vasoconstrictor substances contained in local anesthetic solutions.

Analgesics

Analgesics should be given in the lowest possible dose and for the shortest duration possible to control pain. In dentistry, adjunctive therapy (incision, drainage, and curettage) should be used first.

♦ ASPIRIN

ASA: No

Studies in animals have shown that aspirin can cause a variety of birth defects involving the eyes, central nervous system (CNS), gastrointestinal tract, and skeleton. In humans, controlled studies have not been able to demonstrate that aspirin use during pregnancy increases the incidence of birth defects. During the third trimester, aspirin can prolong gestation, complicate delivery, decrease placental function, or increase the risk of maternal or fetal hemorrhage. Premature closure of the patent ductus arteriosus may occur (see Chapter 5). These effects have been reported with chronic high-dose aspirin use. Abuse of aspirin may increase stillbirths or neonatal death.

♦ NONSTEROIDAL ANTIINFLAMMATORY DRUGS

NSAIDs: No

The nonsteroidal antiinflammatory agents (NSAIDs) produce effects similar to aspirin; therefore if they are given near term, the outcome on the fetus would be expected to be the same as aspirin's effects. They can delay delivery and make it more difficult and can constrict the ductus arteriosus. NSAIDs also potentiate vasoconstriction if hypoxia exists. All NSAIDs carry a warning to avoid use during pregnancy. For ibuprofen and naproxen, studies in animals have not shown adverse effects on the fetus. Diflunisal (category C), but not naproxen (category B), has been shown to be teratogenic in rabbits in large doses. Ibuprofen is the NSAID of choice for the nursing mother.

♦ ACETAMINOPHEN

APAP: Yes

Although no controlled studies in humans have been done, acetaminophen (APAP) is generally considered to be safe in pregnancy. In large doses, it may be associated with fetal renal changes similar to those that occur in adults.

♦ OPIOIDS

Doses used by addicts have been demonstrated to produce problems. The opioids, with the exception of codeine, have not been associated with teratogenicity. Retrospective studies have associated the use of codeine during the first trimester with fetal abnormalities involving the respiratory, gastrointestinal, cardiac, and circulatory systems and with inguinal hernia and cleft lip and palate (Figure 24-1). These studies suggest that codeine or other opioids should not be used indiscriminately during the first trimester. Whether the birth defects associated with codeine are related to its ubiquitous use or to some difference it possesses is not known. Near-term administration can produce respiratory depression in the infant. If the mother is addicted, the infant will experience withdrawal symptoms after birth. The use of codeine in limited quantities for a limited duration of time is common in clinical practice. Although opioids appear in breast milk when analgesic doses are administered, the small amounts appear to be insignificant. By properly timing the doses of analgesic, the dose the infant receives is reduced further. The infant should be observed for signs of sedation and constipation.

TABLE 24-3   DENTAL DRUG USE DURING PREGNANCY,[a] FOOD AND DRUG ADMINISTRATION (FDA) CATEGORIES,[b] AND NURSING SAFETY

| Dental Drug | TRIMESTER | | FDA Category | Comments | NURSING | |
	First	Second/Third			OK?	Comment
Local Anesthetics						
Lidocaine	Yes	Yes	B	First-choice anesthetic; fetal bradycardia near term	Yes	Central nervous system changes
Mepivacaine	Yes	Yes	C	Fetal bradycardia near term; no animal testing	Yes	Central nervous system changes
Bupivacaine	No	No	C	Embryocidal in rabbits; high lipid solubility	No	Central nervous system changes
Vasoconstrictors						
Epinephrine	Yes	Yes	C	Vasoconstriction can produce hypoxia; limit to cardiac dose	Yes	Hyperactivity or irritability
Analgesics						
Aspirin	No	No	C/D	Bleeding; near-term dystocia and prolonged gestation, delayed parturition, premature closure of patent ductus arteriosus; treatment of certain pregnancy problems	Yes, caution	Occasional low dose poses minimal hazard; chronic high dose may present problems; infant may have inhibition of prostaglandins
Nonsteroidal antiinflammatory drugs (NSAIDs)	No	No	B-C/D[c]	See aspirin B=ibuprofen, naproxen, ketoprofen C=etodolac, tolmetin, diflunisal, mefenamic acid, nabumetone, oxaprozin	No	Avoid NSAIDs; ibuprofen may be used when more information is available
Acetaminophen	Yes	Yes	B	Teratogenic at overdose levels	Yes	Present in milk in small amounts (peak 1-2 hr); no documented problems
Opioids	Yes	Yes	B[d]/C[e]	Respiratory depression near term; use low-dose, short duration; high doses contraindicated	Yes	Small doses, no problem; large doses (addict), sedation, poor feeding, constipation
Penicillins/Cephalosporins						
Penicillin V	Yes	Yes	B	Safe, especially penicillin V	Yes	Allergy, diarrhea
Amoxicillin, ampicillin	Yes	Yes	B	Safe	Yes	Allergy, diarrhea
Augmentin[f]	Yes	Yes	B	Safe	Yes	Allergy, diarrhea
Cephalosporins	Yes	Yes	B	Safe	Yes	Allergy, diarrhea
Macrolides						
Erythromycin	Yes	Yes	B	Safe, except estolate form (cholestatic jaundice)	Yes[g]	Present in milk; diarrhea
Clarithromycin	Avoid	Yes	C	Teratogenic in mice and monkeys	Yes	Insufficient information
Azithromycin	Avoid	Yes	B	Unlikely to need in dentistry	Yes	Insufficient information
Tetracyclines						
Tetracycline	No	No	D	Stains teeth; affects bones	No	Tooth staining questionable
Doxycycline	No	No	D	Stains teeth; affects bones	No	Tooth staining questionable
Minocycline	No	No	D	Stains teeth; affects bones	No	Tooth staining questionable

Continued.

TABLE 24-3   DENTAL DRUG USE DURING PREGNANCY,[a] FOOD AND DRUG ADMINISTRATION (FDA) CATEGORIES,[b] AND NURSING SAFETY—cont'd

| Dental Drug | TRIMESTER | | FDA Category | Comments | NURSING | |
	First	Second/Third			OK?	Comment
Others						
Clindamycin	Yes	Yes	B	Very low risk of pseudomembranous colitis	Yes/No[g]	Diarrhea; pseudomembranous colitis
Metronidazole	No	Yes, caution	B	Only if alternatives do not exist	No	Express and discard milk
Antifungals						
Nystatin	Yes	Yes	B	Not absorbed into systemic circulation from gastrointestinal tract	Yes	Not absorbed into systemic circulation from mouth or gastrointestinal tract
Clotrimazole, topical	No	Yes, caution	B	Poorly absorbed topically; abnormal liver function	Yes	No proof of problems
Miconazole, topical			B	No link with fetal abnormalities	Yes	No proof of problems
Ketoconazole, systemic	No	No	C	Embryotoxic in rats	Yes	No proof of problems
Antivirals						
Acyclovir	No	No	B	Limited experience	No	Concentrated in milk
Penciclovir	Probably		B	Topical		Inadequate information
Antianxiety Agents						
Nitrous oxide (with oxygen)	No	Yes, caution	D	Ensure adequate oxygen intake; female operators should avoid chronic exposure[h]	Yes	Nitrous oxide excreted via the lungs; amount in milk is negligible
Benzodiazepines[i]			D/X			
Alprazolam	No	No	D	Floppy infant syndrome; cleft lip; neural tube defects; do not use in dentistry	No	Chronic use by nursing mother can lead to infant lethargy and weight loss; slower metabolism may get accumulation of drug and its metabolites.
Diazepam	No	No	D	Floppy infant syndrome; cleft lip; neural tube defects; withdrawal syndrome	No	Chronic use by nursing mother can lead to infant lethargy and weight loss; slower metabolism may get accumulation of drug and its metabolites.
Halazepam	No	No	D		No	
Lorazepam	No	No	D	Floppy infant syndrome; anal atresia	No	
Midazolam	No	No	D		No	
Estazolam	No	No	X		No	
Quazepam	No	No	X		No	
Temazepam	No	No	X	Cleft lip	No	
Triazolam	No	No	X		No	

[a]Do not administer any drug that is not absolutely necessary; potential risk to the fetus must be weighed against the benefit to the woman; consult the patient's health care provider before using drugs.
[b]See Table 24-2 for definition of FDA categories.
[c]Category D in third trimester of pregnancy.
[d]Oxycodone, meperidine, hydrocodone.
[e]Codeine.
[f]Augmentin = amoxicillin + clavulanic acid.
[g]References differ.
[h]Check levels in the dental operatory, minimize risk, increase ventilation exchanges.
[i]Clorazepate, flurazepam, oxazepam—no category.

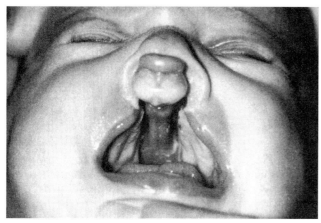

FIGURE 24-1

A 3-week-old female infant with a typical bilateral cleft lip and palate deformity. Certain drugs used during pregnancy, including opioids and benzodiazepines, have been known to cause this deformity. (From Sanders RC, Blackman LR, Hogge WA: *Structural fetal abnormalities,* ed 2, Philadelphia, 2002, Mosby.)

Antiinfective Agents

Antiinfective agents should only be used when a definite indication for their use exists. Prophylactic use, use when no indication exists, and use when an infection can be locally treated are inappropriate.

◆ AMOXICILLIN

The most common antiinfective agent used in dentistry is amoxicillin. It is generally agreed that the amoxicillin is safe to use during pregnancy. Using amoxicillin for a dental infection that is not controlled by local measures would be acceptable. Amoxicillin appears in breast milk, and infants should be observed for signs of diarrhea, candidiasis, and allergic reactions.

◆ ERYTHROMYCIN

Erythromycins, other than the estolate form, also appear to be safe for use during pregnancy. The estolate form (Ilosone) should not be used in pregnant women because it has been associated with reversible hepatic toxicity in the mother. Erythromycin is concentrated in breast milk but has not been documented to produce problems.

◆ CEPHALOSPORINS

The first- and second-generation cephalosporins have not been associated with teratogenicity. These cephalosporins should be used in dentistry only if a specific indication exists.

◆ TETRACYCLINES

All tetracyclines, including tetracycline and doxycycline, are contraindicated during pregnancy because of the potential for adversely affecting the fetus. They cross the placenta and are deposited in the fetal teeth and bones. Deciduous teeth may become stained (see Color Plate 15), and fetal bone growth inhibited. Hepatotoxicity can occur in the pregnant woman treated with large doses of tetracycline. Whether the amount excreted in milk, after it is complexed with the calcium in milk, can produce problems in the nursing infant is not known.

◆ CLINDAMYCIN

Clindamycin should be used for dental infections during pregnancy for susceptible anaerobic infections not sensitive to penicillin. It is also indicated for prophylaxis of endocarditis in penicillin-allergic patients. No adverse fetal problems have been reported. Because clindamycin is excreted in breast milk if it is given to nursing mothers, the infant should be monitored for diarrhea.

◆ METRONIDAZOLE

In animals, metronidazole can produce birth defects. Metronidazole should be used carefully during the first trimester. It would be difficult to encounter a dental situation in which the risk to the fetus would not be greater than the benefit to the mother. Because animal studies have shown metronidazole to be carcinogenic, the nursing mother should only be given metronidazole if the breast milk is expressed and discarded during treatment and for 48 hours after the last dose.

◆ NYSTATIN

Nystatin is safe to use during pregnancy to treat oral *Candida* infections. When applied topically or taken orally, it is not absorbed into the systemic circulation. It may also be used by either the pregnant woman or the nursing infant to treat thrush.

◆ CLOTRIMAZOLE

Small amounts of clotrimazole are absorbed from topical administration of this agent. No occurrences of abnormality have been reported, but nystatin is safer.

◆ KETOCONAZOLE

Ketoconazole is classified by the FDA as a category C drug. It has been shown to be teratogenic in rats, producing an abnormal number of digits (syndactyly [Figure 24-2] and oligodactyly). Dystocia during delivery has been demonstrated in animals. Ketoconazole appears in breast milk and may increase the chance that kernicterus (jaundice) may occur in the nursing infant. If ketoconazole must be used, breast milk must be expressed and discarded during therapy and for 72 hours after cessation of therapy. Fluconazole, like ketoconazole, is also scheduled as category C.

Antianxiety Agents

◆ NITROUS OXIDE–OXYGEN MIXTURE

Operating room personnel exposed to trace amounts of nitrous oxide (N_2O) have a significantly higher incidence of spontaneous abortion and birth defects in their children, regardless of whether the man or woman was exposed. These data suggest that methods for reducing the environmental exposure, especially chronically, should be explored and implemented. Pregnant dental health care workers should have knowledge of the levels of N_2O that are present in the dental offices in which they practice.

◆ BENZODIAZEPINES

First-trimester use of the benzodiazepines (chlordiazepoxide and diazepam) has been reported to increase the risk of congenital malformations. Cleft palate and lip and neural tube defects (Figure 24-3) have been seen. Other benzodiazepines may be associated with this increase in risk also. Temazepam and triazolam are FDA pregnancy category X drugs, and alprazolam, halazepam, and lorazepam are category D drugs. Benzodiazepines are indicated during pregnancy only for the treatment of status epilepticus (no dental use).

Chronic ingestion of the benzodiazepines can produce physical dependence in the infant. Floppy infant syndrome, or neonatal flaccidity, has been seen at birth, with inadequate sucking reflex or apnea. Use of benzodiazepines in the nursing mother, which may accumulate in the neonate because of slower metabolism, may cause sedation and feeding difficulties. Therefore if they are needed, the infant should be monitored for sedation.

♦ ALCOHOL

Pregnancy + alcohol = FAS

Although alcohol is not a dental drug, it is mentioned here because the evidence for the teratogenicity of alcohol is strong. Fetal alcohol syndrome (FAS) is the syndrome associated with the changes that occur in an infant exposed to excessive alcohol intake by the mother. FAS involves abnormalities in three areas: growth retardation (prenatal or postnatal), CNS abnormalities (neurologic or intellectual), and facial dysmorphology (e.g., microcephaly, microphthalmia or short palpebral fissures, and flat maxillary area or a thin lip [Figure 24-4]).

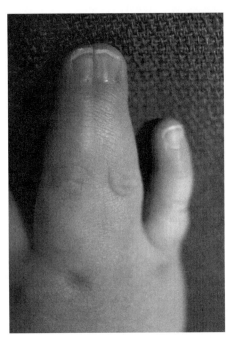

FIGURE 24-2
Complete simple syndactyly. Administration of the drug ketoconazole to pregnant women has been shown to cause this deformity. (From Canale ST, Beaty JH: *Campbell's operative orthopaedics,* ed 11, Philadelphia, 2007, Mosby.)

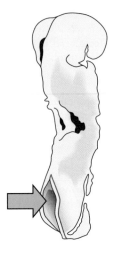

FIGURE 24-4
A child with fetal alcohol syndrome. (From Zitelli BJ, Davis HW: *Atlas of pediatric physical diagnosis,* ed 5, Philadelphia, 2007, Mosby.)

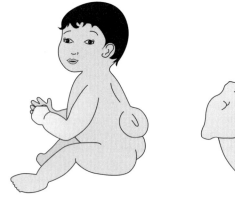
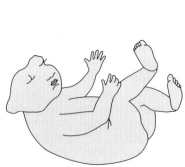

FIGURE 24-3
Neural tube defects include spina bifida and anencephaly. Administration of benzodiazepines during pregnancy can cause neural tube defects. (From Schlenker E, Long S: *Williams' essentials of nutrition & diet therapy,* ed 9, St Louis, 2007, Mosby. Redrawn from Centers for Disease Control and Prevention, Atlanta.)

Infants born to mothers who drank throughout pregnancy show more tremors, hypertonia, restlessness, crying, and abnormal reflexes compared with control groups after birth.

Pregnant dental patients should be encouraged to abstain from the ingestion of alcohol. No safe threshold level for the pregnant woman is known. Well-documented studies show that adverse effects on the fetus are dose related and can extend for years after the birth of the baby. The dental health care worker, as a health care professional, is in a position to remind the pregnant woman to care for her oral cavity and also her baby's development.

DENTAL HYGIENE CONSIDERATIONS

1. The dental hygienist should ask appropriate questions during the medication/health history regarding pregnancy and lactation.
2. The information that the dental hygienist obtains will help avoid the use of specific drugs if the patient is pregnant and lactating.
3. Pregnant women should not be x-rayed because x-rays are harmful to the developing fetus.
4. The dental hygienist should consult with the appropriate reference in order to determine the FDA pregnancy category of a drug before it is prescribed to a pregnant or nursing mother.
5. Pregnant women may require a semi-supine position in the dental treatment chair. The dental hygienist should work with the patient in order to determine the better position.
6. Mothers who are nursing should nurse just prior to receiving medication if medication is necessary.
7. Always check blood pressure and pulse.
8. Appointments should be planned for the second trimester when there is less risk for nausea and vomiting.
9. Stress the importance of oral health care because pregnancy can lead to gingival inflammation.
10. Review the information in Box 24-1.

CLINICAL SKILLS ASSESSMENT

1. Describe the proper method for the dental hygienist to obtain information about possible pregnancy or breastfeeding patients. State the information to be obtained.
2. Explain the three trimesters and the special risks for each one.
3. Define *teratogenicity* and describe why identifying drugs that produce it is so difficult.
4. Explain the FDA pregnancy categories and state their significance.
5. Determine the factors that are important when a woman who is breast feeding is to receive drugs.
6. For the commonly used dental drugs, such as local anesthetics, antibiotics, and analgesics, state the agents in each group that are the least safe.
7. Describe two activities that the dental health care worker should perform before giving a pregnant woman any medications to minimize future legal problems.

⊖volve

Please visit http://evolve.elsevier.com/Haveles/pharmacology for review questions and additional practice and reference materials.

25 Drug Abuse

LEARNING OBJECTIVES

1. Define addiction, dependence, tolerance, and withdrawal in relation to drug abuse.
2. Name several types of central nervous system depressants that are commonly abused and outline the typical pattern of abuse, treatment, adverse reactions, management of overdose and withdrawal, and dental treatment implications of each.
3. Identify several types of central nervous system stimulants that are commonly abused.
4. Describe the pattern of abuse and treatment options associated with tobacco use, and summarize the role of the dental health care worker in tobacco cessation.
5. Discuss ways in which the dental health care worker can identify patients or colleagues who may be abusing drugs.

Dental health care workers may become involved with drug abuse in a variety of ways. Drugs that can be abused include both legal and illegal drugs. Patients seen in the dental office may be abusing drugs. Another interaction with the abusing patient involves the "potential" patient. Potential patients call the dental office, complain of pain, and request a prescription. Employees working in the dental office, including the dentist, dental hygienist, dental assistant, receptionist, bookkeeper, or other employees, may abuse drugs. Friends and relatives, as well as their friends and relatives, may abuse drugs. In our society, drug abuse, especially in adolescents, is epidemic. Wherever there are people, drug abuse can occur. Therefore the dental health care worker should become familiar with the various types of drugs commonly abused and their patterns of abuse. It is important to be able to recognize the problem in others. Because drug abuse is also a community issue, the dental health care worker should have a heightened awareness of the potential for patients to present with abuse problems (a high index of suspicion but not unrealistically high). The proper awareness is only learned with experience.

Alcohol and tobacco: worst public health problems

Alcohol and tobacco abuse causes more medical problems than all the other drugs of abuse combined. If no one in the United States used tobacco or drank alcohol, half of the filled hospital beds would be empty.

The idea of using drugs to produce profound effects on mood, thought, and feeling is as old as civilization. Only the kinds of substances used for this purpose have changed. Abuse has assumed a much bigger role in society because the forms of drugs used today are much stronger and have a much faster onset of action. This quick reinforcement produces abuse more quickly. For example, natives in Colombia have chewed coca leaves for many years as part of their culture, with little inappropriate use. Purifying cocaine and making it into a powder form to be "snorted" increased its abuse. When cocaine was "free based," it became easier to abuse, but the chemical reaction was dangerous. The most recent adaptation of cocaine, making it into "rocks," has increased abuse of the drug even more by making it available to smoke in convenient, small, reasonably priced doses. As is common with drugs of abuse, the potential for abuse is greatly increased when a drug is very potent, has a quick onset of action, is inexpensive, and is easy to distribute, making it the perfect drug of abuse.

Agents used for their psychoactive properties (capable of changing behavior or inducing psychosis-like reactions or both) can be divided into those that also have therapeutic value (opioids and sedative-hypnotics) and those that have no proven therapeutic value (psychedelics). Some agents may move from one category to the other. For example, marijuana, an agent previously considered to be worthless, is now claimed to be useful in the treatment of the nausea associated with cancer chemotherapy and for glaucoma. However, more controlled studies are needed to determine whether this claim is true.

GENERAL CONSIDERATIONS

Abuse of a drug is defined as the use of a drug for nonmedical purposes, almost always for altering consciousness. Both legitimate and illegitimate drugs may be abused. Whether a drug has an abuse potential is determined by the drug's pharmacologic effect. In contrast, the *misuse* of a drug means using the drug in the wrong dose or for a longer period than prescribed. The difference between these two uses is subtle.

Definitions

Terms relating to abuse that are used in this chapter are defined as follows:

*   *Abstinence syndrome:* A state of being free of drugs that is the goal of any treatment program.
*   *Addiction:* This vague term, although still used, should be replaced with dependence. Addiction is the pattern of abuse that includes compulsive use despite complications (medical or social) and frequent relapses after "quitting."
*   *Dependence:* A combination of either physical or psychological manifestations (withdrawal) occurring in a drug-dependent person when the drug is removed.
*   *Drug abuse:* Self-administration of a drug in a socially unacceptable manner, resulting in negative consequences. A component of abuse is that harm is being produced from using the drug.
*   *Drug dependence:* A state, which may be physical, psychological, or both, that occurs as a consequence of the interaction between a drug and a patient. It is characterized by a compulsion to take the drug to obtain its effects or to prevent the abstinence syndrome. Tolerance may occur.
*   *Enabling:* The behavior of family or friends that associate with the addict that results in continued drug abuse. This inappropriate coping mechanism requires family therapy.
*   *Habituation:* Physiologic tolerance to or psychological dependence on a drug, short of addiction.
*   *Misuse:* Use of the drug for a disease state in a way considered inappropriate.
*   *Physical/physiologic dependence:* The state in which the drug is necessary for continued functioning of certain body processes. In a dependent person, discontinuing the drug produces the abstinence syndrome, sometimes called *withdrawal* (physiologic reactions).
*   *Psychological dependence:* The state in which, following withdrawal of the drug, there are manifestations of emotional abnormalities and drug-seeking behavior. Craving is present, but there is no physiologic dependence.
*   *Tolerance:* With repeated dosing, the dose of a drug must be increased to produce the same effect. Or, the same dose of a drug, with consecutive dosing, produces less effect.
*   *Withdrawal:* The constellation of symptoms that occurs when a physically dependent person stops taking the drug.

Psychological Dependence

Psychological dependence is a state of mind in which a person believes that he or she is unable to maintain optimal performance without having taken a drug. Psychological dependence can vary in severity from mild desire (e.g., for a morning cup of coffee) to compulsive obsession (e.g., for the next dose of cocaine). Although some highly abused drugs have only psychological dependence, the "need" to use these drugs can be as strong as or stronger than drugs with a physical dependence. Other examples include benzodiazepines, opioids, and amphetamines.

Physical Dependence

Physical dependence refers to the altered physiologic state that results from constantly increasing drug concentrations. The presence of physical dependence is established by the withdrawal or abstinence syndrome, a combination of many drug-specific symptoms that occur on abrupt discontinuation of drug administration. Withdrawal symptoms are often the opposite of the symptoms of use of the drug, for example, excessive parasympathetic action (e.g., diarrhea, lacrimation, and piloerection ["goose flesh"]) when withdrawing from the opioids.

Tolerance

Tolerance: body gets "used to" drug

Tolerance is characterized by the need to increase the dose continually to achieve the desired effect or the giving of the same dose, which produces a diminishing effect. The type of tolerance referred to in this discussion of abuse of psychoactive drugs is *central* (functional or behavioral) *tolerance,* that is, a definite decrease in the response of brain tissue to constantly increasing amounts of a drug. (One can think of the brain becoming "stronger" [less responsive] to "withstand" the large doses it must tolerate.) In terminal patients, this tolerance requires ever-increasing doses of opioids even if the pain remains constant. The doses reached over time with the terminally ill would be fatal to a patient without tolerance.

Tolerance of metabolic origin (dispositional or metabolic tolerance) is caused by an accelerated rate of metabolism of the drug and is excluded in this discussion. Metabolic tolerance is an insignificant factor in the tolerance observed in humans to most of the psychoactive drugs.

Addiction, Habituation, and Dependence

Terminology not clear

Addiction and *habituation* are terms that have been misused almost as much as the drugs they attempt to characterize. Any use of these terms must be preceded by an adequate definition. In both addiction and habituation, the desire to continue using the drug is present, but in addiction, dependence is also present. Habituation and addiction are really only degrees of misuse or abuse of drugs. It has been recommended that these terms be replaced by the term dependence, a state of psychological or physical desire to use a drug.

Drugs that produce tolerance and physical dependence are grouped according to their ability to be substituted for one another. For example, if a person is addicted to heroin, an opioid, then other opioids, such as morphine, can prevent withdrawal. However, a barbiturate cannot be substituted for an opioid and vice versa. Therefore the opioids and barbiturates are separate groups of dependence-producing drugs. The phenomenon of substitution to suppress withdrawal between different drugs is called *cross-tolerance* or *cross-dependence.* It is observed among members of the same drug group but not among different drug groups. Cross-tolerance may be either partial or complete and is determined more by the pharmacologic effect of the drug than by its chemical structure.

Most characteristics of drug abuse are determined by the individual drug involved, but the following generalizations can be made:

- When comparing drugs in the same group, the time required to produce physical dependence is shortest with a rapidly metabolized drug and longest with a slowly metabolized drug.
- The time course of withdrawal reactions is related to the half-life of the drug. The shorter the half-life, the quicker the withdrawal is.

Approximately 80% of incarcerated (jailed) individuals are there because of drug abuse problems.

Many drugs have been abused extensively, and whether abuse can occur is a function of a particular drug's effects on neurotransmitters (combined with some genetic component within the user). At various times, sniffing airplane glue, inhaling propellant, smoking banana peels, smoking peyote (contains mescaline), and ingesting morning glory seeds have been attempted. The problems and treatment of drug abuse are less related to the drugs themselves, although they can cause definite problems, than to the "inner person" of the patient involved in this type of behavior and his or her genetic predisposition. To treat abuse, a multifactorial approach is needed: counseling, education, self-help groups, and an intense desire to stop.

| "Huffing" volatile substances |

Propellant that is included in paint cans is preferred. The procedure is called "huffing" because the contents are sprayed into a plastic bag and fumes are repeatedly inhaled. Abuse of paint can easily produce irreversible damage to the liver and brain.

This chapter discusses the properties of the specific groups of agents abused and the differences among the groups. The abusable drugs are divided into the following groups: central nervous system (CNS) depressants ("downers"), CNS stimulants ("uppers"), and hallucinogens. Some drugs, depending on the dose, may fall in more than one group. For example, marijuana may be classified as either a CNS depressant or a hallucinogen. Table 25-1 lists the common drugs of abuse by categories.

CENTRAL NERVOUS SYSTEM DEPRESSANTS

CNS depressants include alcohol, opioids, barbiturates, benzodiazepines, volatile solvents (glue and gasoline), and nitrous oxide (abused mainly in dentistry).

Ethyl Alcohol

| Alcoholism affects 1 in 10. |

Ethyl alcohol, or ethanol (ETH-an-ol), is a sedative agent used socially. Because it is legal, its availability makes it the most often abused drug. Abuse of alcohol, called *alcoholism,* is the number one public health problem in the United States and is associated with many major medical problems. The incidence of alcoholism in the United States is about 10% (i.e., 1 in 10).

TABLE 25-1   DRUGS OF ABUSE BY CATEGORY

Drug Group	Most Common Examples	Other Examples
Opioids	Heroin	Morphine Codeine Meperidine Hydromorphone
Stimulants	Cocaine Methamphetamine	Amphetamines Methylphenidate Nicotine
Depressants (sedative-hypnotics)	Ethanol Benzodiazepines Inhalants Nitrous oxide*	Barbiturates Nonbarbiturate sedatives
Hallucinogens	Lysergic acid diethylamide (LSD)	Mescaline Phencyclidine (PCP)
Other	Marijuana	Caffeine

*In dentistry because of availability.

Many "accidental" deaths are associated with the use of alcohol. Two-fifths of traffic fatalities involve alcohol. More than 50% of gunshot wounds in teenagers are preceded by abuse of alcohol. The best use of resources for addiction would be to deal with alcoholism as soon as it can be identified.

♦ PHARMACOKINETICS

Ethyl alcohol is rapidly and completely absorbed from the gastrointestinal tract. Peak levels while fasting occur in less than 40 minutes. Food delays absorption and reduces the peak levels. Alcohol is oxidized in the liver to acetaldehyde, which is then metabolized to carbon dioxide (CO_2) and water (H_2O) (Figure 25-1).

Its metabolism follows zero-order kinetics, so a constant amount of alcohol is metabolized per unit of time regardless of the amount ingested. Because of its zero-order kinetics, excessive intake of alcohol can produce a prolonged effect. It is also excreted from the lungs (alcohol breath) and in urine.

♦ ACUTE INTOXICATION

With mild intoxication, impairment of judgment, emotional lability, and nystagmus occur. When intoxication is moderate, dilated pupils, slurred speech, ataxia, and a staggering gait are noted. If intoxication is severe, seizures, coma, and death can occur. Treatment includes fluids and electrolytes, thiamine (B_6), sodium bicarbonate, and magnesium.

♦ WITHDRAWAL

| Delirium tremens (DTs) |

Withdrawal from alcohol use occurs after the use of alcohol. The more alcohol consumed and the more time spent consuming, the more violent the withdrawal syndrome is (Figure 25-2). Stage 1 usually begins 6 to 8 hours after drinking has stopped and includes withdrawal, psychomotor agitation, and autonomic nervous system hyperactivity. Stage 2 withdrawal includes hallucinations, paranoid behavior, and amnesia. Stage 3 includes disorientation, delusions, and grand mal seizures. It takes 3 to 5 days after cessation of drinking alcohol for stage 3 to occur.

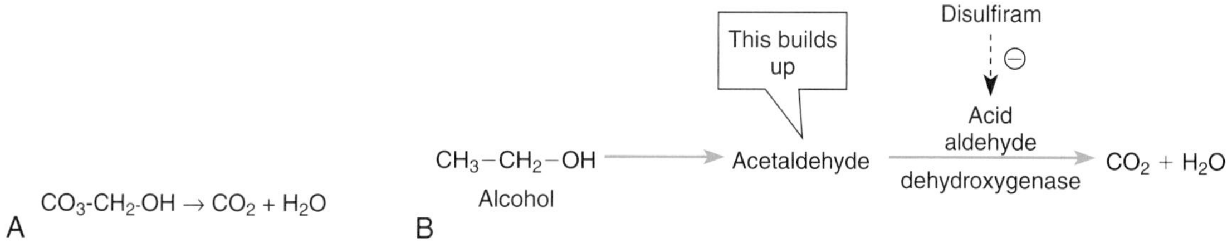

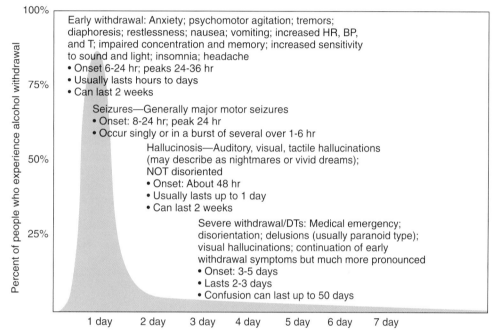

FIGURE 25-1

A, Metabolism of alcohol. **B,** Effects of disulfiram on alcohol metabolism.

FIGURE 25-2

Alcohol withdrawal syndrome. (From Stuart GW, Laraia MT: *Principles and practice of psychiatric nursing,* ed 7, St Louis, 2001, Mosby.)

A cross-tolerant benzodiazepine (e.g., chlordiazepoxide; see Chapter 11) may be used to prevent withdrawal symptoms. Withdrawal from alcohol is termed *delirium tremens (DTs)* because the patient will often experience shaky (tremor) movements. Alcohol withdrawal can be life threatening if not properly treated.

◆ CHRONIC EFFECTS

The chronic medical effects of alcoholism can include deficiency of proteins, minerals, and water-soluble vitamins. Impotence, gastritis, esophageal varices, arrhythmias, and hypertension have been reported. If a pregnant woman is using ethanol chronically, fetal alcohol syndrome can occur (see Figure 24-4). The infant is retarded in body growth and has a small head (microencephaly), poor coordination, underdevelopment of the midface, and joint anomalies. More severe cases include cardiac abnormalities and mental retardation. Chronic alcohol use increases the risk of cancer of the mouth, pharynx, larynx, esophagus, and liver, which may occur with tobacco use to make the risk higher than with alcohol alone. The liver can be affected with alcoholic hepatitis and amnesic syndrome (Wernicke-Korsakoff syndrome), and peripheral neuropathy can occur.

BOX 25-1 CAGE: A SELF-TEST FOR ALCOHOLISM

- Have you ever felt you ought to **C**ut down on your drinking?
- Have people **A**nnoyed you by criticizing your drinking?
- Have you ever felt bad or **G**uilty about your drinking?
- Have you ever had a drink first thing in the morning to steady your nerves or get rid of a hangover (**E**ye-opener)?

More information on CAGE can be obtained by reading Ewing JA: Detecting alcoholism: the CAGE, *JAMA* 252:1905-1907, 1984.

◆ ALCOHOLISM

Alcoholism is a disease in which the alcoholic continues to drink despite the knowledge that drinking is producing a variety of problems (Box 25-1). There is a genetic link for alcoholism; children of alcoholics are at a much greater risk for becoming alcoholics. In the future, genetic testing may be able to identify at-risk children and target that population for intense educational and social intervention for prevention.

"Red flags" for alcohol abuse include drinking at an inappropriately early time, shaking when not drinking, blackouts when drinking, and being told that you drink too much. Missing work and problems in personal relationships are also strong warning signs.

♦ TREATMENT

Alcoholics Anonymous has the best results.

Alcoholics Anonymous. Alcoholics Anonymous, the most successful group for treating alcoholism, is a self-help organization made up of recovering alcoholics. The members (who are recovering alcoholics) give support to alcoholics who are attempting recovery. In most alcoholics, inpatient detoxification is usually not required. In fact, inpatient treatment does not give the alcoholic any experience in recovery in the "real world." Outpatient psychiatric treatment can help provide some insight for alcoholics.

Drug Treatment. Alcoholics who are motivated and socially stable can be given disulfiram (dye-SUL-fi-ram) (Antabuse). Occasionally, employers will insist on the ingestion of disulfiram as a condition of employment.

Because disulfiram inhibits the metabolism of aldehyde dehydrogenase, a buildup of acetaldehyde occurs. Acetaldehyde produces significant side effects if alcohol is ingested. These include vasodilation, flushing, tachycardia, dyspnea, throbbing headache, vomiting, and thirst. The reaction may last from 30 minutes to several hours. Certain drugs that produce the disulfiram-like reaction (e.g., metronidazole) may cause a minor version of these symptoms with alcohol intake.

Naltrexone (ReVia), an oral opioid antagonist, is an old drug with a new use. Originally, it was indicated to prevent relapse in the opioid-dependent patient. Its new use is to reduce alcohol craving. Because naltrexone is partially effective in decreasing craving from alcohol, the logical conclusion is that alcohol stimulates some of the opioid receptors (among other receptors). More detailed knowledge of the receptors affected by alcohol may increase the chance of developing other agents to manage this disease. Other agents that might be useful are related to other neurotransmitters such as dopamine or serotonin.

♦ DENTAL TREATMENT OF THE ALCOHOLIC PATIENT

The dental health care worker must have an index of suspicion for alcoholism in patients treated in the dental office. The great majority of alcoholics look exactly like our neighbors, not like those characterized in old movies (e.g., unshaven, shaky). All health care workers have been given the charge to identify and assist patients in obtaining treatment.

The dental treatment of the alcoholic patient includes some modifications, depending on the severity of the disease process. Most alcoholic patients have poor oral hygiene. Check for the sweet musty breath and painless bilateral hypertrophy of parotid glands characteristic of alcoholism. Cirrhosis of the liver can occur when alcoholics continue to abuse alcohol (Figure 25-3). The major problem in these patients is a failure of the liver to perform adequately. Because of hepatic failure, the liver is able

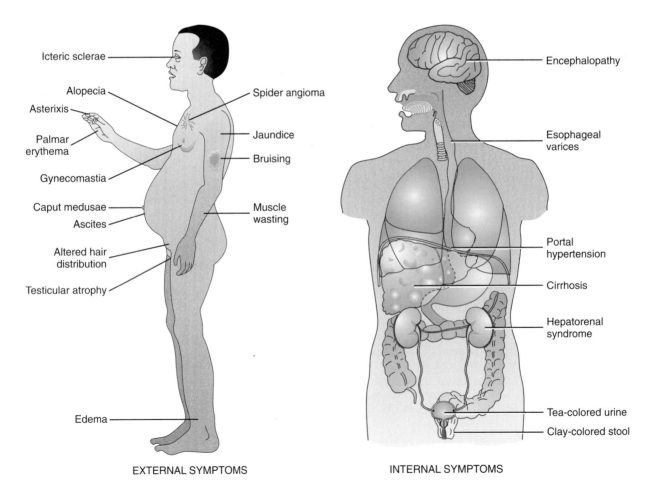

EXTERNAL SYMPTOMS   INTERNAL SYMPTOMS

FIGURE 25-3
Clinical manifestations of cirrhosis. (From Mahan LK, Escott-Stump S: *Krause's food, nutrition, & diet therapy,* ed 12, St Louis, 2008, Saunders.)

to store less vitamin K and the conversion of vitamin K to the coagulation factors is reduced. The outcome of these effects is a deficiency in coagulation factors II, VII, IX, and X (vitamin K–dependent factors) with resulting bleeding tendencies. The patient's international normalized ratio (INR) can be elevated to 6 or more without the presence of other concomitant medications. Thrombocytopenia secondary to portal hypertension and bone marrow depression magnifies the hemostatic deficiency, sometimes resulting in spontaneous gingival bleeding. With the presence of esophageal varices, spontaneous bleeding can occur. Later in liver failure, the abdomen becomes distended with fluid (the patient appears 9 months pregnant).

Oral complications of alcoholism include glossitis, loss of tongue papillae, angular/labial cheilosis, and *Candida* infection. Healing after surgery may be slow, and bleeding may be difficult to stop.

Because alcohol and tobacco use and abuse predispose a patient to oral squamous cell carcinoma, the dental health care worker should check any oral lesions carefully. Special attention should be paid to leukoplakia and ulceration (especially on the lateral border of the tongue or the floor of the mouth).

With reduced liver function, the liver has difficulty metabolizing drugs usually metabolized in the liver. The levels of drugs metabolized by the liver, such as amide local anesthetics and oxidized benzodiazepines, will not fall as rapidly as in normal patients. Dose reductions are necessary because of diminished liver function. The signs of potential advanced alcoholic liver disease are listed in Box 25-2.

The dental health care worker should have an index of suspicion so that alcoholics can be identified. The dental worker should smell the patient's breath, palpate the parotid glands, expect poor oral hygiene, and evaluate the patient's bleeding tendency. Those with cirrhosis and severe hepatic disease will have greatly prolonged prothrombin times and may require vitamin K a few days before a surgical procedure in which bleeding is expected. Table 25-2 lists the dental management of the alcoholic patient.

BOX 25-2 SIGNS OF ADVANCED ALCOHOLIC LIVER DISEASE

Head Area
- Edema/puffy face
- Parotid gland enlargement
- Advanced periodontal disease
- Sweet, musty breath odor
- Ecchymoses, petechiae, bleeding

Rest of the Body
- Memory deficit
- A lot of injuries
- Spider angiomas
- Jaundice
- Ankle edema
- Ascites
- Palmar erythema
- White nails
- Transverse pale band on nails

Modified from Little JW, Falace D, Miller C, et al: *Dental management of the medically compromised patient*, ed 7, St Louis, 2008, Mosby.

TABLE 25-2 DENTAL MANAGEMENT OF THE ALCOHOLIC PATIENT

Condition	Comments	Management
Bleeding abnormalities		Platelets during and after chronic alcohol abuse
		Thrombocytopenia secondary to congestive splenomegaly, folate deficiency, bone marrow EtOH toxicity; quickly reverse if stop drinking; begins up to 2-3 days and increases 20,000-60,000/day
		Impaired aggregation decreased TXA$_2$, increased bleeding time (like ASA or NSAIDs); improves 2-3 weeks after stopping
		Decreased hemostasis vitamin K–dependent clotting factors missing
If cirrhosis and decreased liver function, clotting factors not being made (vitamin K-dependent)	LFT test—AST	Give vitamin K, give whole blood (fresh clotting factors)
		PT prolonged
		Use local hemostatic procedure
Gastrointestinal Tract Problems		
Stomach bleeding (varices)	Avoid NSAIDs, ASA	Topical
Drug interactions		??Acute intake—high levels
		Chronic intake—increased metabolism
Acute alcohol use		Chronic alcoholism
Enzyme-induced drugs metabolized by liver are metabolized faster, leading to lower blood levels of drugs metabolized by the liver	Raise drug level	Liver does not function properly; therefore drugs metabolized by liver are not metabolized as fast and levels increase
		Metabolism decreased
Tylenol levels 4 gm; ASA, NSAIDs	4 gm usual	Less with some EtOH, none with more

Data from Glick M: Medical considerations for dental care of patients with alcohol-related liver disease, *J Am Dent Assoc* 128:61-72, 1997; and Mandel L, Hamele-Bena D: Alcoholic parotid sialadenosis, *J Am Dent Assoc* 128(10):1411-1415, 1997.
EtOH, Alcohol; *TXA$_2$*, thromboxane A; *ASA*, aspirin; *NSAIDs*, nonsteroidal antiinflammatory drugs; *LFT*, liver function test; *AST*, aspartate aminotransferase; *PT*, prothrombin time.

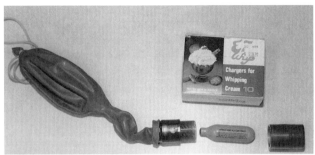

FIGURE 25-4
Whippet assembly for recreational misuse of nitrous oxide (N₂O). (From Clark M, Brunick A: *Handbook of nitrous oxide and oxygen sedation,* ed 3, St Louis, 2008, Mosby.)

Nitrous Oxide

Nitrous oxide (N_2O) is an incomplete general anesthetic readily available in many dental offices (see Chapter 10). It is abused primarily by dentists, dental hygienists, and dental assistants. Food service employees sometimes become N_2O abusers because it is available in the aerosol in canned whipping cream products. Misuse often begins as "therapeutic" use only, progressing to abusive or "recreational" use at a later stage.

◆ ABUSE PATTERN

N_2O is available in the dental office in tanks and as a propellant for whipping cream (Figure 25-4). The availability of this gas to dental office personnel probably accounts for its unique abuse pattern.

Abuse of N_2O can result in psychological but not physical dependence. Inhalation of 50% to 75% produces a "high" for 30 seconds followed by a sense of euphoria and detachment for 2 to 3 minutes. Tingling or warmth around the face, auditory illusions, slurred speech, and a stumbling gait can occur. The typical chemically dependent dentist (with N_2O as the drug of choice) is a 40-year-old white man who has often abused illicit drugs and primarily uses alone.

◆ ADVERSE REACTIONS

General. Adverse reactions include dizziness, headache, tachycardia, syncope, and hypotension. N_2O impairs the ability to drive or operate heavy machinery. Other effects of N_2O use include hallucinations and religious experiences. Equilibrium, balance, and gait are affected. With chronic use, it can produce chronic mental dysfunction and infertility.

If 100% N_2O is inhaled, nausea, cyanosis, and falling may occur. Without oxygen, pure N_2O can produce hypoxia that results in death. Dentists who have self-administered N_2O have been found dead in their dental chairs with the mask still attached to the face.

Myelopathy with abuse may be irreversible

Myeloneuropathy. Chronic use or abuse can lead to myelopathy (sensory and motor) resulting in a combination of symptoms pathognomonic for N_2O abuse. Initial symptoms include loss of finger dexterity and numbness or paresthesia of the extremities. Position and vibration sensory neurons are lost. Other sensations, such as to pain, light touch, and temperature, may be lost. Later, Lhermitte's sign, clumsiness, and weakness can be demonstrated. Neurologic deficiencies include extensor plantar reflex and polyneuropathy (slow conduction velocity in nerves). The neurologic deficiency is similar to that of spinal cord degeneration in pernicious anemia. The neurologic problems from vitamin B_{12} deficiency are improved by parenteral vitamin B_{12}. Whether B_{12} improves N_2O myelopathy is controversial. If the abuse of N_2O is discontinued soon enough, clinical improvement can occur. However, with an increase in abuse the myelopathy is often irreversible.

Opioid Analgesics

Heroin, methadone (Dolophine), morphine, hydromorphone (Dilaudid), meperidine (Demerol), oxycodone (Percodan), and oxycodone sustained release (OxyContin) are currently the most popular abused opioids. Opioids used as analgesics are discussed in Chapter 6, which focuses on the pharmacology of the opioids themselves. It should be noted that opioids sold illegally on the street may be adulterated. They may contain other unknown agents or diluters and often contain inactive filler so the doses can be more easily divided.

In addition to being analgesics, opioids produce a state described as complete satiation of all drives in some people. The opioids elevate the user's mood, cause euphoria, relieve fear and apprehension, and produce a feeling of peace and tranquility. They also suppress hunger, reduce sexual desire, and diminish the response to provocation. Undoubtedly, initial abuse is reinforced by this "positive" experience. Other side effects include slowed respiration, constipation, urinary retention, and peripheral vasodilation.

With the development of physical dependence, however, the driving motivation to obtain the drug becomes more and more negative. Fear of the withdrawal syndrome begins to override other motivation. At this point, the addict may resort to criminal activity and violence to support the drug habit. These activities are not direct actions of the drug but are related to opioid dependence.

◆ PATTERN OF ABUSE

Heroin is the opioid most commonly administered parenterally. The signs and symptoms of an acute overdose are fixed, pinpoint pupils, depressed respiration, hypotension and shock, slow or absent reflexes, and drowsiness or coma. Tolerance develops to most of the pharmacologic effects of the opioids, including the euphoric, analgesic, sedative, and respiratory depressant actions. However, tolerance does not develop to miosis or constipation.

The symptoms and time course of the withdrawal syndrome are determined by the specific drug abused and the dose of drug used. Withdrawal usually begins at the time of the abuser's next scheduled dose. The first signs of withdrawal from heroin are yawning, lacrimation, rhinorrhea, and diaphoresis, followed by a restless sleep. With further abstinence, anorexia, tremors, irritability, weakness, and excessive gastrointestinal activity occur. The heart rate is rapid, the blood pressure is elevated, and chills alternate with excessive sweating. Without treatment, symptoms disappear by about the eighth day after the last dose of heroin.

◆ MANAGEMENT OF ACUTE OVERDOSE AND WITHDRAWAL

Triad: respiratory depression, pin point pupils (P³), and coma

If the triad of **narcotic** overdose (respiratory depression, pinpoint pupils, and coma) is present, naloxone (Narcan) should be administered immediately. If there is no response, it is unlikely that the depressed respiration is caused by opioid overdose.

In the past, immediate withdrawal reaction from an opioid sold on the street was only moderately distressing to the patient because of the poor quality and dilution of these drugs. Recently, high-quality heroin has reached the streets, and overdoses are more common and the withdrawal more intense. Some addicts go "cold turkey" because the daily cost of their habit has risen too high. After withdrawal, they begin using again, but a smaller dose (therefore less expensive) is needed to produce the desired effect.

Patients in withdrawal can be made comfortable with methadone, a long-acting opioid that can replace heroin and then be gradually withdrawn. A phenothiazine or benzodiazepine is often administered for relief of tension. Long-term rehabilitation programs use several treatment approaches such as methadone maintenance. These include substitution of a physiologically equivalent drug (e.g., methadone) in high doses, gradual weaning from methadone, or use of a long-acting opioid antagonist (e.g., naltrexone) (see Chapter 6). Other psychotropic agents may be helpful in managing the alcoholic patient because of the high incidence of comorbidity of psychiatric conditions.

♦ DENTAL IMPLICATIONS

The following should be considered when treating a dental patient who abuses opioids (narcotics).

Pain Control. Because an opioid abuser develops tolerance to the analgesic effects of any opioid, treating pain with opioids is ineffective and can cause a recovering addict to begin using opioids again. It is best to alleviate the cause of the pain first and prescribe nonsteroidal antiinflammatory drugs (NSAIDs) for analgesia.

Be alert for "shoppers."

Prescriptions for Opioids. Opioid abusers often come to the dental office requesting an opioid for severe pain ("shopping"). Often, the drug abuser suggests the name or partial name of a specific opioid or states allergies to several less potent agents.

Increased Incidence of Disease. Certain diseases that can be transmitted by use of needles for injections have a higher incidence in opioid abusers. These include hepatitis B, human immunodeficiency virus (HIV) producing acquired immune deficiency syndrome (AIDS), and sexually transmitted diseases. Infections caused by the use of nonsterile solutions and instruments can produce osteomyelitis and abscesses in the kidneys and heart valves. Intravenous drug abusers have about a 30% chance of developing cardiac valve damage over a 3-year period.

Chronic Pain. The dental health care worker will occasionally encounter dental patients with chronic pain. There are two ways in which these patients present to the dental office: a patient with symptoms of chronic dental-related pain (temporomandibular joint disorder or trigeminal neuralgia) or a patient reporting an elongation of the period of pain related to normal dental treatment (e.g., patient gets several refills of opioids for a root canal and no pathology can be identified). Patients who have pain for a much longer time than normal deserve a workup for chronic pain. Opioids are usually not effective in the management of chronic pain. If the dentist begins providing prescriptions for opioids to some patients, it is difficult to stop writing these prescriptions for the patient. The patient may state, "I hurt real bad." Another subtle lever that may increase the chance that the dentist would prescribe more opioids is the unsettling feeling that he or she has not performed some dental treatment correctly. Sometimes mild references to malpractice can magnify this worry. One should not be "blackmailed" into prescribing opioids if one feels uncomfortable. One should just state the office policy, for example, "The policy of this office is that no refills for an opioid (narcotic) analgesic are given without an additional office visit. It is important to identify the cause of the pain so that it can be alleviated."

♦ OPIOID STREET DRUGS

Opioids available on the street change with time and are different in different parts of the country. The dental health care worker should be aware that most drug abusers misuse more than one substance and that street drugs are often adulterated.

An illicitly produced meperidine derivative that produced classic opioid effects contained 1-methyl-4-phenyl-1, 2, 3, 6-tetrahydropyridine (MPTP). This powerful neurotoxic agent has a toxicity unrelated to its opioid effects. It produces classic and permanent (irreversible) Parkinson's disease by destroying the cells in the substantia nigra (they make dopamine) within a very short period. This contaminant has become a valuable research tool because it can induce Parkinson's disease in animals, providing an animal model for research of drugs for treatment of Parkinson's disease.

Sedative-Hypnotics

Sedative-hypnotics include barbiturates; alcohol; meprobamate (Miltown); methaqualone (Quaalude; not made legally now, called "ludes"); chloral hydrate; benzodiazepines, such as chlordiazepoxide (Librium) and diazepam (Valium); and N_2O. Although their chemical structures vary greatly, their pharmacologic actions and pattern of abuse are similar.

Initial symptoms resemble the well-known symptoms of alcohol intoxication: loss of inhibition, euphoria, emotional instability, belligerence, difficulty in thinking, poor memory and judgment, slurred speech, and ataxia. With increasing doses, drowsiness and sleep occur, respiration is depressed, cardiac output is decreased, and gastrointestinal activity and urine output are diminished. Paradoxic reactions can range from elation to excessive stimulation. The mechanism of excitement with a CNS depressant is related to an increased sensitivity to blocking of the inhibitor fibers, leaving the excitatory fibers unopposed. With additional CNS depression, the excitatory fibers are also depressed, resulting in sedation.

♦ PATTERN OF ABUSE

Addict's usual dose becomes closer to fatal dose with increasing tolerance.

The CNS depressant drugs are generally taken orally, often in a combination with some of the other drugs of abuse. With an acute overdose, respiratory and cardiovascular depression occur, leading to coma and hypotension. The pupils may be unchanged or small, and lateral nystagmus is seen. Confusion, slurred speech, and ataxia are always present. Compared with opioids, the CNS depressants have a slower onset of tolerance and physical dependence. Tolerance to the sedative effect is not accompanied by a comparable tolerance to the lethal dose. With prolonged misuse, emotional instability, hostile and paranoid ideations, and suicidal tendencies are common.

Although the withdrawal syndrome for all CNS depressants is similar, its time course depends on the half-life of the drug abused. The first signs of withdrawal are insomnia, weakness, tremulousness, restlessness, and perspiration. Often nausea and vomiting, together with hyperthermia and agitation, occur. Delirium and convulsions may culminate in cardiovascular collapse and loss of the temperature-regulating mechanism.

Another troubling abuse of the sedative-hypnotics involves administering them to other people to control them. Old movies have demonstrated the "slipping of a Mickey Finn" (chloral hydrate) to knock a person out ("knock-out drops"). A recent similar practice involves using a short-acting benzodiazepine, flunitrazepam or Rohypnol (nickname is "Ruffies") to make an unsuspecting young woman excessively sedated. After the woman becomes semiconscious, her partner would take sexual advantage of her and commit rape. This is often referred to as "date rape." Because of the excessive sedation and the amnesia produced by the flunitrazepam, recounting or even remembering what happened is difficult. Therefore prosecution would be unlikely because it would be difficult to prove whether the action was consensual.

◆ MANAGEMENT OF ACUTE OVERDOSE AND WITHDRAWAL

The most important consideration with an acute overdose of a CNS depressant is support of the cardiovascular and respiratory systems. An airway must always be established and maintained. Early gastric lavage after intubation and dialysis can assist in removal of some drugs. CNS stimulants are harmful and should not be given.

In contrast to withdrawal from opioids, withdrawal from CNS depressants can be life threatening and the patient should be hospitalized. The treatment of withdrawal from any CNS depressant includes (1) replacement of the abused drug with an equivalent drug and (2) gradual withdrawal of the equivalent drug.

The drug usually substituted for the abused drug is a long-acting benzodiazepine such as chlordiazepoxide or diazepam. The substitute drug is then gradually withdrawn over a period of weeks; during this time, the patient receives psychotherapy.

CENTRAL NERVOUS SYSTEM STIMULANTS

The CNS stimulants include cocaine, the amphetamines, caffeine, and nicotine.

Cocaine

Cocaine is a CNS stimulant with local anesthetic properties when applied topically. It is used primarily for its stimulant action by "sniffing," "snorting," or intravenous injection. The most recent variant is a free-base form that is smoked and goes by the street name of "crack" or "rock." It is more pure and potent, and the resulting intoxication is far more intense than that of snorted cocaine. It acts much quicker and is much more euphoric and addicting. Cocaine induces intense euphoria, a sense of total self-confidence, and anorexia. Because of its short duration of action, the effects of cocaine last only a few minutes. Paranoia and extreme excitability cause some cocaine users to perform violent acts while under its influence. The paranoia produced by cocaine causes people to be unpredictable. The senseless violent acts sometimes committed by cocaine users cause society to fear cocaine abusers. Unpredictable actions are

feared the most. Psychological dependence becomes intense, but neither tolerance nor withdrawal has been shown. Cocaine's medical use is on mucous membranes (the inside of the nose) in which it produces local anesthesia and vasoconstriction to reduce hemorrhage. There is no appropriate dental use of cocaine. Although cocaine abuse is greatly publicized, the proportion of the population using cocaine is relatively small (compared with alcohol and tobacco).

Amphetamines

◆ PATTERN OF ABUSE

Drugs in the amphetamine class include methamphetamine (Desoxyn), dextroamphetamine (Dexedrine), diethylpropion (Tenuate), and methylphenidate (Ritalin). Another member of this group is phentermine (Fastin), which is the *phen* in Phen-Fen (a diet drug combination removed from the market). Because methamphetamine produces a much longer duration of effect than cocaine, "meth" use is spreading across the nation. Many meth laboratories (labs) have been raided, but more pop up immediately. The manufacture of methamphetamine can be carried out with common chemistry lab equipment and a precursor drug (ephedrine) that can be bought over the counter. Because of this, ephedrine is no longer available for purchase and products containing pseudoephedrine are now stocked in the actual pharmacy. Persons, over the age of 18, can only purchase a limited quantity of pseudoephedrine each year and most sign a log verifying the purchase. Unfortunately, these meth labs are explosive, smell bad (distinctive odor), and have been found in many residential neighborhoods.

The sympathomimetic CNS stimulants are abused for their ability to produce a euphoric mood, a sense of increased energy and alertness, and a feeling of omnipotence and self-confidence. Other effects include mydriasis, increased blood pressure and heart rate, anorexia, and increased sweating.

CNS stimulants are taken orally, parenterally (intravenously or "skin popping"), intranasally, or by inhalation (smoking). With prolonged use, tolerance develops to the euphorigenic effect and toxic symptoms appear, including anxiety, aggressiveness, stereotyped behavior, hallucinations, and paranoid fears.

Signs and symptoms of an acute overdose include dilated pupils (sympathetic autonomic nervous system stimulation), elevated blood pressure, rapid pulse, and cardiac arrhythmias. The patient may exhibit diaphoresis, hyperthermia, fine tremors, and hyperactive behavior. Oral adverse reactions include xerostomia and bruxism.

Although tolerance develops to the central sympathomimetic effect, no tolerance develops to the tendency to induce toxic psychoses at higher doses. Modest levels of abuse over a long period do not produce withdrawal reactions except fatigue and prolonged sleep, but large doses can precipitate a withdrawal syndrome consisting of aching muscles, ravenous appetite with abdominal pain, and long periods of sleep. This is followed by profound psychological depression and sometimes even suicide. During this period, abnormal electroencephalographic (EEG) results have been recorded.

◆ MANAGEMENT OF ACUTE OVERDOSE AND WITHDRAWAL

Treatment of an overdose of a CNS stimulant is symptomatic. It may include a phenothiazine for psychotic symptoms, a short-acting sympathomimetic-blocking agent if hypertension is severe, and a tricyclic antidepressant if severe depression occurs.

The most serious sociologic problem with stimulant abuse is the induction of mental abnormalities, especially in young abusers. Experimental evidence suggests that amphetamine psychoses can be induced in previously unaffected volunteer subjects. The psychoses are dose related, and repeated dosing can reproduce the psychoses.

Caffeine

Caffeine, the most widely used social drug in the world, is contained in coffee, tea, cola drinks, and other drinks named to reflect the effect of their contents. Its action on the CNS is stimulation, which is why many people use these beverages. Caffeine toxicity can occur with as little as 300 mg of caffeine (contained in two to three cups of coffee). With five cups or more of caffeine daily, physical dependence can occur. Although many people do not consider it a drug, a withdrawal syndrome can be identified that begins around 24 hours after the last cup of coffee. It consists of headache, lethargy, irritability, and anxiety. Tolerance develops to the effects of caffeine, and some persons continue to use caffeine even when it produces harm. Table 25-3 lists the caffeine content of several beverages.

Tobacco

◆ NICOTINE

Awareness of the toxicity from chronic smoking and chewing tobacco has increased dramatically over the past 2 decades. The CNS-active component of tobacco is nicotine, but a large number of components of the gaseous phase of tobacco smoke contribute to its undesirable effects: carbon monoxide, nitrogen oxides, volatile nitrosamines, hydrogen cyanide, volatile hydrocarbons, and many others.

◆ PATTERN OF ABUSE

> Cigars are the new "dumb craze."

Approximately 25% of the adult American population smokes. Children commonly begin smoking between 11 and 14 years of age. In some geographic areas, more teenage girls than teenage boys smoke. The newest "craze" is cigar smoking; it is portrayed as glamorous, and famous movie stars are observed smoking cigars. Smokers claim that the most desirable effects of smoking are increased alertness, muscle relaxation, facilitation of concentration and memory, and decreases in appetite and irritability. These are consistent with the effect of nicotine on the CNS. In addition, nicotine produces an increase in blood pressure and pulse rate and induces nausea, vomiting, and dizziness as a result of stimulation of the chemoreceptor trigger zone. Smokers are tolerant to these latter effects, but such tolerance does not last long. The first cigarette of the day may induce a certain degree of dizziness and nausea. Chronic use of tobacco is causally related to many serious diseases, including coronary artery disease and oral and lung cancers.

◆ SMOKELESS TOBACCO

In some communities, more than one-fourth of high school males use chewing tobacco. Oral mucosal changes include chronic gingivitis, leukoplakia, and precancerous lesions. In these patients, an extremely thorough oral examination should be done at each prophylaxis. Education concerning the oral health hazards that smokeless tobacco poses should also be included.

◆ MANAGEMENT AND WITHDRAWAL

The withdrawal syndrome that occurs after cessation of chronic tobacco smoking varies greatly from person to person. The most consistent symptoms are anxiety, irritability, difficulty in concentrating, and cravings for cigarettes. Drowsiness, headaches, increased appetite, and sleep disturbances are also common. The syndrome is rapid in onset (within 24 hours after the last cigarette) and can persist for months.

The syndrome of withdrawal from tobacco can be suppressed to some extent by administration of nicotine chewing gum (Nicorette, Nicorette DS) or nicotine patches (NicoDerm, Nicotrol, and Habitrol; Table 25-4). These products do reduce the irritability and difficulty in concentrating but appear to be less effective in controlling insomnia, hunger, and the craving for tobacco. The most important dental side effect of the use of nicotine gum is dislodging dental fillings. Another form of nicotine replacement is the nasal spray Nicotrol NS. A potential problem with the nasal spray is that the rapid rise in blood level more closely mimics the effect of using tobacco.

◆ BUPROPION

Another approach to treating tobacco cessation involves the use of bupropion (Wellbutrin, Zyban), which is an antidepressant, to reduce craving. Dentists can prescribe bupropion but should encourage concomitant treatment modalities (e.g., behavior modification). The recommended dosage schedule is 150 mg daily (qd) for 3 days, followed by 150 mg twice a day (bid) for an additional 2 to 3 months if the patient is experiencing success.

TABLE 25-3 CAFFEINE CONTENT OF SELECTED CAFFEINE-CONTAINING BEVERAGES (MG)	
Beverage	Caffeine (mg)
Cup of coffee—brewed	100-150/5 oz
Decaffeinated coffee	2-4/5 oz
Cup of tea—brewed	60-75/5 oz
Cola drink	60-105/12 oz
Mountain Dew	55/12 oz (0)*
Jolt	71/12 oz
Chocolate, milk	3-6/oz
Chocolate, bittersweet	25/oz
No-Doz	100 mg/tablet

oz, Ounce.
*In Canada.

TABLE 25-4 NICOTINE-CONTAINING PRODUCTS	
Vehicle	Product
Patch	Habitrol, NicoDerm, Nicotrol, ProStep
Gum	Nicorette DS
Nasal spray	Nicotrol NS

Refills should not be indicated on the original prescription because the dental health care worker should talk with the patient by phone before authorizing a refill (see Chapter 17).

◆ VARENICLINE

The newest approach to treating tobacco cessation involves the use of varenicline (CHANTIX), Varenicline is a nicotine-receptor blocker that binds to the nicotine receptor and prevents the nicotine from tobacco from reaching its receptor site. By binding to this receptor, varenicline limits the amount of dopamine that is released in the brain. It is thought that stimulation of nicotinic receptors releases dopamine, which accounts for the feeling of pleasure that is often associated with tobacco use. Varenicline is dosed daily for the first three days of therapy and is then dosed twice daily for the remaining course of therapy. Varenicline is taken after meals with a full glass of water. A normal course of therapy is 12 weeks. The most common side effects include nausea, sleep problems, constipation, gas, vomiting, and changes in mood and behavior. It cannot be used in conjunction with other smoking cessation drug products.

◆ THE DENTAL HEALTH CARE WORKER'S ROLE IN TOBACCO CESSATION

Dental health care workers are in a special situation to be helpful in promoting tobacco cessation because of their role in encouraging patients to change habits (e.g., floss, brush teeth, and use fluoride). Smoking cessation is another habit change (behavior modification). The dental health care worker is in a position to point out some of the oral manifestations of nicotine and tobacco abuse firsthand in the patient's own mouth. The National Cancer Institute currently has a program for dental personnel that includes a variety of patient education devices.* Every dental office should offer its patients help in smoking cessation.

PSYCHEDELICS (HALLUCINOGENS)

The psychedelic agents are capable of inducing states of altered perception and generally do not have any medically acceptable therapeutic use. The drugs in this section include lysergic acid diethylamide (LSD) and phencyclidine (PCP), but many other agents, including psilocybin, dimethyltryptamine (DMT), 2,5-dimethoxy-4-methylamphetamine (STP), methylenedioxyamphetamine (MDMA), and mescaline (peyote), also fall into this class. Clearly, the agents discussed in this section represent only a fraction of those released on the illicit drug market. These hallucinogens are often mislabeled or adulterated with substances such as strychnine.

Psychedelics affect perceptions in such a way that all sensory input is perceived with heightened awareness; sounds are brighter and clearer, colors are more brilliant, and taste, smell, and touch are more acute. Psychedelic-induced dependence is psychologic, and tolerance develops within a short time. These two characteristics combined with the unpredictable nature of the response favor periodic rather than continuous abuse of psychedelic drugs. Prolonged use can cause long-lasting mental disturbances varying from panic reactions to depression to schizophrenic reactions.

*National Cancer Institute: 800-4-CANCER.

Lysergic Acid Diethylamide

LSD is the most potent hallucinogen; only micrograms are required for an effect. In addition to its psychogenic actions, LSD has sympathomimetic effects, including tachycardia, rise in blood pressure, hyperreflexia, nausea, and increased body temperature.

An overdose of LSD produces symptoms that include widely dilated pupils, flushed face, elevated blood pressure, visual and temporal distortions, hallucinations, derealization, panic reaction, and paranoia. Because the user does not lose consciousness and is highly suggestible, treatment is to provide reassurance ("talking the user down"). Rarely, chlorpromazine has been used to treat the situation in an emergency. Flashbacks, commonly precipitated by marijuana use, can occur years after ingesting LSD. LSD is currently making another comeback.

Phencyclidine

PCP (or angel dust), originally developed as an animal tranquilizer, was popular in the 1970s. It inhibits the reuptake of dopamine, serotonin, and norepinephrine. Although it has anticholinergic properties, hypersalivation is produced. It is a powerful CNS stimulant with dissociative properties. Users may exhibit sweating and a blank stare. Changes in body image and disorganized thought have led to bizarre behavior and psychosis. Elevation of blood pressure and pulse and muscle movement and rigidity occur. It is abused alone or as an adulterant to other street drugs.

Marijuana

Marijuana (marihuana, cannabis) is derived from the hemp plant, and its active ingredient is tetrahydrocannabinol (tet-ra-hi-dro-can-NAB-i-nol) (THC). Marijuana can be administered orally or by inhalation (smoking), and its effects include an increase in pulse rate, reddening of the conjunctivae (bloodshot eyes), and behavioral changes. Slight changes in blood pressure and pupil size and hand tremors have been noted. With normal doses, euphoria and enhanced sensory perception occur. This is followed by sedation and altered consciousness (a dreamlike state).

Studies of the influence of marijuana on driving have concluded that the drug impairs motor and mental abilities required for safe driving. For example, the perception of time and distance is distorted and reflexes are decreased. A more common adverse reaction is apprehensive, nervous, and panic-stricken feelings that the user is losing his or her mind. This reaction responds to friendly reassurance. Psychological dependence on marijuana is determined by the frequency of use. Physical dependence, tolerance, and withdrawal symptoms are rare.

Of particular interest to the dental health care worker is the fact that a high level of marijuana abuse may cause xerostomia. It has been noted anecdotally that some marijuana users develop gingivitis. Heavy marijuana smoking can lead to chronic bronchitis and precancerous changes in the bronchioles. THC is known to reduce intraocular pressure and has been used in the treatment of resistant glaucoma. It is also effective as an antiemetic to treat the nausea associated with cancer therapy.

IDENTIFYING THE DRUG ABUSER

"Shoppers" interact with many health care workers in an attempt to obtain controlled substances for illegitimate uses. Some references suggest that shoppers can be identified by the presence of poor hygiene, long-sleeved shirts, scars along veins, sunglasses, abrupt changes in behavior, moodiness, and behaving as though they were under the influence of an intoxicant, although usually this is not the case.

Most shoppers are excellent storytellers and actors with convincing histories and the presence of a pathologic dental condition. They look and behave like a typical patient. They may suggest specific drugs or give a history of allergy to analgesics they do not want. One should note the patient's response to the mention of drugs that the dental provider is going to prescribe. This can be a tip-off that the patient is hoping for a more potent drug.

> Abusers have more STDs and blood-borne infections.

Intravenous drug abusers are more likely to contract sexually transmitted diseases (STDs) and are more likely to have hepatitis (hepatitis B virus [HBV] and hepatitis C virus [HCV]) or be a carrier, be HIV positive, or have AIDS and to be infected with multidrug-resistant tuberculosis and to have altered heart valves.

The dental office should not stock many controlled substances because it can become the target of robberies and burglaries. Addicts searching for drugs can be violent. The location of the supply of controlled substances must be under lock and key and in an inconspicuous place.

THE IMPAIRED DENTAL HEALTH CARE WORKER

When dental health care workers abuse drugs, they can present a danger to the patients being treated.

A professional who is abusing drugs, like most abusers, is in denial, and confrontation by staff, relatives, and friends is often ineffective. The dentist's dental practice deteriorates and mood swings, including depression, occur. Often, suicide is thought to be the only recourse.

Any dental health care worker who observes or suspects that another worker is abusing drugs should report the person to the appropriate "impaired professional committee" for their profession. Most state boards currently have committees to work with any impaired dental professional (those that have abused alcohol or drugs). The committee's goal is to assist the dental health care worker in becoming a functioning practitioner again. The objective of these committees is not to punish the worker to make the person lose his or her license. These committees can also investigate a suspicion of abuse. The difficulty in self-regulation is the silent practitioners who do not want to get involved.

DENTAL HYGIENE CONSIDERATIONS

1. Conduct a detailed medication and health history as well as an extraoral and clinical exam for evidence of substance abuse.
2. Monitor the patient's blood pressure and heart rate at each visit.
3. Perform an oral cancer screen, evaluate salivary flow, and recommend anticaries agents as necessary.
4. Monitor for caffeine stains and educate the patient about the high risk for stains with caffeine consumption.
5. Educate the patient regarding the risks of tobacco, especially smokeless tobacco.
6. Avoid aspirin and NSAIDs in patients with alcohol abuse issues.
7. Acetaminophen should be avoided if there is liver damage due to alcohol abuse.
8. Opioid analgesics should be avoided in patients recovering from substance abuse.
9. Vasoconstrictors should not be used in patients who are actively using cocaine.
10. Recommend nonalcoholic mouthrinses.
11. Always be on the lookout for the drug abuser or "shopper."

CLINICAL SKILLS ASSESSMENT

1. Define the following terms:
   a. Psychological dependence
   b. Tolerance
   c. Physical dependence
   d. Withdrawal syndrome
   e. Addiction
   f. Abstinence
   g. Abuse
2. What physical effects occur at low and high doses of caffeine consumption?
3. Can one build tolerance or become "addicted" to caffeine?
4. What are the symptoms associated with caffeine withdrawal?
5. What is caffeine toxicity and what are its signs and symptoms?
6. What factors influence the metabolism of alcohol?
7. What are the physiologic effects of alcohol?
8. What are the chronic, long-term effects of alcohol consumption?
9. Is caffeine effective in treating acute alcohol intoxication? What should be done?
10. Describe the long-term problems associated with cigarette smoking. Mention several organs that are affected.
11. Discuss the use of smokeless tobacco in adolescents and their idols (think baseball).
12. State oral changes that can occur with smokeless tobacco.
13. Describe the increased use of cigars and hypothesize about probable causes.
14. Describe the dental health care worker's role, if any, in a dental office tobacco cessation program. Could a community role for the dental health care worker be planned?
15. What are some of the products available to people to help them stop smoking or using other smokeless tobacco products?

26 Natural/Herbal Products and Dietary Supplements

LEARNING OBJECTIVES

1. Discuss why people choose herbal products over traditional medicine.
2. Discuss the federal legislation governing herbal and dietary products.
3. Discuss Good Manufacturing Practice and the standardization of herbal products.
4. Explain the adverse effects associated with herbal products and their impact on oral health care.
5. Explain the drug interactions associated with herbal products and their impact on oral health care.
6. Discuss the herbal supplements that are used in oral health care.
7. Explain the dental hygiene considerations associated with the use of herbal products.

Herbal medicine, also called *botanical medicine* or *phytomedicine*, refers to the use of a plant's seeds, berries, roots, leaves, bark, or flowers for medicinal purposes. Long practiced outside of conventional medicine, herbalism is becoming much more commonplace in Western medicine. More aggressive marketing of the purported health benefits of herbal and dietary supplements has dramatically increased their use during the last decade. Herbal supplements are available without a prescription, which eliminates the cost and time of visiting a health care professional that can prescribe conventional medicine (Figure 26-1). Others have turned to herbal supplements because of cultural influences, a sense of taking control of one's health, distrust of physicians, and a lack of health insurance. Also, improvements in analysis and quality control, as well as advances in clinical research show their value in the treatment and prevention of disease.

> Patients do not always report supplement use.

The recent trend in the use of natural or herbal substances has been an exponential rise in the use of these products and the number of people using them. As a result, dental hygienists need to inquire about the use of these products as part of the health history/medication review.

During this growth period, concerns have been raised about adequate safety and efficacy research and about a lack of uniform product standardization. Because they are considered to be natural products or dietary supplements, manufacturers do not have to prove efficacy in treating or preventing a specific disease nor can they make that claim. However, they can state that the herbal or natural product can be used for general health and well-being. Because they are considered natural products or dietary supplements, most patients do not consider them to be medicine, especially since a prescription is not necessary for their use. Dental hygienists should make it a point to ask about herbal or dietary supplement use because many patients will fail to mention them.

Much of what is known about herbal products or supplements has been compiled by the German Commission E, which is an expert panel composed of physicians, pharmacists, pharmacologists, and biostatisticians. This commission was originally established by the German Federal Health Agency (equivalent to the Food and Drug Administration [FDA]) to review and analyze the world literature on plant-based products. *Commission E Monographs* contain information regarding

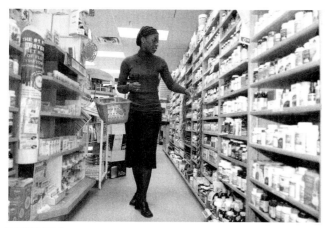

FIGURE 26-1
Herbal supplements are widely available without a prescription—in grocery stores, drug stores, and health food stores. (Copyright 2009 JupiterImages Corporation.)

the chemistry, pharmacology, toxicology, traditional uses, and if available, data on clinical trials, epidemiologic studies, and patient case records on herbal products. These monographs are considered to be the most authoritative guide to herbal therapy available today. An English translation is available and is titled *The Complete German Commission E Monographs: Therapeutic Guide to Herbal Medicines.*

LIMITED REGULATION

Dietary Supplement Health and Education Act

More than 20,000 herbal (botanical) and other natural products are available in the United States. The term *natural* has been associated with herbal products because they are primarily derived from plant sources. Herbal products are marketed as dietary supplements in the United States and are not required to comply with safety and efficacy regulations imposed on drug products. Manufacturers cannot make claims of curing conditions, but they can make claims of improving structure or function. The FDA can allow a qualified health claim if there is scientific evidence to support the claim. Before 1994, the FDA attempted to propose stricter regulations for the herbal supplement industry. However, aggressive lobbying by the dietary supplement industry and thousands of letters from the general public to Congress blocked the proposed regulations.

| FDA must prove product is unsafe. |

Today, herbal products are regulated by the Dietary Supplement Health and Education Act (DSHEA). which exempts vitamins, minerals, and botanical products from meaningful FDA regulation. Before this act, manufacturers had to prove that the herbal product was safe and effective. Today, the FDA must prove that the product is unsafe. The manufacturer only needs to notify the FDA of any efficacy claims. Changes in the Federal Food, Drug and Cosmetic Act in 2006 now require the supplement industry to report all serious dietary supplement–related adverse drug effects to the FDA. In 2007, the FDA drafted regulations that would require supplement manufacturers to test for purity and to ensure that their products do not contain contaminants and to verify that the contents

within the package matched the labeling information. These regulations were approved in August of 2007 and will be phased in over the next 3 years and be completely in place by the end of 2010.

Package Labeling

Other aspects of the DSHEA prevent the use of therapeutic claims on the label. All herbal products must be labeled as a dietary supplement. These products cannot have labels such as "for treatment of hypertension." However, the labels can contain claims of effects on the structure or function of the body. Thus a natural product could be said to "increase immunity" without a comment about what that might mean to a person's health. Another rule is that information may be provided that may not be necessarily scientific, but it cannot be false or misleading. Again, the responsibility for proof of misleading labeling is in the hands of the FDA.

The DSHEA required that the following phrase must be included on each natural product's label: "This product is not intended to diagnose, treat, cure, or prevent any disease." This phrase is also required in the advertising of these herbal products. (It is said really quickly in TV ads.) Another requirement is that "information" must be physically separate from the natural product. The product would be on one shelf and the information would be placed in another aisle. It is unclear what benefit separating the information from the product would serve other than getting the Act passed. Health food store employees help customers obtain the literature and associate it with the products to determine their purchase choices.

SAFETY OF HERBAL AND NUTRITIONAL PRODUCTS

Many consumers consider herbal products to be nontoxic or free of side effects because they are often called "natural" remedies. Most of the herbal products available contain ingredients that produce profound pharmacologic effects. Some products may have potential therapeutic effects, and the vast majority cause adverse effects and drug interactions. Since 1994, the FDA has investigated over 800 reports of adverse reactions with over 100 different ephedra alkaloid-containing products. Adverse effects included insomnia, nervousness, tremor, headaches, hypertension, seizures, arrhythmias, heart attack, stroke, and death. More than 50% of the adverse effects were reported in people under the age of 40, while another 25% occurred in people 40 to 49 years of age. In 2004, following reports of cardiovascular events with ephedra (Ma-Huang), the FDA issued a regulation prohibiting the sale of all dietary supplements containing ephedrine alkaloids and warned consumers to stop taking the product. A Utah supplement company challenged the ban stating that the FDA was trying to regulate a food supplement as a drug. Unfortunately, a federal judge ruled in favor of the supplement company.

| Treat herbal products as drugs. |

Because some of these products have pharmacologically active ingredients, the dental health professional should acknowledge this and treat the herbal product as a drug. Any use of herbal products by the patient should be noted in the patient's chart. Table 26-1 lists examples of selected herbal products, their adverse effects, and implications for the dental hygienist.

TABLE 26-1   SELECTED NATURAL HERBS: ADVERSE EFFECTS AND DENTAL HYGIENE IMPLICATIONS

Herbal Supplements	Adverse Effects	Dental Hygiene Implications
Feverfew	Oral mucosal irritation, ulcerations	Potential to cause ulcerations. Check oral cavity for ulcerations.
Ephedra (Ma-Huang)	Tachycardia, hypertension	Monitor blood pressure and pulse rate.
Niacin, yohimbe	Postural hypotension	Raise the chair to the sitting position slowly. Have the patient dangle their legs over the side of the treatment chair for a few minutes and then slowly get out of the treatment chair.
Chaparral, comfrey, kava (oral dose forms)	Hepatotoxicity, bleeding	Reduces the metabolism of many drugs. Patient may require lower doses of those drugs because of potential for increased bleeding during procedures. Monitor the patient for clotting.
Angelica, clove, feverfew, garlic, ginkgo, ginseng, red clover, high doses of vitamin E	Bleeding	Potential for increased bleeding during procedures. Monitor the patient for clotting.
Coenzyme Q-10, echinacea, milk thistle, pomegranate, wormwood	Allergic reactions	Watch for and alert the patient to the possibility of skin rash, stomatitis, angioedema, shortness of breath.

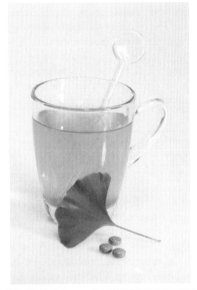

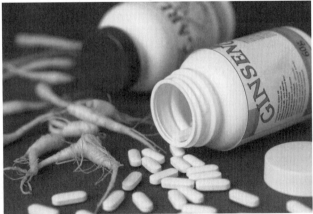

FIGURE 26-2
Herbal products can interact with more conventional drugs and create serious adverse reactions. For example, both ginkgo biloba and ginseng can increase the risk of bleeding when taken in conjunction with antiplatelet or anticoagulant agents. (Copyright 2009 JupiterImages Corporation.)

DRUG INTERACTIONS

Herbal products can interact with conventional drugs and cause disastrous results. The principal concerns associated with these interactions are increased risk for toxicity and a reduced therapeutic effect. The dental health professional should be aware of this possibility. Several drug-herbal product interactions have been identified and validated. Garlic, gingko biloba, and feverfew can increase the risk for bleeding when taken in conjunction with antiplatelet drugs or anticoagulants (Figure 26-2). Ma huang contains ephedrine and can increase heart rate when given with sympathomimetic drugs. St John's wort can induce the 3A3/4 isoenzyme of the cytochrome P-450 system and can increase the metabolism of many different drugs. Table 26-2 lists examples of drug-herbal product interactions and implications for the dental hygienist.

Unfortunately, there is little information regarding drug interactions with herbal supplements. Much of this is based on the inherent uncertainties regarding herbal products. In many instances, the purity and potency of the product is unknown, the dose is not standardized, package labeling is incomplete or inaccurate, or the product may contain more than one active ingredient. If a patient is taking conventional medicine and herbal supplements and a perceived drug interaction occurs (toxicity or decreased therapeutic effect), it is difficult to determine what was actually responsible for the effect. Until herbal products are standardized and labeling is accurate and comprehensive, it will be difficult to obtain accurate information on possible interactions.

Reliable scientific sources of information regarding herbal supplements are available and are reviewed in Box 26-1.

STANDARDIZATION OF HERBAL PRODUCTS

Standardization is the process by which one or more active ingredients of an herb are identified and all batches of the herbs produced by a single manufacturer contain the same amount of active ingredient specified on the label. Consumers expect

TABLE 26-2   SELECTED HERBAL SUPPLEMENTS AND DENTAL HYGIENE IMPLICATIONS

Herbal Supplements	Interacting Drug	Dental Hygiene Implications
Cranberry	Opioid analgesics, antidepressants, some antibiotics	Large amounts of cranberries can reduce urinary pH and potentially increase the excretion of these drugs
Black cohosh, butterbur, Echinacea purpurea	Acetaminophen, NSAIDs, macrolide antibiotics, azole antifungals	Additive hepatotoxicity Avoid the use of herbal supplements with these drugs
Coleus forskolin, goldenseal, gota kola, hawthorn, melatonin, nettle root, passion flower, valerian root	Benzodiazepines, barbiturates, CNS depressants, opioids	Potential to lower blood pressure Monitor blood pressure at each visit Watch for orthostatic hypotension Potential to increase the risk for sedation Remind the patient of this risk
Dong quai	Antihypertensives, opioids, benzodiazepines, CNS depressants, barbiturates, aspirin, warfarin	Increased risk for postural hypotension Monitor blood pressure Raise the patient slowly from the supine to sitting position Have them dangle their legs over the side of the treatment chair for several minutes before getting up Increased bleeding Monitor the patient for clotting
Bilberry fruit, bromelain, chamomile, Cordyceps, coenzyme Q-10, evening primrose, garlic, ginger, ginseng, ginkgo, feverfew, Guggul, horse chestnut, kava, licorice, oil of clove, tumeric	Warfarin, heparin products, aspirin, clopidogrel, NSAIDs	Increased bleeding Monitor the patient for clotting Advise the patient to stop the herbal supplements 2 weeks before procedures that result in bleeding
Guar gum	Penicillins	Decrease absorption of the penicillins Use the gum 1 hour after taking the penicillin product
St John's wort	Induces the CYP 3A3/4, CYP 1A2, and CYP2 isoenzymes Many drug interactions	Advise the patient of enhanced sedation with CNS depressants Increased potential for photosensitivity when used with tetracycline Advise patients to use sunblock and stay out of the sun Increased use for serotonin syndrome if used with tramadol or meperidine
Yohimbe	Indirect-acting sympathomimetics	Risk for hypertension Monitor blood pressure and pulse

CNS, Central nervous system; *CYP*, cytochrome; *NSAIDs*, nonsteroidal antiinflammatory drugs.

that all prescription and nonprescription drug products are standardized and what is printed on the label is actually in the drug in the container. However, consumers may not expect the same level of standardization with an herbal supplement because herbal supplements are considered food products or because they just assume that standardization has taken place. A major consequence of a lack of standardization is the variability of the quantity of the known or supposed active ingredient. In a study of 44 feverfew products, 32% contained less than the minimum 0.2% of parthenolide, which is proposed as the necessary primary active ingredient and concentration. Another 23% did not contain any detectable levels of parthenolide.[1]

GOOD MANUFACTURING PRACTICE

Good Manufacturing Practice (GMP) standards were introduced by the FDA in 2003 to ensure that dietary supplements be devoid of adulterants, contaminants, and impurities and that package labels accurately reflect the identity, purity, quality, and strength of what's actually inside the package. Package labeling should also include both active and all inactive ingredients

present in the formulation. It was not until 2007 that GMP standards mandated that manufacturers establish quality-control procedures that would prevent mislabeled or underfilled bottles; variations in tablet size, color, and potency; and the prevention of contamination with drugs, bacteria, pesticides, glass, lead, and other potential contaminates. These regulations require manufacturers of herbal supplements to test their products for purity and provide accurate labeling information for consumers. However, testing is left to the discretion of the manufacturer, and the FDA does not inspect all manufacturing facilities for compliance. Only those manufacturers that have demonstrated unsafe practices are subject to more frequent inspections. If a supplement is found to be contaminated or mislabeled, the FDA considers it to be adulterated or misbranded. Larger companies were to comply with these regulations by 2008, and companies with less than 20 employees have until 2010. Despite these much needed standards, manufacturers are not obligated to prove their products safe or effective.

Rather than wait for the GMP standards to be implemented, the U.S. Pharmacopeia began testing herbal supplements for quality. A "seal of approval" is given to products that

> Manufacturers are not required to prove their products are safe or effective.

BOX 26-1 **SCIENTIFIC SOURCES OF INFORMATION FOR HERBAL SUPPLEMENTS**

Journals
- *American Journal of Chinese Medicine*
- *Journal of Alternative and Complementary Medicine: Research on Paradigm, Practice, and Policy*
- *Alternative Therapies in Clinical Practice*
- *Alternative Therapies in Health and Medicine*
- *Alternative Medicine Review*
- *Focus on Alternative and Complementary Therapies*
- *Journal of Herbal Pharmacotherapy*

Databases
- Alternative and Allied Medicine Database
- Centralized Information Services for Complementary Medicine
- Cochrane Complementary Medicine Field
- Natural Products Alert
- Natural Medicines Comprehensive Database

Websites
- Research Council for Complementary Medicine: www.rccm.org.uk
- American Botanical Council: www.herbalgram.org
- National Institute of Health, National Center for Complementary and Alternative Medicine: http://nccam.nih.gov
- The Cochrane Library: www.cochrane.co.uk
- Center for Food Safety and Applied Nutrition: http://vm.cfsan.fda.gov
- International Bibliographic Information on Dietary Supplements: http://dietary-supplements.info.nih.gov/databases/ibids.html
- Micromedex Internet Healthcare Services: www.micromedex.com/products/hcs/
- Office of Dietary Supplements: http://.ods.od.nih.gov/databases/ibids/html
- American Herbal Products Association: www.ahpa.org
- Facts and Comparisons: www.drugfacts.com
- healthfinder: http://healthfinder.gov

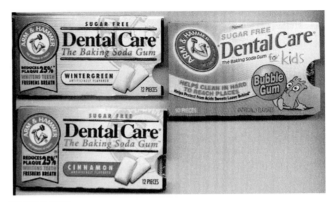

FIGURE 26-3
Xylitol-containing products, such as sugar-free gum with xylitol, can help prevent caries. (From Darby ML, Walsh MM: *Dental hygiene: theory and practice*, ed 3, St Louis, 2010, Saunders.)

meet their standards, which are very similar to the GMP. The U.S. Pharmacopeia requires that manufacturers pay for the testing. The Federal Trade Commission (FTC) has forced some herbal supplement manufacturers to remove advertisements with false or unsubstantiated claims.

HERBAL SUPPLEMENTS USED IN ORAL HEALTH CARE

Herbal supplements are used in several different oral health care products. They include essential oils (EO) that are used in mouth rinses (thymol, eucalyptol, or menthol), xylitol, acemannan, oil of cloves, and triclosan.

Acemannan

Acemannan hydrogel is an extract of the aloe vera plant leaf that has immunomodulating properties. It is available as an OTC topical patch to reduce the healing time of aphthous ulcerations. It is thought to cause the ulceration to heal at a faster rate. Acemannan hydrogel was found to be as effective as both prescription and nonprescription products in healing aphthous ulcerations.

Essential Oil Mouth Rinse

Over 20 mouth rinses that contain the EOs thymol, eucalyptol, and menthol have been approved by the American Dental Association (ADA). EOs are proposed to have a bacteriostatic effect on oral pathogens known to cause plaque and gingivitis. Clinical trials have shown that EOs are effective in protecting against plaque and gingivitis.

Oil of Cloves (Eugenol)

Oil of cloves has been used for many years as a topical analgesic for dental pain. This nonprescription product is used empirically by dental professionals. There are no published trials that confirm its efficacy. Its proposed mechanism of action is unclear, but it is thought that pulpal nerves are affected in some way to deaden pain.

Triclosan

Triclosan is an herbal-based product that has been shown to significantly reduce plaque and gingivitis when compared to placebo dentifrice. One triclosan-containing product has received the ADA's Seal of Acceptance for its antigingivitis effect.

Xylitol

Xylitol is a naturally occurring sweetener derived from plants that can be extracted from birch bark, raspberries, plums, and corn fiber. Its sweetness is comparable to sucrose, but it has one fewer carbon than sucrose and cannot be metabolized by *Streptococcus mutans* to form acids. As a result, xylitol consumption reduces *S. mutans* levels leading to antibacterial and cariostatic effects (Figure 26-3). Xylitol's antibacterial effects inhibit the ability of microbes to adhere and grow in plaque.

REFERENCES

1. Heptinstall S, Awang DVS, Dawson BA, et al: Parthenolide content and bioactivity of feverfew (*Tanacetum parthenium* (L.) Schultz-Bip.): estimation of commercial and authenticated feverfew products, *J Pharm Pharmacol* 44:391-395, 1992.

DENTAL HYGIENE CONSIDERATIONS

Dental hygienists need to know about these products for the following reasons:

1. Identify clinical considerations for commonly used herbal products.
2. Make personal choices in the use of herbal products based on evidence.
3. Find out about undisclosed medical conditions that the patient may be self-treating with herbal products. By knowing the indication(s) for the herb, the dental health care worker can be alerted to the presence of unreported diseases. (For example, if a patient is taking St John's wort, he or she may be treating depression.)
4. Identify adverse effects associated with herbal products.
5. Identify drug interactions with drugs that might affect the patient.
6. Identify sources of oral health care implications of herbal products.

CLINICAL SKILLS ASSESSMENT

1. What is the Dietary and Supplement Health and Education Act and how does it regulate herbal products?
2. List four herbal supplement–drug interactions and their impact on oral health care.
3. What is the process of standardization of herbal products?
4. What is Good Manufacturing Practice and how does it relate to herbal supplements?
5. What is acemannan and how is it used in oral health care?
6. What is the role of essential oil mouth rinse in oral health care?
7. What is the role of triclosan in oral health care?
8. What is the role of xylitol in oral health care?

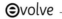volve

Please visit http://evolve.elsevier.com/Haveles/pharmacology for review questions and additional practice and reference materials.

Compilation of the Top 200 Generic and Branded Drugs of 2008 by Total Prescriptions

Rank*	Drug Name†	Generic Name	Total Prescriptions	Pharmacologic Group	Indication‡
1	Hydrocodone/acetaminophen	Hydrocodone/acetaminophen	121,266	Analgesic, opioid/nonopioid	Pain
2	Lisinopril	Lisinopril	69,805	ACE inhibitor	HTN, CHF
3	Simvastatin	Simvastatin	60,152	HMG-CoA reductase inhibitor	Hyperlipidemia
4	Levothyroxine	Levothyroxine	58,607	Thyroid agent	Hypothyroidism
5	Amoxicillin	Amoxicillin	52,063	Antibiotic, penicillin	Infection
6	Azithromycin	Azithromycin	49,280	Antibiotic, macrolide	Infection
7	Lipitor	Atorvastatin	49,043	HMG-CoA reductase inhibitor	Hyperlipidemia
8	Hydrochlorothiazide	Hydrochlorothiazide	47,080	Diuretic, thiazide	HTN, edema
9	Alprazolam	Alprazolam	43,586	Benzodiazepine	Anxiety
10	Atenolol	Atenolol	40,918	β-Adrenergic blocker	HTN
11	Metformin	Metformin	40,055	Antidiabetic	Diabetes, type 2
12	Metoprolol succinate	Metoprolol succinate	38,900	β-Adrenergic blocker	HTN, CHF, angina
13	Furosemide oral	Furosemide oral	37,451	Diuretic, loop	HTN, edema
14	Metoprolol tartrate	Metoprolol tartrate	29,663	β-Adrenergic blocker	HTN, CHF
15	Sertraline	Sertraline	29,483	SSRI	Depression, OCD, PTSD, social phobia, PMDD
16	Omeprazole	Omeprazole	29,174	Proton pump inhibitor	GERD, PUD
17	Zolpidem tartrate	Zolpidem	28,324	Sedative-hypnotic	Insomnia
18	Nexium	Esomeprazole	26,856	Proton pump inhibitor	GERD, PUD
19	Lexapro	Escitalopram	26,267	Antidepressant, SSRI	Depression
20	Oxycodone/acetaminophen	Oxycodone/acetaminophen	26,243	Analgesic, opioid/nonopioid	Pain
21	Singulair	Montelukast	25,787	Leukotriene receptor antagonist	Asthma
22	Ibuprofen	Ibuprofen	25,542	NSAID	Pain
23	Plavix	Clopidogrel	25,148	Platelet inhibitor	ACS
24	Prednisone oral	Prednisone oral	24,755	Corticosteroid, oral	Inflammation
25	Fluoxetine (Prozac)	Fluoxetine	23,271	Antidepressant, SSRI	Depression
26	Synthroid	Levothyroxine	23,113	Thyroid agent	Hypothyroidism
27	Warfarin	Warfarin	22,830	Anticoagulant	Thrombosis
28	Cephalexin	Cephalexin	22,080	Antibiotic, cephalosporin	Infection
29	Lorazepam	Lorazepam	22,043	Benzodiazepine	Anxiety
30	Clonazepam	Clonazepam	21,846	Benzodiazepine	Anxiety, seizures
31	Citalopram HBR	Citalopram HBR	21,567	Antidepressant, SSRI	Depression
32	Tramadol	Tramadol	21,273	Analgesic, opioid-like	Pain
33	Gabapentin	Gabapentin	20,662	Anticonvulsant	Seizures
34	Ciprofloxacin HCl	Ciprofloxacin HCl	20,478	Antibiotic, quinolone	Infection
35	Propoxyphene-N/acetaminophen	Propoxyphene-N/acetaminophen	20,412	Analgesic, opioid/nonopioid	Pain
36	Lisinopril/hydrochlorothiazide	Lisinopril/hydrochlorothiazide	20,375	ACE inhibitor/diuretic, thiazide	HTN
37	Triamterene/hydrochlorothiazide	Triamterene/hydrochlorothiazide	20,363	Diuretic, K-sparing/thiazide	HTN
38	Amoxicillin/potassium clavulanate	Amoxicillin/potassium clavulanate	20,077	Antibiotic, penicillin	Infection
39	Cyclobenzaprine	Cyclobenzaprine	19,874	Muscle relaxant	Muscle spasms
40	Prevacid	Lansoprazole	18,632	Proton pump inhibitor	GERD, PUD
41	Advair Diskus	Fluticasone/salmeterol	17,820	Corticosteroid/β$_2$-adrenergic agonist	Asthma

Rank*	Drug Name†	Generic Name	Total Prescriptions	Pharmacologic Group	Indication‡
42	Effexor XR	Venlafaxine XR	16,910	Antidepressant	Depression
43	Trazodone HCl	Trazodone HCl	16,701	Antidepressant	Depression
44	Fexofenadine	Fexofenadine	16,489	Antihistamine, nonsedating	Allergy
45	Fluticasone Nasal Spray	Fluticasone	16,163	Corticosteroid, nasal	Allergy
46	Diovan	Valsartan	15,684	ARB	HTN, CHF
47	Paroxetine	Paroxetine	15,566	Antidepressant, SSRI	Depression
48	Lovastatin	Lovastatin	15,299	HMG-CoA reductase inhibitor	Hyperlipidemia
49	Crestor	Rosuvastatin	15,125	HMG-CoA reductase inhibitor	Hyperlipidemia
50	Trimethoprim/ sulfamethoxazole	Trimethoprim/ sulfamethoxazole	14,590	Antibiotic, sulfonamide	Infection
51	Vytorin	Ezetimibe/simvastatin	14,559	Antihyperlipidemic/HMG-CoA reductase inhibitor	Hyperlipidemia
52	Cymbalta	Duloxetine	14,422	Antidepressant, SSNRI	Depression
53	Albuterol aerosol	Albuterol aerosol	14,087	β_2-Adrenergic agonist	Asthma
54	ProAir HFA	Albuterol sulfate	13,929	β_2-Adrenergic agonist	Asthma
55	Diazepam	Diazepam	13,870	Benzodiazepine	Anxiety
56	Pravastatin (Pravachol)	Pravastatin	13,619	HMG-CoA reductase inhibitor	Hyperlipidemia
57	Klor-Con	Potassium chloride	13,549	Electrolyte	Hypokalemia
58	Acetaminophen/codeine	Acetaminophen/codeine	13,424	Analgesic, nonopioid/opioid	Pain
59	Alendronate	Alendronate	13,328	Bisphosphonate	Osteoporosis
60	Amitriptyline	Amitriptyline	13,298	Antidepressant, TCA	Depression, chronic pain
61	Diovan HCT	Valsartan/ hydrochlorothiazide	13,196	ARB/diuretic, thiazide	HTN
	Naproxen	Naproxen	13,196	NSAID	Pain, inflammation
62	Fluconazole	Fluconazole	12,996	Antifungal	Fungal infection
63	Levaquin	Levofloxacin	12,898	Antibiotic, quinolone	Infection
64	Enalapril	Enalapril	12,746	ACE inhibitor	HTN, CHF
65	Carvedilol (Coreg)	Carvedilol	12,728	β-Adrenergic blocker	HTN
66	Ranitidine HCl	Ranitidine HCl	12,706	Antihistamine, H2-RA	GERD, PUD
67	Doxycycline	Doxycycline	12,525	Antibiotic, tetracycline	Infection
68	Actos	Pioglitazone	12,518	Antidiabetic	Diabetes, type 2
69	Carisoprodol	Carisoprodol	12,245	Muscle relaxant	Muscle spasms
70	Allopurinol	Allopurinol	12,208	Xanthine oxidase	Gout
71	Methylprednisolone tabs	Methylprednisolone tabs	12,141	Corticosteroid, oral	Inflammation
72	Meloxicam	Meloxicam	12,006	NSAID	Pain, inflammation
73	Amlodipine besylate/ benazepril	Amlodipine besylate/ benazepril	11,762	CCB/ACE inhibitor	HTN
74	Potassium chloride	Potassium chloride	11,713	Electrolyte	Hypokalemia
75	Flomax	Tamsulosin	11,576	α_1-Adrenergic blocker	BPH
76	Seroquel	Quetiapine	11,509	Antipsychotic	Schizophrenia
77	Clonidine	Clonidine	11,425	α_2-Adrenergic agonist	HTN
78	Zetia	Ezetimibe	11,046	Antihyperlipidemic	Hyperlipidemia
79	TriCor	Fenofibrate	10,997	Fibric acid derivative	Hyperlipidemia
80	Celebrex	Celecoxib	10,759	COX-2 inhibitor	Pain
81	Nasonex	Mometasone	10,463	Corticosteroid, nasal	Allergy
82	Premarin tabs	Estrogens, conjugated tabs	10,442	Estrogen	Hormone replacement
83	Lantus	Insulin Glargine	10,259	Insulin	Diabetes, type 1 and 2
84	Promethazine tabs	Promethazine tabs	10,181	Antihistamine, H1-RA	Nausea, sedation
85	Viagra	Sildenafil	10,112	Phosphodiesterase inhibitor	ED
86	Yaz	Drospirenone/ethinyl estradiol	9962	Estrogen/progestin	Contraception
87	Lyrica	Pregabalin	9845	Antiseizure, antipain	NPDPN, PHN, adj ther POS, fibromyalgia
88	Isosorbide mononitrate	Isosorbide mononitrate	9249	Nitrate	Angina
89	Adderall XR	Amphetamine/ dextroamphetamine	8799	Adrenergic agonists	ADHD
90	Folic acid	Folic acid	8784	Vitamin	Anemia, megaloblastic
91	Spironolactone	Spironolactone	8569	Diuretic, K-sparing	HTN, edema
92	Glimepiride (Amaryl)	Glimepiride	8567	Antidiabetic	Diabetes, type 2
93	Valtrex	Valacyclovir	8521	Antiviral	Herpes infection
94	Pantoprazole (Protonix)	Pantoprazole	8468	Proton pump inhibitor	GERD, PUD
95	Cozaar	Losartan	8389	ARB	HTN
96	Glyburide	Glyburide	8260	Antidiabetic	Diabetes, type 2

Rank*	Drug Name†	Generic Name	Total Prescriptions	Pharmacologic Group	Indication‡
97	Verapamil SR	Verapamil SR	8215	CCB	HTN
98	Albuterol nebulizer soln	Albuterol nebulizer soln	8183	β₂-Adrenergic agonist	Asthma
99	Cefdinir (Omnicef)	Cefdinir	8011	Antibiotic, cephalosporin	Infection
100	Temazepam	Temazepam	7911	Benzodiazepine	Insomnia
101	Topamax	Topiramate	7888	Anticonvulsant	Seizures
102	Triamcinolone acetonide top	Triamcinolone acetonide top	7878	Corticosteroid, topical	Inflammation
103	Penicillin VK	Penicillin VK	7871	Antibiotic, penicillin	Infection
104	Concerta	Methylphenidate	7863	Stimulant, CNS	ADHD
105	Oxycodone	Oxycodone	7805	Analgesic, opioid	Pain
106	Levoxyl	Levothyroxine	7745	Thyroid agent	Hypothyroidism
107	Metformin ER	Metformin ER	7624	Antidiabetic	Diabetes, type 2
108	Benazepril	Benazepril	7352	ACE inhibitor	HTN
109	Actonel	Risedronate	7261	Bisphosphonate	Osteoporosis, Paget's disease
110	Glipizide	Glipizide	7215	Antidiabetic	Diabetes, type 2
111	Ambien CR	Zolpidem tartrate extended release	7214	Sedative-hypnotic	Insomnia
112	Spiriva inhaler	Tiotropium bromide inhaler	7121	Anticholinergic	COPD
113	Clindamycin systemic	Clindamycin systemic	7112	Antibiotic, lincosamide	Infection
114	Ramipril (Altace)	Ramipril	6964	ACE inhibitor	HTN, CHF
115	Benicar	Olmesartan	6821	ARB	HTN
116	Metronidazole tabs	Metronidazole tabs	6669	Antibiotic	Infection
117	Digoxin	Digoxin	6571	Cardiac glycoside	CHF
118	Metoclopramide	Metoclopramide	6492	Gastrointestinal stimulant	GERD
119	Xalatan	Latanoprost	6251	Prostaglandin, ophth	Glaucoma
120	Benicar HCT	Olmesartan/ hydrochlorothiazide	6235	ARB/diuretic, thiazide	HTN
121	Aricept	Donepezil	6214	Cholinesterase inhibitor	Alzheimer's disease
122	Ortho Tri-Cyclen Lo	Ethinyl estradiol/ norgestimate	6069	Estrogen/progestin	Contraception
123	Hyzaar	Losartan/ hydrochlorothiazide	6021	ARB/diuretic, thiazide	HTN
124	Estradiol oral	Estradiol oral	5983	Estrogen	Hormone replacement
125	Hydroxyzine	Hydroxyzine	5978	Antihistamine, H1-RA	Nausea, vomiting
126	Amphetamine/ dextroamphetamine	Amphetamine/ dextroamphetamine	5921	Adrenergic agonists	ADHD
127	Diclofenac sodium	Diclofenac sodium	5864	NSAID	Pain
128	Gemfibrozil	Gemfibrozil	5825	Fibric acid derivative	Hyperlipidemia
129	Tri-Sprintec	Ethinyl estradiol/ norgestimate	5780	Estrogen/progestin	Contraception
130	Propranolol HCl	Propranolol HCl	5732	β-Adrenergic blocker	HTN
131	Vitamin D	Vitamin D	5706	Vitamin	Vitamin D deficiency
132	Cialis	Tadalafil	5689	Phosphodiesterase inhibitor	ED
133	OxyContin	Oxycodone	5677	Analgesic, opioid	Pain
134	AcipHex	Rabeprazole	5675	Proton pump inhibitor	GERD, PUD
135	Quinapril	Quinapril	5666	ACE inhibitor	HTN, CHF
136	Lunesta	Eszopiclone	5622	Sedative-hypnotic	Insomnia
137	Lamictal	Lamotrigine	5601	Anticonvulsant	Seizures
138	Promethazine/codeine	Promethazine/codeine	5546	Antihistamine, H1-RA/opioid	Common cold, cough
139	Doxazosin	Doxazosin	5525	α₁-Adrenergic blocker	HTN, BPH
140	Mirtazapine	Mirtazapine	5452	Antidepressant, tetracyclic	Depression
141	Detrol LA	Tolterodine	5423	Anticholinergic	Overactive bladder
142	Chantix	Varenicline	5381	Nicotine receptor agonist	Smoking cessation
143	Glipizide ER	Glipizide ER	5354	Antidiabetic	Diabetes, type 2
144	Avapro	Irbesartan	5330	ARB	HTN
145	Phentermine	Phentermine	5250	Stimulant, CNS	Obesity
146	Proventil HFA	Albuterol inhaler	5243	β₂-agonist	Asthma
147	Abilify	Aripiprazole	5221	Atypical antipsychotic	Schizophrenia
148	Acyclovir	Acyclovir	5216	Antiviral	Herpes infection
149	Yasmin 28	Ethinyl estradiol/ drospirenone	5157	Estrogen/progestin	Contraception
150	Budeprion XL	Bupropion	5146	Antidepressant	Depression
151	Meclizine HCl	Meclizine HCl	5116	Antihistamine, H1-RA	Motion sickness

Rank*	Drug Name†	Generic Name	Total Prescriptions	Pharmacologic Group	Indication‡
152	Potassium Chloride E	Potassium Chloride E	5087	Mineral	Hypokalemia
153	Niaspan	Niacin	5083	Vitamin	Hyperlipidemia
154	Nitrofurantoin monohydrate macrocrystals	Nitrofurantoin monohydrate macrocrystals	5070	Antiinfective, urinary	UTI
155	Sulfamethoxazole/ Trimethoprim	Sulfamethoxazole/ Trimethoprim	5038	Antiinfective	Infection
156	Fentanyl transdermal	Fentanyl transdermal	4939	Opioid analgesic	Moderate-to-severe pain
157	Buspirone HCl	Buspirone HCl	4884	Anxiolytic	Anxiety
158	Combivent	Albuterol/ipratropium	4878	β₂-Adrenergic agonist/ anticholinergic	COPD
159	Januvia	Sitagliptin	4868	Dipeptidyl peptidase-4 (DPP-4) inhibitor	Type 2 diabetes
160	Boniva	Ibandronate sodium	4789	Osteoclast inhibitor	Osteoporosis
161	TriNessa	Norgestimate/ethinyl estradiol	4783	Estrogen/progestin	Contraception
162	NuvaRing	Etonogestrel/ethinyl estradiol	4733	Estrogen/progestin	Contraception
163	Cartia XT	Diltiazem ER	4681	CCB	HTN, angina
164	Nifedipine ER	Nifedipine ER	4641	CCB	HTN, angina
165	Risperdal	Risperidone	4633	Antipsychotic	Schizophrenia
166	Glyburide/metformin	Glyburide/metformin	4626	Antidiabetic	Diabetes, type 2
167	Methotrexate	Methotrexate	4623	DMARD	Rheumatoid arthritis
168	Cheratussin AC	Codeine/guaifenesin	4516	Antitussive	Cough
169	Polymagma Plain	Kaolin in alumina gel	4476	Laxative	Constipation
170	Clotrimazole/ betamethasone	Clotrimazole/betamethasone	4405	Topical antifungal/ corticosteroid	Fungal infection
171	Flovent HFA	Fluticasone propionate	4403	Inhaled corticosteroid	Asthma
172	Imitrex oral	Sumatriptan	4400	Serotonin agonist	Migraine headache
173	Mupirocin	Mupirocin	4369	Topical antiinfective	Infection
174	Benzonatate	Benzonatate	4363	Antitussive	Cough
175	Methadone HCl noninjectable	Methadone HCl noninjectable	4348	Analgesic, opioid	Pain
176	Evista	Raloxifene	4313	SERM	Osteoporosis
177	Butalbital/acetaminophen/ caffeine	Butalbital/acetaminophen/ caffeine	4265	Barbiturate/analgesic, nonopioid	Headache
178	Polyethylene glycol	Polyethylene glycol	4260	Bowel evacuant	Bowel preparation
179	Diltiazem CD	Diltiazem CD	4207	CCB	HTN
180	Bisoprolol/ hydrochlorothiazide	Bisoprolol/ hydrochlorothiazide	4192	β-Adrenergic blocker/diuretic, thiazide	HTN
181	Minocycline	Minocycline	4108	Antibiotic, tetracycline	Infection
	Terazosin	Terazosin	4108	α₁-Adrenergic blocker	HTN, BPH
182	Avelox	Moxifloxacin	4086	Antiinfective	Infection, respiratory
183	Depakote ER	Divalproex	4059	Anticonvulsant	Seizures
184	Protonix	Pantoprazole	4044	Proton pump inhibitor	GERD
185	Atenolol/chlorthalidone	Atenolol/chlorthalidone	4023	β-Adrenergic blocker/diuretic	HTN
186	Nabumetone	Nabumetone	4022	NSAID	Pain, inflammation
187	Lidoderm	Lidocaine patch 5%	3860	Anesthetic	PHN
188	Famotidine	Famotidine	3838	Antihistamine, H2-RA	GERD, PUD
189	Tizanidine HCl	Tizanidine HCl	3818	Muscle relaxant	Spasticity
190	Ferrous sulfate	Ferrous sulfate	3816	Mineral supplement	Deficiency
191	Zyprexa	Olanzapine	3813	Antipsychotic	Schizophrenia
192	Namenda	Memantine	3806	NMDA receptor blocker	Moderate-to-severe dementia, Alzheimer's type
193	Tussionex	Chlorpheniramine/ hydrocodone	3789	Antihistamine, H1-RA/opioid	Common cold, cough
194	Thyroid, Armour	Thyroid	3738	Thyroid agent	Hypothyroidism
195	Humalog	Insulin Lispro	3722	Insulin	Diabetes, type 1 and 2
	Methocarbamol	Methocarbamol	3722	Muscle relaxant	Skeletal muscle conditions
196	Finasteride	Finasteride	3705	Antiandrogen	Prostate cancer
197	Phenytoin sodium extended	Phenytoin sodium extended	3631	Anticonvulsant	Seizures

Rank*	Drug Name†	Generic Name	Total Prescriptions	Pharmacologic Group	Indication‡
198	NovoLog	Insulin aspart	3599	Insulin analog	Diabetes
199	Clobetasol	Clobetasol	3590	Corticosteroid, topical	Skin disorders
200	Chlorhexidine gluconate	Chlorhexidine gluconate	3578	Oral rinse	Gingivitis

Data from 2008 top 200 generic drugs by total prescriptions and 2008 top 200 branded drugs by total prescriptions, *Drug Topics* June: 4-6, 10-12.

ACE, Angiotensin-converting enzyme; *ACS*, acute coronary syndrome; *ADHD*, attention deficit hyperactivity disorder; *Adj Ther POS*, Adjunctive therapy for adult patients with partial onset seizures; *ARB*, angiotensin II receptor blocker; *BPH*, benign prostatic hypertrophy; *CCB*, calcium channel blocker; *CHF*, congestive heart failure; *CNS*, central nervous system; *COPD*, chronic obstructive pulmonary disease; *COX-2*, cyclooxygenase 2; *DMARD*, disease-modifying antirheumatic drug; *ED*, erectile dysfunction; *GERD*, gastrointestinal esophageal reflux disease; *HMG-CoA*, 3-hydroxy-3-methylglutaryl coenzyme A; *H1-RA*, histamine$_1$ receptor antagonist; *H2-RA*, histamine$_2$ receptor antagonist (H$_2$-blockers); *HTN*, hypertension; *NMDA*, N-methyl-D-aspartate; *NPDPN*, neuropathic pain associated with diabetic peripheral neuropathy; *NSAID*, nonsteroidal antiinflammatory drug; *ophth*, ophthalmic; *OCD*, obsessive compulsive disorder; *PHN*, postherpetic neuralgia; *PMDD*, premenstrual dysphoric disorder; *PTSD*, post-traumatic stress disorder; *PUD*, peptic ulcer disease; *SERM*, selective estrogen receptor modulator; *soln*, solution; *SSNRI*, selective serotonin and norepinephrine reuptake inhibitor; *SSRI*, selective serotonin reuptake inhibitor; *TCA*, tricyclic antidepressant; *UTI*, urinary tract infection.

*Drugs are ranked from number 1, the most prescribed drug in 2008, to number 200, the least prescribed drug based on the number of prescriptions written.

†Name by which prescribed; if prescribed by generic name, that name is listed in this column.

‡One indication listed; many other indications often exist.

APPENDIX **B** Medical Acronyms

Term	Meaning
5-FU	5-fluorouracil
5-HT	serotonin (5-hydroxy-tryptamine)
AAC	antibiotic-associated colitis
ACE	angiotensin-converting enzyme
ACEI	angiotensin-converting enzyme inhibitor
ACTH	adrenocorticotropic hormone
AD(H)D	attention deficit (hyperactivity) disorder
ADA	American Dental Association
ADHA	American Dental Hygiene Association
ADP	adenosine diphosphate
AHA	American Heart Association
AHF	antihemophilic factor
AIDS	acquired immunodeficiency syndrome
AII	angiotensin II
ALG	antilymphocyte globulin
ALL	acute lymphocytic leukemia
ALT	alanine aminotransferase (formerly called SGPT)
APAP	acetaminophen
APTT	activated partial thromboplastin time
ARA	angiotensin receptor antagonist
ARB	angiotensin receptor blocker
ASA	aspirin
ASA I, II, III, IV	American Society of Anesthesiology*
ASCVD	atherosclerotic cardiovascular disease
AST	aspartate aminotransferase (formerly called SGOT)
ATG	antithymocyte globulin
ATP	adenosine triphosphate
AV	atrioventricular
AZT	zidovudine, azidothymidine
BCG	Bacillus Calmette-Guérin vaccine
BCP	birth control pill
BE	bacterial endocarditis
BMS	bone marrow suppression
BMT	bone marrow transplant
BNDD	Bureau of Narcotics and Dangerous Drugs
BP	blood pressure
BPH	benign prostatic hypertrophy
BT	bleeding time
BUN	blood urea nitrogen
CAT	computed axial tomography
CAD	coronary artery disease
CABG	coronary artery bypass graft
C & S	culture and sensitivity
CBC	complete blood count
CDC	Centers for Disease Control and Prevention
c-GMP	cyclic guanosine monophosphate
CHF	congestive heart failure
CIS	carcinoma in-situ
CK	creatine phosphokinase
CLL	chronic lymphocytic leukemia
CML	chronic myelocytic leukemia
CNS	central nervous system

*Roman numerals indicate planes of anesthesia.

Term	Meaning
COM	catecholamine-O-methyl transferase
COPD	chronic obstructive pulmonary disease
CRH	corticotropin-releasing hormone
CSF	corticotropin-stimulating factor
CVA	cerebral vascular accident
CVS	cardiovascular system
D/C	discontinue
DDAVP	1-deamion-8-d-arginine vasopressin, desmopressin
ddC	zalcitabine
ddI	didanosine
DEA	Drug Enforcement Administration
DIC	disseminated intravascular coagulation
DIP	distal interphalangeal joints
DM	diabetes mellitus, dextromethorphan
DMARD	disease-modifying antirheumatic drug
DNA	deoxyribonucleic acid
DTs	delirium tremens
EACA	epsilon aminocaproic acid
EBV	Epstein-Barr virus
ECG	electrocardiogram
ED$_{50}$	effective dose 50%
EEG	electroencephalogram
ENL	erythema nodosum leprosum
EPA	Environmental Protection Agency
EPS	extrapyramidal syndrome
ESRD	end-stage renal disease
EtOH	ethanol (alcohol)
FAD	flavin adenine dinucleotide
FDA	Food and Drug Administration
FMN	flavin mononucleotide
FTA	fluorescent treponema antibodies
G6PD	glucose-6-phosphate dehydrogenase (NADP+)
GABA	γ-aminobutyric acid
GBV	hepatitis G virus
GCF	gingival crevicular fluid
GI(T)	gastrointestinal (tract)
GU	genitourinary
GVHD	graft versus host disease
HAV	hepatitis A virus
HB$_c$Ag	hepatitis B core antigen
HB$_c$Ab	hepatitis B core antigen
HBIG	hepatitis B immune globulin
HBP	high blood pressure
HB$_s$Ag	hepatitis B surface antigen
HBV	hepatitis B virus
HCTZ	hydrochlorothiazide
HCV	hepatitis C virus, parenteral non-A, non-B hepatitis
HDL	high-density lipoprotein
HDV	hepatitis D virus, delta hepatitis virus
HER2	human epidermal growth factor receptor 2 protein
HEV	hepatitis E virus, epidemic non-A, non-B hepatitis
HGBV-C	hepatitis GB virus C

Term	Meaning
HGV	hepatitis G virus
HIV	human immunodeficiency virus
HPA	hypothalamic pituitary adrenal (axis)
HPV	human papillomavirus
HR	heart rate
HRT	hormone replacement therapy
HSV	herpes simplex virus
HSV-1	herpes simplex virus, type I
HSV-2	herpes simplex virus, type II
HTN	hypertension
HZV	herpes zoster virus
I & D	incision and drainage
IBD	inflammatory bowel disease
IBS	irritable bowel syndrome
ID	intradermal
IDDM	insulin-dependent diabetes mellitus
IDU	idoxuridine
IE	infective endocarditis
IgE	immunoglobulin E
IgG	immunoglobulin G
IgM	immunoglobulin M
IM	intramuscular
IND	investigational new drug
INH	isoniazid
INR	international normalized ratio
ISI	international sensitivity index
IV	intravenous
IVF	in vitro fertilization
IUD	intrauterine device
LD_{50}	lethal dose 50%
LDH	lactic acid dehydrogenase
LDL	low-density lipoprotein
LH	luteinizing hormone
LFT	liver function test
LJP	localized juvenile periodontitis
LSD	lysergic acid diethylamide
MAC	*Mycobacterium avium* (intracellulare) complex
MAO	monoamine oxidase
MAOI	monoamine oxidase inhibitor
MCA	monoclonal antibody
MD	multiple dystrophy
MDM	minor determinate mixture
MDR	multidrug resistant
MHC	major histocompatibility complex
MI	myocardial infarction
MRI	magnetic resonance imaging
MS	multiple sclerosis, morphine sulfate
MTX	methotrexate
N_2O	nitrous oxide
NDA	new drug application
NHL	non-Hodgkin's lymphoma
NIDDM	non–insulin-dependent diabetes mellitus
NMS	neuromalignant syndrome
NNRTI	nonnucleoside reverse transcriptase inhibitor
NPH	neutral protein Hagedorn (insulin)
NPO	nil per os (nothing by mouth)
NREM	nonrapid eye movement
NS	normal saline
NSAIAs	nonsteroidal antiinflammatory *agents*
NSAIDs	nonsteroidal antiinflammatory *drugs*
NTG	nitroglycerin
NTX	naltrexone
N&V	nausea and vomiting
O_2	oxygen
OA	osteoarthritis

Term	Meaning
OB	obstetrics
OCs	oral contraceptives
OCD	obsessive-compulsive disorder
OD	overdose
O&E	observation and examination
OGTT	oral glucose tolerance test
OPV	oral poliovirus vaccine
OSHA	Occupational Safety and Health Administration
OTC	over-the counter
PABA	*para*-amino benzoic acid
2-PAM	pralidoxime
PANS	parasympathetic autonomic nervous system
para 1	unipara (1 child)
PAS	*para*-aminosalicylic acid
PAT	paroxysmal atrial tachycardia
PBP	penicillin-binding protein
PCN	penicillin
PCP	*Pneumocystis carinii*, phencyclidine
PCR	polymerase chain reaction
PD	Parkinson's disease
P/D	packs per day
PDE5	phosphodiesterase type 5
PDT	photodynamic therapy
PG	pregnant
PG(s)	prostaglandin(s)
pH	function of amount of hydrogen ion (log $1/[H^+]$)
PID	pelvic inflammatory disease
PMC	pseudomembranous colitis
PMS	premenstrual syndrome
PO	per os (by mouth)
PPD	purified protein derivative
PPL	penicilloyl polylysine
PT	prothrombin time
PTCA	percutaneous transluminal coronary angioplasty
PTH	parathyroid hormone
PTT	partial thromboplastin time
PTU	propylthiouracil
PUD	peptic ulcer disease
PVD	peripheral vascular disease
PVT	paroxysmal ventricular tachycardia
QRS	ECG effects of cardiac muscle depolarization
RA	rheumatoid arthritis
RAS	recurrent aphthous stomatitis
RBC	red blood cell
RHD	rheumatic heart disease
RNA	ribonucleic acid
R/O	rule out
RPR	rapid plasma reagin
RSV	respiratory syncytial virus
SA	sinoatrial (node)
SANS	sympathetic autonomic nervous system
SAR	structure-activity relationship
SC	subcutaneous
SGOT	serum glutamic-oxaloacetate transferase (AST)
SGPT	serum glutamic-pyruvate transferase (ALT)
SL	sublingual
SLE	systemic lupus erythematosus
SMP-TMX	sulfamethoxazole-trimethoprim
SOB	shortness of breath
SQ	subcutaneous
SSRI	selective serotonin reuptake inhibitor
STD	sexually transmitted disease
STS	serologic test syphilis
SVT	supraventricular tachycardia

Term	Meaning	Term	Meaning
T_3	triiodothyronine	TNM	tumor node metastasis
T_4	levothyroxine	TPA	tissue plasminogen activator
TB	tuberculosis	TPP	thiamine pyrophosphate
TBG	thyroid-binding globulin	TPR	total peripheral resistance
TCA	tricyclic antidepressant	TRH	thyroid-releasing hormone
TCN	tetracycline	TSH	thyroid-stimulating hormone
THC	tetrahydrocannabinol	TT	thrombin time
TI	therapeutic index	Tx	treatment
TIA	transient ischemic attack	TXA	thromboxane
TMD	temporomandibular disease	VLDL	very-low-density lipoprotein
TMJ	temporomandibular joint	VZV	varicella-zoster virus
TNF	tumor necrosis factor	WBC	white blood cell

APPENDIX C Medical Terminology

This appendix does not attempt to provide a course in medical terminology. To cover that subject completely would require an entire book. However, there are many new medical vocabulary words in pharmacology needed to discuss drugs and their effects. In fact, many of these words that sound strange now will seem familiar later. Without this vocabulary, one will find it difficult to comprehend drug reference sources. Because some of the words will be unfamiliar, one should have an opportunity to learn these and other new terms.

When one sees a medical terminology word that one does not know, one should approach the word like a puzzle and attempt to identify any pieces that are known. One should consider whether one has seen a piece before and what it might mean. One should guess what those few letters might mean. Then one should "look up" the drug in a database, medical dictionary, or even the glossary in the appendix. One should write the word on a small card (one third of a 3 × 5 card) and write the definition on the other side. After one has written the definition on the card, one should consider the word parts and identify the little pieces that make up the word. These pieces may be beginning pieces (prefixes), middle pieces (word roots [= core]), or end pieces (suffixes). There are also pieces that mean *no* or *not* or that reverse the word's meaning. These little pieces come from Greek and/or Latin word parts. Now one should look at a couple of words.

Hypertension: (Hyper-) One may have heard someone say "That person is 'hyper-'." It means a lot of, or more of, or too much of. Therefore the piece of the word *hyper-* means excessive. *Tension* refers to tension or blood pressure. So *hypertension* means excessive blood pressure. What would be the definition of *hypotension?*

Dysmenorrhea: Dys- means bad, difficult, or abnormal; for example, teenagers use the phrase to "dys you." *Men-* is a root word meaning monthly and is associated with menstruation. The suffix *-rhea* refers to flowing. From these parts, the definition of this word is the painful flowing menstruation.

The prefix *a-* refers to less or lack of. What is the definition of *amenorrhea?*

If the prefix for the nose is *rhin-* (as in *rhinoceros* nose horns, wild animal, charge), then what does *rhinorrhea* mean?

BOX C-1 A FEW PREFIXES

a- without, absent
brady- slow
hemi- one-half
hyper- above, excessive
intra- within
lith- stone, calculus
pan- all
qua- four; quarter (one fourth of a dollar), *qid* means 4 times a day
sub- under (submarine?)
tachy- fast
tri- tricycle (3-wheeled), *tid* (3 times a day)

BOX C-2 A FEW ROOT OR CORE WORDS

bronch- bronchus
cardi- heart
cephal- head
chol- gall, bile
col- colon
cyan- blue
derm- skin
epitheli- epithelium (outside of skin)
gast- stomach
hem- blood
hepat- liver
leuk- white
lingu- tongue
lip- fat
my- muscle
neph- kidney
neur- nerve
path- disease
pneum- lungs, air
poster- back, behind
proct- rectum
prostat- prostate
stenosis- narrowing
stomat- mouth
thrombo- blood clot
vertebr- spine

BOX C-3 A FEW SUFFIXES

-algia pain
-dynia pain
-ectomy surgical removal
-itis inflammation
-lysis destruction, loosening
-malacia softening
-megaly enlargement
-ologist specialist
-oma tumor
-otomy incision into
-penia fewer (abnormal)
-plasty surgical repair
-ptosis droopy or falling down
-rrhea flow
-scopy visual examination ("scope it out")
-thorax chest

If the suffix *-itis* means inflammation, then what does *rhinitis* mean?

Thyroidectomy: Thyroid refers to the thyroid gland, whereas *-ectomy* means surgical removal. So the word means surgically removing the thyroid gland. How about *tonsillectomy?*

Box C-1 lists a few prefixes, Box C-2 a few core words, and Box C-3 a few suffixes. One can add new word parts as one learns them.

When a new drug group is named, a generic name and a trade name are given. The generic name is longer, and the trade name is short and easier to remember. Sometimes, when more members of a drug group are discovered and marketed, the subsequent drugs in the group are given the same suffix. A few drug suffixes—drug names ending in the same letters that belong to the same group—are listed in Box C-4.

BOX C-4 SUFFIXES FOR DRUGS	
Suffix	Drug Group
-azolam	benzodiazepines
-clovir	antiviral agents
-cycline	antibiotics
-dipine	calcium channel blockers
-ecoxib	cyclo-oxygenase (COX) II–specific antiinflammatory
-floxacin	antiinfective, quinolones
-glinide	hypoglycemic, oral
-glitazone	thiazolidinediones (antidiabetic)
-ifene	antiestrogen
-lukast	leukotriene inhibitor
-mycin	antibiotic
-olol	β-blockers
-prazole	proton pump inhibitor
-pril	angiotensin-converting enzyme (ACE) inhibitors
-sartan	angiotensin II receptor antagonist
-stigmine	cholinergic agent
-triptan	serotonin agonist, migraine
-tron	serotonin antagonist
-[con]azole	antifungal, azoles
-[va]statin	3-hydroxy-3-methylglutaryl (HMG)-CoA reductase inhibitors

APPENDIX D What If ...

This appendix addresses a number of patient-related questions that are among the most common the dental practitioner will encounter in daily practice. The "decision trees" help guide the practitioner through the steps involved in assessing clinical situations quickly and making related treatment decisions.

Topics covered in *"What If"* include drugs safe to use in pregnancy, allergy management, infective endocarditis prophylaxis, and a summary of the relationship between dental treatment, warfarin, and the international normalized ratio.

Allergies discussed include codeine, aspirin, penicillin, sulfites, and latex.

WHAT IF ... THE PATIENT IS PREGNANT?*

Drug Group	Drug Name	OK to Use
Local anesthetics	Lidocaine with epinephrine	Yes
Analgesics	Aspirin	No
	Acetaminophen	Yes
	NSAIDs	No
	Opioids	Yes
Antiinfective agents/ antibiotics	Penicillin	Yes
	Erythromycin	Yes†
	Tetracycline	No
	Doxycycline	No
	Clindamycin	Yes
	Metronidazole	No

NSAIDs, Nonsteroidal antiinflammatory drugs.
*For more details see Chapter 24.
†Avoid erythromycin estolate in pregnancy.

WHAT IF ... THE PATIENT IS ALLERGIC TO ASPIRIN?

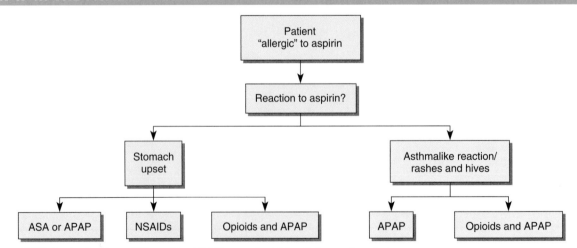

APAP, Acetaminophen; *ASA,* aspirin; *NSAIDs,* nonsteroidal antiinflammatory drugs.

WHAT IF ... THE PATIENT IS ALLERGIC TO PENICILLIN?

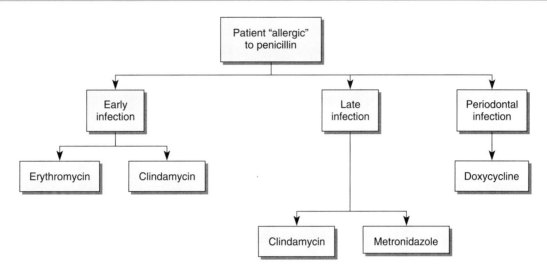

WHAT IF ... THE PATIENT IS ALLERGIC TO SULFITES?

There is a lack of cross-hypersensitivity among the following: "sulfa" drugs, sulfites, sulfur, sulfate, and sulfide. "Sulfa drugs" are used to treat urinary tract infections, and their allergic reaction is usually a rash. Dental patients allergic to "sulfa" drugs may safely be given local anesthetics or a vasoconstrictor that contains sulfites.

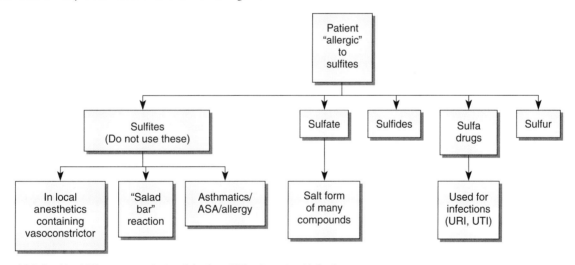

ASA, Aspirin; *URI*, upper respiratory infection; *UTI*, urinary tract infection.

WHAT IF ... THE PATIENT IS ALLERGIC TO CODEINE?

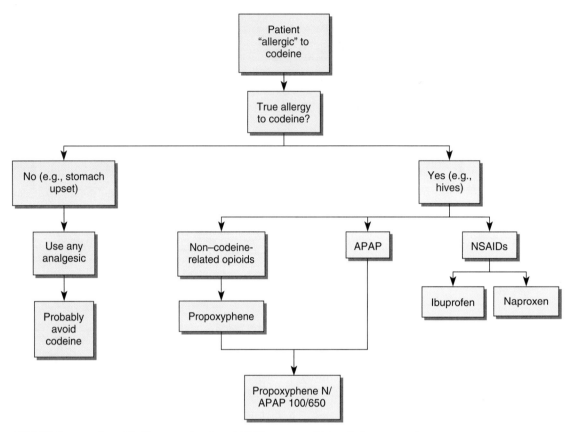

N/APAP, Propoxyphene N with acetaminophen; *NSAIDs*, nonsteroidal antiinflammatory drugs.

WHAT IF ... THE PATIENT IS ALLERGIC TO LATEX?

The increased use of latex-containing products has exposed more people with increasing frequency to latex allergens. Latex comes from the rubber tree and contains natural latex. Patients who are frequently exposed to latex-containing products (e.g., patients with spina bifida) and health care workers who use latex products (e.g., dental professionals) have a greater likelihood of developing allergies.

The extent of the reactions to latex ranges from contact dermatitis to severe anaphylactic reaction with death within a few minutes. If a dental practitioner uses any latex materials in his or her office, then parenteral epinephrine should be readily available.

There is also a cross-hypersensitivity between the foods listed in Box D-1 and latex allergy. If a patient is allergic to the listed fruits, then the dental health care worker should carefully question the patient regarding any reactions to latex-containing products (e.g., balloons, condoms). The patient should also be informed about cross-hypersensitivity that may occur between these fruits and latex. When powdered gloves are used, the latex can be absorbed into the powder and circulated around the room. This airborne latex can float around rooms and can even be stirred up with cleaning. Airborne latex can produce respiratory reactions such as asthma and anaphylaxis.

If a patient has an allergy to latex, he or she should be given the first appointment so that the latex particles have not contaminated the operatory air. The ventilation should be checked and measured for turnovers to make sure that the particles are removed overnight. One should be aware of the occupants of the building because use of latex in another office could inject latex particles into the central heating or cooling.

Manufactured latex products may contain a small amount of natural latex proteins, a very large amount, or somewhere in between. Asking for more information on the latex gloves used in the dental office may reduce the exposure to allergenic proteins.

BOX D-1 FOODS HAVING POTENTIAL FOR CROSS-HYPERSENSITIVITY WITH LATEX HYPERSENSITIVITY	
Apples	Papayas
Avocados	Peaches
Bananas	Pears
Carrots	Pineapples
Celery	Potatoes
Cherries	Rye
Chestnuts	Strawberries
Hazelnuts	Tomatoes
Kiwis	Wheat
Melons	

BOX D-2 DENTAL OBJECTS COMPOSED OF LATEX
All Commonly Used Brands Contain Latex
Gloves
Rubber dam
Local anesthetic cartridges (stopper)
Syringes (black rubber inside)
Bite block
Some May Contain Latex
Strings that hold mask on
Strings that hold gown on
Glasses bridges

When treating a latex-allergic patient, nonlatex equipment should be substituted for any products that contain latex (Box D-2). Newer catalogues contain a wide range of dental-related products (e.g., nonlatex bite blocks, dams, and adhesives for bandages). Books that contain additional information about latex allergy may include infection-control topics.

WHAT IF ... THE CARDIAC PATIENT NEEDS ANTIBIOTICS? (See Chapter 7)

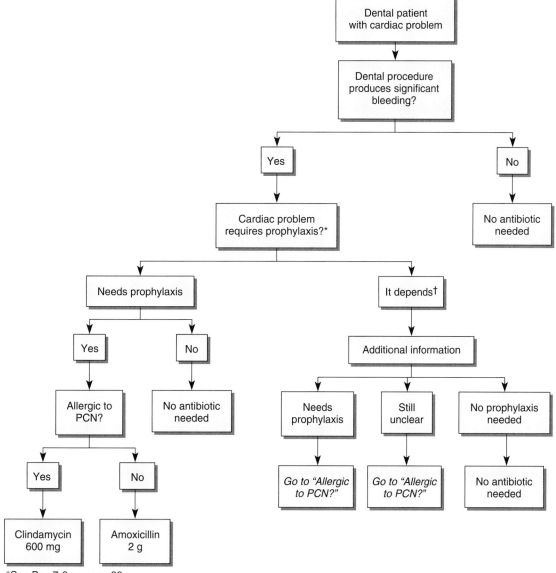

*See Box 7-6 on page 99.
†Includes rheumatic heart disease, mitral valve prolapse, and unspecified murmur.
PCN, Penicillin.

WHAT IF …THE PATIENT WITH PRIMARY TOTAL JOINT REPLACEMENT NEEDS ANTIBIOTICS?
(See Chapter 7)

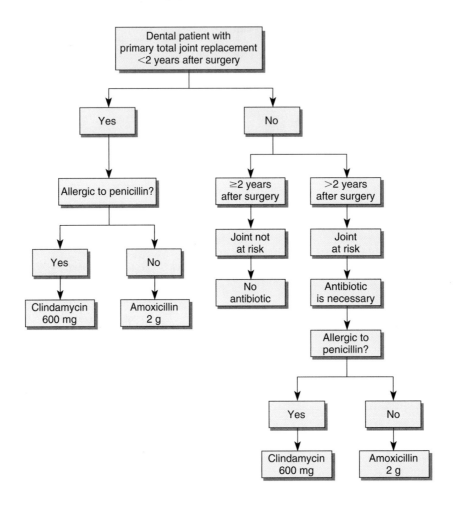

WHAT IF … THE PATIENT IS TAKING WARFARIN (COUMADIN)? (See Chapter 15)

Dental Procedure	OK to Treat if INR <
Periodontal probing	<4
Restorative, simple scaling/root planning endodontics	3.5
Extraction, simple	2.5-3.5
Extraction, multiple	2-3.5
Periodontal surgery	2.5

INR Acceptable (Safe).
INR, International normalized ratio.

APPENDIX E Oral Manifestations: Xerostomia and Taste Changes

BOX E-1 AGENTS THAT PRODUCE XEROSTOMIA (DRY MOUTH)*

Drug Group	Examples	Drug Group	Examples
Adrenergic agents (decongestants, anoretics)	Albuterol (Proventil, Ventolin)	Antidepressants, other	Bupropion (Wellbutrin, Zyban)
	Dextroamphetamine (Dexedrine)		Maprotiline (Ludiomil)
	Dopamine (Intropin)		Mirtazapine (Remeron)
	Ephedrine		Nefazodone (Serzone)‡
	Epinephrine (Adrenalin)		Sibutramine (Meridia)
	Isoproterenol (Isuprel)		Trazodone (Desyrel)
	Metaproterenol (Alupent)		Venlafaxine (Effexor)‡
	Methylphenidate (Ritalin)	Antidepressants, SSRI	Fluoxetine (Prozac)
	Phenylephrine (Neo Synephrine)		Fluvoxamine (Luvox)
	Pseudoephedrine (Sudafed)		Paroxetine (Paxil)
Serotonin amplifiers	Dexfenfluramine (Redux)		Sertraline (Zoloft)
Antiarrhythmics	Disopyramide	Antidepressants, MAO inhibitor	Isocarboxazid (Marplan)
	Procainamide		Phenelzine (Nardil)
	Quinidine		Tranylcypromine (Parnate)
Anticholinergics†	Atropine	Antihistamines	Acrivastine (in Semprex-D)
	Belladonna		Azatadine (Optimine) (ophthalmic)
	Belladonna alkaloids with phenobarbital (Donnatal)		Brompheniramine (Dimetane)
			Carbinoxamine (Clistin)
	Clidinium (in Librax, in Clindex)		Chlorpheniramine (Chlor-Trimeton)
	Dicyclomine (Bentyl)		Clemastine (Tavist)
	Flavoxate (Urispas)		Cyclizine
	Glycopyrrolate (Robinul [Forte])		Cyproheptadine (Periactin)
	Homatropine (Isopto-Homatropine)		Dexchlorpheniramine (Polaramine)
	Ipratropium (IH) (Atrovent)		Dimenhydrinate (Dramamine)
	l-Hyoscyamine (Anaspaz, Levsin)		Diphenhydramine (Benadryl)
	Meclizine (Antivert)		Hydroxyzine (Atarax, Vistaril)
	Methantheline (Banthine)		Levocabastine (Livostin) (opthalmic)
	Methscopolamine (Pamine)		Meclizine (Antivert)
	Oxybutynin (Ditropan)		Methdilazine
	Propantheline (Pro-Banthine)		Olopatadine (Patanol) (ophthalmic)
	Scopolamine (hyoscine)		Phenindamine
Antiparkinsonian	Amantadine (Symmetrel)		Promethazine (Phenergan)
	Benztropine (Cogentin)		Tripelennamine (PBZ)
	Biperiden (Akineton)		Triprolidine (Actidil)
	Ethopropazine (Parsidol)	Antihistamines, nonsedating	Cetirizine (Zyrtec)
	Levodopa + carbidopa (Sinemet)		Fexofenadine (Allegra)
	Pergolide (Permax)		Loratadine (Claritin)
	Procyclidine (Kemadrin)	Antihypertensives	Calcium channel blockers
	Selegiline (Eldepryl) [AKA deprenil and deprenyl]		Bepridil (Vascor)
			α_1-antagonist
	Trihexyphenidyl (Artane)		Prazosin (Minipres)
Anticonvulsants	Carbamazepine (Tegretol)		Doxazosin (Cardura)
	Gabapentin (Neurontin)		Terazosin (Hytrin)
Antidepressants, tricyclic	Amitriptyline (Elavil)		α_2-agonist
	Amoxapine (Asendin)		Clonidine (Catapres)§
	Clomipramine (Anafranil)		Guanabenz (Wytensin)
	Desipramine (Norpramin, Pertofrane)		Guanfacine (Tenex)
	Doxepin (Sinequan, Adapin)		Methyldopa (Aldomet)
	Imipramine (Tofranil)		Peripheral α antagonists
	Nortriptyline (Aventyl)		Guanethidine (Ismelin)
	Protriptyline (Vivactil)		Guanadrel (Hylorel)
	Trimipramine (Surmontil)		Reserpines

Continued.

BOX E-1	AGENTS THAT PRODUCE XEROSTOMIA (DRY MOUTH)—cont'd		
Drug Group	**Examples**	**Drug Group**	**Examples**
Antipsychotics,† phenothiazines	Chlorpromazine (Thorazine)	Cardiac glycoside	Digoxin
	Clozapine (Clozaril)	Diuretics	**Thiazides**
	Droperidol (Inapsine)		Hydrochlorothiazide (HCTZ)
	Fluphenazine (Prolixin)		**Loop**
	Haloperidol (Haldol)		Bumetanide (Bumex)
	Loxapine (Loxitane)		Furosemide (Lasix)
	Mesoridazine (Serentil)		**Combinations**
	Methdilazine (Tacaryl)		Dyazide
	Molindone (Moban)		Maxzide
	Pimozide (Orap)	Antiemetics	Metoclopramide (Reglan)
	Prochlorperazine (Compazine)		Dronabinol (Marinol)
	Promazine (Sparine)		Ondansetron (Zofran)
	Promethazine (Phenergan)		Oxybutynin (Ditropan)
	Quetiapine (Seroquel)	Miscellaneous	Caffeine
	Risperidone (Risperdal)‡		Cromolyn (Intal)
	Thioridazine (Mellaril)		Ergotamine (Ergostat, in Cafergot)
	Thioxanthenes		Nicotine (smoking cessation)
	Trifluoperazine (Stelazine)		**Vitamin A analogues**
	Triflupromazine (Vesprin)		Isotretinoin (Accutane)
Benzodiazepines/ sedative-hypnotics	**Benzodiazepines**	Muscle relaxants	Carisoprodol (Soma)
	Alprazolam (Xanax)		Chlorzoxazone (Parafon Forte)
	Chlordiazepoxide (Librium)		Cyclobenzaprine (Flexeril)
	Clonazepam (Klonopin)		Methocarbamol (Robaxin)
	Clorazepate (Tranxene)		Orphenadrine (Norflex)
	Diazepam (Valium)	Opioids	Codeine
	Estazolam (ProSom)		Meperidine
	Flurazepam (Dalmane)		Morphine
	Halazepam (Paxipam)		Oxycodone
	Lorazepam (Ativan)		Pentazocine
	Midazolam (Versed)		Propoxyphene
	Oxazepam (Serax)		Tramadol
	Prazepam (Centrax)		
	Quazepam (Doral)		
	Temazepam (Restoril)		
	Triazolam (Halcion)		
	Others		
	Phenobarbital		
	Zolpidem (Ambien)		

MAO, Monoamine oxidase; *SSRI*, selective serotonin reuptake inhibitor.
*See Box 13-1 and Box 13-2 for other oral effects of drugs.
†More likely than others to produce xerostomia.
‡Less likely to cause xerostomia.
§Most likely to produce xerostomia.

BOX E-2   AGENTS THAT ALTER TASTE

Drug	Taste Effects	Drug	Taste Effects
ACE inhibitors		Mesna	B
Aceon		Metaproterenol	B
Acetazolamide	M	Methazolamide	M
Adenosine	M	Methimazole	A
Albuterol	C	Methylergonovine	F
Allopurinol	N	Metronidazole	M, C
Al(OH)$_3$	Chalky	Moexipril (ACE inhibitor)	A
Amiodarone	U	Moricizine	B
Amoxapine	U, A	Nedocromil	U
Ampicillin	N	Norfloxacin	B
Antineoplastics	N	Nortriptyline	U
Antithrombin III	F	Ofloxacin	A
Aspirin	N	Omeprazole	A
Auranofin	M	Pamidronate	L
Aurothioglucose	M	Penicillamine	N
Aztreonam	A	Pentamidine	B, M
Benazepril	C	Perindopril	D
Benzocaine	N	Perindopril erbumine	A
Bepridil	A	Phytonadione	C
Bitolterol	A	Pirbuterol (Maxair)	C
Budesonide	B, L	Pravastatin	A
Calcifediol	M	Propafenone	L
Calcitriol	M	Protirelin	B
Carboprost tromethamine	A	Protriptyline	U
Ceftriaxone	A	Propylthiouracil	L
Chlorhexidines	C, L	Quinapril	C
Cidofovir	A	Quinidine	B
Clarithromycin	A	Quinine	B
Clofazimine	A	Ramipril	A
Clofibrate	N	Ranitidine/bismuth	D
Clomipramine	U	Rifabutin	P
Cyclophosphamide	N	Ritonavir	A
Gold salts	N	Simvastatin	U
Griseofulvin	N	Sodium phenylbutyrate	A
Interferon alfa-2a	M, C	Succimer	B
Interferon alfa-n3	M, C	Terbinafine	A
Iodinated glycerol	M	Terbutaline	B
Iron dextran complex	M	Tetracycline	N
Potassium iodide	M	Trazodone	B
Labetalol	A	Triazolam	A
Levamisole	P	Tricyclic antidepressants	N
Lithium	A	Ursodiol	U, M
Lomefloxacin	A	Valsartan	A
Losartan	A	Vinblastine	M
Lovastatin	A	Vinorelbine	M
Mechlorethamine	M		

A, Abnormal; *ACE*, angiotensin-converting enzyme; *B*, bad; *C*, change; *D*, disturbance; *F*, foul; *L*, loss; *M*, metallic; *N*, not specified; *P*, perversion; *U*, unpleasant.

APPENDIX F Children's Dose Calculations

CALCULATION OF CHILDREN'S DOSE

The patient's weight is the usual basis for determining drug dose, although not the ideal method. The following lists various methods for determining a child's dose based on an adult dose.

Clark's Rule

$$\frac{\text{Weight (lb)} \times \text{Adult dose}}{150} = \text{Infant dose}$$

Fried's Rule

$$\frac{\text{Age (mo)} \times \text{Adult dose}}{150} = \text{Infant dose}$$

Young's Rule

$$\frac{\text{Age (yr)} \times \text{Adult dose}}{\text{Age (yr)} + 12} = \text{Child dose}$$

Cowling's Rule

$$\frac{\text{Age (at next birthday)} \times \text{Adult dose}}{24} = \text{Child dose}$$

Surface Area Rule

$$(0.7 \times \text{Weight in lb}) + 10 = \% \text{ Adult dose}$$

$$(1.5 \times \text{Weight in kg}) + 10 = \% \text{ Adult dose}$$

Because weight may vary in children of the same age, a better method of calculating a child's or an infant's dose is based on body surface area. This method requires the use of a table or nomogram from which the body surface of the child can be determined. The child's body surface is a function of the height and weight of the child. The surface area formula is a convenient and more accurate formula than those based on the age or weight of the child.

Another method used to determine the child's dose is to follow a suggested pediatric dosage schedule prepared by the manufacturer. These doses are usually given in terms of milligrams of drug per kilogram of body weight per 24 hours (occasionally dose to give every 6 hours). This is especially common for antibiotic agents. It is important to note that the 24-hour dose calculated must be divided into the number of doses to be given daily. The manufacturer's recommendations probably provide the most accurate suggestions.

Example: What is the dose of amoxicillin for rheumatic heart disease prophylaxis for a 50-lb child? (See Chapter 7.)

$$\text{Dose} = 50 \text{ mg/kg of body weight}$$

1. Change pounds to kilograms: Divide by ≈ 2 equals 25 kg for a 50-lb child

$$\frac{2.2 \text{ lb}}{1 \text{ kg}} = \frac{50 \text{ lb}}{x \text{ kg}}$$

$$x = \frac{50 \text{ lb}}{2.2} = 23 \text{ kg}$$

2. Multiply dose in milligrams per kilograms by number of kg = mg = dose

$$\frac{50 \text{ mg}}{\text{kg}} = \frac{x \text{ mg}}{23 \text{ kg}}$$

$$x = (50 \times 23) \text{ mg}$$

Glossary

abscess accumulation of pus in a body tissue, usually caused by a bacterial infection

acetic acid substance produced when acetylcholine is broken down

acetylcholinesterase enzyme that destroys acetylcholine; inactivates effect

acromegaly enlargement of peripheral body parts such as head, face, hands, feet; secondary to metabolic disorder

active transport movement of ions or molecules across cell membrane; uses energy to accomplish; can be against a gradient

addiction dependence on a substance (e.g., alcohol or other drugs) or an activity to the point that stopping is very difficult and causes severe physical and mental reactions

adrenal medulla center portion of the adrenal gland; secretes epinephrine

adverse effect unwanted effects of a drug

adverse reaction unwanted effects of a drug

affective disorder mental disorder involving abnormal moods and emotions, includes depression and bipolar affective disorder (manic-depressive disorder)

afferent coming back to center; for example, nerves from periphery to CNS

afterload load against which the heart beats

agranulocytosis sudden drop in white blood cell count that is accompanied with a high fever

akathisia motor restlessness; muscular quivering

akinesia loss (or difficulty) of voluntary movement

allergy hypersensitivity reaction caused by an antigen-antibody reaction

alopecia baldness or loss of hair, mainly on the head

amblyopia dimness of vision without apparent physical deficit or disease

ampules sterile sealed glass containers, broken before use

anabolic steroid drug similar to testosterone that builds muscles and strengthens bones

anaphylactic shock serious allergic reaction resulting in difficulty breathing, low blood pressure, and death

anaphylaxis hypersensitivity reaction that produces difficulty breathing; life threatening

anesthesia loss of sensation in a certain part of the body (local/general)

angiotensin-converting enzyme inhibitor (ACEI) drug group used to treat high blood pressure

anorexia reduced appetite, not hungry; food aversion

antacid drug that neutralizes stomach acids; used to treat indigestion, heartburn, and acid reflux

anticoagulant prevents blood coagulation

antiemetic prevents vomiting

antisialagogue a treatment for excessive salivation

antithyroglobulin antibodies to thyroglobulin

anxiolytic action of antianxiety agents; reduces anxiety

apnea breathing stops, for either a short or a long period; drug- or disease-induced

arachidonic acid precursor of prostaglandins and leukotrienes

arrhythmia loss of rhythm; refers to irregular heartbeat

arteriosclerosis thickening and hardening of artery walls; atherosclerosis

artery a large blood vessel that carries oxygenated blood from the heart to tissues and organs in the body

arthralgia pain in joint

arthritis osteoarthritis: inflamed joints with pain and stiffness; rheumatoid arthritis: autoimmune disease of joints characterized by inflammation, pain, stiffness, and redness

arthus type of immediate hypersensitivity produced when an antigen is administered to a previously sensitized rabbit

ascorbic acid chemical term for vitamin C

asthma disorder characterized by bronchial constriction and inflamed airways; difficulty breathing

ataxia cannot coordinate voluntary muscle activity; caused by disorders in the brain or drugs such as alcohol or CNS depressants

atherosclerosis lipid deposits inside arteries; location of clogging of blood vessels

atony lack of tone; relaxation

atrial fibrillation the atria beat rapidly and inconsistently; irregular heartbeat

attention deficit disorder (ADD) a disorder present in children and adults, characterized by learning and behavior problems, inability to pay attention, and sometimes hyperactivity

aura a sensation that sometimes comes before a migraine headache or seizure; may include sensations of movement or discomfort or emotions

autocoids substances produced by some cells that change the function of other cells (e.g., histamine)

autoimmune reaction that consists of destruction that occurs because of the immune response of the body to itself

bacillus any bacteria that is rod shaped; responsible for many diseases, such as diphtheria, tetanus, and tuberculosis

bacteremia condition in which bacteria are present in the bloodstream; may occur after minor surgery or infection and may be dangerous for people with a weakened immune system or abnormal heart valves

bacteriostatic term used to describe a substance that stops the growth of bacteria, such as an antibiotic

barbiturates group of sedative-hypnotic drugs that reduce activity in the brain; are habit-forming and possibly fatal when taken with alcohol

bacillus Calmette-Guérin vaccine used to protect against tuberculosis

bile fluid made in the liver and stored in the gallbladder; aids in digestion

bipolar disorder illness in which the patient goes back and forth between opposite extremes; the most notable bipolar disorder is manic-depressive disorder, which is characterized by extreme highs and lows in mood

bladder organ to collect and store urine until it is expelled

blood clot semisolid mass of blood that forms to help seal and prevent bleeding from a damaged vessel

bradycardia slow heart rate, usually below 60 beats per minute in adults

bronchodilator drug that increases the diameter of the bronchioles, improves breathing, and relieves muscle contraction or build-up of mucus

bronchospasm temporary narrowing of the airways in the lungs, either as a result of muscle contraction or inflammation; may be caused by asthma, infection, lung disease, or an allergic reaction

bundle of His bundle of conduction tissue located between the atrium and the ventricles

calcium mineral in the body that is the basic component of teeth and bones; essential for cell function, muscle contraction, transmission of nerve impulses, and blood clotting

calcium channel blocker (CCB) drug used to treat chest pain, high blood pressure, and irregular heartbeat by preventing the movement of calcium into the muscle

cancer group of diseases in which cells grow unrestrained in an organ or tissue in the body; can spread to tissues around it and destroy them or be transported through blood or lymph pathways to other parts of the body

candidiasis yeast infection caused by the fungus *Candida albicans;* occurs vaginally and orally

canker sore small, painful sore, usually occurs on the inside of the lip or cheek or sometimes under the tongue; most likely an autoimmune reaction, many triggers; aphthous stomatitis

cardiac arrest cessation of the heart beat; results from a heart attack, respiratory arrest, electrical shock, drug overdose, or a severe allergic reaction

cardiopulmonary resuscitation (CPR) administration of heart compression and artificial respiration to restore circulation and breathing

cardiovascular system the heart and blood vessels that are responsible for circulating blood throughout the body

cellulitis skin infection caused by bacteria (usually streptococci); characterized by fever, chills, heat, tenderness, and redness; if dental, treat aggressively

cerebrospinal fluid clear, watery fluid circulating in and around the brain and spinal column

cerebrovascular disease disease affecting any artery supplying blood to the brain; may cause blockage or rupture of a blood vessel, leading to a stroke

chemotherapy treatment of infections or cancer with drugs that act on disease-producing organisms or cancerous tissue; may also affect normal cells; antibiotics or antineoplastics

cholesterol substance in body cells that plays a role in the production of hormones and bile salts and in the transport of fats in the bloodstream

cholinergic stimulated, activated, or transmitted by choline

chronic obstructive pulmonary disease (COPD) combination of the lung diseases emphysema and bronchitis, characterized by blockage of airflow in and out of the lungs

cleft lip birth defect in which the upper lip is split vertically, often associated with cleft palate

cleft palate birth defect in which the roof of the mouth is split, extending from behind the teeth to the nasal cavity; often occurs with other birth defects such as cleft lip and partial deafness

colitis inflammation of the large intestine (the colon), which usually leads to abdominal pain, fever, and diarrhea with blood and mucus

congenital present or existing at the time of birth

conjugation the addition of glucuronic or sulfuric acid to certain toxic substances to terminate their biological activity and prepare them for excretion

contraindication an aspect of a patient's condition that makes the use of a certain drug or therapy an unwise or dangerous decision

cycloplegia spasm of accommodation

cretinism congenital disease due to the absence or deficiency of normal thyroid secretion; characterized by physical deformity, dwarfism, mental retardation, and goiter

defibrillation short electric shock to the chest to normalize an irregular heartbeat

delusions false beliefs; remain even when evidence to the contrary exists

dependence reliance on drug to feel "normal"

depolarization change in polarity (e.g., positive to negative)

depression feelings of hopelessness, sadness, and a general disinterest in life; in most cases, there is no known cause; may be a result of neurotransmitter abnormality

dermatitis inflammation of skin

diabetes insipidus output of large amounts of dilute urine; results from lack of antidiuretic hormone

diabetes mellitus (DM) disease with abnormal glucose use; insulin lacking or does not work properly; many complications (e.g., periodontal disease)

diaphoresis perspiration (sweating)

dietary fiber constituent of plants that cannot be digested, which helps maintain healthy functioning of the bowels (e.g., bran flakes)

diffusion random movement of molecules in solution or suspension, distributes molecules to different compartments (parts of body); moves from a higher concentration to a lower concentration

direct-acting acts by stimulation of the receptor

distribution how a drug moves around the body (where it goes)

diuretic drug that increases the amount of water in the urine, removing excess water from the body; used in treating high blood pressure and fluid retention

DNA (deoxyribonucleic acid) responsible for passing genetic information in nearly all organisms

drug substance that affects the body; used to treat diseases

duration the time it takes for a drug's effect to cease

dwarfism undersized, abnormal; body parts not in proportion

dynorphin endogenous opioid ligand; stimulates kappa receptor

dysgeusia impairment and/or perversion of taste

dysmorphology study of abnormal tissue development

dyspepsia "upset stomach"

dysphoria unpleasant feeling

dyspnea difficulty breathing

dysrhythmia abnormal rhythm

dystocia difficult childbirth

dystonia abnormal tone of tissue; can be hyper- or hypo-

dysuria difficult or painful urination

ectopic out of place (e.g., heart beats from outside the conduction tissues)

ectopic foci location where ectopic events occur

edematous edema (fluid retention) present

efferent conveying or conducting away from an organ or part

efficacy maximal amount of beneficial effect resulting from a treatment

electrocardiogram (ECG) graphic record of heart's nerve action potential

electroconvulsive therapy (ECT) sending electricity through patient's brain; treatment of depressed patient, neuromuscular blockers prevent convulsions

emboli a mass, such as an air bubble, a detached blood clot, or a foreign body, that travels through the bloodstream and lodges so as to obstruct or occlude a blood vessel

embolism blockage of a blood vessel by an embolus—something previously circulating in the blood (e.g., blood clot, gas bubble, tissue, bacteria, bone marrow, cholesterol, or fat)

emphysema chronic disease in which the small air sacs in the lungs (the alveoli) become damaged; characterized by difficulty breathing

endocarditis inflammation of the inner lining of the heart, usually the heart valves; typically caused by an infection

endocrine gland gland that secretes hormones into the bloodstream

endorphin group of chemicals produced in the brain; reduce pain and positively affect mood

endothelium smooth muscle lining blood vessels and heart

enkephalin endogenous opioid ligand; stimulates delta receptor

enteral by way of the gastrointestinal tract

enuresis involuntary urine release

enzyme chemical, originating in a cell, that regulates reactions in the body

epilepsy disorder of the nervous system in which abnormal electrical activity in the brain causes involuntary effects (e.g., seizures)

epinephrine hormone produced by the adrenal glands in response to stress, exercise, or fear; increases heart rate and opens airways to improve breathing; also called adrenaline

epinephrine reversal with high doses of epinephrine, the α effect predominates and leads to an increase in blood pressure and a reflex decrease in heart rate (like norepinephrine); when the dose is lower, β effects predominate (α receptors are less sensitive), β_1 increases heart rate, β_2 produces vasodilation and reflex tachycardia

erythema redness of skin

estrogens a group of hormones (produced mainly in the ovaries) that are necessary for female sexual development and reproductive functioning

estrogen replacement therapy treatment with synthetic estrogen drugs to relieve symptoms of menopause and to help protect women against osteoporosis and heart disease

ethanol ethyl alcohol

ethyl alcohol alcohol with two carbons (ethyl); form of alcohol in alcoholic beverages

euthyroid normal thyroid

excretion removal of wastes from the body

exophthalmos eyeballs that protrude, caused by hyperthyroidism

expectorant medication used to promote the coughing up of phlegm from the respiratory tract

extrapyramidal refers to part of brain outside the nerve tracks (shaped like pyramids); related to adverse reactions of the antipsychotics; parkinsonian-like

facilitated diffusion movement of agent across cell membranes mediated via a protein

fetal alcohol syndrome combination of defects in a fetus as a result of the mother drinking alcohol during pregnancy

fibrillation rapid, inefficient contraction of muscle fibers of the heart caused by disruption of nerve impulses

fight or flight effects that occur when the sympathetic autonomic nervous system is stimulated

fluoride halogen added to municipal water to decrease caries; mineral that helps protect teeth against decay

flushing transient erythema

folic acid a water-soluble vitamin that is converted to a coenzyme essential to purine and thymine biosynthesis

Food and Drug Administration (FDA) government organization responsible for approval of prescription drugs

free base releasing base from salt form, used to change one form of cocaine into another more desirable form (before rock cocaine)

friable easily breakable, easy to crumble

fungus group of organisms that include yeasts and molds, toadstools, and *Candida*

gagging reflex gagging that occurs when a foreign body touches the mucous membranes in the back of mouth; sometimes occurs with alginate impressions or fluoride trays

gastritis inflammation of the mucous membrane lining of the stomach; causes include viruses, bacteria, and use of alcohol and other drugs

gastroparesis some paralysis of stomach muscles; common with diabetes

generic drug nonproprietary name (not trade name)

genital herpes an infection caused by the herpes simplex virus, which causes a painful rash of fluid-filled blisters on the genitals; transmitted through sexual contact

geographic tongue disorder of tongue, different colored patches visible, lesions move; lesions look like continents on a world map

gestation period between fertilization of an egg by a sperm and birth of a baby

giantism (gigantism) abnormal growth of body or its parts

gingivitis inflammation of the gums, typically caused by a build-up of plaque resulting from poor oral hygiene

gland group of cells or an organ that produces substances that are secreted or excreted

glaucoma (wide angle) disease with elevated pressure in eye; treated with ophthalmic drops; 95% of glaucoma cases

glaucoma (narrow-angle) disease with elevated pressure in eye because of narrow angle; treated with emergency surgery; 5% of glaucoma cases

glossitis tongue inflammation

glossodynia painful (or burning) tongue

glossopyrosis same as glossodynia

gluconeogenesis hydrolysis of glycogen to glucose (make glucose)

glucose sugar that is the main source of energy for the body

glucuronidation process of combining a drug with glucuronic acid; product is more water soluble, more easily excreted

glutamate form produced by adding glutamic acid; inhibitor neurotransmitter in central nervous system

glycogenolysis breaking down glycogen

glycoside structure produced when sugar condenses with other radicals

goiter enlargement of the thyroid gland, which produces a swelling on the neck

gout disorder marked by high levels of uric acid in the blood; usually experienced as arthritis in one joint

gradient rate of change of variable, especially concentration of drug in two different places

grand mal type of seizure occurring with epilepsy, producing loss of consciousness, involuntary jerking movements

graves' disease hyperplasia of thyroid gland; exophthalmos common

gynecomastia swelling of male breasts; can be side effect of drug

H₂ (histamine) blocker blocks acid production produced by histamine; used to treat acid reflux and ulcers

hallucination perception that occurs when there is actually nothing there to cause it (e.g., hearing voices when there are none)

hapten substance that cannot cause antibody production alone; combines with larger molecule that acts as a carrier to stimulate formation of antibodies

Hashimoto's disease lymphocytes enter thyroid, diffuse goiter; hypothyroidism produced thyroiditis

heart attack see "Myocardial infarction"

heart block disorder of the heart caused by a blockage of the nerve impulses throughout the heart that alters heartbeat; may lead to dizziness, fainting, or stroke

heart failure the heart cannot pump effectively

heart rate rate at which the heart pumps blood; units = heartbeats per minute

heart valve structure at each exit of the four chambers of the heart that allows blood to exit but not to flow back in

heartburn burning sensation experienced in the center of the chest up to the throat; caused by gastroesophageal reflux disease (GERD)

Heimlich maneuver maneuver in which fist of treating person is placed on abdomen of choking person above navel and is forcefully pushed; used to remove object lodged in throat

hematuria blood in the urine; can be caused by kidney infection

hemoglobin pigment in red blood cells that is responsible for carrying oxygen; hemoglobin bound to oxygen gives blood its red color

hemolysis breakdown of red blood cells in the spleen; can cause jaundice and anemia if the red blood cells are broken down too quickly

hemolytic destruction of blood cells; liberates hemoglobin

hemophilia inherited disorder; blood lacks a protein needed to form blood clots, leads to excessive bleeding

hemorrhage blood loss through broken vessel wall

hemorrhoid bulging vein near the anus; often caused by childbirth or straining during bowel movements

hemostasis stop bleeding

hepatic microsomal enzymes enzymes in the liver that are responsible for metabolizing drugs; mixed function oxidases

hepatic related to the liver

hepatitis inflammation of the liver, which may or may not be caused by a viral infection; can be caused by poisons, drugs, or alcohol

hepatitis A caused by the hepatitis A virus; usually transmitted by contact with contaminated food or water

hepatitis B caused by the hepatitis B virus; transmitted through sexual contact or contact with infected blood or body fluids

hepatitis C transmitted through sexual contact or contact with infected blood or body fluids

hepatitis D causes symptoms when hepatitis B is present

hernia bulging of an organ or tissue through a weakened area in the muscle wall

heroin a white, bitter, crystalline compound that is derived from morphine and is a highly addictive narcotic

herpes simplex infection that causes blisterlike sores on the face, lips, mouth, or genitals

hiatal hernia part of the stomach bulges up into the chest cavity through the diaphragm

high-density lipoprotein (HDL) protein found in the blood that removes cholesterol from tissues; "good cholesterol"

histamine chemical released during allergic reactions, causing inflammation; causes production of acid in the stomach and narrowing of the bronchioles

hives common term for urticaria; an itchy, inflamed rash that results from an allergic reaction

hormone replacement therapy (HRT) use of natural or artificial hormones to treat hormone deficiencies

hormone produced by a gland or tissue; released into the bloodstream; controls body functions such as growth and sexual development (e.g., insulin)

huffing illegal use of hydrocarbon inhalants (e.g., paint, gasoline); inhalant is deposited in a plastic bag and the user breathes in and out

human immunodeficiency virus (HIV) a retrovirus that attacks helper T cells of the immune system and causes acquired immunodeficiency syndrome (AIDS); transmitted through sexual intercourse or contact with infected blood

hypercalcemia abnormally high levels of calcium in the blood; can lead to disturbance of cell function in the nerves and muscles

hypercapnia increase in the arterial level of carbon dioxide; abnormal

hypercholesterolemia an abnormally high level of cholesterol in the blood, which can be the result of an inherited disorder or a diet that is high in fat

hyperglycemia abnormally high levels of blood glucose; usually as a result of untreated or improperly controlled diabetes mellitus

hyperlipidemia lipid levels in the blood are abnormally high, including hypercholesterolemia

hyperlipoproteinemia elevation of the lipoproteins in the blood

hyperplasia increase in the number of cells in an organ or tissue

hyperprolactinemia increased level of prolactin in blood; abnormal

hyperpyrexia elevated body temperature; side effect of aspirin overdose

hypertension abnormally high blood pressure, even when at rest

hyperthermia elevated body temperature

hyperthyroidism overactivity of the thyroid gland, causing nervousness, weight loss, hair changes

hyperuricemia elevated blood level of uric acid; associated with gout

hypoglycemia low blood sugar

hypoprothrombinemia low level of prothrombin in blood

hypotension abnormally low blood pressure

hypothyroidism underactivity of the thyroid gland; causing tiredness, cramps, a slowed heart rate, and possibly weight gain

hypoxia reduced level of oxygen in tissues or body

iatrogenic term used to describe a disease, disorder, or medical condition that is a direct result of medical treatment

idiopathic something that occurs of an unknown cause

idiosyncratic peculiar characteristic; may be caused by a drug ileum lowest section of the small intestine, which attaches to the large intestine

immune system cells, substances, and structures in the body that protect against infection and illness

immunity resistance to a specific disease because of the responses of the immune system

immunosuppressant inhibits the activity of the immune system; used to prevent transplant organ rejection and for disorders in which the body's immune system attacks its own tissues (rheumatoid arthritis, psoriasis)

impetigo contagious skin infection caused by bacteria, usually occurring around the nose and mouth; commonly occurring in children; common causative organisms include streptococci and staphylococci

implant organ, tissue, or device surgically inserted and left in the body

impotence inability to acquire or maintain an erection of the penis

incontinence inability to hold urine or feces

incubation period period from when an infectious organism enters the body to when symptoms occur

indirect-acting acts either before or after the receptor (e.g., cause release of neurotransmitter, blocks metabolism of neurotransmitter)

induction increase in production (e.g., enzymes in the liver); time from the start of general anesthesia until surgical anesthesia occurs

infection disease-causing microorganisms that enter the body, multiply, and damage cells or release toxins

inflammation redness, pain, and swelling in an injured or infected tissue

inflammatory bowel disease (IBD) general term for two inflammatory disorders affecting the intestines; also known as *Crohn's disease* and *ulcerative colitis*

influenza viral infection; characterized by headaches, muscle aches, fever, weakness, and cough; commonly called the "flu"

infusion introduction of a substance, such as a drug or nutrient, into the bloodstream or a body cavity

inhaler device used to introduce a powdered or misted drug into the lungs through the mouth; usually to treat respiratory disorders such as asthma

inhibition reduces an effect (e.g., liver enzymes)

injection use of a syringe and needle to insert a drug into a vein, muscle, or joint or under the skin

innervation nerves that are connected to tissue

inotropic influencing contraction of muscle (especially cardiac)

insomnia inability to sleep, difficulty falling or remaining asleep

insulin shock reaction that occurs when blood sugar is too low; excessive insulin is one factor

insulin hormone made in the pancreas that plays an important role in the absorption of glucose (the body's main source of energy) into muscle cells

interferon protein produced by body cells that fights viral infections and certain cancers

international normalized ratio (INR) laboratory value that adjusts the prothrombin time ratio to take into account the difference in the potency of prothrombin used in different laboratories; used to monitor warfarin use, calculated by taking the PT ratio to the power of the international sensitivity index (ISI);

$$\left(\frac{PT_{test}}{PT_{normal}}\right)^{ISI}$$

international sensitivity index (ISI) factor that is used to convert an individual's PT to an INR; corrects for variability in sensitivity of prothrombin used in different laboratories

intestine long, tubular organ extending from the stomach to the anus; absorbs food and water, passes the waste as feces

intrauterine device plastic device inserted into the uterus that helps to prevent pregnancy

intravascular within blood vessels

intrinsic term used to describe something originating from or located in a tissue or organ

intubation passage of a tube into an organ or structure; used to refer to the passage down trachea for artificial respiration (e.g., during general anesthesia)

invasive describes something that spreads throughout body tissues such as a tumor or microorganism; also describes a medical procedure in which body tissues are penetrated

iodine element for the formation of thyroid hormones

Iodine-131 radioactive iodine; used to treat hyperthyroidism

iron mineral necessary for the formation of important biologic substances such as hemoglobin, myoglobin, and certain enzymes

iron-deficiency anemia type of anemia caused by a greater-than-normal loss of iron resulting from bleeding, problems absorbing iron, or a lack of iron in the diet

ischemia condition in which a tissue or organ does not receive a sufficient supply of blood

jaundice yellowing of the skin and whites of the eyes because of the presence of excess bilirubin in the blood; usually a sign of a disorder of the liver

jock itch fungal infection in the groin area

Kaposi's sarcoma skin cancer that is characterized by purple-red tumors that start at the feet and spread upward on the body; commonly occurs in people who have AIDS

kidney an organ that is part of the urinary tract; responsible for filtering the blood and removing waste products and excess water as urine

lacrimation secretion of tears

larynx the voice box; the organ in the throat that produces voice and also prevents food from entering the airway

leukocyte white blood cell

leukopenia abnormally low number of white blood cells in the circulating blood

leukoplakia an abnormal condition characterized by white spots or patches on mucous membranes, especially of the mouth and vulva

lipid-lowering agents drugs taken to lower the levels of specific fats called *lipids* in the blood to reduce the risk of narrowing of the arteries

lipids group of fats stored in the body and used for energy

lipolysis breakdown of fats

lipoproteins substances containing lipids and proteins; comprising most fats in the blood

liver failure final stage of liver disease, in which liver function becomes so impaired that other areas of the body are affected, most commonly the brain

liver largest organ in the body, producing many essential chemicals and regulating the levels of most vital substances in the blood

low-density lipoprotein (LDL) type of lipoprotein that is the major carrier of cholesterol in the blood, with high levels associated with narrowing of the arteries and heart disease lumbar spine lower part of the spine between the lowest pair of ribs and the pelvis; made up of five vertebrae

lungs two organs in the chest that take in oxygen from the air and release carbon dioxide

luteinizing hormone (LH) hormone produced by the pituitary gland that causes the ovaries and testicles to release sex hormones and plays a role in the development of eggs and sperm

lymph milky fluid-containing white blood cells, proteins, and fats; plays an important role in absorbing fats from the intestine and in the functioning of the immune system

lymphadenopathy disease that affects lymph nodes; often refers to swelling of lymph nodes; associated with infection

lymphocyte white blood cell that is an important part of the body's immune system, helping to destroy invading microorganisms

lymphokines substances that are released by lymphocytes; involved in immune response

lymphomas group of cancers of the lymph nodes and spleen that can spread to other parts of the body

lysis destruction of blood cells, bacteria; caused by immune reaction

macroangiopathy disease of larger blood vessels

macrophages mononuclear cells with phagocytic action

magnesium mineral that is essential for many body functions, including nerve impulse transmission, formation of bones and teeth, and muscle contraction

malignant hyperthermia acute rise in body temperature, muscle rigidity; caused by change in body's muscle metabolism; can be fatal

malignant cells that exhibit uncontrolled growth, such as a cancerous tumor

mandible lower jaw

mania mental disorder characterized by extreme excitement, happiness, overactivity, and agitation; usually refers to the high of the highs and lows experienced in manic-depressive disorder

manic-depressive disorder mental disorder characterized by extreme mood swings, including mania and depression, or a continuing shift between the two extremes

marijuana plant containing the active ingredient tetrahydrocannabinol; hallucinogen, sedative

mast cell cell present in most body tissues that releases substances in response to an allergen, which causes symptoms such as inflammation

measles illness caused by a viral infection, causing a characteristic rash and a fever; primarily affects children

medulla the soft center part of an organ or body structure (e.g., medulla oblongata [brain], renal medulla [kidney])

megaloblastic anemia anemia resulting from the lack of vitamin B$_{12}$ or folic acid

melanoma skin tumor composed of cells called melanocytes

meningitis inflammation of the protective membranes that cover the brain, called *the meninges;* usually caused by infection by a microorganism (meningitis caused by bacteria is life threatening; viral meningitis is more mild)

menopause the period in a woman's life when menstruation stops, resulting in a reduced production of estrogen and cessation of egg production

menstrual cycle periodic discharge of blood and mucosal tissue from the uterus, occurring from puberty to menopause in a woman who is not pregnant

menstruation shedding of the lining of the uterus during the menstrual cycle

mescaline active ingredient in peyote (cactus); a hallucinogen

metabolic tolerance with chronic use, drug produces less effect because of metabolic change

metabolism process by which the body changes a drug chemically to make it easier to excrete

metabolite compound that is produced when a drug is metabolized

metastasis spreading of a cancerous tumor to another part of the body; through the lymph, blood, or across a cavity; also sometimes refers to a tumor that has been produced in this way

metered-dose inhaler (MDI) inhaler that gives a specific amount of medication with each use

methadone maintenance program to treat opioid addicts (heroin) by administering a high dose of oral methadone; usual doses of heroin then cannot produce euphoria

methemoglobinemia the presence of methemoglobin in the blood due to conversion of part of the hemoglobin to this inactive form

microangiopathy disease of small capillaries

microcephaly small head; abnormal

microorganism any tiny, single-cell organism (e.g., bacterium, virus, or fungus)

microphthalmia small eyes; abnormal

migraine headache severe headache, usually accompanied by vision problems and/or nausea and vomiting, that typically recurs

mineral substance that is a necessary part of a healthy diet (e.g., potassium, calcium, sodium, phosphorus, and magnesium)

minipill oral contraceptive containing only progesterone (no estrogen)

miosis constriction of pupil

mitral valve prolapse common condition in which the mitral valve in the heart is deformed, may cause blood to leak back across the valve; may be characterized by a heart murmur and sometimes chest pain and disturbed heart rhythm

mitral valve valve in the heart that allows blood to flow from the left atrium to the left ventricle but prevents blood from flowing back in

molecule smallest unit of a substance that possesses its characteristics

monoamine oxidase enzyme that destroys single amines

monoamine oxidase inhibitor substance that works by blocking an enzyme that breaks down stimulating chemicals in the brain; used to treat depression

morbidity state of being ill or having a disease

mortality death rate; measured as the number of deaths per a certain population; may describe the population as a whole or a specific group within a population (e.g., infant mortality)

mucous membrane soft, pink cells that produce mucus; found in respiratory tract (including mouth), eyelids, and urinary tract

mucus slippery fluid produced by mucous membranes that lubricates and protects the internal surfaces of the body

multiple sclerosis disease in which the protective coverings (myelin) of nerve fibers in the brain are gradually destroyed; symptoms vary from numbness to paralysis and loss of control of bodily function

muscarinic receptors that are activated by muscarine, contained in certain mushrooms; anticholinergics block this action

muscle relaxants group of drugs used to relieve muscle spasm and to treat conditions such as arthritis, back pain, and nervous system disorders such as stroke and cerebral palsy

myalgia muscle pain

myasthenia gravis disease in which the muscles, mainly those in the face, eyes, throat, and limbs, become weak and tire quickly; caused by the body's immune system attacking the receptors in the muscles that pick up nerve impulses

mycobacterium genus of slow-growing bacterium; resistant to the body's defense mechanisms and responsible for diseases such as tuberculosis and leprosy

mydriasis dilation of the pupils

myeloma cancerous cells in the bone marrow

myocardial infarction (MI) heart attack; heart vessel becomes clogged, severe pain in the chest experienced; can be fatal

myocardium heart muscle

myopathy a muscle disease

myxedema a condition characterized by thickening of the skin, blunting of the senses and intellect, and labored speech, associated with hypothyroidism

myositis inflammation of muscle

narcolepsy frequent and uncontrollable episodes of falling asleep; excessive sleepiness

narcotic analgesics pain relievers that bind to opioid receptors in the brain; inhibit ascending pain fibers, alter response to pain; often causes tolerance and dependence

narcotic addictive substance that blunts the senses; with increased doses causes sedation, coma, and death; called opioids

nausea feeling the need to vomit

necrosis death of tissue cells

negative feedback secretion of hormone 1 inhibits the release of hormones 2 and 3 that stimulate the secretion of hormone 1, for example, give prednisone (hormone 1), which inhibits CRF (hormone 2) and ACTH (hormone 3), both of which stimulate release of hydrocortisone

neonate newborn infant from birth to 1 month of age

neoplasm tumor

nephritis inflammation of kidney(s), caused by an infection, an abnormal immune system response; a metabolic disorder

nerve action potential changes in voltage (via ions) that transmits the nerve impulse along the nerve fiber

nerve fibers that transmit electrical messages between the brain and most body areas; convey information both ways

nerve block preventing transmission of pain from an area of the body by injecting a local anesthetic near a nerve

neuralgia pain along the course of a nerve

neuromuscular junction synapse between the nervous innervation and the somatic (voluntary) muscles

neuropathy disease, inflammation, or damage to the nerves connecting the brain and spinal cord to the rest of the body

neurosis mental illness with anxiety; stimulates useless action (e.g., counting things); relatively mild emotional disorders (e.g., mild depression and phobias)

neurotransmitters chemicals that are released after excitation of the presynaptic neuron; cross synapse to excite the postsynaptic neuron

neutropenia deficiency of white blood cells

neutrophil white blood cell in granulocyte group

nicotinic receptors that are activated by nicotine; contained in cigarettes

nitrates drugs that produce widespread vasodilation; used to treat angina pectoris and heart failure, reduce preload and afterload

nocturnal enuresis bedwetting at night

nonsteroidal antiinflammatory drug (NSAID) drug group that relieves pain and reduces inflammation; not corticosteroids (e.g., ibuprofen)

norepinephrine hormone that regulates blood pressure by causing vasoconstriction of the blood vessels

nystagmus persistent, rapid, rhythmic, involuntary movement of the eyes; used by police to check for the effect of drugs

obesity condition in which there is an excess of body fat; used to describe those who weigh at least 20% more than the maximum amount considered normal for age, sex, and height

obsessive-compulsive disorder action that must be repeated to make person comfortable (e.g., hand washing)

oligodactyly fewer than five digits

onset time it takes for a drug's effect to begin

opacities not transparent

opportunistic infection infection by organisms that would be harmless to a healthy person but cause infection in those with a weakened immune system (e.g., persons with AIDS or chemotherapy patients)

optic pertaining to the eyes

oral used in or taken through the mouth

oral contraceptives pills that prevent pregnancy; contain a progesterone and an estrogen

organophosphate organic compounds that combine with acetylcholinesterase, in activating it, called *irreversible cholinesterase inhibitors;* used as insecticides and war gases

orthopnea breathing difficulty experienced while lying flat; can be a symptom of heart failure or asthma

orthostatic hypotension when a person stands up from the supine position, and the blood pools in the lower extremities and the blood flow to the brain is greatly reduced, causing dizziness and potential fainting; common side effect of some antihypertensives

osteoarthritis disease that breaks down the cartilage that lines joints, especially weight-bearing or malaligned joints; leads to inflammation, pain, and stiffness

osteomalacia loss of minerals and softening of bones because of a lack of vitamin D; called *rickets* in children

osteoporosis condition in which bones become less dense and more brittle and fracture more easily

otitis media inflammation of the middle ear caused by infection from the nose, sinuses, or throat

ototoxicity harmful effect that some drugs have on the organs or nerves in the ears, which can lead to hearing and balance problems

outpatient treatment medical attention that does not include an overnight stay at a hospital

ovaries two almond-shaped glands located at the opening of the fallopian tubes on both sides of the uterus; produce eggs and the sex hormones estrogen and progesterone

over-the-counter (OTC) medication that can be purchased without a provider's prescription

overdose excessively large dose of a drug; can lead to coma and death; used to commit suicide

ovulation development and release of the egg from the ovary, which usually occurs halfway through a woman's menstrual cycle

oxidation chemical reaction that adds oxygen; can damage cells (free radicals)

oxygen gas that is colorless, odorless, and tasteless; essential to almost all forms of life

oxytocin hormone from the pituitary gland; causes contraction of the uterus and stimulation of milk flow

pacemaker small electronic device that is surgically implanted to stimulate the heart muscle to produce a normal heartbeat

palate roof of the mouth

palliative treatment treatment that relieves the symptoms of a disorder without curing it

pallor abnormally pale skin; usually refers to the skin of the face

palpebral fissures eyelid folds

palpitation abnormally rapid and strong heartbeat

pancreas gland that produces enzymes that break down food and hormones (insulin and glucagon) that help to regulate blood glucose levels

pancreatitis inflammation of the pancreas; one cause is alcohol abuse

panic disorder attacks of anxiety, made worse by stress; patient focuses on avoiding situations in which it occurs

paralysis inability to move a muscle

paralytic ileus ilium motility reduced or absent; often caused by general anesthetics

paranoia mental disorder involving delusions (e.g., "the FBI is following me")

parasympathetic pertaining to that part of the autonomic nervous system consisting of nerves and ganglia that function in opposition to the sympathetic system

parathyroid glands small glands located in the neck that produce a hormone that regulates the levels of calcium in the blood

parenteral introduction of a substance into the body by any route other than the digestive tract; often used to mean an injection

Parkinson's disease lack of brain dopamine; leads to muscle stiffness, weakness, and trembling

parkinsonism symptoms include restlessness, tremors, rigidity, and lack of facial expression

paroxysmal sudden onset of symptoms (e.g., paroxysmal tachycardia)

partial seizure abnormal electrical discharge in the cortex of the brain, affecting certain functions

pathogen substance capable of causing a disease; usually refers to a disease-causing microorganism

pedal relates to feet (check for pitting edema in feet for congestive heart failure)

peptic ulcer disease (PUD) erosion in the lining of the esophagus, stomach, or small intestine; most related to the presence of *Helicobacter pylori*

perception nerve impulse going to central nervous system

peripheral resistance opposition to flow of blood through the vessels, varies with vessel diameter; total peripheral resistance

peripheral vascular disease (PVD) narrowing of blood vessels in the legs or arms; causing pain and possibly tissue death (gangrene) as a result of a reduced flow of blood to areas supplied by the narrowed vessels

pernicious anemia anemia resulting from deficiency (failure to absorb) of vitamin B_{12} caused by a deficiency of intrinsic factor (IF) (autoimmune disease); abnormal red blood cells are produced (macrocytic, megaloblastic)

petit mal complete seizure characterized by loss of consciousness for brief periods, posture retained (do not fall)

peyote cactus that contains mescaline; a hallucinogen

pharmacokinetic movement of a drug within the body

pharmacologist specialist in pharmacology

pharmacology science of drugs and their properties

pharyngitis inflammation of the throat (the pharynx); causing sore throat, fever, earache, and swollen glands

pharynx throat; the tube connecting the back of the mouth and nose to the esophagus and windpipe

pheochromocytoma tumor that secretes epinephrine

phobia persisting fear of and desire to avoid something

phocomelia defective development of arms and/or legs; foot or hand connected to body (flipperlike)

photophobia abnormal sensitivity of the eyes to light

pigmentation coloration of the skin, hair, and eyes by melanin

piloerection hair on body standing up

pituitary gland gland located at the base of the brain; releases hormones that control other glands and body processes

placebo inactive substance given in place of a drug; required to adequately test drugs (total effect of the drug equals the effect that a patient taking the drug gets minus the effect that the placebo produces)

placebo effect the positive or negative response to a drug that is caused by a person's expectations of a drug rather than the drug itself

placenta organ formed in the uterus during pregnancy that links the blood of the mother to the blood of the fetus; provides the fetus with nutrients and removes waste

plaque patch of differentiated tissue on body; fatty deposits in an artery cause narrowing of the artery and heart disease; dental plaque: coating on the teeth, consisting of saliva, bacteria, and food debris, which causes tooth decay; demyelinated patch (e.g., multiple sclerosis)

plasma fluid part of the blood (no cells); contains nutrients, salts, and proteins

platelet adhesiveness stickiness of platelets; if reduced, retards clotting

platelet megakaryocyte fragment shed into blood; plays an important role in blood clotting, contains no nucleus; adhesiveness affected by aspirin

Plummer's disease hyperthyroidism from nodular toxic goiter

pneumonia inflammation of the lungs, alveoli filled with exudate; most cases are caused by a bacterial or viral infection; symptoms include fever, shortness of breath, and the coughing up of phlegm

polyp mass of tissue that bulges outward from the surface, growth occurs on mucous membranes such as the nose and intestine; bleeds easily and can become cancerous

polyuria excessive production of urine; can be a symptom of a disease, commonly diabetes

posterior describes something that is located in or relates to the back of the body

postural hypotension unusually low blood pressure that occurs after suddenly standing or sitting up

potassium a mineral that plays an important role in the body, helping to maintain water balance, normal heart rhythm, conduction of nerve impulses, and muscle contraction

potency the pharmacological activity or relative strength of a compound

precocity development occurs early; used to refer to early puberty

preganglionic fibers nerve fibers that precede the ganglia, especially in autonomic nervous system

preload force pushing into the heart

priapism penile erection; painful and persistent

progesterone female sex hormone; plays role in reproduction, thickens uterine lining

prostate gland organ located under the bladder that produces a large part of the seminal fluid

prostatic hypertrophy enlarged prostate gland, common in older men

proteins large molecules made up of amino acids that play many major roles in the body, including forming the basis of body structures such as skin and hair, and important chemicals such as enzymes and hormones

prothrombin agent involved in clotting

prothrombin time (PT) time in seconds that it takes for the patient's blood to clot when combined with thromboplastin and calcium

pruritus itching

psoriasis skin disorder characterized by patches of thick, red skin often covered by silvery scales

psychoactive has effect on mood

psychosis mental disorder in which a serious inability to think, perceive, and judge clearly causes loss of touch with reality

pulse changes in diameter of blood vessel caused by the heart beat; synonymous with the heart rate

Purkinje fibers part of the conduction system of the heart located in the ventricles

quinidine-like has effects on cardiac muscle similar to quinidine

Raynaud's syndrome disease involving constriction of blood vessels of extremities

reaction effect of brain on interpretation of nerve impulse received to central nervous system

rebound congestion vasoconstrictor given, results in vasoconstriction; vasoconstrictor repeated; vasoconstrictor stopped, results in vasodilation (stuffy nose)

receptor structural protein molecule that binds with specific agents (ligands)

retraction cord cord used around tooth to separate tissue from tooth, improves accuracy of impression; many contain epinephrine

sacral part of the vertebral column near the pelvis, includes the coccyx

salicylate a salt or ester of salicylic acid

salicylism reaction to an overdose of aspirin

salivation secretion of saliva

schizophrenia category of psychosis

semen fluid containing secretions from the prostate gland and sperm, which is expelled on ejaculation

sialadenitis inflammation of salivary gland

side effect unwanted effect of a drug

silent killer refers to lack of symptoms; hypertension

sinus channels that carry fluid

somatic relating to body or trunk of body

sphygmomanometer instrument that inflates with a gauge to measure blood pressure

Starling's law cardiac output and stroke volume increases with an increase in end-diastolic pressure up to a point, then the heart fails

subdiaphragmatic below the diaphragm

sublingual gland salivary gland located below the tongue

sublingually under the tongue

submaxillary gland salivary gland in lower jaw

supraventricular referring to the atrium (part of heart above ventricles)

synaptic cleft space between nerve cells or between nerve cells and effector organ (space between)

syncope fainting, loss of consciousness

syndactyly fusion or webbing of fingers or toes; fewer digits

tachycardia increase in heart rate

tachyphylaxis with repeated administration, the body quickly has a decrease in response

tardive dyskinesia voluntary muscle performance; irreversible; side effect of antipsychotics

temporomandibular joint (TMJ) joint of the lower jaw

teratogenicity abnormal fetus, *terato* means "monster"

tetraiodothyronine thyroid hormone, T_4

therapeutic effect desired effect of a drug

therapeutic index LD_{50}/ED_{50}; used to compare safety of drugs

thrombocytopenia abnormal decrease in the number of blood platelets

thrombophlebitis inflammation of the venous vessels

thromboplastin substance present in tissues and platelets that is necessary for blood coagulation

thyroidectomy thyroid removal

thyrotoxicosis produced by excessive thyroid hormone

tinnitus ringing of the ears

tolerance process of becoming less responsive to a drug over time; the need for larger amounts of a drug to produce the same effect

toxic of, relating to, or caused by a toxin or other poison

tracheotomy surgical opening of trachea; emergency procedure for choking

transferases enzymes that move one-carbon groups from one substance to another

tremors muscle movement producing shaking; involuntary

trigeminal neuralgia pain in the trigeminal (side of face) nerve

triglycerides type of fat found in blood; risk factor for atherosclerosis

triiodothyronine thyroid hormone; T_3

type I diabetes chronic disease that is caused by a total lack of insulin production and primarily occurs in people less than 20 years of age; can only be treated with insulin

type II diabetes chronic disease that occurs mainly in people older than 40 years, overweight persons; treated with diet changes and oral drugs that reduce glucose levels in the blood; known as type II diabetes; insulin may be needed in some patients

unipolar depression mental disorder with only depression as a component (in contrast to bipolar in which there is depression and elation alternating)

urethral refers to urethra, canal between bladder and outside of body

urinary retention retain urine in bladder; associated with prostatic hypertrophy

urination excretion of urine

urticaria itching wheals; hypersensitivity reaction caused by foods, drugs, emotions, or physical agents

vagus vagal nerve; parasympathetic autonomic nervous system stimulates vagus (produces bradycardia)

vasoconstriction blood vessels narrow

vasodilation blood vessels widen

vasomotor collapse fainting

ventricular arrhythmia abnormal rhythms originating from ventricles

vesicles sac containing something; in autonomic nervous system vesicles store neurotransmitters

viscous thick

volume depleted amount of water in body (a lot in blood) too low

von Willebrand's disease disease with tendency to bleed, prolonged bleeding time; inherited

withdrawal the act or process of ceasing to use an addictive drug; the physiological and mental readjustment that accompanies such discontinuation

xerostomia reduced saliva (dry mouth)

Drug Index

Index entries followed by "f" indicate
figures; "t" tables; "b" boxes.

Index

A

Abbreviations, 9t, 11
Abortion
   and exposure to nitrous oxide, 132-133
   midtrimester, prostaglandin effects, 239
   vitamin E effects, 159
Absorption of drug
   from injection site, 17
   ionization effects on, 17
   oral absorption, 17
Abstinence syndrome, 309
Acetaminophen
   See also Nonopioid (nonnarcotic)
      analgesics.
   in pregnancy, 302
   and warfarin interaction, 99
Acetylcholine as neurotransmitter, 14
Acetylsalicylic acid. *See* Nonopioid
   (nonnarcotic) analgesics.
Acquired immunodeficiency syndrome
   (AIDS)
   combination of drugs, 110
   nonnucleoside reverse transcriptase
      inhibitors, 110
   nucleoside reverse transcriptase inhibitors,
      109-110
   with opioid abuse, 315, 319
   opportunistic infections, 109-110, 109t
   protease inhibitors, 110
Action potential, 14-15
Acyclovir, 107-109
Addiction
   to drugs, 309
   to opioid analgesics, 69-70
Addison's disease, 242, 245
Adequate intake (AI), 149b
Administration routes of drugs. *See* Drug
   action and handling.
Adrenal cortex, 241
Adrenal gland, corticosteroid effects in
   crisis, 244, 247
α_1-Adrenergic blockers, 204
β-Adrenergic blocking agents, 194, 200-201
   drug interactions, 201
   for heart failure, 189
Adrenocortical insufficiency, acute, 294
Adrenocorticosteroids
   adverse reactions, 243-244, 246-247
   classification of, 241-242
   definitions of, 242
   dental implications, 246-248, 246b
   in infections, 28-29
   mechanism of action, 242-243
   mechanism of release, 241, 242f

Index entries followed by "f" indicate
figures; "t" tables; "b" boxes.

Adrenocorticosteroids *(Continued)*
   pharmacologic effects, 243, 243f, 244b
   routes of administration, 242, 242t
   steroid supplementation, 247-248, 247f
   synthetic products, 246, 246t
   topical use, 248
   uses
      dental, 245
      medical, 245
Adrenocorticotropic hormone (ACTH),
   241-242, 250
Adverse reactions
   of acetaminophen, 61-62
   of acetylsalicylic acid, 53-54
   of acyclovir, 107
   of alpha$_1$-adrenergic blockers, 204
   of aminoglycosides, 93
   of angiotensin-converting enzyme
      inhibitors (ACEIs), 202-203,
      203b
   of anticonvulsant agents, 215-217
   of antihistamines, 237
   of antihypertensive agents, 205, 205b
   of antiinfective agents
      allergic reactions, 81
      costs, 81
      dose forms, 81
      drug interactions, 81
      gastrointestinal tract, 81
      in pregnancy, 81
      superinfection, 81
   of antineoplastic drugs, 272-274, 273t
   of antipsychotic agents
      agranulocytosis, 227
      anticholinergic effects, 227
      extrapyramidal effects, 226-227
      metabolic effects, 227
      orthostatic hypotension, 227
      sedation, 226
      seizures, 227
   of ascorbic acid, 150
   of barbiturates, 143
   of benzodiazepines, 139-140
   of calcium, 163
   of calcium channel blocking agents,
      201-202
   of carbamazepine, 217
   of cephalosporins, 91-92
   of cimetidine, 285
   of clindamycin, 89
   clinical manifestations of
      drug interactions, 30
      fetal development, 29-30
      hypersensitivity, 30-31
      idiosyncrasy, 31
      interference with natural defense
         mechanisms, 31

Adverse reactions *(Continued)*
      local irritation, 30
      nontarget tissues, 29
      target tissues, 29
   of cyanocobalamin, 155
   definitions and classifications
      drug allergy, 28-29
      idiosyncratic reactions, 28-29
      interference with natural defense
         mechanisms, 28-29
      side effects, 28-29
      toxic reaction, 28-29
   of erythromycin, 86
   of folic acid, 154
   of general anesthetics, 129, 129t
   of herbal products, 321
   of histamine, 235
   of isoniazid, 97
   of ketoconazole, 105
   of leukotriene modifiers, 281-282
   of local anesthetics, 116-117
      allergy, 117
      local effects, 117
      malignant hyperthermia, 117
      maximum safe dose, 116t
      in pregnancy and nursing, 117
      toxicity, 116-117
   of metronidazole, 90
   of niacin, 153
   of nitroglycerin, 193
   of nitrous oxide, 132, 314
   of NSAIDs, 58
   of opioid analgesics, 68-70, 69t
   of penicillins, 83-84
   of phenytoin, 219-220, 219f
   of pyridoxine, 154
   of quinolones, 95
   of riboflavin, 153
   of rifampin, 97
   of selective serotonin reuptake inhibitors,
      231
   of statins, 206
   of sulfonamides, 94
   of tetracyclines, 87-88
   of thiamine, 151
   of thiazides, 199-200, 200t
   toxicologic evaluation, 31-32, 31f
   of tricyclic antidepressants, 228-230,
      230f
   of valproate, 218
   of vancomycin, 93
   of warfarin, 99
Age and weight, and drug effects, 25-
   27
Agonists in drug action, 15
Agranulocytosis with antipsychotic agents,
   227